NE Spring 2001

not a 'great' book!
not clear. not
continuous in
thought -
very confusing
+ disorderly

AF616521

# MEDICAL NUTRITION

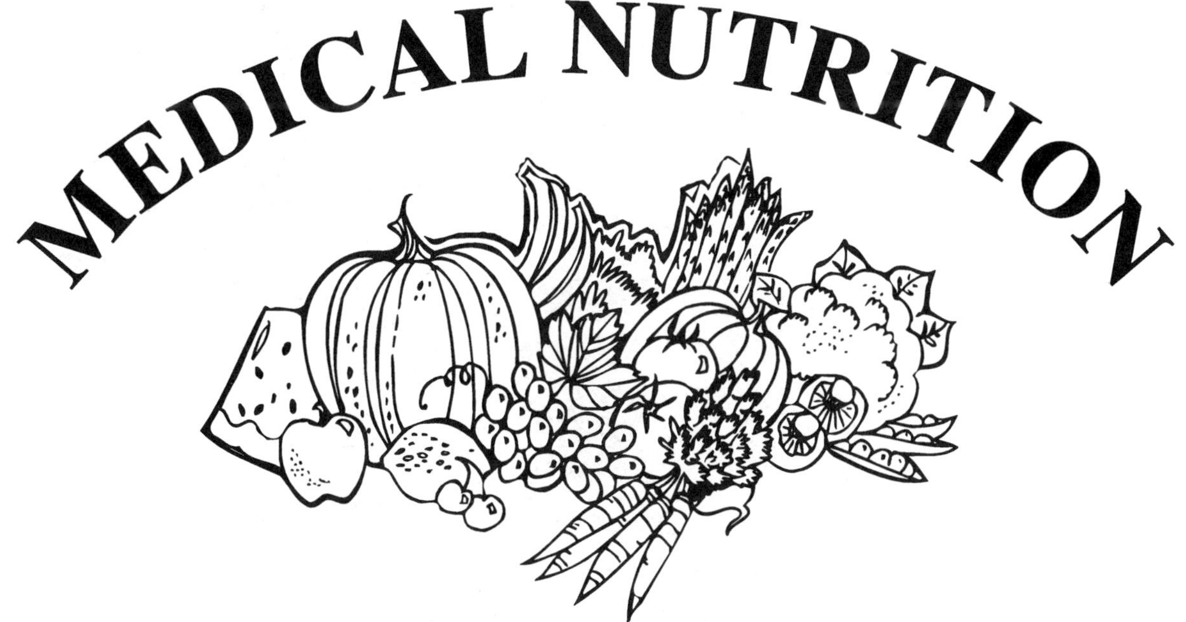

# FROM MARZ

## 2nd Edition

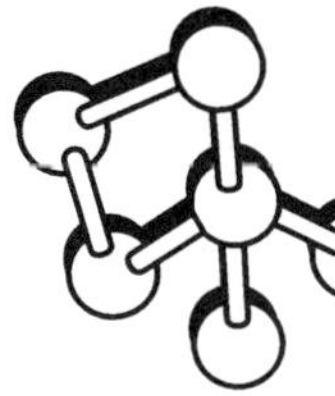

**Russell B. Marz, N.D., M.Ac.O.M.**
**naturopathic physician**

# Medical Nutrition From Marz
# 2nd edition

(A Textbook in Clinical Nutrition)

Russell B. Marz, N.D., M.Ac.C.O.M.
Assistant Clinical Professor
National College of Naturopathic Medicine
Oregon College of Oriental Medicine
Portland, OR

Published by Omni-Press
2002 S.E. 50th Ave.
Portland, OR 97215
1-800-424-OMNI
Omni-Press is an imprint of Quiet Lion Press
Printed by Malloy Lithography Inc. cover and binding
5411 Jackson Rd.; Ann Arbor Michigan, 48103-1865

# Medical Nutrition From Marz
## 2nd edition

Copyright October 1, 1999
Russell Bennett Marz, N.D., M.Ac.O.M.

All rights reserved. No part of this book may be reproduced or transmitted in any form or by any means, electronic or mechanical, including photocopying, recording, or any information storage and retrieval system, without permission in writing from the author. For information contact Omni-Press (503) 233-9553.

Printed in the United States of America
1st edition-1992
2nd edition-1997 & 1999
ISBNI-882550-28-5-case bind
ISBNI-882550-28-5-29-3-Rep cover

**ACKNOWLEDGEMENTS**

I would like to thank my Mom for directing me down the path of nutritional science and Dad for inspiring me toward perfection. In addition I would like to thank Greg Pais and Chris Meletis for their exhaustive efforts in the first edition. Others who deserve honorable mention are Tim Henwood who helped with many of the computer graphics as well as his indefatigable patience in answering countless computer questions and rescuing my computers from certain death on more than one occasion, Paul Crabtree, who through his expertise and patience, also saved my computers from their death bed as well as answering the million questions concerning hard drive problems and computer incompatibilities. A special thanks also must be given to Jonathan Merritt who single handedly recreated the entire text in a more readable and up to date format as well as proofing and re-proofing the frequently revised chapters of the book. In addition to all this he lent his moral support and was instrumental in creating the index. Others who deserve mention are Ellen Carlin who has been a long standing cheerleader and a precision editor who can turn around a proof faster than I could handle them, Phuong Ha who donated software and expertise on both soft and hard ware, and Lisa Carberry who added her encouragement and time in the editing department. Finally my ace finisher was Tess Yevka whose meticulous attention to detail and organization was instrumental in me finally finishing the book. Her knowledge of Pagemaker® and Freehand® was invaluable and she did many of the illustrations, or else helped tidy up or finish many of the ones I started.

Lastly I would like to thank the students at the National College of Naturopathic Medicine for pushing me to my limits and inspiring me to write this second edition (a special mention should go to the class of 1998 who waited so patiently for the book to finally arrive long long overdue). I want to also mention Jonathan Wright, Alan Gaby, Joe Pizzorno, Michael Murray, Melvin Werbach, and Kirk Hamilton for much of the information in this book. Without their work I would not have had the opportunity to even write this book. Other pioneers in the field who I been influenced by are Steve Austin, Tejaswini Yayathi, Maria Linder, Weston Price, Roger Williams, David Horrobin, Abram Hoffer, Jeff Bland, William Crook, James Breneman, Linus Pauling, Marshall Mandell, Doris Rapp, Theron Randolph, Roy Walford, Steven Levine, Paris Kidd, A.L. Willis and many others whom I apologize for not remembering.

**DEDICATION**

In special recognition I would like to acknowledge my wife Gwenevere and my son Emil who had to bear the brunt of my routine all night jam sessions at the computer and with my books. They unfortunately had to suffer through my mental and physical absence doing so with the utmost of tolerance believing my tall tales that the book was, "going out tomorrow", time and time again. I am delighted that they can read this knowing that I am not downstairs still hammering away at the multiple computers.

**Table of Contents Alphabetized**

## *PREFACE TO SECOND EDITION*

*Medical Nutrition From Marz,* 1st edition served a very useful purpose since it was used mostly as a teaching textbook for students of naturopathic medicine at the National College of Naturopathic Medicine in Portland, Oregon. I am very grateful to all the students who sat through my classes and gave me much needed comments on my first text. Certainly without them I would have never taken on such a task. It has been 5 years since the first edition came out and the time seemed ripe to embark upon an update and revision of the first edition. Because of the popularity of the first edition and the inspiring nature of my students, I have undertaken the task of writing the 2nd edition. I especially want to thank the class of '98 for their patience and understanding in waiting for this second edition. The entire text has been rewritten and reformatted with several new sections added, such as amino acids, minerals, select diseases, and an expanded infant nutrition section. It is my hope that the countless revisions and editing have made this text more user friendly.

Medical Nutrition is a relatively new science. Its roots are varied–arising primarily from the 19th century philosophy of "Nature Cure." The principles of "Nature Cure" are very simple: "*follow the laws of nature and the body will heal itself," or "vis medicatrix naturae,"* (the healing power of nature). By restoring the delicate balance of essential nutrients in the body, we can allow its natural homeostatic mechanisms to bring the body to health. The body's natural instinct is to be well and it strives to reach optimal health. This is its own innate survival mechanism.

In today's conventional western model of medicine, we tend to look at the body as being either healthy or diseased. In recent years we have come to realize that we have a vaster potential for health than we have ever before recognized. We have seen people in certain parts of the world live, with very little disease or sickness, to ripe old ages. These people have begun to tap into their "*health potential*." The study of these progenitors of optimal health and the factors that have contributed to their long-lived vitality is the burgeoning science of longevity. Extending one's life span, with a high degree of wellness, is a direct consequence of optimizing health.

What are all the factors that bring about disease processes and adversely effect longevity? These factors are varied, arising from mental, physical and spiritual planes. To truly understand and achieve optimal health, all of these factors must be examined and followed correctly. Our mental well-being has a tremendous effect on our health. Psychoneuroimmunology is a relatively new science that explores the effects of a *"positive outlook"* on our immune system. Of course, a positive outlook can also be effected by our physical health. If we aren't well physically, we may easily develop a poor mental outlook that may then further debilitate our physical health. Correspondingly, if we have optimal physical health, the chances are that our mental state will be positive and that our immune system will be empowered. Thus each plane interacts and influences the others either toward optimal health or disease. This book focuses mainly on the physical plane and how it effects our spiritual and mental well-being in the quest for optimal health.

How do essential nutrient's –which include vitamins, minerals, amino acids, negative ions, light, fiber etc.–(I am using the term *essential nutrients* loosely here as negative ions, light and fiber are not technically considered essential nutrients)–effect our optimal health? Truly it seems that there are a great many nutrient interactions that have positive effects on our health. It is becoming more clear that there are many synergistic effects between nutrients and that looking at them individually will not give the entire picture. I believe that we should rethink the term essential nutrients to include those items that act synergistically with other nutrients and are necessary for optimal health. It has only been in the last century that essential vitamins and minerals were discovered. Unfortunately, the health and lives of many people were lost before the essential need for these nutrients was accepted. There was much controversy over the causes of the deadly diseases such as pellagra, scurvy, and beriberi. Most scientists of the early 20th century refused to believe that a deficiency of minute substances could bring on the onset of disease. Then, as now, bacteria and viruses were the popular targets as the causes of disease. It is my contention that many of the diseases that we see today are a direct result of a deficiency or an imbalance in our essential nutrients. We are constantly finding out more about interactions between nutrients and how they may play a vital role in our health.

For instance, why did some people die and others survive when the bubonic plague swept through Europe? Some evidence suggests that the survivors, in general, had greater intakes of vitamin C and other vital nutrients that are involved in enhancing one's immunity. We may ask the same questions concerning many of the diseases that we see today including diabetes, heart disease, and cancer, diseases that are rampant today.

Certainly genetics comes into play, but I believe if you supply the body with the correct essential nutrients, the body does not have to succumb to its genetic predisposition. Current nutritional research is showing that certain conditions or diseases can be ameliorated by specific nutrients. In addition, it has been shown that there is an association between certain diseases and low levels of certain nutrients.

Studies have shown that many diseases that we see today are relatively new and are, most probably, a direct result of the way we live. We are exposed to incredible amounts of environmental toxins. There are no places left on earth that have been spared from the effects of our polluting hands. Cars, factories, mercury amalgams, radon, herbicides, pesticides, tobacco smoke, drugs (including prescription drugs such as birth control pills, anti-cancer agents, and antibiotics), ultraviolet radiation, and many more insults on our health have increased our requirements for certain nutrients far beyond what we previously needed to provide us with optimal health. Antioxidant nutrients, in particular, have been associated with the prevention of many diseases including cancer, atherosclerosis, autoimmune diseases, birth defects, psoriasis, asthma, allergies, aging and many more. We have overburdened our bodies, and, in particular, our livers with numerous endo and exotoxins. It has reached the point where most people are not receiving adequate antioxidant nutrients to optimally protect their cells. We have much work to do to bring our toxic exposure down. In the meantime, we need to increase our intake of antioxidant nutrients if we are to maintain our health.

Another major problem that has developed is the deficiency of trace minerals in the foods that we eat. Modern agricultural practices have led to the depletion of the soil so that vital trace minerals such as selenium, chromium, vanadium, boron, molybdenum, germanium, silica and more are significantly depleted in our foods. John Hamaker and Donald Weaver give an excellent discussion of the value of trace minerals to plants and humans in their book *Survival of Civilization*, 1982. For plants, the lack of trace minerals means a lack of vitality and a higher susceptibility to drought and disease. For humans it means suboptimal health and the development of new diseases.

In addition to the lose of minerals from our soil, vitamins are being lost in the storage, transportation, processing and preparation of foods. As the list below shows, a high percentage of people in the U.S. are deficient in many vital nutrients.

| **Nutrient** | **% deficiency in U.S. Population** |
|---|---|
| Folate | 50-90% |
| B-6 | 80% |
| Magnesium | 75% |
| Calcium | 68% |
| Iron | 57% |
| Vitamin A | 50% |
| Vitamin B-1 | 45% |
| Vitamin C | 41% |
| Vitamin B-2 | 34% |
| Vitamin B-3 | 33% |
| Vitamin B-12 | 34% |

These deficiencies are based upon RDAs and do not take into consideration our exposure to environmental factors that have created an even greater need for some of these nutrients. An excellent example of this is Alan Gaby's book, *The Drs' Guide to Vitamin B-6,* in which he points out numerous environmental contaminants which act as antagonists to vitamin B-6 and how we may be seeing an epidemic in vitamin B-6 deficiency.

The intent of this book is to highlight those deficiencies that may be related to certain diseases. The nutritional physical in the appendix is one of the ways I have tried to get the clinician to look at nutrients and their deficiencies. The first edition mostly focused on the diseases and how to treat them nutritionally. The intent of this 2nd edition is basically to diversify the reading audience. The beginning of the book, covering introduction to nutrition along with digestion, absorption and metabolism is designed for the beginning student and its purpose is to introduce some basic concepts in digestive physiology and at the same time introduce some alternative nutritional concepts. This basic section is different from conventional texts in nutrition in that it points out certain possible clinical applications as related to alternative nutrition. It scientifically points out why RDAs may not be clinically useful in the treatment of some of the conditions that we see today. The section on digestion and absorption tries to put some light on the burgeoning science of food sensitivities and their causes. In addition it points out how prolonged bowel transit times may have clinical significance in many areas of health. Many of these alternative concepts are becoming more mainstream due to advances in research techniques that has enabled many authors access to ever increasing bodies of knowledge throughout the world. Many of the illustrations, tables and diagrams are designed to be used as overheads in teaching classrooms. They provide excellent teaching aids for the instructor or lecturer to illustrate key or technical concepts.

The first part of this book, as mentioned above, is devoted to digestion, absorption, carbohydrates, fats, proteins, and energy metabolism. The next section in this book is devoted to amino acids, minerals, fat and water soluble vitamins. Vitamins are discussed with regard to their history, metabolism, function, requirements, optimal intakes, sources, therapeutics, and toxicity. In this section a thorough understanding of each vitamin can be gained. This knowledge can be used to treat conditions not specifically listed under therapeutics. Every effort has been made to thoroughly document the clinical applications of each vitamin, and when key studies are available, they are usually presented with abstracts directly under the condition being discussed. This is done so the clinician can easily and immediately check the reference to the therapeutic use of a particular nutrient.

Following the section on macro and micro nutrients, the book covers selected diseases or conditions. The diseases have been selected in an order that I hope provides some continuity with the body. A brief description of each disease is followed by both an allopathic and naturopathic etiology, signs & symptoms, diagnosis (including alternative and conventional diagnostic tests) and treatment. By simultaneously looking at both points of view, the clinician/reader is able to make a more clear assessment of the condition and thus prescribe/access the most ideal treatment. Some of the diagnostic tests described are quite conventional while others are relatively new and innovative relative to the field of nutrition. These newer tests tend to reflect a much broader or alternative look at the disease. I have taken some liberties to discuss my feelings on certain diagnostic procedures both pro and con.

In the section on the treatment of the disease, a discussion of diet recommendations is provided first followed by the use of vitamins, minerals, amino acids, and other nutritional treatments. Botanical treatments have, for the most part, been omitted; however, there is a large gray area where botanicals are really foods or nutrient-related substances and invariably they are discussed with each condition. There are a few botanicals that may be mentioned for certain conditions. When mentioned under a certain disease or condition they are usually important and extremely effective in regard to treatment. Certainly this book does not attempt to address the enormity of the subject of herbs and I apologize for being so terse and simplified when it comes to botanicals. Mostly only the herb is listed but not with regard to the form in which it is to be given, nor the dosage, or frequency.

One last point concerning the treatment of disease, as it appears in this book, needs to be stated. Naturopathic medicine, which this author practices, has traditionally precluded the use of specific nutrients in the treatment of disease. In my thinking, it is rare that any condition can be optimally treated with one nutrient, one herb, or one type of medicine (I am sure some homeopaths, chiropractors or other health care professionals might disagree). Naturopathic nutrition is by nature an eclectic art. Often different nutrients have synergistic effects with each other. I often combine many different types of therapy —botanicals, acupuncture, manipulation, homeopathic, and general immunological support— to heal my patients/clients. To look at just one nutrient in the treatment of diseases is like cooking with one spice. Just as it takes many herbs and spices to make a delicious casserole it too also takes a variety of nutrients combined in the correct ratios to create a successful treatment protocol. It is up to the clinician to decide what nutrients and/or dietary changes will be most effective for the treatment of a specific disease. Most diseases and ailments present themselves simultaneously with a myriad of other seemingly unrelated signs and symptoms and, hence, must be treated together as a whole picture. In addition, one nutrient may be far more effective for one individual than for another with the same disease. Every one has his/her own genetic weaknesses, miasms and strengths.

Finally, it may appear that there is much talk about vitamins, pills, powders, etc. in the treatment plans. It is not my intention for all of the nutrients listed under therapeutics to be used in the treatment of one patient's disease. The skill and art of the clinician should come into play to be able to use the **least number of remedies in the smallest dosages**. Generally if a certain dose of a nutrient is used and it is working, it is wise to decrease the dose until the smallest effective dose is reached. I believe that the least invasive treatment should always be used first (*primum no nocere*, first do no harm). In addition it should also be pointed out that the first order of treatment should always be dietary. Whatever can be accomplished dietarily should be done first before any supplemental therapy is undertaken. After all the use of nutrient supplements is in many cases no more different than using prescription drugs, especially when they are used in high doses. One significant difference would be where drugs usually have side effects that they are trying to minimize, nutrient therapy often has side benefits which is something that is very welcome.

Generally speaking the use of nutrients to treat disease is relatively quite safe, unlike conventional allopathic treatments. There are times, however, where vitamin and mineral therapy might be contraindicated (as in infants or toddlers) and homeopathic remedies might be the best treatment of choice for a particular condition. There may be times, however, when even if the correct remedy is given the patient may not respond. This may be due to the fact that the patient may not be "*biochemically ready*" for the healing energy of the remedy. This could also apply to many of the other healing modalities such as acupuncture, manipulation, herbs and even pharmaceuticals. It may also be the case that the correct remedy or treatment may prime the patient into responding to a nutritional therapy. This is why the eclectic approach, or what has sometimes been referred to sarcastically as the "shotgun treatment" , may be the most effective treatment plan. Combining modalities often creates a synergy. Thus, someone who has a multifactorial disease can be treated uniquely with several different modalities which all enhance the effectiveness of each treatment and leads the patient to optimal health.

*Listed here are the most common causes of death in the U.S. in 1991. As can be seen, the top six out of eight causes (marked with *) make up 71.3% of all deaths, of which diet plays a significant role. Certainly we can improve the morbidity and mortality statistics in the U.S. to reflect the level of knowledge that we have to prevent these conditions.*

**The Ten Leading Causes of Death in the United States in 1991**

| Rank | Cause of Death | Number | % of Total Deaths |
|---|---|---|---|
| 1* | Heart Disease | 720,862 | 33.2 |
| 2* | Cancer | 514,657 | 23.7 |
| 3* | Stroke | 143,481 | 6.6 |
| 4 | Chronic obstructive lung disease | 90,650 | 4.2 |
| 5* | Unintentional injury | 89,347 | 4.1 |
| 6 | Pneumonia & flu | 77,860 | 3.6 |
| 7* | Diabetes mellitus | 48,951 | 2.3 |
| 8* | Suicide | 30,810 | 1.4 |
| 9 | AIDS | 29,555 | 1.4 |
| 10 | Homicide & legal intervention | 26,513 | 1.2 |

FromPublic Health Service DHHS: Health, U.S., 1993. DHHS (PHS)Publ # 94-1232. Washington, DC, DHHS, 1994. Also from Public Health Service, DHHS: TheSurgeon General's Report on Nutrition and Health. DHHS (PHS) Publ # 88-50211. Washington, DC, DHHS, 1988.

# AN INTRODUCTION TO NUTRITION

Nutrition is the study of how a living organism ingests, digests, absorbs, transports, utilizes, and excretes food substances which are necessary for the survival of the organism. This book tries to address the subject from a holistic overview–i.e., looking at a person's unique biological makeup (taking into consideration genetics, environmental factors including prenatal nutrition, and pollution exposure) and attempting to optimize a person's nutritional status. In the past, nutrition has been concerned with describing major dietary constituents and naming gross deficiencies associated with the lack of these specific nutrients. The following is a more realistic view of the current status of nutrition as it now applies to western civilization:

> "Gone are the days when instruction in nutritional science was adequately represented by a description of the chemistry of the major constituents of the diet, the diseases associated with gross insufficiency of each nutrient, and the amounts needed to prevent these deficiency diseases. Not only have florid deficiencies become rare events in Western medicine, but interest has been aroused in much more subtle and pervasive relationships of long-term nutritional habits to chronic conditions such as atherosclerosis, hypertension, cancer and osteoporosis, and in the role of nutrition as a therapeutic weapon in the treatment of patients postoperatively and in other clinical settings."
>
> Hamish N. Munro, M.D.
> *Nutritional Biochemistry and Metabolism*
> *with Clinical Applications*
> by Maria C. Linder, Ph.D.

In contrast to our current system of medicine which, for the most part, regards nutrition as an extraneous science to be relegated to dietitians, I have tried to make nutrition the focal point in the treatment of all diseases. We can look back in our history and discover that some of our greatest minds have felt an inherent value in the treatment of disease through the use of food.

*"Leave your drugs in the chemist's pot if you can cure the patient with food."*
Hippocrates, *the father of medicine,* 420BC

In this book I have tried to present the specific nutrients found in foods and to explain how they can affect disease both in their prevention and treatment. Furthermore, I have tried to expand ideas on nutrition to include the optimization of health. This concept has led to what is now called the science of longevity. What is our true potential? To what age are we genetically programmed to live? Is this something that is fixed in stone or do we have the capability to live beyond our genetic markers? Certainly we have not come close to our potential, considering the vast knowledge that we possess in the field of health and disease.

The illustration on the following page demonstrates our current health care system. It represents the two extremes of the state of our health. On one end of the spectrum, we have "death," and on the other, "optimal health." Most people tend to be where the arrow points upward. They are ambulatory (in the vertical position) but nowhere near optimal health. As they age, they gradually come closer to the center of the continuum-toward the line that marks the point where they become horizontal. They need more severe medical interventions such as surgery or hospitaliza-

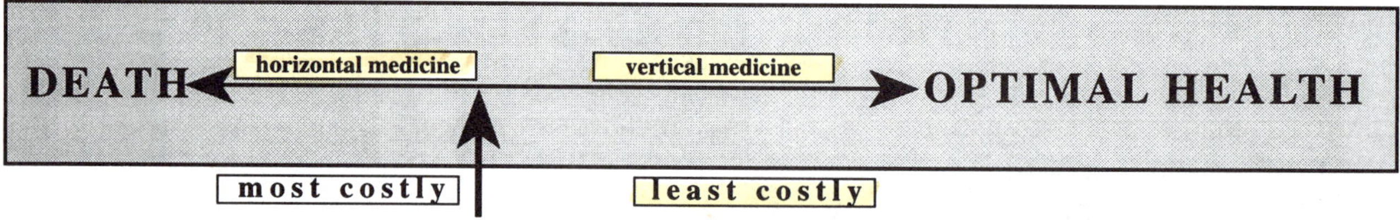


tion. In fact, it has been demonstrated that 25% of all Medicare expenditures are for medical care in the last half year of life. These heroic and costly methods of health care have resulted in 76.8 billion dollars per year spent for the treatment of heart disease, and 14.4 billion dollars per year spent on the treatment of nutritionally preventable cancers. According to Metropolitan Life Insurance statistics, in 1989 coronary bypass surgeries alone accounted for 10.1 billion dollars in medical expenses. Considering all the political rhetoric concerning governmental subsidies for health care, it seems obvious that if we spent more money on the environment and on sound nutritional programs for the poor and the sick, on school lunch programs and nutritional education, we would receive a pay-back far exceeding our wildest dreams in terms of health care benefits and savings.

## Historical Background

Nutrition is a relatively new science only recently recognized as a distinct discipline since 1934. The first professional organization, the *American Institute of Nutrition*, emerged from the basic sciences of chemistry, physiology and biology.

In 1747 Dr. James Lind, a British physician, conducted the first nutritional experiment on board his ship. This involved treating the disease scurvy with foods containing the essential nutrient ascorbic acid (see vitamin C).

In the 18th century ***Antoine Laurent Lavoisier***, who later became known as the "Father of Nutrition," studied how food was used for energy. He was the first person to study the relationship between heat production, oxygen use, and carbon dioxide expired in the body.

In the early 1800's, scientists determined that organic compounds contained the elements carbon, hydrogen, and nitrogen. One scientist, Liebig, found that a food's nutritive value was a function of its nitrogen content. He also proposed that an adequate diet must provide what he called *plastic* foods (protein) and fuel foods (carbohydrates and fat). In 1871 a French chemist, Dumas, tried to produce a synthetic milk of carbohydrate, fat and protein in the same proportion as found in cow's milk. When infants did not survive on this formula, he concluded that there was some naturally occurring nutritive substance in human milk which was lacking in his formula.

## The Discovery of Vitamins

In 1912 Casimir Funk proposed an extraordinary hypothesis that pellagra, beriberi, scurvy and rickets were all deficiency diseases not caused by airborne or insect-carried bacteria. The scientific consensus of the time, fifty years after Louis Pasteur's first famous experiment proving that bacteria were in the air and could contaminate sterile media, was that beriberi was caused by a bacteria and pellagra by a fly carrying a "pellagra microbe." Funk knew that there was a "vital for life" nutrient which had a nitrogen carrying component and thus coined the word "**vita-mine**"(*vita* in Latin meaning "essential for life" and *amine* signifying a nitrogen-containing compound). Later, when it was found that there were vitamines that did not contain a nitrogen-containing group, the "e" at the end of the word was dropped and the final name became **"vitamin"** which is now a household term.

## Definitions related to nutritional science

**FDA** (Food and Drug Administration)–This agency is responsible for overseeing the safety and wholesomeness of our food supply. It is also responsible for making sure that herbicides, pesticides, and antibiotics used on or with plants or animals will not result in undue risk to the consumer. In addition, it is responsible for the safety of additives in foods and for any contaminants that might also be present there. Lately, the FDA has become more involved with the safety of food supplements and their labeling. It has become immersed in the regulation of herbs, amino acids, minerals and vitamins, as well as with the safety of pharmaceuticals. As far as the billion dollar nutritional supplement business goes, its regulations can have a major financial impact on this industry.

The FDA has been caught in a political nightmare trying to regulate both the nutritional supplement and pharmaceutical industries. It is also in the position of trying to defend itself against allegations that some of its administrative members are owners of pharmaceutical companies who have vested interests in many of its decisions. The FDA is, however, required to regulate the myriad array of new drugs which have been introduced on an already flooded market.

With recent raids on some alternative medical clinics, some people feel that the FDA has been acting more like the *Gestapo* than a consumer protection agency. On the other hand, with all the fantastic claims that have been made about an enormous number of nutritional supplements and with the introduction of an incredible number of new nutritional products, they are faced with a real crisis. People want to be left with the choice to choose their own supplements and they also want to be protected against fraudulent claims that may do them harm.

**Organic**–This term has always been a rather ambiguous one that really had no enforceable definition in the past. Currently, the expression, **"certified organic,"** means that the food has been organically raised or grown without inorganic herbicides, pesticides, or fertilizers and then processed in accordance with the California Organic Foods Act of 1990. Furthermore, the soil must not have had any of these chemicals added to it for at least 5 years prior to planting for the food to earn the label, "certified organic."

In the U.S. each year 1.2 billion pounds of pesticides and herbicides are sprayed or added to crops. This does not include all the herbicides and pesticides that have been banned in this country but are added to foods grown in other countries. This amounts to about 13-14 pounds of chemicals per person per year in the U.S.! It has been estimated that 80% of all breast cancer may be due to environmental toxins. Even though organic food is supposed to be grown without synthetic herbicides or pesticides, there may be a contamination problem from neighboring farms which still use these chemicals. There may also be residual contamination from years past. According to the Natural Resources Defense Council, a public-interest environmental group, 17% of the carrots analyzed in 1984 still contained detectable traces of DDT, a pesticide that was banned from this country in 1973!

**Nutrient**–A nutrient is a chemical substance in food that provides energy, forms new body components, or assists in the function of various bodily processes.

**Essential Nutrient**–An essential nutrient is one that must be ingested in the diet because it cannot be synthesized by the body quickly enough or in sufficient quantities to meet bodily needs for survival.

**Functions of nutrients in the body**

- Supply energy
- Promote growth and repair of body tissues
- Regulate body processes

**6 main nutrient categories**

- Carbohydrates
- Lipids (fats)
- Proteins
- Vitamins
- Minerals
- Water

**Note**–Not all nutrients are necessarily essential even though they perform some of the above functions and fit into one of the 6 main categories.

## Essential nutrients

(nutrients with * are often deficient or sub-optimal in diet)

|  | Minerals | Vitamins |
|---|---|---|
| **Carbohydrates** | **Minerals** | **Vitamins** |
| glucose | *Macroelements* | *Fat soluble* |
| | *calcium | *vitamin A |
| **Fats** | *magnesium | *Beta carotene |
| linoleic acid | phosphorus | @vitamin D (cholecalciferol) |
| *linolenic acid | sodium | *vitamin E (tocopherol) |
| | *potassium | *vitamin K (phytonadione) |
| **Proteins** | sulfur | |
| **(amino acids)** | chlorine | *Water soluble* |
| 1) isoleucine | | thiamin |
| 2) leucine | *Microelements* | riboflavin |
| 3) lysine | •iron | *niacin/niacinamide |
| ~4) methionine | *selenium | *pantothenic acid |
| 5) phenylalanine | *zinc | *pyridoxine |
| 6) tryptophan | copper | cobalamin |
| 7) threonine | *boron | biotin |
| 8) valine | manganese | *folate |
| #9) histidine | cobalt | *vitamin C (ascorbic acid) |
| #10) glutamine | molybdenum | |
| #11) arginine | iodine | |
| | *chromium | **Water** |
| | vanadium | |
| | tin | |
| | nickel | |
| | silica | |
| | arsenic | |
| | lead | |
| | cadmium | |
| | fluorine | |
| | aluminum | |
| | lithium | |

* These nutrients may not be at optimal daily intake levels although apparently sufficient in diet.

\# These nutrients may be essential in childhood or in times of stress.

@ Vitamin D can be synthesized in the skin if enough sunlight exposure; hence may not be essential.

• Iron may be stored in higher than normal amounts in genetically susceptible individuals leading to certain health risks.

~ Methionine may be too high in our western diets leading to increased incidence of homocysteinuria.

**Note**–Many of the above trace minerals have some degree of toxicity. Some have very low levels of toxicity and others only require small amounts to be toxic. Therapeutically, the more toxic the trace minerals, the more narrow the range from a therapeutic dosage to a toxic one.

## Conventional Nutrition vs Alternative Nutrition

We have seen a definite trend in "conventional nutritional" practices to embrace some of the "alternative nutritional" perspectives. Although conventional nutritional teachings have been very slow, for fear of being labeled "unscientific" , to adapt many of the recent alternative approaches, we have seen medical schools teach classes in the alternative healing arts, including alternative nutrition. While conventional nutrition is very conservative in its approach to the use of nutritional supplements to treat disease, the recommendations for folic acid supplements for prospective moms to prevent neural tube defects in newborns are now widely endorsed. It took close to ten years to adapt such a basic recommendation because of the resistance to prescribing vitamin supplements.

With the wide use of vitamin, mineral, amino acid, herbal and enzyme supplements, it is really essential that today's health care practitioner have a good knowledge of the claims that have been made, as well as the studies that are being cited, in support of such claims. It is important to remember that the so-called scientific approach and statistical analysis do not always give a fair and complete evaluation of a particular treatment. Statistics, in their analytical approach, exclude the subset of the population that may respond very well to a particular treatment because the results may not show statistical significance for a wider population. If we could somehow isolate this subset of the participants who responded well in the study, we might reach quite different conclusions. The problem is, of course, how to isolate this subset of the population that might respond particularly well. Thus, what we see is that today's practitioner must be acutely aware that there may be ways to determine biochemical individuality in regard to who will respond to a particular therapy versus who will not. It is the goal of this book to shed some light on the variety of evaluations that could be made of a single patient by looking at a number of diagnostic criteria, both conventional and nonconventional.

### How do we assess nutritional requirements for the general population?

**RDAs–Recommended Dietary Allowances**–*This represents the known nutritional needs of 97.5% of the population.* It is calculated by taking the mean requirement of a nutrient and then increasing the amount by **two** standard deviations. This figure also includes a margin of safety to account for nutrient losses that might occur in the cooking and storage of food, the range of requirements in the population, and to provide a buffer under stress conditions. Other factors considered were the stability of the nutrient, the body's ability to store the nutrient, the range of observed requirements, the availability of the nutrient in the North American diet, the possible hazards from an excessive intake, and the difficulties involved in establishing precise requirements.

## Mathematical Gaussian Distribution of Nutrient Requirements

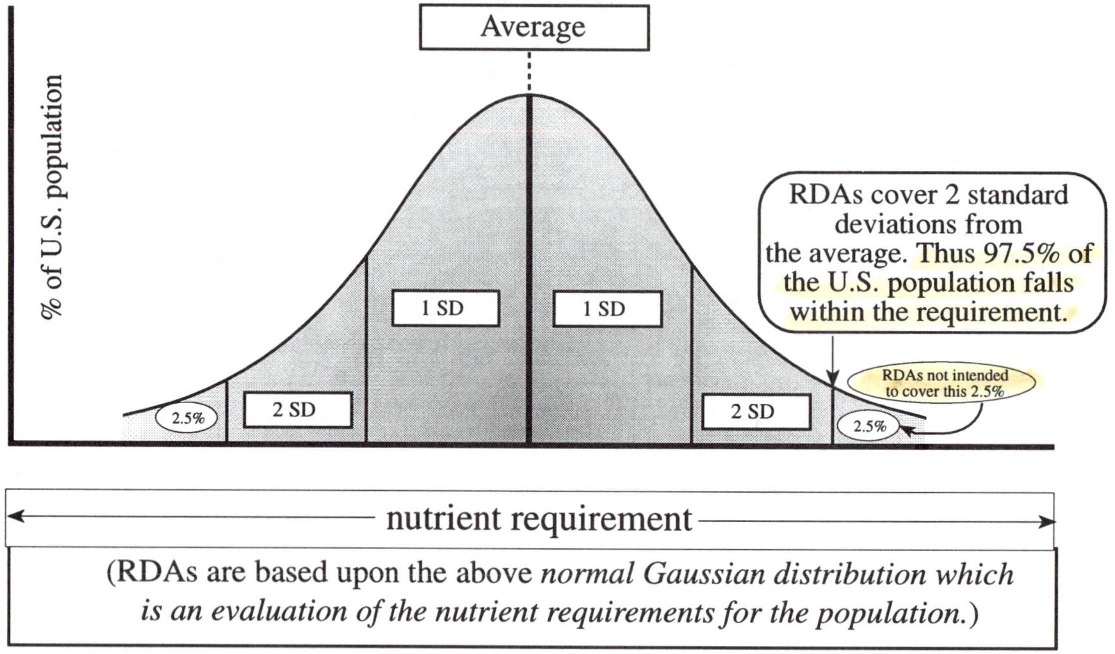


(RDAs are based upon the above *normal Gaussian distribution which is an evaluation of the nutrient requirements for the population.*)

**What the RDAs do <u>not</u> cover:**

1) disease states (including malabsorption states, digestive problems, chronic infections)
2) environmental pollutants
3) genetic metabolic defects
4) increased requirements due to the use of both prescription and nonprescription medications

**Note–USRDAs**–United States Recommended Daily Allowances–Because the RDAs take into consideration different requirements according to age, the USRDAs were established for uniform labeling purposes. It is an abbreviated version of the RDAs and involves only one standard for everyone over age 4 with the exception of pregnant and lactating women.

**Problems with RDAs**

1) As mentioned previously, the RDAs are basically established for healthy populations. Special additional requirements may be needed for problems such as premature birth, inherited metabolic disorders, infections, chronic diseases, digestive problems (especially malabsorption syndromes), and the use of medications, both prescription and nonprescription. In addition, environmental pollutants, anti-metabolites, excessive stress, and excessive dietary constituents, such as certain fats, proteins, carbohydrates, food additives, and naturally occurring food toxins, can also increase the requirements for many nutrients.

2) RDAs assume that nutrient requirements in normal healthy people are distributed according to the mathematical Gaussian (so-called "normal") distribution which is shown in the above diagram. Below are possible alternative distributions which may more accurately represent the reality due to biochemical individuality and to some of the previously mentioned factors.

3) RDAs assume that standard deviations for nutrient requirements are generally about 15% of the mean (thus 2 standard deviations higher than the mean would cover about 97% of the healthy population). This 15% standard deviation is based largely on an assumed biological measurement and of a finding for nitrogen losses in male college students deprived of protein. The study below was done with animal and human requirements of a number of selected amino acids, calcium and vitamin B-1 (thiamin). From examining just this small sampling we can plainly see that there is a tremendous variation in the requirements for these nutrients. If we were to examine **all** of the current existing essential nutrients, it stands to reason that we would also find a tremendous variation in the requirement for many of these nutrients as well. The average range in this study was about a 4-fold variation. This is twice what the Food and Nutrition Board has assumed based on protein requirements.

**Ranges of Requirements for selected Nutrients**

| Nutrient | Amt required | Range of Differences | # of subjects |
|---|---|---|---|
| Tryptophan | 82-250mg | 3.0 fold difference | 50 |
| Valine | 375-800mg | 2.1 fold difference | 48 |
| Phenylalanine | 420-1,100mg | 2.6 fold difference | 38 |
| Leucine | 170-1,100mg | 6.4 fold difference | 31 |
| Lysine | 400-2,800 | 7.0 fold difference | 55 |
| Isoleucine | 250-700mg | 2.8 fold difference | 24 |
| Methionine | 800-3,000mg | 3.7 fold difference | 29 |
| Threonine | 103-500mg | 4.8 fold difference | 50 |
| Calcium | 222-1,018mg | 4.6 fold difference | 19 |
| Thiamin | 0.4-1.59mg | 3.9 fold difference | 15 |

The only conclusion that we can make from this study is that there are probably a number of nutrients that have higher than a 7.0 fold range of variation in their requirement among the population and a number of nutrients that have a lower than 2.1 fold requirement range. In addition, if we very conservatively estimate that there is about 3% of the healthy population that is not covered by the RDA for a particular nutrient, is it acceptable to run a 3% deficiency risk for each of 19 different nutrients for which there are RDAs?

**Summary**–Considering how widespread chronic fatigue, depression, hyperactivity, allergies, arthritis, cancer, cardiovascular disease, diabetes, and gastrointestinal problems are, it seems likely that the RDAs are not applicable to the majority of Americans and should only be used as a very general guideline.

**Optimal Daily Intake** (ODI)–This is a term I would like to employ to describe a level of intake that takes into consideration a person's genetic background, their environment–both in their home and their place of employment (or where they spend the majority of the day)–as well as their daily habits such as smoking, drinking, stress levels, prescription medications and other factors unique to them. In considering all of these factors, the ODI would reveal an optimal level of intake for the individual. Each person has individual optimal requirements which depend on his or her unique biological makeup and living situation. Because of the large divergence in requirements among people, establishing an average intake level can be very difficult. It thus becomes a more useful term for individuals rather than for the general population. In addition, the minimal toxic dose needs to be taken into consideration with each nutrient. The **Optimal Daily Intake** usually falls between the RDA and the toxic dose.

**Toxic Daily Dose** (TDD)–This is the dosage at which, over a period of time, someone will likely develop toxicity symptoms. This dose varies from person to person and is dependent on the biochemical individuality, level of health, and toxic environmental exposure level of the individual. For example, an alcoholic might have a much lower TDD to vitamin A (vitamin A toxicity can affect the liver) compared to a healthy individual who is not challenging an otherwise healthy liver. It is a dose that is designed to cover the vast majority of individuals. It should be noted, as in the previous example of the alcoholic, that there may be some individuals who may exhibit toxicity from a daily dose below the TDD. It is assumed that the many factors involved are also taken into consideration when evaluating this dose. The toxic daily dose is meant to describe toxicity that will usually manifest over a period of months rather than over a few days.

## Notes

# DIGESTION, ABSORPTION AND METABOLISM

## Digestion

In order for food to be utilized by the body it must undergo a breakdown process. Food that is in the intestines is actually outside the body. The body must break down food into particles small enough to pass across the intestinal wall in order to be absorbed into the blood. The process by which food gets broken down into these small particles is called **digestion**. The **digestive tract** refers to the 30 feet (9m) of intestine that runs from the mouth to the anus.

Although this process begins in the mouth, the actual preparation begins in the brain where certain cues trigger the brain to send messages to the digestive system to start secreting numerous enzymes. This point can not be overemphasized. The act of thinking about, preparing, and, hopefully, sitting down to eat food is essential for the proper secretion of many enzymes which come from the mouth, stomach, pancreas, gall bladder, liver and intestines.

## The Alimentary System

The alimentary canal, which is part of the alimentary system, is a tube that is, for practical purposes, considered external to the body. It begins in the mouth and ends at the anus. The alimentary tract includes the alimentary canal and its appendage organs such as the liver, pancreas, and gall bladder.

The function of the alimentary system is to receive, macerate, and transport foodstuffs. In addition, it is responsible for secretion of digestive enzymes, hydrochloric acid, mucus, bile, and other materials. Lastly, it digests foods, absorbs and transports products of digestion, and then transports, stores and excretes waste products.

## Digestion and Absorption

Digestion of foods, which starts in the mouth, is accomplished via the physical act of chewing and the mixing of various enzymes from the mouth, stomach, pancreas, gall bladder, and the intestines themselves. The enzymes used to break down foods are classified as *exoenzymes* (enzymes which are synthesized within cells of various organs and then released into the lumen) and *endoenzymes* (those enzymes which are synthesized inside the cells in the lipoprotein membranes of the mucosal cells and attach to food particles as they enter the cells). Normally 92-97% of the standard American diet (SAD) is digested and absorbed. Water, monosaccharides, vitamins, minerals, and alcohol are usually absorbed intact in their original form. However there are considerable instances where larger molecules can get absorbed from the GI tract, possibly triggering an antibody response, thus leading to various types of allergies. Excessive production of cortisol secretion (from excessive stress), inflammatory conditions such as colitis, celiac disease, and gastritis, as well as allergies, parasites and the use of certain medications (NSAIDS, aspirin, and cortisone) can all lead to an increased permeability called *"Leaky Gut Syndrome."*

> ***"Leaky Gut Syndrome" can lead to allergies and systemic food reactions due to an excessive absorption of macro (large) molecules.***

# Food Allergy and Digestion

*The Small Intestine*

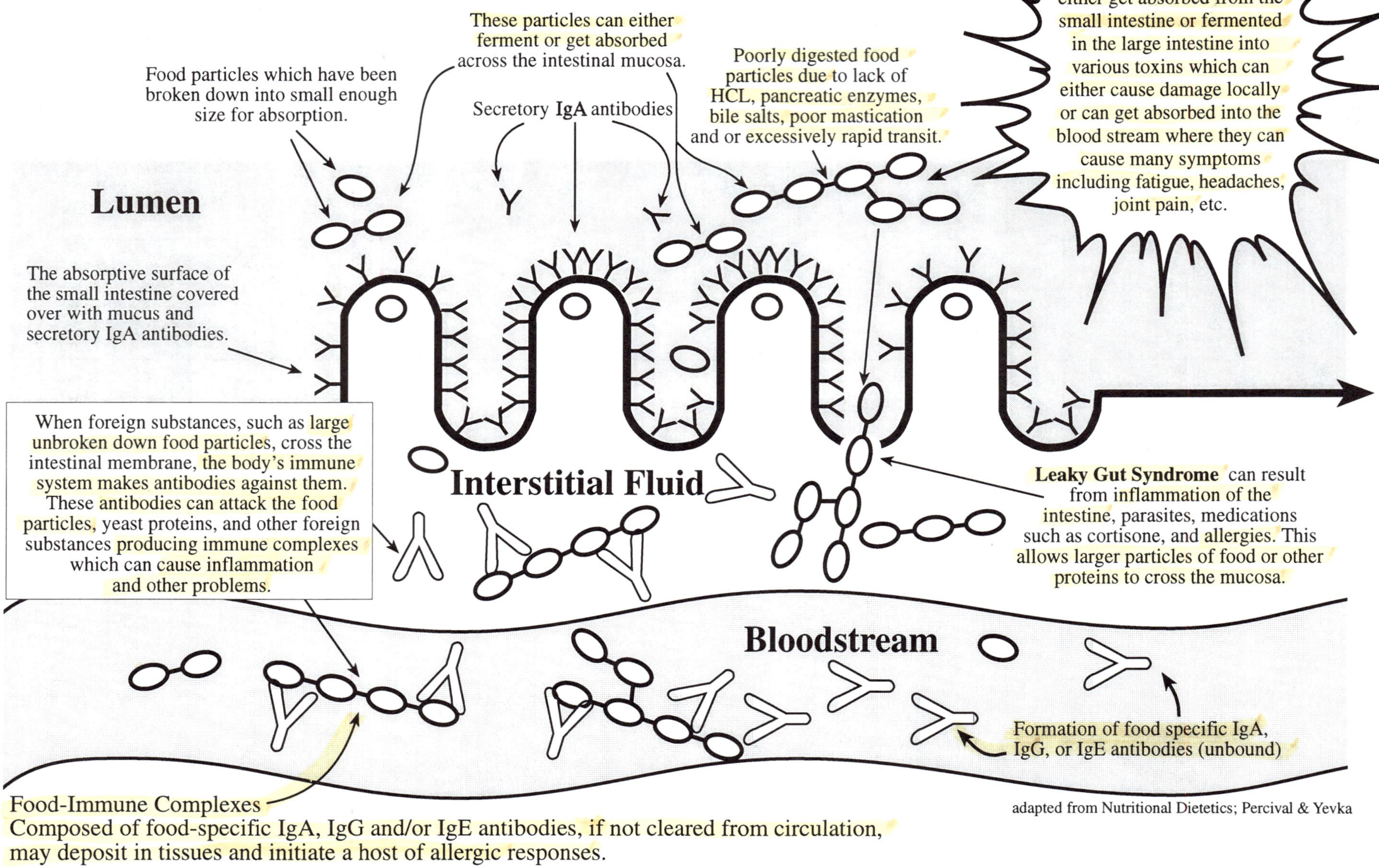

Food particles which have been broken down into small enough size for absorption.

These particles can either ferment or get absorbed across the intestinal mucosa.

Secretory **IgA** antibodies

Poorly digested food particles due to lack of HCL, pancreatic enzymes, bile salts, poor mastication and or excessively rapid transit.

These larger particles may either get absorbed from the small intestine or fermented in the large intestine into various toxins which can either cause damage locally or can get absorbed into the blood stream where they can cause many symptoms including fatigue, headaches, joint pain, etc.

**Lumen**

The absorptive surface of the small intestine covered over with mucus and secretory IgA antibodies.

When foreign substances, such as large unbroken down food particles, cross the intestinal membrane, the body's immune system makes antibodies against them. These antibodies can attack the food particles, yeast proteins, and other foreign substances producing immune complexes which can cause inflammation and other problems.

**Interstitial Fluid**

**Leaky Gut Syndrome** can result from inflammation of the intestine, parasites, medications such as cortisone, and allergies. This allows larger particles of food or other proteins to cross the mucosa.

**Bloodstream**

Formation of food specific IgA, IgG, or IgE antibodies (unbound)

Food-Immune Complexes
Composed of food-specific IgA, IgG and/or IgE antibodies, if not cleared from circulation, may deposit in tissues and initiate a host of allergic responses.

adapted from Nutritional Dietetics; Percival & Yevka

Regulators of GI contractile and secretory activity are found locally within the gut wall, enteric nervous system, and the external system of nerve fibers from the autonomic nervous system. Mucosal receptors are sensitive to the chemical composition of chyme and HCL, as well as the physical stimulus of stretching via food, *especially fiber.* These stimuli send impulses to the muscle and secretory cells of the GI tract via transmitters of the ***submucosal and myenteric plexuses***. These transmitters include enkephalin, somatostatin, serotonin, bombesin, and neurotensin.

Autonomic innervation is supplied by 2 routes:

**1)** **sympathetic fibers** that run along vessels generally inhibit digestive activity

**2)** **parasympathetic fibers** via the vagus nerve ("the wanderer")–Generally, parasympathetic fibers stimulate enzymatic activity and motility.

## The Mouth

The act of thinking about, smelling, and looking at food stimulates the flow of a thin mucus-like fluid that comes from three sets of salivary glands located under the tongue, and at the back angle of the jaw (sublingual, submandibular, and parotid glands). These secretions, totaling 1.5 liters of fluid per day, contain the enzyme, *alpha amylase* (ptyalin), which is responsible for the beginning of starch digestion. These secretions are known as *saliva.*

The function of this fluid is:

1) to lubricate food so it may be more easily swallowed;

2) to provide starch-splitting digestive enzymes (salivary amylase or ptyalin).

The chewing process in the mouth essentially breaks down food into smaller particles. This enables the digestive juices of the intestines to more easily penetrate the food and break it down still further. People who do not chew food well because they eat too quickly or because they have problems with their teeth or jaw may put an excessive burden on the other digestive organs of the body. This, in turn, may lead to various types of pathologies. During the secretion of saliva, digestion is continued through the tearing, crushing and grinding of the food. The proper chewing of food cannot be over emphasized, for it is here that many people start having problems with digestion, especially if enzyme secretion is weak.

## The Esophagus

The esophagus is a 10-12 inch muscular tube which connects the oropharynx with the stomach. Once food has been sufficiently chewed up and lubricated, the tongue rolls up the food into a small ball called a **bolus**. This bolus is placed by the tongue on the top of the esophagus. Upon the initiation of swallowing, a small flap called the epiglottis covers the top of the trachea, thus preventing food from going into the lungs. Food travels down the esophagus by the action of **peristalsis**. Peristalsis is the rhythmic contraction and relaxation of the smooth muscles of the digestive tract. Peristalsis starts in the esophagus. Its function is to move the food, reduce the size of the food particles and further mix the bolus with digestive enzymes.

## The Stomach

Food enters into the stomach from the esophagus as **chyme**. Chyme refers to the alkaline mixture of food and saliva that comes from the esophagus. Chyme passes into the stomach through a special muscular opening called the **lower esophageal sphincter** (LES) or the cardiac sphincter.

This is the area of the esophagus which is tightly surrounded by the diaphragm.

Once chyme enters into the stomach, it stimulates the release of the hormone **gastrin**. Gastrin, once released into the blood from the stomach, stimulates the parietal cells of the stomach to release **hydrochloric acid (HCL)**. Distention of the stomach, as well as the thought of eating food (cephalic phase of digestion), also stimulates the stomach to secrete HCL and pepsin. In addition, **intrinsic factor** gets released from the parietal cells. Intrinsic factor is a substance that must combine with vitamin B-12 from food in order to be absorbed in the ileum of the small intestine.

The **normal pH of the stomach is between 1-2** when it is empty of food. This represents more than a million-fold concentration of acid in the stomach as compared to the blood. The stomach, particularly the parietal cells, expends very large amounts of energy in order to concentrate these hydrogen ions.

The purpose of this high concentration of HCL is:

1) To kill any parasites, bacteria or viruses that may be ingested with either food or water;
2) To aid in the digestion of proteins;
3) To digest foods containing vitamin B-12, freeing this B-12 so that it may combine with intrinsic factor and get absorbed in the distal ileum;
4) To make the duodenal pH more acidic which, in turn, makes it much more conducive to absorbing many of the B vitamins;
5) To keep minerals such as iron in the reduced form in order to enhance their absorption.

Physically, the stomach breaks down foods via its peristaltic activity. Active chemical breakdown begins in the central area of the stomach. An average of 2 to 2.5 liters per day of enzyme filled fluid is secreted by the stomach. The following enzymes and related compounds are also secreted:

- **HCL**–This strong acid is primarily responsible for protein digestion. It also enhances mineral absorption, is essential for vitamin B-12 absorption, and is important in regulating the pH of the small intestine which in turn regulates the bacterial flora.
- **Intrinsic factor**–This important protein molecule, which is secreted by the parietal cells, is responsible for the binding and absorption of vitamin B-12.
- **Pepsinogen**–This protein molecule is secreted by the chief cells of the stomach, which is then cleaved by HCL into the active **pepsin** enzyme. It is a potent enzyme responsible for protein digestion. It has an optimum pH of between 1-3 and becomes denatured above pH 5. It breaks down peptides containing aromatic amino acids.
- **Gastric lipase**–This is a weak enzyme which, to a small extent, digests lipids.
- **Mucus**–Mucus is released into the stomach by specialized cells of the stomach for protection. Its secretion is regulated by chemical and physical stimulants such as alcohol and fiber. It is, in part, regulated by prostaglandins, hormones that are synthesized from essential fatty acids in the diet.
- **Gastrin**–is a small peptide hormone secreted from the wall of the stomach in response to the presence of food in the stomach. Gastrin stimulates the release of HCL in the stomach along with certain foods such as coffee and alcohol. Foods with calcium tend to stimulate gastrin. HCL, through negative feedback, inhibits its secretion.

## Gastric emptying

Generally the stomach takes 1-5 hours to empty, depending upon the types of foods eaten. Carbohydrates empty the most rapidly, then proteins and finally fats. In a mixed diet, the emptying time is generally prolonged.

As food particles get digested in the stomach via peristalsis and enzymatic action, some of the resulting chyme leaves the stomach from the pylorus through the action of gastrin. Gastrin acts to alternately relax the pylorus and stimulate the pyloric pump which promotes stomach emptying. Factors which inhibit gastric emptying involve the **enterogastric reflex**. The enterogastric reflex is a neurological signal from the duodenum to the pylorus to constrict the pylorus; thus, preventing food from leaving the stomach.

The following are factors that regulate this enterogastric reflex:

1) How much distention is in the duodenum;
2) How much irritation through acidity or other factors is occurring in the duodenum;
3) How concentrated the chyme entering into the duodenum is;
4) How many protein breakdown products as well as, but to a lesser extent, fats are entering into the duodenum.

Fats entering into the duodenum stimulate the release of several hormones including cholecystokinin and gastric inhibitory peptide. These hormones act to delay gastric emptying, the purpose of which is to allow more time for the breakdown of fats in the digestive tract. It thus appears that fats entering into the duodenum have the most pronounced effect on keeping food in the stomach.

## The Small Intestine

Food gradually enters into the small intestine from the stomach through a muscular opening called the **pyloric sphincter**. The small intestine is where the final digestion and absorption of food takes place. The small intestine is about 7 meters (20 feet) in length and has a diameter of about 1 to 1.5 inches. The surface area of the small intestines, because of the villi and microvilli, is comparable to the size of a tennis court (225 square meters)! This is necessary to help digest and absorb foods efficiently. Enzymes necessary to digest fats, proteins and carbohydrates are secreted by the pancreas into the duodenum. The pancreas releases its enzymes into the duodenum in response to chyme entering into the small intestine. Chyme entering into the small intestine stimulates the release of the hormone **secretin** from the intestinal wall. Besides enzymes, the pancreas also secretes bicarbonate, an alkalizing agent which helps neutralize the acid going into the duodenum. In addition, **bile salts** are secreted into the duodenum from the gall bladder in response to fats entering the duodenum. These bile salts are originally synthesized in the liver from cholesterol and are then stored at a high concentration (12x higher than the liver) in the gall bladder. They are necessary for the digestion and absorption of fats and fat soluble nutrients (i.e., vitamins A, D, E, and K).

Many of the carbohydrates digested by enzymes from the pancreas must be broken down one step further by **disaccharide enzymes**, which are found in the brush border of the small intestine (see diagram on carbohydrate metabolism pg. 33). Without these final carbohydrate digesting enzymes, the carbohydrates are not broken down in particles sufficiently small enough to be absorbed into the bloodstream. As a result, bacteria in the intestine can ferment these unabsorbed carbohydrates; thereby resulting in gas, bloating and diarrhea. For instance, lactose intolerance is a condition in which there is not sufficient lactase enzyme to break down the milk sugar, lactose. As a result, the normal bacteria of the intestines ferments this sugar, causing the bloating, gas, and diarrhea indicative of lactose intolerance.

The small intestine is divided into the duodenum, then the jejunum, and finally the ileum. Most digestion takes place in the duodenum, while absorption takes place predominantly in the jejunum. Most of the enzymes in the small intestine come from the pancreas. The gall bladder adds a significant amount of digestive juices as well.

**The pancreas secretes the following digestive enzymes:**

- **Trypsin**–A protein enzyme used for protein synthesis, it is produced by the cleavage of trypsinogen in the duodenum by the action of enterokinase, an enzyme located on the brush border of duodenal enterocytes. Once formed, trypsin can activate other secreted trypsinogen and also other peptidase precursors from the pancreas.
- **Chymotrypsin**–An enzyme produced from chymotrypsinogen which has been cleaved by HCL, chymotrypsin is responsible for the digestion of proteins with an aromatic amino acid moiety, leucine, and glutamine.
- **Carboxypolypeptidase**–Digests the terminal amino acid of a protein.
- **Ribonuclease**–Hydrolyzes RNA to form mononucleotides.
- **Deoxyribonuclease**–Hydrolyzes DNA to form mononucleotides.
- **Elastase**–Hydrolyzes fibrous proteins to form peptides and amino acids.
- **Lipase**–Hydrolyzes fats to form fatty acids and glycerol.
- **Cholesterol esterase**–Hydrolyzes cholesterol to form cholesterol and fatty acid esters.
- **Alpha amylase**–Hydrolyzes starch and dextrins to form dextrins and maltose.
- **Phospholipase A2**–This enzyme is secreted in an inactive form and becomes active through the action of trypsin. Mixed micelles containing phospholipids are digested by phospholipase A2. Requiring bile salts for the hydrolyzation of dietary phospholipids, it is also responsible for digesting cell membranes which are composed of phospholipids.
- **Colipase**–is activated by trypsin and becomes very active when quantities of fat are present.

**The small intestine secretes the following digestive enzymes**:

- **Secretin**–A hormone secreted into duodenal mucosa in response to acid in the small intestine, it reduces resting pressure of the LES. It reduces gastric and duodenal motility and stimulates pepsinogen secretion. It also inhibits gastric stimulated gastric acid secretion and increases the mucus output of Brunner's glands. Lastly, it increases the output of water and bicarbonate, while increasing certain enzymes secreted from the pancreas along with insulin release.
- **Sucrase**–An enzyme secreted from the mucosal brush border, sucrase is responsible for breaking sucrose into fructose and glucose.
- **Alpha dextrinase**–Secreted from the brush border, it is responsible for the breakdown of dextrins into glucose.
- **Maltase**–Secreted from the brush border, it is responsible for the breakdown of maltose into two glucose molecules.

- **Lactase**–Secreted from the brush border, it is responsible for the breakdown of lactose into galactose and glucose.
- **Cholecystokinin-pancreozymin**–Secreted from the duodenal mucosa, it increases motility, causes contraction of the gallbladder, stimulates enzyme secretion of pancreas, potentiates the effect of secretin on pancreas and slows gastric emptying.
- **Gastric inhibitory polypeptide (GIP)**–Secreted from the small intestine, it inhibits gastrin-stimulated HCL and also stimulates insulin secretion.
- **Enteroglucagon and glucagon**–Secreted from the pancreas, it inhibits pancreatic enzyme secretion and also motility. It also increases gluconeogenesis and glycogenolysis.
- **Vasoactive intestinal polypeptide (VIP)**–Released via neurons in the small intestine, VIP is stimulated to be released by fat, alcohol, and HCL from the stomach.
- **Somatostatin**–From the antrum of the stomach, the duodenum, this hormone is released in response to HCL and amino acids. It functions to inhibit gastrin release and inhibit HCL secretion. It also inhibits release of insulin and glucagon and decreases pancreatic enzyme production.

## Absorption

Absorption is the process by which the smallest broken down units of food get transported across the intestinal mucosa and into the bloodstream or lymphatic system. After digestion is completed, the process of absorption begins. Nutrients must first be bound to certain carrier molecules for carrier facilitated diffusion or active transport. They must then cross through the unstirred water layer (UWL, see next page). Once absorbed into the blood, they are carried by the portal vein to the liver. All nutrients or other substances that get absorbed (besides fats) must first get transported to the liver. The liver then further metabolizes the substance so that it may be more effectively accommodated by the body. If it is a toxic substance, it may get metabolized into a more harmless compound. In Chinese medicine/physiology this is a similar action that the spleen performs, separating the pure from the impure. Nutrients that get absorbed into the lymphatic system (most fats), end up in the general circulation via the thoracic duct near the heart. All nutrients that get transported to cells from the bloodstream must first pass into the interstitial fluid or extracellular fluid.

Nutrients are absorbed in 3 ways:

1) **Passive diffusion**–This requires no energy by the body. It is simply a way in which nutrients flow from an area of higher concentration to an area of lower concentration.

2) **Carrier-facilitated diffusion**–This method is a partially active transport that usually requires the services of protein carrier molecules to transport active nutrients to the intestinal mucosa. One example is the transportation of vitamin B-12 across the ileum through the use of the protein carrier molecule intrinsic factor.

3) **Active transport**–This method is an active process requiring energy from the body in order to transport nutrients or substances usually from an area of lesser concentration to an area of higher concentration. Examples of this include the process by which HCL ions are pumped into the stomach where they are a million times more

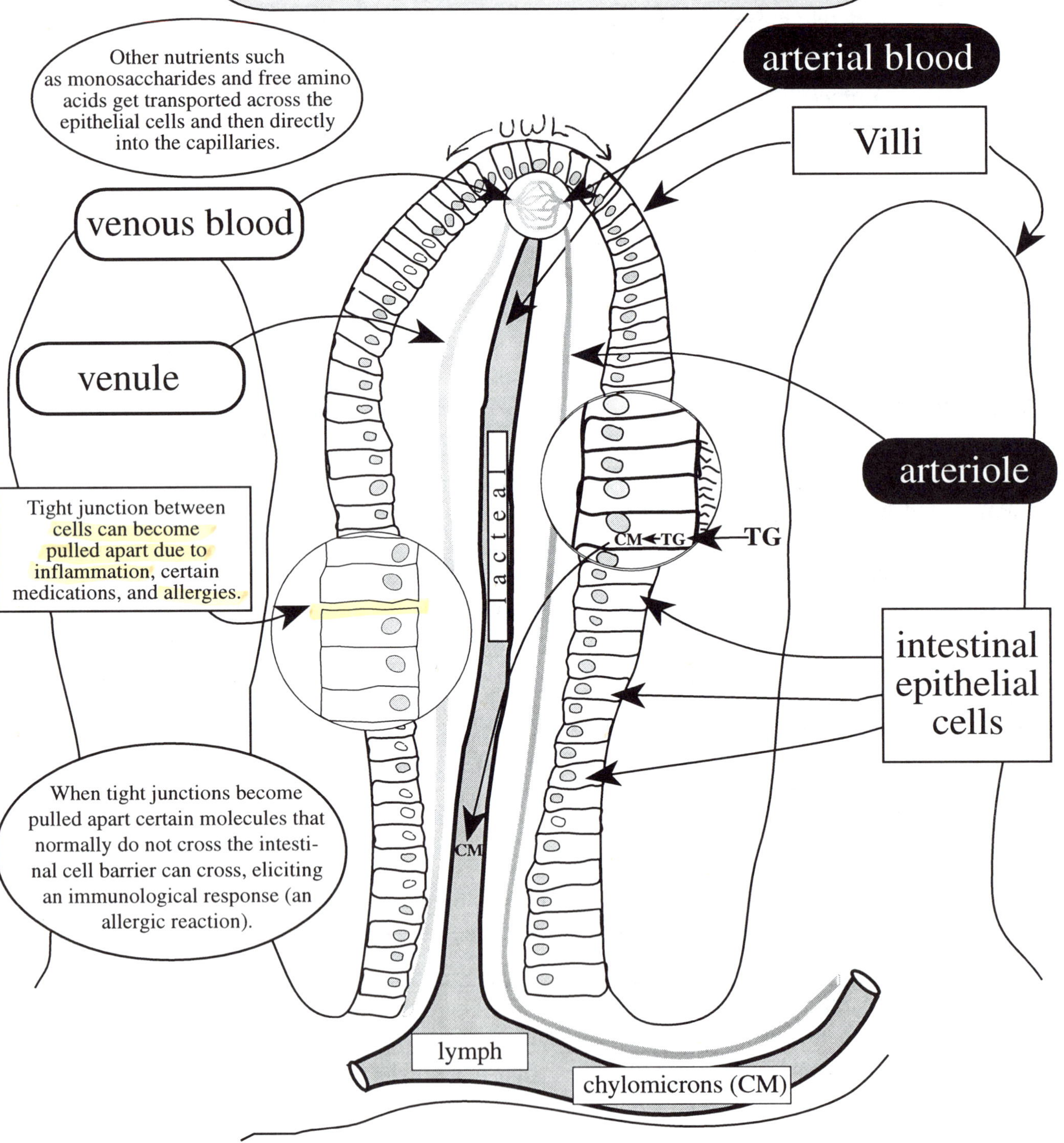
Micelles in the lumen of the GI tract are first broken down into free fatty acids and then transported into the epithelial cells where they are then reassembled into chylomicrons (CM) so they can then be transported into the lymph. From the lymph they enter into the blood via the thoracic duct. Chylomicrons give the blood a milky appearance.
Other nutrients such as monosaccharides and free amino acids get transported across the epithelial cells and then directly into the capillaries.
arterial blood
Villi
UWL
venous blood
venule
arteriole
Tight junction between cells can become pulled apart due to inflammation, certain medications, and allergies.
lacteal
CM
TG
intestinal epithelial cells
When tight junctions become pulled apart certain molecules that normally do not cross the intestinal cell barrier can cross, eliciting an immunological response (an allergic reaction).
lymph
chylomicrons (CM)

concentrated than in the blood; or when magnesium ions are transported into the heart muscle where they are concentrated at a level 18x that of the bloodstream.

**Unstirred water layer(UWL)**–Between the absorptive brush border and the lumen of the small intestine there is a thin area of fluid which acts as a barrier to various molecules. It is here that micelles dissociate into bile salts and free fatty acids. The UWL is water soluble and micelles are able to transport lipid soluble fatty acids through this liquid barrier and up to the brush border so that they can be absorbed across the cell membrane.

## Absorption of various nutrients

*Cholesterol absorption*–Cholesterol is normally found in foods as cholesterol esters. It is first digested by the enzyme *pancreatic cholesterol esterase*. Once the ester forms are hydrolyzed, cholesterol is formed into micelles and ferried across the UWL.

*Fat soluble vitamins*–Once cleaved from foods, they must also be made into micelles to be transported into the brush border for absorption. If no fats are present, then no micelles are formed and fat soluble nutrients may become deficient.

*Water soluble vitamins*–Most of the water soluble vitamins get absorbed in the proximal small intestine by passive diffusion. The exception is vitamin B-12 which must combine with intrinsic factor and then be actively transported across the mucosa in the distal ileum. There are a number of different factors which can effect the absorptive rate including fiber, fats, proteins, medications, parasites, and damage to villi to name a few.

*Minerals* get absorbed across the small intestinal mucosa in various stages. In the first, the *intraluminal stage,* minerals interact with the acid in the stomach and the chemical composition of the food. Cations are most affected, whereas small anions, such as fluoride, are not influenced by either pH or the chemical composition of the diet and are easily absorbed. Cations are readily soluble in the acidic pH of the normal stomach, but once they enter into the small intestine, where the pH is much more alkaline, they may form insoluble soaps. In the small intestine various chelating agents such as amino acids, simple sugars, and other compounds make the minerals available for the next stage.

The 2nd, the *translocation stage*, involves the actual passage of cation minerals across the enterocyte membranes either by active transport or facilitated diffusion. The concentration gradient plays a role in how well minerals are transported across the cell membrane. The final mobilization stage involves the actual passage of the mineral from inside the intestinal enterocyte to the bloodstream. Some minerals, like iron and zinc, are sequestered within the cell by proteins. They are in equilibrium with free minerals and the rate of passage across the membrane is determined by how big the free pool is. There is often competition between minerals for absorption, but sometimes minerals, such as magnesium and calcium, help each other get assimilated by the body.

*Metals* bind to protein carriers to be transported across cell membranes. Some metals, such as iron, require specific protein carriers such as transferrin, while others require more general protein carriers such as albumin. Metals requiring specific carriers usually tend to be only partially saturated. This is probably a way the body has to buffer itself against toxicity.

**Malabsorption** usually refers to inadequate absorption of nutrients from the intestinal tract. There are a multitude of etiologies for malabsorption, including inflammatory bowel disease, parasites, medications, antacids, celiac disease, anything that causes chronic diarrhea (numerous medications including antibiotics, excessive sugar intake, magnesium overload), pancreatic insufficiency, allergies. Malabsorption may be chronic or acute and can show up during a nutritionally oriented physical by examining the fingernails, hair, skin, mouth, tongue, eyes, etc. (see *Nutritional Physical* in the appendix). There are various lab tests that can evaluate the causes of malabsorption.

- *Lactulose and mannitol intestinal permeability*–Administration of two sugars, lactulose and mannitol, with subsequent urine collection can reveal both malabsorption and/or increased intestinal permeability (see Celiac disease chapter).
- *Heidelberg test*–This measures the acidity of the stomach. It uses a capsule that is tethered with a thread and then is swallowed down into the stomach. It can read the pH of the fluids and transmit a signal up to a meter to determine the pH. The stomach is repeatedly challenged with sodium bicarbonate and pH is monitored to see how quickly the stomach reacidifys.
- *Hair analysis* may be somewhat helpful in giving an overall view of how well one is absorbing minerals. If numerous mineral levels appear low on the test, it may indicate malabsorption if other things are ruled out.

When checking for malabsorption during a history, questions regarding whether stools appear frothy or greasy may give important clues. ***Steatorrhea*** is a condition that occurs when fat is not being digested or absorbed and ends up in the stools. Sometimes other food components may end up in the stool as "malabsorbed." There are several labs around the country that evaluates stools for malabsorption or maldigestion including Great Smokies Lab in North Carolina, Meridian Labs in Kent, WA, Diagnostechs and National BioTech Labs, both in Seattle, WA (see appendix at end of book).

**Clinical Note**–Sometimes larger molecules get absorbed from the GI tract, due to excessive cortisol secretion, inflammation of GI tract (caused by allergies, parasites, the use of certain medications like NSAIDS and aspirin). This may result in an immune reaction showing many different symptoms. This phenomenon is sometimes referred to as "leaky gut syndrome" (see diagram on page 10, also allergies chapter).

## The Large Intestine

The main function of the large intestine is to absorb water, electrolytes, and, to a minor extent, some vitamins that are synthesized in the area itself. 80-90% of the fluid of chyme gets reabsorbed by the large intestine, leaving about 5-200ml to be excreted in the feces. The colonic contents move at a rate of approximately 5cm/hour. Most of the nutrients have been absorbed by the time food reaches the large intestine. The remaining mass consists mostly of indigestible dietary fiber and water. There are certain compounds produced in the large intestine. Large amounts of mucus are normally secreted by the mucosa of the large intestine to protect its epithelial cells from physical trauma and bacterial toxins. Bicarbonate ions, secreted in exchange for absorbed chloride ions, help neutralize the acidity of the secretions of the bacteria. The large intestine is about 5ft long, and as the remaining semisolid food passes through it, water gets absorbed out. By the time the mass reaches the anus, the consistency becomes semisolid or **feces** as it is called.

The time it takes for food to reach the anus from the mouth is known as *Bowel Transit Time* (BTT). The longer the period of time, the greater the types of pathologies–such as diverticulitis, allergies, abnormal gut flora, precancerous lesions, etc.–that may develop. Dr. Dennis Burkett, a British research physician, traveled to Africa in 1974 and studied the people of Uganda and other cultures in Africa. He found that the higher the intake of fiber and the shorter the BTT, the lesser the incidence of colon cancer. In his comparisons with western cultures, the people in the areas which had the highest intake of fiber had virtually no diverticulosis, diverticulitis, or heart disease.

> **Clinical note**–A simple technique that can be employed to evaluate the approximate bowel transit time is to take 6 charcoal capsules after dinner and examine the next few bowel movements to see when the stools turn black. Ideally, we like to see most of the blackness appear in the first bowel movement after taking the charcoal and for there to be no charcoal after 24 hours. A longer transit time may indicate elimination problems and an increased susceptibility to absorption of endotoxins from the gut.
>
> One simple test that evaluates whether there is putrefication in the intestines is called the *urinary indican test.* This test measures the conversion of aromatic amino acids into indican in the intestines. The more indican found in the urine, the more that is being made in the intestines and the more endotoxins might be manufactured in the intestines. It should be noted that a diet high in the aromatic amino acids tyrosine and tryptophan can cause an increased production of indican, as well as constipation, without indicating putrefication.
>
> An ideal bowel transit time is around 17 hours. A delayed bowel transit time of 48 hours or more may lead to increased risk of colon cancer and general "autotoxicity." This term describes systemic symptoms that may arise as a result of absorption of various types of putrefication products that may form as a result of abnormal bacteria or an extended exposure to normal bacteria.

Bacteria in the intestines digest some food matter that was not broken down by enzymatic action higher in the intestines. Some bacteria break down indigestible fibers into short chain fatty acids such as butyrate. Butyrate is a 4 carbon chain fatty acid that has been found to be protective against colon cancer. Certain nutrients, such as vitamins K, vitamin B-12, B-1, and B-2, can be synthesized and absorbed, sometimes in significant amounts, directly in the large intestine.

The feces consists of 75% water and 25% solids. About 1/3 of the solid matter is made of dead bacteria. Undigested dietary fiber, epithelial cells, and dried components of digestive juices make up another 1/3. Inorganic solids and fats comprise the remaining 30% of the solid matter with the final 3% being made of protein.

Defecation is the act of peristaltic action removing feces through the anus and occurs as often as once every meal to once every week or so. A delayed or prolonged BTT may lead to hemorrhoids, diverticulosis, diverticulitis, increased risk of cancer of the colon, as well as allergies and **auto toxicity.**

**Microclot Test** - This is a test that measures abnormal fermentation in the GI tract and the presence of endotoxins. This procedure involves drawing blood and mixing it with a special lipopolysaccharide. After incubating for a period of 24 hours a number of microclots will form depending upon how well the liver is clearing endotoxins or how many endotoxins are being produced in the GI tract. The higher the number of microclots, the greater the amount of endotoxins is being produced and/or the less the liver is able to clear them. (Juhlin L & Shelly W *Microclot generation (MCG) test in disease.* ACTA Med Scand. 210:305-307, 1981)

**Chymex Test** - Another test used to evaluate fermentation in the GI tract is the Chymex Test. Chymex is a synthetic peptide that contains the molecule para amino benzoic acid (PABA). The test involves swallowing this compound, and in normal digestion, the pancreatic enzyme chymotrypsin cleaves off PABA. In normal subjects, when PABA is cleaved, it gets conjugated by the liver and then excreted via the kidneys in urine. The amount of PABA recovered is in direct proportion to the function of the pancreas. Normally over 80% of the PABA is recovered in 6 hours. A decreased recovery may indicate pancreatic insufficiency.

## Metabolism

Once nutrients have been absorbed from the GI tract to the blood, they must enter into the interstitial fluid and then into the cells. All the chemical changes that occur in a nutrient once it is absorbed into the blood are known as **metabolism**.

The waste products of cellular metabolism and unused nutrients are released into the extracellular fluid. They enter the capillaries, then the veins of the bloodstream and are eventually excreted from the body, primarily through the lungs and the kidneys. Almost all of the carbon dioxide produced in the body and 10% of the water are excreted through the lungs.

The kidneys act as an efficient and selective filtering system for the bloodstream. They are capable of concentrating waste products of metabolism in the urine and excreting them. They also allow excesses of nutrients, such as water-soluble vitamins, to leave the body. However, as the blood gets filtered through them, the kidneys will reabsorb practically all of the glucose or protein, both of which the body must save or retain. For other nutrients, such as sodium, the kidneys will reabsorb the amounts needed to maintain normal blood and tissue levels and will release the rest in the urine. The kidneys are extremely sensitive, regulating the nature and amount of the metabolites excreted, usually in response to hormones and the body's need for particular nutrients.

Nutrients are lost from the body:

1) **Through the skin**–Nutrients are lost either in perspiration (usually electrolytes) or via sloughing off of epithelial cells (minerals and proteins).
2) **Through the feces**–These are undigested or unabsorbed nutrients such as calcium, carotenoids, iron, etc. Cells lining the gastrointestinal tract are completely replaced every 3 days and there are specific nutrients that the body relies on to replace these cells.
3) **Through the urine**–Many excess water-soluble vitamins are lost through the urine after they have been absorbed. Nitrogenous waste from protein catabolism in the form of urea is lost here as well.
4) **Through the breath**.

The nutrients that do not get excreted will be returned from the capillaries back to the liver.

In fact, all of the nutrients absorbed from the GI tract are first transported to the liver through the portal vein. In this manner, any toxic substance that gets absorbed must first be filtered through the liver before it can travel around in the bloodstream and into tissues of the body. The liver is one of the most critical organs of metabolism since thousands of metabolic reactions take place here. From the liver, the modified nutrients travel back to the heart where they can then be transported around the body for more metabolic activities.

## Anabolism

When the primary products of digestion are used to build structural, storage, enzymatic, or other components of the body, this is known as *anabolism*; thus, anabolism is the building up of body materials, both structural and functional.

## Catabolism

When the body breaks down primary components of digestion, various tissues or compounds of the body, this is known as *catabolism*. This is very important for supplying compounds for energy production, as in deamination of amino acids, or for supplying compounds for tissue or enzyme synthesis, as well as numerous other metabolic activities.

## Notes

---

# CARBOHYDRATES (CHO)

Carbohydrates include starch, which is found in vegetables and both whole grain and refined cereals; cellulose or fiber in whole grains, fruits and vegetables; and various sugars found in fruits, vegetables, milk products, and sweeteners. Since 1900, we have seen a progressive decline in carbohydrate consumption, especially complex carbohydrates. Today about 40% of calories in the average American diet come from carbohydrates. This represents a decrease of about 30% since 1900 (Glinsmann, et.al. 86). About 60% of absorbable carbohydrates is currently in the form of polysaccharides (25% of total calories). In 1900, 75% of ingested carbohydrates were in the polysaccharide form (57% of total calories).

The average American consumes a total of 126 lbs of added caloric sweeteners per year (65 lbs are added sucrose and 40 lbs are added high fructose corn-syrup). This represents about 1/2 lb of sugar per day per person (with 28% of this contained in soft drinks). As of 1996 it has been calculated that 19% of all calories consumed per day come from simple carbohydrates which represents 41 teaspoons of table sugar per day!

In some undeveloped countries 80% of calories come from carbohydrates, especially from complex carbohydrates. This means that very high amounts of fiber are being consumed. It is interesting to note that in those undeveloped areas with high carbohydrate diets, many of the degenerative diseases that are so common in developed countries today do not exist.

## Complex Carbohydrates Versus Simple Carbohydrates

Complex carbohydrates are forms of carbohydrates that contain mostly starches or long chains of mono and disaccharides as well as the natural fibrous moieties that originally were found with the food. It takes time for the body to digest these forms of carbohydrates. This has numerous physiological effects on the body. Complex carbohydrates tend to allow the body time to know that it has had enough to eat. They also have various effects on cholesterol because of the fiber.

Simple carbohydrates, on the other hand are forms that have been refined to contain more of the simple sugar molecules. Usually, part or all of the germ and fibrous components of the plant have been removed during this process. Many of the nutrients that are required to metabolize the starches in the grain are discarded. The result is a food that burns quickly but lacks some of its natural chemical and physical characteristics. In addition, over time, they can deplete those nutrients which were removed during the milling process.

Plants may store carbohydrate as 3 major forms:

1) monosaccharides, a simple carbohydrate;
2) disaccharides, a simple carbohydrate;
3) polysaccharides, complex carbohydrates which include starch, cellulose or fiber (fiber is known as indigestible CHO).

## Monosaccharides

Mostly composed of hexoses (6 carbons rings), this is the simplest form of sugar from which almost all complex carbohydrates are formed. There are 3 hexose monosaccharides of nutritional importance: glucose, galactose and fructose. They are usually found bonded to each other with special bonds and in different combinations.

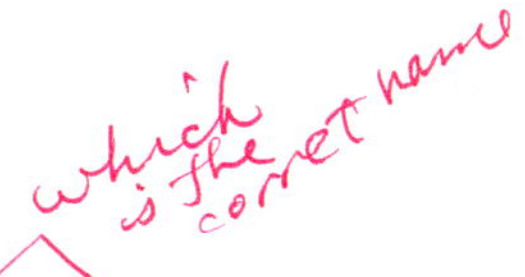



**Glucose** (dextrose)–This monosaccharide molecule is supplied to all the tissues of the body. Also known as "blood sugar," glucose is found in fruits, vegetables, syrups and honey. These foods only provide a small amount (~ 18gms) of glucose per day. Glucose is the main source of energy for the central nervous system (CNS) and red blood cells (RBCs). The CNS requires about 140 gms per day, while RBCs need 40 gms per day. The additional glucose comes from the breakdown of more complex carbohydrates, from certain amino acids, and from the glycerol moiety of triglycerides. Glucose is the only form of CHO carried by the blood. Tissues throughout the body rely on glucose as their major source of energy. Normally the body tries to maintain blood glucose levels of 100mg/dl. This value, taken at least 5 hours after eating, is known as the fasting glucose level.

**CLINICAL NOTES**

**Hyperglycemia**–blood glucose levels above 160mg/dl. This can arise if there is not enough insulin or if the insulin present is not able to adequately bind onto the insulin receptor sites. Lack of binding may be a result of competition with other molecules for the receptor site or damage to the actual receptor sites. When glucose levels rise above 160mg/dl (as an individual value), the kidneys can not reabsorb the glucose fast enough and some of the sugar spills into the urine. The body tries to dilute this glucose (high osmolality) by adding water which results in more frequent urination. More urination results in dehydration and subsequent increased thirst. Transient increases in blood sugar usually go undetected even if these sporadic increases have been going on for years. *It is very important to realize that transient high levels of blood glucose usually do not cause any symptoms.*

**Hypoglycemia**–blood glucose levels below 60mg/dl. When blood glucose levels drop below 60mg/dl, a ravenous feeling of hunger may ensue. This is often accompanied by weakness, trembling, headaches, palpitations, sweating, and light-headedness. There is significant individual variation in these symptoms and they may occur at different blood glucose levels even in the same person at different times. There may be symptoms that relate to large fluctuations in glucose as well as to changes in insulin or cortisol levels. Hypoglycemia is not a disease, but, rather, a symptom (similar to fever). There are two types of hypoglycemia, spontaneous or reactive. Spontaneous hypoglycemia refers to a condition in which there is always an excess of insulin which results in chronically low blood glucose levels. Reactive hypoglycemia refers to a drop in blood glucose due to a prolonged period of time between meals, an excessive ingestion of simple carbohydrates, an allergic reaction to a food, or consumption of alcohol without eating while expending energy. An excessive amount of simple CHO causes an increased secretion of insulin which results in lowered blood glucose. Postprandial (post= after, prandial= meal) hypoglycemia is another term used for hypoglycemia which occurs following a meal or snack (usually 2-4 hours after eating).

**Galactose**–This monosaccharide, found in lactose or milk sugar, has been shown to be important in the production of certain beneficial bacteria in the gut, especially in infants. An inborn error in metabolism (galactosemia) can occur, in which the body cannot metabolize galactose. This usually results in cataract formation in the eyes.

**Fructose**–This is the sweetest of all the sugars with a sweetness value of 173 compared to sucrose at 100. It has been touted as an excellent sugar for diabetics since it does not raise glucose levels like other sugars. While this may be true, there are other problems associated with fructose consumption. Studies have shown a link between fructose and heart disease as well as other problems related to diabetes and allergies.

> **NOTE**–The *Maillard* or *browning reaction* takes place in foods–such as pastries, doughnuts, cookies, puffed and flaked cereals–which contain lysine and simple sugars. The simple sugar needs to be a reducing sugar, such as fructose. When the food is heated, the fructose sugars caramelize. In this process simple sugars hook unto the lysine moiety. This makes the body unable to hydrolyze the protein chain which contains the caramelized lysine molecule. When these peptides are absorbed, they may trigger an immune response. In addition, if lysine levels are already borderline low, these foods can cause a lysine deficiency. For further information, see the amino acid chapter on lysine.

## Pentoses

This is a general class of 5 carbon sugars which include ribose, a monosaccharide which makes up the vitamin riboflavin and the coenzymes made from it. It is also an essential moiety of RNA and DNA. Although essential in the body, it is not an essential nutrient since the body can synthesize ribose from glucose.

## Disaccharides

These sugars require disaccharidase enzymes found in the small intestine brush border for digestion into monosaccharides.

| | |
|---|---|
| Sucrose–100/100 sweetness– | made of glucose and fructose (table sugar) |
| Maltose–32/100 sweetness– | made of 2 glucose molecules |
| Lactose–16/100 sweetness– | made of glucose and galactose |

## Polyhydroxy Alcohols

These are alcohol forms of sucrose, mannose and xylose. They include sorbitol, mannitol and xylitol. Although they retain some of the sweetness of the original sugars they are absorbed more slowly from the GI tract and hence have a lower glycemic index. Xylitol is often used in sugarless chewing gum because cariogenic bacteria are unable to use it as a substrate.

## Alternative sweeteners

In the U.S. saccharin, aspartame and acesulfame K are approved non calorie sweeteners Sucralose, alitame and cyclamates are currently seeking approval by the FDA. Stevia rebaudiana is a naturally occurring plant which possess great sweetening properties yet has a zero glycemic index. Although used safely for many years in other countries, Stevia was banned by the FDA between 1991 and 1995 because of inadequate testing. Because Stevia is a plant that anyone can grow it appears that this ban was probably politically motivated. Extracts of Stevia can be as high as 300x sweeter than sucrose. In addition, it may actually be protective against dental carries.

Honey is a carbohydrate which comes from the nectar of flowers. It is carried back to the hive by honey bees who treat the nectar with an enzyme invertase. This enzyme breaks down the sucrose molecules into fructose and glucose. Its sweetness may range from 57-122% of sucrose. Although honey is 41% fructose it still contains 34% glucose which will rapidly increase blood sugar levels (glycemic index of 126). In addition, the low temperatures that honey is normaly processed at allows spores of Clostridium botulinum to survive and in the GI tract of an infant may germinate and produce toxins. Honey should thus not generally be fed to young infants. Nutritionally honey has small amounts of trace minerals and vitamins that aren't found in other sweeteners.

## Polysaccharides

Amylopectin–branched chains of glucose units.

Amylose–long straight chains of glucose units

## Starch

Found only in plants, it occurs in both *amylose* and *amylopectin* forms. The chemical and physical characteristics of starch are determined by the proportion of each form. Starch granules vary in both size and shape as they are enclosed within the plant cell wall. They are insoluble in cold water and will swell and form a gel when cooked. Cooking also causes the cell membranes to rupture and make the starch available for enzymatic digestive breakdown.

Dextrins are formed from the hydrolysis of starch. They are soluble intermediate polysaccharide products that are sweeter than the original starch molecule.

## Physiological Responses to Carbohydrates

**Glycemic index**– This refers to the rate blood glucose levels rise after the ingestion of a particular food (usually a mixed carbohydrate, fat and protein food) in comparison to an equivalent amount of pure glucose. Glucose alone is given the standard reference of 100. Sometimes the pure glucose is replaced with white bread as a standard. Interesting studies have shown that certain complex carbohydrates such as potato has a considerably higher glycemic index than ice cream. This is probably due to the fat content of the ice cream which has a moderating effect on how quickly the blood sugar will rise (see glycemia index of foods under Diabetes mellitus).

**Energy yield of carbohydrates**= *4 Kcal per gram.*

**Gluconeogenesis** is the synthesis of glucose from noncarbohydrate sources such as amino acids and glycerol moiety of lipids.

**Glycogenolysis** is the breaking down of glycogen to supply needed glucose. This usually comes from either muscle tissue or the liver.

**Dietary essential**–To prevent ketosis it is necessary to consume approximately 50-100 gms of CHO per day.

## Fiber

Fiber related carbohydrates–Fiber or roughage are compounds of plant origin that cannot be broken down by normal digestive enzymatic breakdown processes.

**The average consumption of fiber per day in the U.S. is ~ 12gms/day.**

This represents an average intake which is only 20% of the average intake in 1880. Recommendations by the National Institute of Health are 35 grams per day of fiber. *I recommend 35-50 grams per day.*

**Crude fiber**–This is the amount of undigested material left after a food has been subjected to the digestive action of both acid and alkali in the laboratory. This undigested material is primarily cellulose. It is the fiber which is responsible for the structural framework of plants such as carrots, broccoli, peas, and eggplants. Cellulose is found in fruits, vegetables, whole grains, wood, and plant foliage. Data concerning fiber content of foods has for years reported crude fiber or cellulose (because it is much easier to measure). In reviewing tables for fiber it is important to know how the fiber was measured.

**Dietary fiber**–This is the amount of undigested material left after normal body digestive action. This value is generally *3-5 times greater than the estimates for crude fiber, and can vary greatly from food to food.* Carbohydrates which compose dietary fiber (not included as crude fiber) include hemicelluloses, pectins, and lignins. These fibers tend to absorb water and form gels, thus making stools soft and bulky. Pectins, in particular, have been found to bind onto toxic substances in the colon rendering them harmless. Dietary fiber can further be classified as soluble and insoluble.

> **Note**–Dietary fibers, as measured by most tables (especially the USDA tables) and charts, are quite low in their values for fiber content of foods. As previously explained, digestion of fibrous foods with strong alkali and acid in the laboratory breaks down many of the more delicate soluble fibers, thus decreasing the measured fiber quantity (this yields crude fiber). Some newer techniques yield only slightly higher values. On the other hand, a few tables have included certain starches which falsely elevate the measured fiber content. It is thus important to know how the table or source specifically measured the fiber content in a food. Currently the most advanced techniques, those that yield the most accurate results for the evaluation of fiber in foods, are the AOAC (Association of Analytical Chemists) and the Uppsala techniques. The table compiled in this chapter primarily uses these techniques in measuring the fiber content of foods (see pgs 28 & 29).

### Properties of Fiber

**Soluble fiber**–These fibers include pectins, gums, mucilages, and some hemicelluloses. Pectins are found primarily in fruits (such as apples & oranges), and vegetables (carrots). Soluble fiber also occurs in oat bran, barley, and legumes. Soluble fibers are hydrophilic and tend to form gels in the GI tract. They act as substrate for fermentation by bacteria in the colon. They also bind bile salts and prevent them from being reabsorbed from the ileum.

**Insoluble fiber**–These fibers consist of cellulose and hemicelluloses. They function in plants as supportive structural material. Lignins are a major component of trees and shrubs and provide structure to their woody nature. The major dietary source of insoluble fibers is found in the bran moiety of grains. Insoluble fibers function to increase the bulk of the stools and stimulate normal GI motility. They also dilute the concentration of colonic toxins that may be present. They are effective in preventing the formation of diverticulosis which is characterized by a weakening of the intestinal wall and small protrusions due to excessively hard or firm stools. Diverticulosis affects 30 million Americans.

### Functions of Fiber

1) Fiber stimulates chewing which, in turn, is a stimulus for parotid, mandibular, sublingual glands and, eventually, gastric secretions.
2) Fiber's hydrophobic and bulky nature provides *satiety.*
3) By increasing volume of the stools, fiber *decreases intraluminal colonic pressure.*
4) Fiber dilutes the intestinal contents and thus *dilutes endotoxins* within the gut.
5) Fiber decreases the bowel transit time, thus allowing less time for fermentation to occur.
6) By decreasing the bowel transit time, fiber reduces the time exposure to endotoxins.

7) Fibers also provide substrate for colonic bacteria which provide short-chain fatty acids–acetate, propionate, and butyrate. Butyrate has an inverse relationship to colon cancer. These short-chain fatty acids can provide a significant number of calories.
8) Soluble fiber delays gastric emptying and slows the rate of digestion and absorption of nutrients, thus maximizing absorption.
9) Soluble fiber lowers serum cholesterol. A study in Finland involving 21,930 men showed that for every 10gm of fiber eaten per day, the risk of dying from a heart attack dropped 17%.
10) Fiber functions to slow absorption of glucose. It also increases insulin sensitivity. This effect is found with certain forms of soluble fiber.
11) Lastly, fiber increases the excretion of endogenous estrogens by binding them and allowing the body to excrete them out the stools. Women who are on vegetarian diets and who have higher intakes of fiber generally excrete 2-3x more estrogens than women on omnivorous diets. In addition, certain fibers can bind estrogen receptors, thus preventing estrogen from binding, and thereby decreasing their ability to stimulate certain estrogen dependant tumors.

**Adverse Affects**

High fiber foods may contain phytic acid and oxalates, two substances which may lead to problems associated with decreased absorption of minerals such as iron, zinc, calcium, and magnesium. This is because they tend to form water insoluble salts (see saponification of fats under fat). Phytic acid is found in insoluble fibrous types. Phytic acid readily binds onto these minerals and prevents their absorption. Cooking causes a breakdown of phytic acid and renders it harmless (heat must exceed 180 degrees Fahrenheit). Also, leavening bread or soaking fibrous foods in water allows the enzyme, phytase, to break down phytic acid, thus rendering it harmless. This activation of phytase usually only happens with certain grains such as wheat, rye, barley, and buckwheat when they are allowed to soak for 45 minutes or more at 100 degrees F. Other grains or legumes containing phytates need to be sprouted to inactivate the phytates. It should be noted that as people consume foods with a higher fiber content, and thus higher phytic acid content, they seem to be able to develop the ability to break down the phytic acid in the GI tract. This was proven by the Scottish people who primarily subsisted on oats, a food with a significant amount of phytic acid. They were able to break down phytic acid in their intestines. Thus, the only time phytic acid might really present a problem is when one is "adapting" to a diet that is high in phytates or if the diet is particularly deficient in iron, zinc, calcium, or magnesium.

Phytic acid may have some benefits in the diet since it can also bind certain heavy metals such as lead and cadmium. Furthermore, it may have the benefit of protecting the teeth against dental caries.

In addition to phytic acid, oxalic acid, which is found in green leafy vegetables–such as turnip greens, kale, mustard greens, collards, beet greens, rhubarb, and spinach–can bind onto minerals and cause them to be excreted in the stools. This may be significant in people who subsist largely on green leafy vegetables, especially if their calcium intake is low. Oxalate is also found in black tea.

With the wide consumption of a variety of foods in the U.S., phytic acid and oxalic acid should not cause a problem except for the rare individual.

(See the table on page 30 concerning phytates and oxalates in foods.)

## Dietary Fiber Content of Foods in Edible Portions (table CHO-1)

* = Upsala technique    ** = AOAC technique    no stars indicates another technique

| FOOD ITEM | Portion | Total Fiber in Grams |
|---|---|---|
| **Vegetables** | | |
| alfalfa sprouts | 1 cup raw (104gms) | 1.4* |
| artichoke | 1 medium (120gms) | 6.4* |
| asparagus | 1/2 cup (106gms) | 1.9* |
| beets, fresh | 1 cup diced (170gms) | 3.6* |
| broccoli, fresh mostly flowers | 1 cup (156gms) | 5.2** |
| brussels sprouts, fresh | 1/2 cup (78gms) | 3.2* |
| cabbage | 1 cup (73gms) | 3.4* |
| carrots | 2 large (110gms) | 2.0* |
| cauliflower fresh | 1 cup (100gms)_ | 2.3* |
| celery, raw | 1 cup chopped (100gms) | 1.6** |
| collard greens | 1 cup cooked (162gms) | 4.8* |
| cucumber | raw 1 medium 100gms) | 1.0** |
| eggplant, fresh | 1 cup (96gms) | 2.4* |
| green beans, fresh | 1 cup (110gms) | 2.8* |
| kale, raw | 1 cup chopped (164gms) | 3.2* |
| lettuce, iceberg | 2 cups chopped (100gms) | 1.7** |
| lettuce, Romaine raw | 2 cups chopped (100gms) | 1.0** |
| mushrooms, American | 1/2 cup (156gms) | 2.0* |
| okra | 1/2 cup sliced | 2.1* |
| onions | 1/2 cup (105gms) | 1.6* |
| parsnips | 1 cup | 3.9 |
| peas, green | 1/2 cup cooked (64gms) | 3.7 |
| peppers, green | 1 cup (100gms) | 1.7* |
| potato, white | 1 medium baked | 4.4 |
| pumpkin | 1 cup cooked mashed | 2.0 |
| rutabaga | 1/2 cup (85gms) | 1.9 |
| *Sea vegetables* | | |
| arame | 1/4 cup dry( 7.8gms) | 0.8 |
| hijiki | 1/4 cup (7.8gms) | 1.0 |
| kombu | 2 strips (7.8gms) | 0.1 |
| nori | 1 sheet (2.5 gms) | 0.0 |
| wakame | 7.8gms | 0.0 |
| sauerkraut | 1/2 cup (73gms) | 1.9 |
| spinach, raw | 1 cup chopped (180gms) | 4.2* |
| squash, acorn winter/ butter. | 1 cup (204gms) | 4.9** |
| sweet potato or yams | 1 small c skin (120gms) | 3.6** |
| turnips, cooked | 1 cup | 4.1 |
| water chestnuts | 1/2 cup (70gms) | 0.8* |
| zucchini | 1/2 cup (90gms) | 0.7* |

| FOOD ITEM | Portion | Total Fiber in Grams |
|---|---|---|
| **Fruit** | | |
| apple | 1 med-large apple & skin | 5.0 |
| apricots | Raw 4 pitted medium | 2.1 |
| apricots | dried 1/2 cup | 15.6 |
| avocado | 1 medium | 4.7 |
| banana | 1 medium (59gms) | 3.2 |
| blackberries | 1 cup (150gms) | 9.9* |
| blueberries | 1 cup (150gms) | 4.3* |
| cantaloupe | 1/4 medium (162gms) | 1.1* |
| cherries | 20 medium | 3.0 |
| dates, dried | 1/2 cup ~8 med. 63gms | 10.8* |
| figs, dried | 1/2 cup 41/2 med 100gms | 7.6 |
| grapefruit, fresh | 1 medium (200gms) | 2.6* |
| grapes, fresh | 15 small fruit (75gms) | 0.7* |
| guava | 2 medium | 10.6 |
| honey dew melon | 1/4 medium (380gms) | 2.2 |
| kiwi | 2 medium (100gms) | 3.4** |
| mango | 1 medium | 3.1 |
| olives, ripe | 100gms | 3.0** |
| orange | 1 medium (135gms) | 2.3* |
| orange juice | 100gms frozen conc. | 0.8** |
| papaya | 1 medium | 4.0 |
| peach | 1 medium (157gms) | 2.7* |
| pear | 1 large (242gms) | 6.8* |
| pineapple | 1 cup (156gms) | 1.4* |
| prunes, dried | 6 medium (50gms) | 3.6* |
| raisins, dried | 1/4 cup or 4T(175gms) | 7.2* |
| raspberries | 1 cup 124gms | 5.2* |
| strawberries | 1 cup (188gms) | 2.8* |
| tomato | 1 large (123gms) | 1.0* |
| watermelon | 11/4 cups (200gms) | 0.8* |

NOTE-the above data was in part compiled by Dr. Judith Marlett, professor at the University of Wisconsin, Madison, using the Upsala & Assoc of Official Analytical Chemists (AOAC) methodologies. It represents the most accurate data to date concerning the actual fiber content of food, carefully avoiding digestion of some of the more delicate soluble fiber fractions (thus falsely lowering actual values), while not including non-fiber starches which can artificially elevate the fiber readings of foods.  January 1996

| FOOD ITEM | Portion | Total Fiber |
|---|---|---|
| **Grains** | | **(in Grams)** |
| all bran cereal | 1 cup | 8.0 (insol) |
| amaranth, whole | 1 cup | 6.7 |
| barley | 1 cup cooked | 0.8 |
| buckwheat (not a grain) | 1 cup cooked | 5.0 |
| corn | 1/2 cup (83gms) | 1.6* |
| cornmeal | 1/4 cup dry | 5.0 |
| cous cous | 1/3 cup dry | 9.0 |
| ***Flours*** | | |
| oat flour whole | 100gms | 9.6 |
| rice, brown | 100gms | 4.6 |
| rice, white | 100gms | 2.4 |
| rye | 100gms | 14.6 |
| semolina | 100gms | 3.9 |
| triticale | 100gms | 14.6 |
| wheat, white | 100gms | 2.7 |
| wheat, whole | 100gms | 12.6 |
| Oatmeal rolled oats | 1 cup dry | 8.0 |
| popcorn | 1/2C = 1qt popped=107g | 15.0** |
| Quinoa (not a grain) | 1 cup cooked | 4.6 |
| rice brown | 1 cup cooked | 4.5 |
| rice white | 1 cup cooked | 1.5 |
| rice wild | 1 cup cooked | 5.0** |
| Rye, Cream of | 1/3 cup dry (37gms) | 5.0 |
| Bran Muffin | 1 medium | 2.5 |
| French bread | 1 slice | 1.0 |
| wheat germ | 3 Tablespoons (18gms) | 2.5 |
| ***Cereals (commercial)*** | | |
| Cherrios/Oatios New M | 1 cup (30gms) | 3.0 |
| Corn Flakes or *Prod 19* | 1 cup (30gms) | 1.0 |
| Fiber 1 General Mills | 1/2 cup (30gms) | 13.0 |
| Grape Nuts Post | 1/2 cup (58gms) | 5.0 |
| Kashi puffed cereal | 2 cups (50 gms) | 4.0 |
| Millet Rice oatbran flake | 3/4 cup (30gms) | 3.0 |
| Nutrigrain wheat Kellogg's | 1 cup (30gms) | 4.0 |
| Post 100% bran | 1/2 cup (45gms) | 12.0 |
| Quaker Oat Bran | 1 cup (46gms) | 5.6 |
| Rice Crispies Kellogg's | 11/4 cup (30gms) | 1.0 |
| Shredded Wheat Nabisco | 2 medium biscuits (46 g) | 5.0 |
| Total or *wheaties* | 1 cup (30gms) | 3.0 |
| Nutty Rice Perkies | 3/4 cup (57gms) | 2.0 |
| Uncle Sam cereal | 1 cup | 10.0 |

| FOOD ITEM | Portion | Total Fiber |
|---|---|---|
| **Crackers (commercial)** | **& Pasta** | **(in Grams)** |
| Ak-Mak (4 sections) | 5 sections (28gms) | 3.5 |
| Kavli Rye crackers | 3- ( 8 x 4.5")very thin 15g | 2.0 |
| Popcorn (unpopped) | 1/4 cup | 6.0 |
| Rice cake (brown) | 2 medium sized cakes | 4.0 |
| Ritz crackers | 12 crackers | 1.6 |
| Ry-Krisp | 2 triple crackers | 1.6 |
| Tortilla corn | 1 average | 1.2 |
| Wheat thins | 12 crackers | 4.5 |
| whole wheat Triscuit | 5 crackers 28gms) | 2.6* |
| ***Noodles*** | | |
| udon (buckwheat) | 3/4 cup (50gms) | 2.7 |
| saghetti, regular durum semolina | 3/4 cup (50gms) | 1.2 |
| spaghetti, spinach | 3/4 cup (50gms) | 5.3 |
| spaghetti, whole wheat | 3/4 cup (50gms) | 5.9 |
| | | |
| **Dairy Products & eggs** | any type/any amount | 0.0 |
| **Meats** | any type/any amount | 0.0 |
| | | |
| **Legumes and Nuts** | | |
| almonds | 12 whole nuts (16 gms) | 2.5 |
| black beans | 1/2cup 120gms) | 4.0 |
| black-eyed peas | 1/4 cup dry (37gms) | 10.0 |
| brazil nuts | 6 large nuts | 3.0 |
| cashews | 1/4 cup (35gms) | 2.1** |
| chickpeas | 1/2 cup cooked | 5.5 |
| filberts | 1/4 cup (35gms) | 2.2** |
| kidney beans | 1/2 cup cooked | 9.7 |
| lentils | 1/2 cup cooked (83gms) | 3.4** |
| lima beans | 1/2 cup (88gms) | 3.7** |
| peanut butter | 3 Tablespoons (100gms) | 6.6** |
| peanuts | 1/4 cup (36gms) | 2.9** |
| pecans | 1/4 cup (27gms) | 1.8** |
| pinto beans | 1/2 cup | 4.8 |
| pistachio nuts | 1/4 cup (31 gms) | 3.4** |
| sesame seeds | 2 tablespoons | 1.2 |
| soybeans, cooked | 1/2 cup | 2.6 |
| split green peas | 1/4 cup dry (45gms) | 7.0 |
| sunflower seeds | 1/4 cup 4 T (37gm) | 2.5** |
| tofu | 100gms | 1.2** |
| walnuts | 1/4 cup chopped (31 gms) | 1.6** |

## Calcium, Magnesium, phosphorus phytates & oxalates in selected foods–100gms

| Food item | | Calcium | Magnesium | Phosphorus | Phytate | Oxalate |
|---|---|---|---|---|---|---|
| **Dairy products**-- cheeses | | 750 | 45 | 479 | | 0 |
| | Eggs | 48 | 11 | 183 | | 0.6 |
| | Milk | 118 | 113 | 93 | | .07 |
| | Yogurt (2/5th C) | 111 | 9 | 79 | | |
| **Meats** | Beef chopped | 10 | 28 | 214 | | 0.4 |
| | Chicken, roast | 9 | 19 | 169 | | 1.1 |
| | Haddock | 20 | 289 | 197 | | 0.2 |
| | Oysters | 94 | 24 | 143 | | |
| | Sole | 4 | 30 | 64 | | |
| **Grains** | Barley, whole | 11 | 37 | 70 | 216 | |
| | Buckwheat, flour 1c | 40 | 229 | 330 | 192 | |
| | Corn flakes | 3 | 10 | 70 | | 5.6 |
| | Corn grits | 0 | 3 | 11 | | 41 |
| | Oatmeal (1/2c dry) | 10 | 24 | 80 | 127 | 1.0 |
| | Rice, brown (1/2c cook) | 10 | 42 | 80 | 225 | |
| | Rice, white(1/2c cook) | 3 | 30 | 100 | 70 | |
| | Rye, whole flour 1c | 24 | 76 | 211 | 236 | |
| | Wheat bran 11/2c | 66 | 549 | 900 | 1000 | |
| | Wheat germ 1c | 51 | 362 | 1294 | 550 | 269 |
| | White wheat flour | 100 | 24 | 87 | 30 | 4.9 |
| | Whole wheat | 99 | 78 | 229 | 240 | |
| | Wholewheat bread (2 slice) | 50 | 40 | 104 | 51 | |
| | Wheat bread, white | 40 | 11 | 88 | 6 | |
| **Fruit & Vegs.** | Apple | 2 | 5 | 2 | | |
| | Beets | 15 | 37 | 23 | | 122 |
| | Broccoli | 80 | 24 | 61 | | ? |
| | Cabbage | 55 | 20 | 26 | | 1.0 |
| | Cauliflower | 24 | 15 | 56 | | 1.0 |
| | Collard greens 1c cook | 28 | 7 | 9 | | 74 |
| | Kale | 160 | 37 | 60 | | 89 |
| | Leeks 1 c cook | 32 | 14 | 18 | | 89 |
| | Lettuce | 23 | 10 | 21 | | 17 |
| | Okra 9 pods | 58 | 51 | 51 | | 145 |
| | Orange | 15 | 12 | 15 | | 6.2 |
| | Parsley 11/2c raw | 120 | 45 | 49 | | 100 |
| | Peas, sweet boiled | 23 | 27 | 80 | 91 | 1.0 |
| | Peas, sweet sprouted | 20 | 20 | 80 | 28 | 1.0 |
| | Potato, sweet | 32 | 23 | 63 | | 56 |
| | Potato peeled, white | 7 | 22 | 43 | | 23 |
| | Potato whole, white | 7 | 34 | 43 | | 23 |
| | Raspberries, black | 28 | 17 | 18 | | 53 |
| | Rhubarb | 27 | 10 | 8 | | 260 |
| | Spinach | 100 | 76 | 51 | | 779 |
| | Strawberries | 18 | 11 | 20 | | 1.9 |
| | Swiss chard 1c cook | 60 | 84 | 35 | | 645 |
| | Tomato | 12 | 10 | 27 | | 5.3 |
| **Legumes** | Pecans 1c | 39 | 138 | 314 | | 202 |
| | **Peanuts, roasted 2/3c** | 76 | 160 | 446 | 529 | 187 |
| | Sunflower seed 3/4c | 126 | 382 | 750 | 803 | |
| | Soybean meal | 92 | 78 | 220 | 426 | 207 |
| | Mung beans | 13 | 22 | 56 | 81 | |
| | Mung beans, sprout | 13 | 22 | 56 | 32 | |
| | Lentil beans 1/2c cook | 19 | 36 | 178 | 87 | |
| | Lentil sprouts raw 11/3c | 25 | 33 | 146 | 41 | |
| | Garbanzo beans 2/3c cook | 48 | 47 | 166 | 124 | |
| | Garbanzo beans, sprouted | | | | 73 | |
| **Miscellaneous** | Ovaltine | 126 | 33 | | | 46 |
| | Tea, black -weak | 2.8 | 0.6 | 0 | | 46 |
| | Tea, strong | 5.2 | 2.5 | 0 | | 83 |
| | Chocolate, bitter | 78 | 292 | 385 | | 124 |
| | Cocoa, dry powder 1/3c 100g | 80 | 420 | 400 | | 623 |

### Miscellaneous

**Sorbitol** is a sugar alcohol which occurs naturally in fruits such as apples, pears, peaches and in several vegetables. It is absorbed from the intestine at about 1/3rd the rate of glucose. Because it may delay hunger signs, it is used in weight loss products. It is also used in chewing gum because it is much less cariogenic. It can cause problems with cataracts in the lens of the eye.

**Modified food starches** are synthetic starches designed to give foods properties such as thickening, stability in acid and at high temperatures, and varied textures. These properties are important in the processing of foods such as dressings, pie fillings, canned soups, gravies, canned puddings, and baby food.

**Carrageenan** comes from algae and is a gum which is used as a thickening agent in many processed foods.

**Mannitol**, which exists in fruit and is poorly digested, yields about 50% of the caloric value of glucose. It does get absorbed but more slowly than glucose.

**Xylitol** is absorbed about 20% as fast as glucose. It is used in chewing gum because cariogenic bacteria are unable to use it as a substrate.

**Clinical note**–The botanical *Gymnema sylvestre* has been used to treat insulin dependant diabetes mellitus because it stimulates the beta cells of the pancreas to produce more insulin. The dried or fresh leaf can also be chewed to alter the perception of sweetness. For several hours after chewing on a small amount of the herb, the taste sensation of sweet totally disappears. This may be useful for someone who is addicted to sugary foods.

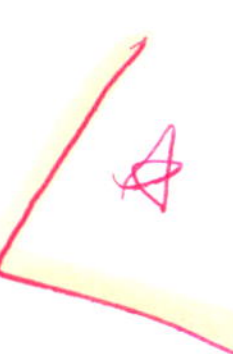

## Alcohol

Though most alcohol is produced from carbohydrates, it is chemically related to fats. It is usually fermented from glucose found in foods such as fruit and cereal grains. Data estimates that alcohol consumption is about 1 oz of pure alcohol per person per day assuming that 1/3 of the population over 14 years old does not drink. Calculating 7 calories per gram of alcohol yields about 200 Cal per day. For 3% of the population over 15 years old, estimates are that alcohol contributes over 100 Cal per day. Ethanol is a small water soluble molecule that does not require any digestion. Absorption begins immediately in the mouth and stomach. 80% of the alcohol gets absorbed in the small intestine and is immediately distributed into various tissues of the body.

Alcohol is immediately metabolized by the liver through the action of the enzyme alcohol dehydrogenase. This enzyme converts alcohol into a form that can be used for energy production. Alcohol is a preferred source of energy over fatty acids and glucose. The fact that alcohol spares other carbohydrate sources means that it indirectly contributes to fat storage. Alcohol absorption can be modified by various drugs, but it is not affected by physical exercise or caffeine.

### Milling of cereals

Certain toxins, such as lead, tend to concentrate in the endosperm, which is the part of the grain that is left after milling. Other potentially toxic substances–such as cadmium, which exerts its toxic effects by replacing zinc in various biochemical pathways–tend to concentrate in the inner layers of the grain (as part of the endosperm). Zinc, which tends to neutralize the negative effects of the cadmium, is found primarily in the outer layers of the grain. Thus, milling effectively removes most of the zinc, while leaving the remaining toxic cadmium behind.

**NOTE**

In India, the traditional milling process only removes 5-10% of the grain, primarily cellulose which is devoid of most of the nutrients. In addition, phytic acid, which is normally found in high amounts in the cellulose, gets removed, thus making, in some ways , a more nutritious product than whole wheat. More of the nutrients are available. Furthermore breads that are made from this type of wheat are lighter and have more delicate flavor.

AN ENLARGED VIEW OF A WHEAT KERNEL

**Endosperm**–This represents most of the volume of the grain kernel. It is the "starchy" part of the grain. It contains the gluten, which is made up of gliadin and glutenin, and is the part of the grain that is used to make white flour products.

**Bran**–This is the outer layer or husk covering and contains all of the fiber as well as some protein and trace minerals. It is removed during the milling process.

**Germ**–The germ or embryo contains protein and the highest concentration of B vitamins, trace minerals and essential fatty acids. This is where the vitamin E is found, which is vital for the protection of the nutrients against oxidative damage. It is removed during the milling process.

The Endosperm
The Bran
The Germ

## Enrichment

Because of the loss of nutrients during the milling process, the government, in its effort to prevent nutrient deficiencies, decided to replace some of the lost vitamins and minerals. This process, called *"enrichment,"* replaces only thiamin, riboflavin, niacin and iron. Thus, most of the vital vitamins and minerals are lost for good. This sets up the potential for widespread sub optimal nutrient intake in the U.S.

DISTRIBUTION OF NUTRIENTS IN CEREAL GRAIN (EXPRESSED AS A % OF TOTAL)

| part of grain | protein | total mineral | thiamin (B-1) | riboflavin (B-2) | niacin (B-3) | pyridoxine (B-6) | pantothenic acid (B-5) |
|---|---|---|---|---|---|---|---|
| Endosperm | 72 | 20 | 3 | 32 | 12 | 6 | 43 |
| Bran | 19 | 68 | 33 | 42 | 86 | 73 | 50 |
| Germ | 8 | 12 | 64 | 26 | 2 | 20 | 7 |

Adapted from *Introductory Nutrition* by Helen Guthrie

## SUMMARY OF CARBOHYDRATE METABOLISM

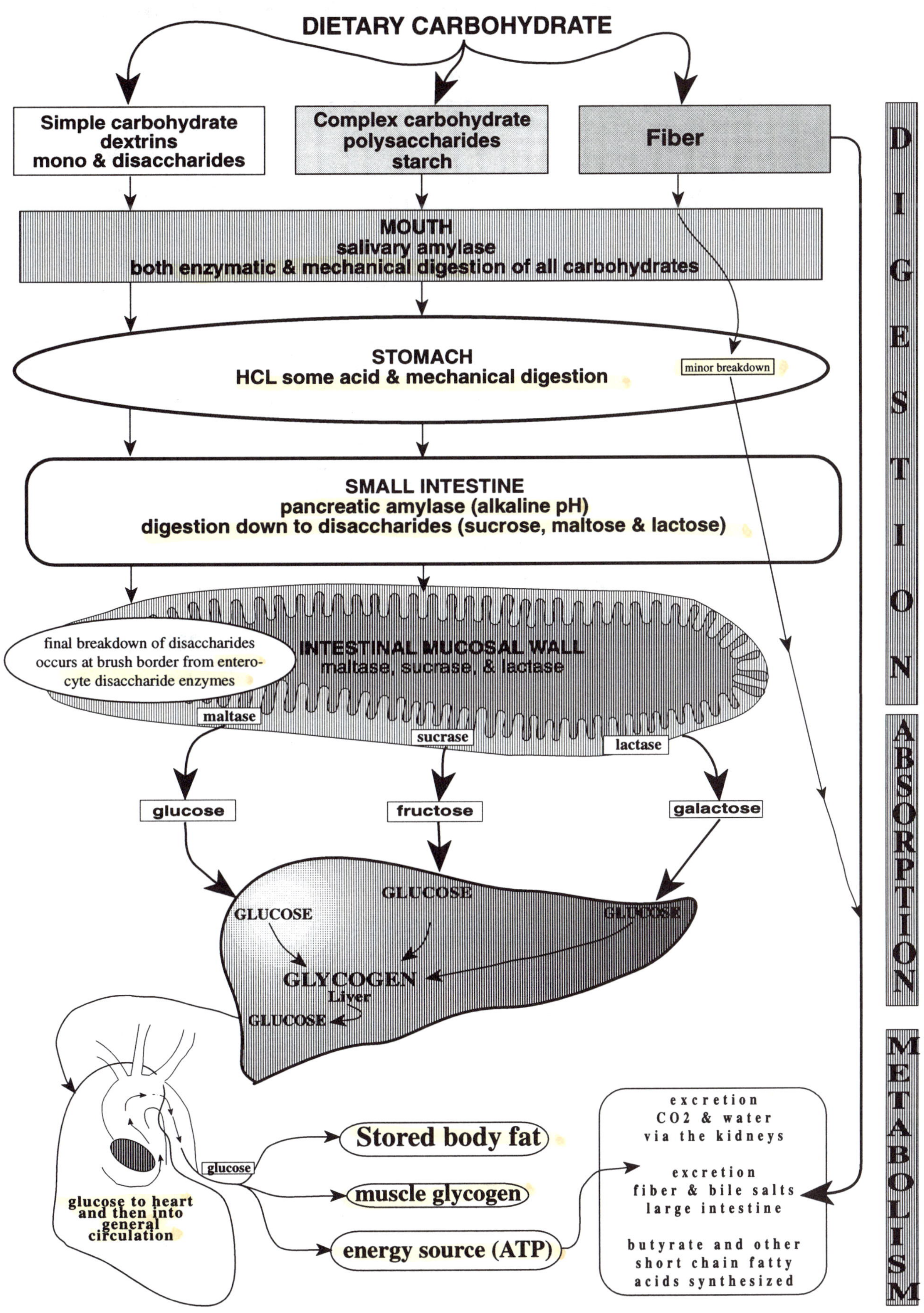

**(for more information on carbohydrate metabolism see chapter on Diabetes)**

**Notes**

---

# FATS or LIPIDS

- The average consumption of fats in the U.S. comprises approximately 38% of the total caloric intake in the diet. This is a reduction from the mid 1960's when the amount was 43%. Butter and fat have been replaced by oils, margarine, and shortening, all from vegetable sources. In 1910 the average American consumed 25% less fat than Americans consume today. Cholesterol intake has remained about the same, averaging about 500mg/day in 1910 and 480mg/day in 1979. In the late 1940's we reached a cholesterol consumption high of 570mg/day. The ingestion of trans-fatty acids has reached about 6% of total fats.
- Increased ingestion of fat along with decreased fiber has been linked to the increased incidence of certain forms of cancer and atherosclerosis. The National Research Council has recommended a reduction in the consumption of fats to 30% of calories. My recommendation is that no more than 20% of calories should come from fats, depending upon physical activity, family history of CVD, and possibly blood type.

## I. Major Classes of Lipids

**1) Simple lipids**–Most natural fats consist of 98-99% triacylglycerol (triglycerides). This is the form in which fat is stored for fuel and, by far, the most abundant form in foods and tissues. Unsaturated FAs have a bent configuration and make the TG more fluid whereas the saturated FAs are straight and make the TG more rigid or solid.

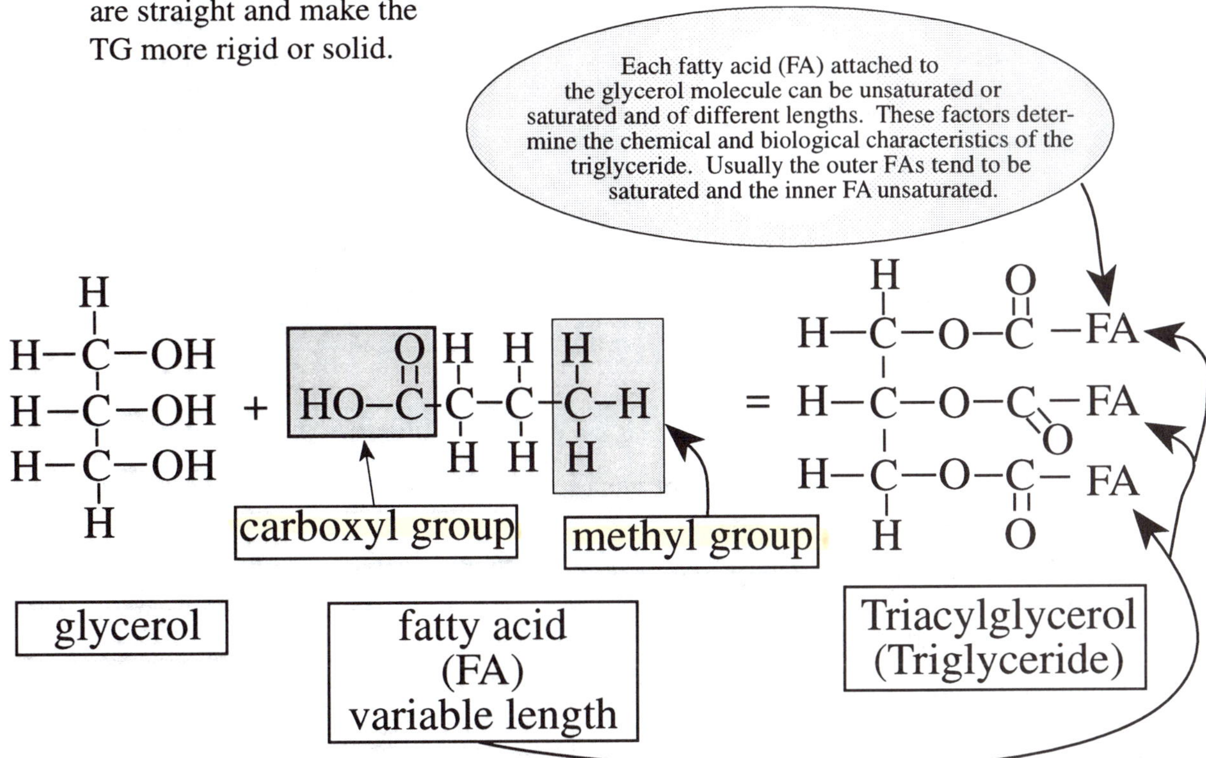


**Basic Triglyceride Chemistry**

**2) Compound lipids**

Phospholipids
- lecithins
- cephalins found in cell membranes and myelin sheaths
- sphingomyelins

Glycolipids–compounds of fatty acid combined with CHO and a N base
- Cerebrosides
- Gangliosides

Sulfolipids–sulfur containing lipids

Lipoproteins: (lipids and proteins)
- Apolipoproteins

Lipopolysaccharides

**3) Derived lipids**–Derived lipids include fatty acids and derivatives such as prostaglandins. Prostaglandins are very important hormones which have much clinical significance, especially in relation to diet. Essential fatty acids along with cholesterol are used to form prostaglandins.

**Mono and diglycerides**

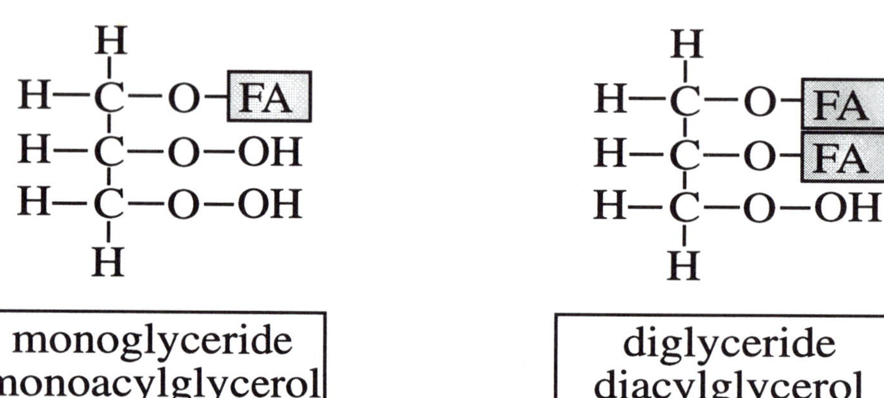


**4) Sterols**

Cholesterol–not found in the plant world ?
Ergosterol–found only in plants
Steroid hormones–testosterone, estrogen, cortisol, DHEA
Vitamin D
Bile salts–made from cholesterol in the liver

**5) Miscellaneous lipids**

Carotenoids and vitamin A
Vitamin E
Vitamin K

## II. Nomenclature of Fatty Acids

- The term used for a specific fatty acid is based on the number and placement of double bonds in the fatty acid chain.
- The location of the first double bond, as counted from the methyl end of the fatty acid, is designated by the "omega."
- Chain length may vary from 4-30 carbon atoms. The first number represents the number of carbons in the chain and the 2nd number represents the number of double bonds in the chain. The last number after the ω indicates the carbon number on which the first double bond occurs when measured from the methyl end of the fatty acids.

Fatty acids are named according to the placement of their double bonds along the carbon chain. Omega 3 fatty acids are named because their first double bond occurs on the 3rd carbon when counting from the methyl end of the chain. These fats are found in certain nuts & seeds (walnuts, hemp, pumpkin), other oil containing foods such as, canola, soy and various fish (especially cold water fish). Omega 3 fatty acids have been found to have properties which protect the body against a number of different disease processes including cancer, cardiovascular disease, and inflammatory conditions.

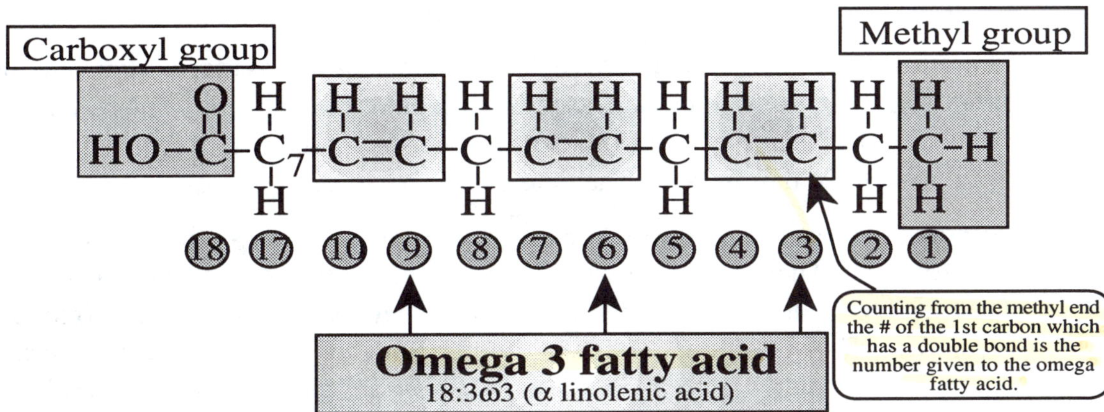


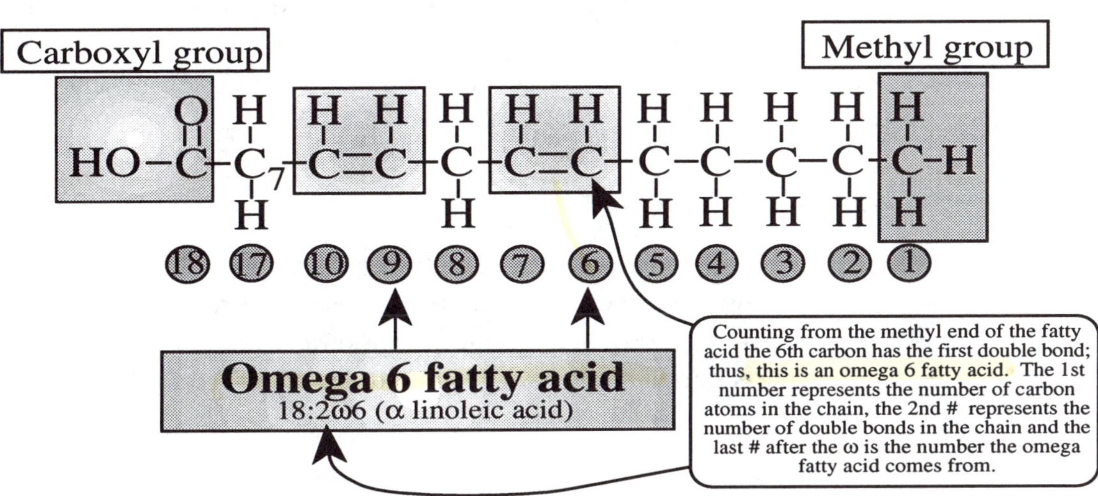

1) **Short-chain- fatty acids** < 6 carbons–These fatty acids include butyrate, caprylic acid, and propionate. They are responsible for maintaining proper bacterial flora and have been shown to be protective against cancer. They are made from the bacterial breakdown of certain fibers.

2) **Medium-chain** = 8 to 12 carbons–These fatty acids are important for people who have compromised digestion and absorption because they can be absorbed directly into the circulation (see diagram).

3) **Long-chain** = 14 to 27 carbons, with chain length averaging 16 to 18 carbons–Long-chain fatty acids include both essential and nonessential fatty acids such as arachidonic acid and linoleic acid. They are involved in synthesizing prostaglandins and other prostanoids.

## III. Properties of Fatty Acids (saturated vs unsaturated)

1) **Saturated fatty acids** (SFA)–These fatty acid chains do not have any double bonds. They are considered nonessential and come mostly from animal products such as dairy and meat. They have been implicated in cardiovascular disease and other inflammatory conditions.

2) **Unsaturated fatty acids** (USFA)–This is a general term describing many fatty acids with different properties. These fatty acids contain at least one double bond in their structure and may include essential fatty acids.

3) **Monounsaturated fatty acids** (MUFA)–They are fatty acids that contain only one double bond. They are considered nonessential, although they appear to have some beneficial properties such as protection from cancer (because of their stability) and also protection from cardiovascular disease. They are found in *olive oil.*

4) **Polyunsaturated fatty acids** (PUFA)–PUFAs are fatty acids which contain at least two double bonds. They have been associated with protection against cardiovascular disease. They tend to be unstable and susceptible to oxidative damage, forming free radicals and peroxides. They are found in all cell membranes throughout the body. Certain PUFAs have been associated with an increase in cancer and, as their intake increases, requirements for antioxidant nutrients also increase. Certain other PUFAs, like omega 3 fatty acids, have been shown to be protective against cancer and cardiovascular disease. PUFAs are found in nuts, seeds, whole grains and, in small amounts, in dairy and meats. Wild animals, who are more active than domestic animals, have a higher content of PUFAs in their tissues.

## IV. Essential Fatty Acids (EFAs)

1) **Linoleic acid** (LA)–This is an essential fatty acid that is a PUFA and also a USFA. Various prostaglandin hormones are made from these fatty acids which can be found in virtually all tissues in the body. This is an omega-6 fatty acid. It is found in nuts, seeds and whole grains. A deficiency of LA results in dermatitis and other hormonal abnormalities.

2) **Alpha Linolenic acid** (LNA)–This is another essential fatty acid which was once thought nonessential because it can be made from linoleic acid. Recent research has shown that it has

its own properties which can not entirely be supplied through LA. LNA is classified as an omega 3 fatty acid. Currently, the ratio of omega 6 to omega 3 fatty acids is about 18 to 1. It has been calculated that thousands of years ago (hunters and gatherers before agriculture), when people consumed a primarily vegetarian diet, the ratio between omega 6 to omega 3 oils was a more balanced 5 to 1.

## V. Essential Fatty Acid Deficiency

An essential fatty acid deficiency results in dermatitis, stunted growth and other symptoms relating to hormone imbalances. More research has shown that many people may have suboptimal intakes of these important fats. Trans-fatty acids act as antagonists to EFAs and increase the requirements for them in the diets.

## VI. Triacylglycerols (Triglycerides orTGs)

1) **Properties**–They are composed of 1 glycerol molecule and 3 fatty acids (see diagram). They comprise a general class of fats which includes many types of fatty acids, both saturated and unsaturated. Triacylglycerol may have mixed fatty acid chains attached to it; that is, it could have both saturated fatty acids and unsaturated fatty acids.

2) **Reactions of TGs (include peroxidation, hydrogenation, saturation, saponification, and emulsification).**

**Peroxidation of fatty acids**

Fatty acids are susceptible to oxidation by the nature of their carbon bonds. Generally speaking, the more double bonds a fatty acid has, the more unstable the molecule and the more susceptible it will be to oxidative attack. Certain factors tend to facilitate the production of free radicals or oxidative products. Temperature, light, oxygen and the presence of certain cofactors such as iron and copper may speed up the oxidative process. The more unsaturated a fatty acid is (the more double bonds), the more susceptible the oil or fat is to oxidation. During the process of oxidation, various oxidized products are formed such as peroxides, hydroxyl radicals and various other free radicals. Once these peroxides and free radicals start to form, they in turn oxidize other fats creating a cycle of oxidation (known as propagation). This process is different from hydrogenation because it does not result in trans-fatty acids being formed. Foods that have a significant amount of USFA should be kept cold and away from light and air. These would include items such as nuts, seeds, whole grains, oils, fish, and other foods containing oil.

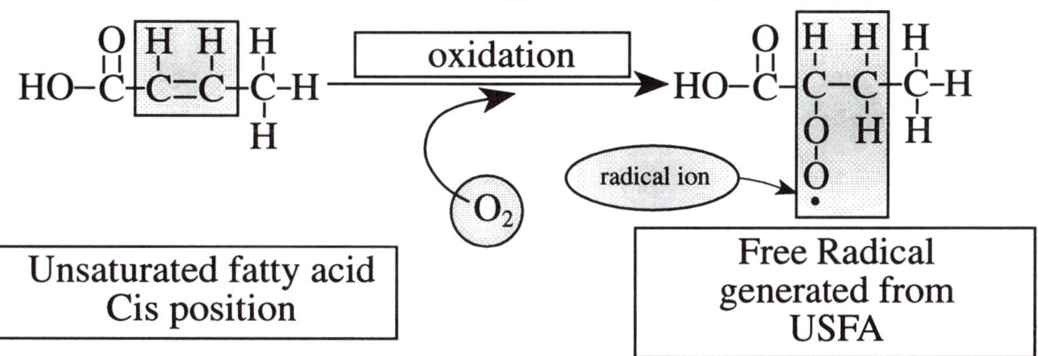

## Hydrogenation

Hydrogenation involves the use of an unsaturated fatty acid such as corn or safflower oil. Hydrogen gas is bubbled through the oil in the presence of a nickel catalyst. The net result is a conversion of the USFA into SFA. The more solid the product is at room temperature, the more saturated the oil has become. Hydrogenated oil is also known as vegetable shortening or margarine. Crisco is a product that is highly hydrogenated and very saturated. Margarines that come in a tub rather than a stick are less hydrogenated or less saturated. During the process of hydrogenation, some of the double bonds break and reform again. Some of the double bonds that reform do so in an unusual confirguration known as a *trans-configuration*. Recent studies in Europe have shown an increased incidence of breast cancer associated with an increase in trans-fatty acid consumption.

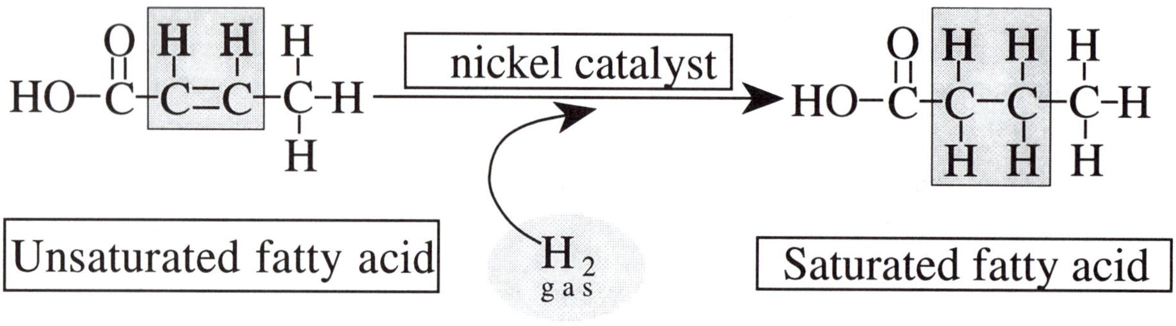

## Trans-fatty acid formation

Trans-fatty acids (TFAs) are unsaturated fatty acids that are formed during the commercial production of hydrogenated oils. In nature, unsaturated fatty acids only exist as the cis configuration. During the process of hydrogenation, some of the double bonds break apart and then reform again. During the reformation a % of the double bonds, some of the hydrogens, reattach in the trans-configuration. It has been shown in some studies that these trans-fatty acids cause increases in cholesterol and LDL cholesterol even more so than saturated fats. Furthermore, these trans-fatty acids get incorporated into all cell membranes around the body. Further research needs to be done regarding the effects that these foreign fatty acids have on membrane characteristics such as permeability and membrane receptor binding. They also act as antagonists to essential fatty acids and can interfere with important prostaglandin production.

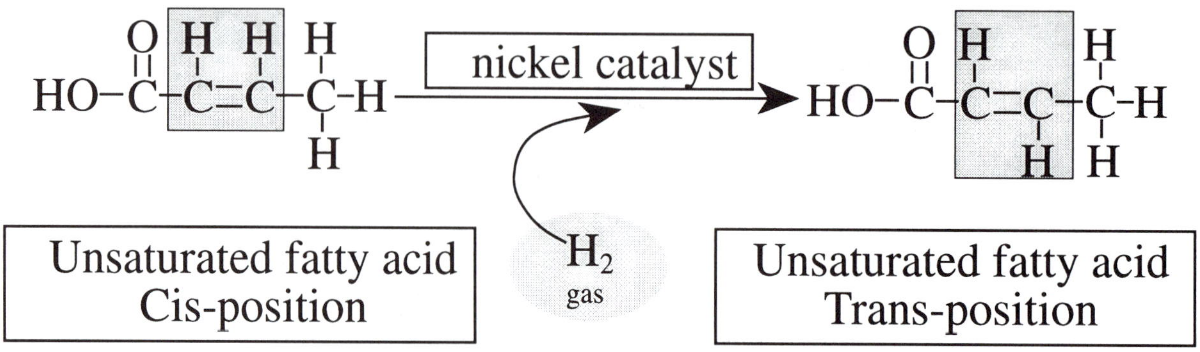

# Emulsification of fat by bile salts

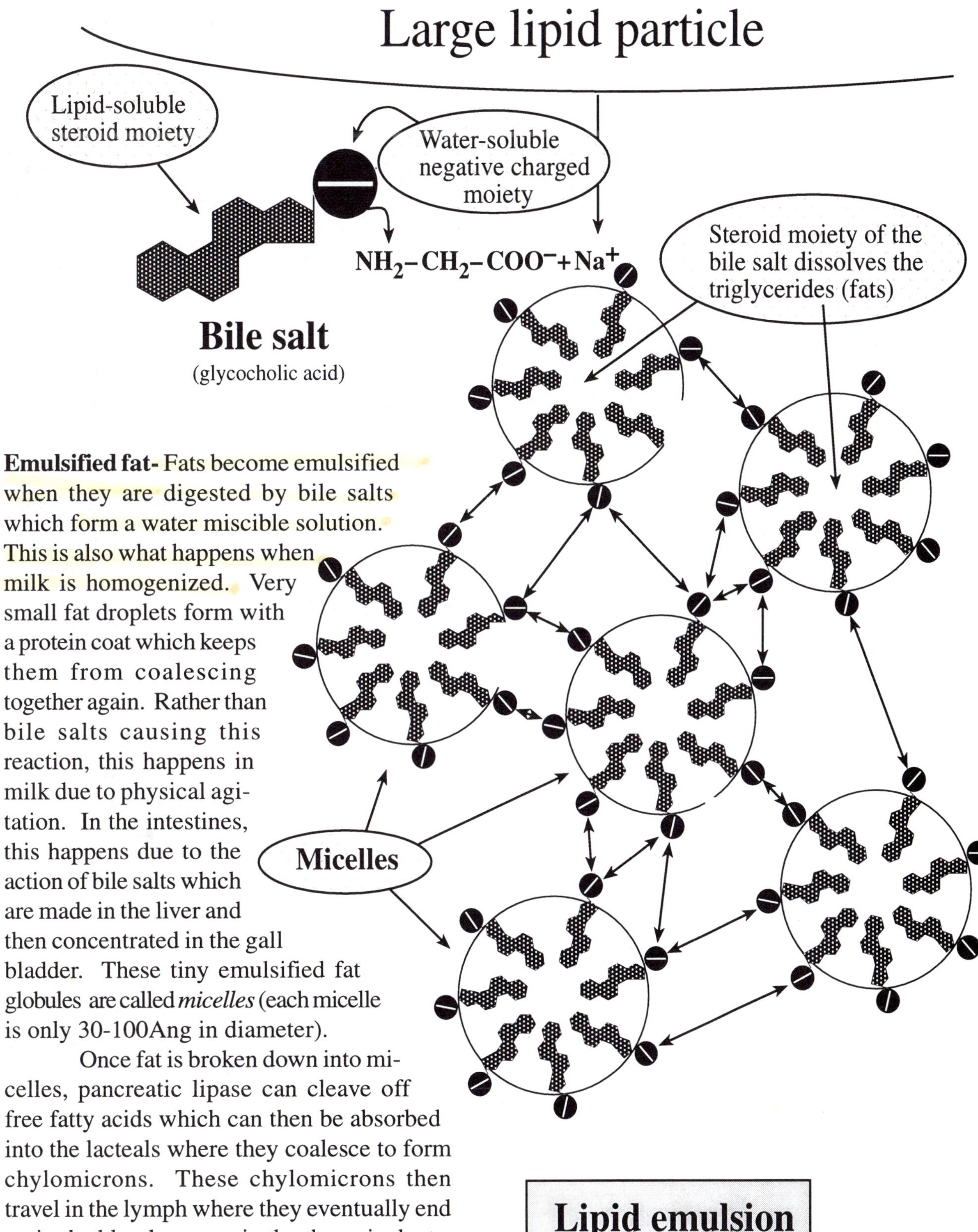


**Emulsified fat-** Fats become emulsified when they are digested by bile salts which form a water miscible solution. This is also what happens when milk is homogenized. Very small fat droplets form with a protein coat which keeps them from coalescing together again. Rather than bile salts causing this reaction, this happens in milk due to physical agitation. In the intestines, this happens due to the action of bile salts which are made in the liver and then concentrated in the gall bladder. These tiny emulsified fat globules are called *micelles* (each micelle is only 30-100Ang in diameter).

Once fat is broken down into micelles, pancreatic lipase can cleave off free fatty acids which can then be absorbed into the lacteals where they coalesce to form chylomicrons. These chylomicrons then travel in the lymph where they eventually end up in the bloodstream via the thoracic duct.

**Saponification–**This is a chemical process using alkali to cleave FA's off TG's. The free fatty acids that are formed bind with sodium or potassium to form insoluble soaps.

3) **Medium chain triglycerides** (MCT)–MCTs are more water soluble and can be absorbed directly into the blood stream without first having to go into the lacteals. They are often prescribed for people who have fat malabsorption due to some intestinal pathology. They can be found in elemental diets as well as other enteral feeding formulas.

4) **Short chain triglycerides–**These TG's, because of their size and solubility, can get absorbed directly into the blood stream. In the colon they have numerous protecting effects against colon cancer and damage to the endothelium.

## VII. Derived and Compound Lipids

1) **Monoglycerides and diglycerides–**These are breakdown products of triglycerides. They tend to be more water soluble depending upon the chain length. They are often added to foods in various forms to emulsify, stabilize and enhance the texture of different food products like ice cream, candies, chocolates and bread products.

2) **Phospholipids–**Phospholipids and cholesterol have their chief function in the formation of all interior and exterior cell membranes. In our current understanding of cell membrane anatomy, these lipids provide a semifluid matrix within which various protein derivatives are suspended (see diagram). The lipid matrix is composed of an inner layer and an outer layer. The inner layer is made of an inner phospholipid region made of cholesterol and fatty acids, and an outer region of polar groups off of the fatty acids which are soluble in water. This membrane phospholipid is composed of specific fatty acids which are determined by what you eat. These fatty acids are responsible for the characteristics of the cell membrane. In addition, they are also used as a source of substrate for the formation of prostaglandins, leukotrienes and thromboxanes, which are essential for normal body functions.

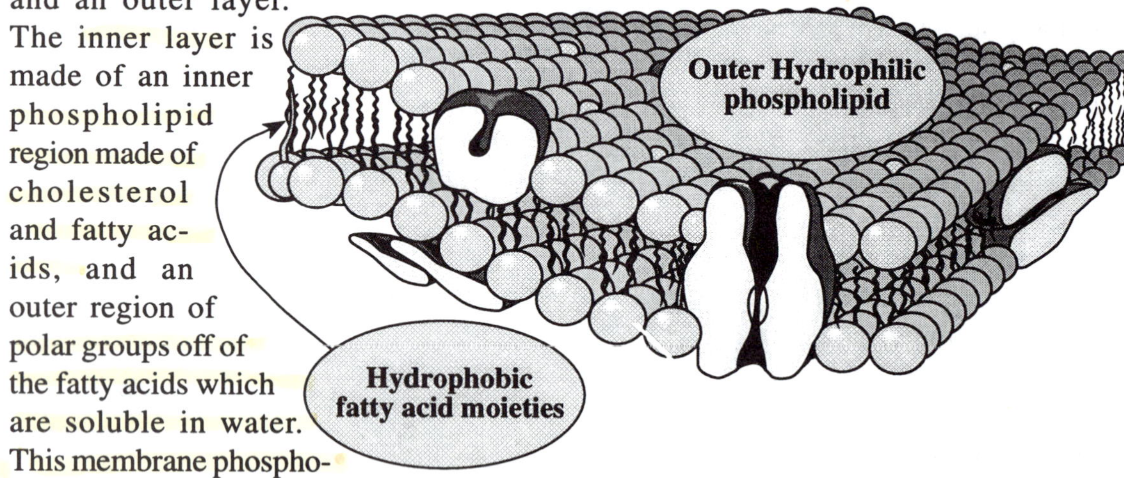


3) **Lecithin–**Lecithin-cholesterol acyltransferase (LCAT) transports fatty acids from lecithin to cholesterol to form cholesteryl ester. It is considered to be responsible for much of the cholesteryl ester in plasma lipoproteins.

4) **Sphingomyelins, Lipontols and cephalins–**These phospholipids are incorporated into various cell membranes in the nervous system.

## VIII. Sterols

1) **Cholesterol**–The body uses cholesterol to make various steroid hormones. If cholesterol is absent from the diet, the liver will synthesize it. It is therefore not considered essential. In the skin 7 Dehydrocholesterol is irradiated to make the active form of vitamin D (cholecalciferol) and in the adrenal glands (in both the cortex and medulla) various hormones are produced. These include epinephrine, norepinephrine, aldosterone, progesterone, estrogens and androgens both in the liver and gonads. Another steroid hormone precursor, dehydroepiandrosterone (DHEA), is made in the adrenals and is one of the building blocks for all the other hormones. It has been the subject of much study. More recently it has been used therapeutically for hypoadrenal function, in the treatment of unexplained fatigue, autoimmune diseases, and many other conditions.

2) **Phytosterols**–These compounds are a group of lipids found in plants, some of which competitively inhibit the absorption of cholesterol. Another sterol, ergosterol, is a precursor to vitamin D.

## IX. Lipid digestion, absorption, and metabolism

Lipid digestion begins in the mouth and stomach where lingual lipase and gastric lipase act to break down the triglycerides found in foods. These 2 enzymes are rather weak, however, and only a small amount of fat digestion occurs by the time fat reaches the small intestine. Primarily fat digestion occurs in the proximal small intestine through the action of bile salts released from the gall bladder in response to chyme reaching the duodenum. Without bile salts, as when the gall bladder has been removed, fat digestion is severely hampered. Bile salts (see diagram of emulsification of fats page 41) break down larger fat globules into tiny water soluble particles called *micelles.* Once formed, they can be broken down at the brush border of the intestines through the action of pancreatic lipase, which acts to cleave off fatty acids from the triglycerides found inside the micelles (see diagram page 41).

Once acted upon by pancreatic lipase, the micelles release free fatty acids, mono and diglycerides. The free fatty acids are carried across the intestinal epithelial cells and reformed back into chylomicrons whereupon they enter into the lacteals. From the lacteals they travel through the lymph system up to the thoracic duct, located in the upper area of the neck, where they enter into the general circulation. Small and medium chain length fatty acids, which have been cleaved from micelles, can enter directly from the small intestine into the bloodstream because they are more water soluble. All blood from the intestines goes first to the liver before it enters into the general circulation.

The fatty acids can be utilized as fuel by virtually all tissues in the body except the brain, RBC's, the skin, and the renal medulla. The muscles utilize fatty acids as a major source of energy even when glucose is available. Glycerol gets oxidized by only a couple of tissues in the body. When fatty acids are used for energy it is under the control of *hormone sensitive lipase (HSL),* which is responsible for cleaving fatty acids and glycerol from fat cells. Free fatty acids are then carried into the circulation by albumin for transport to the liver. Glycerol diffuses back into the plasma because it can only be oxidized in the liver and kidney cells.

In the liver, fatty acids are Beta oxidized, a process that cleaves fatty acids, 2 carbons at a time. As oxidation proceeds, shorter fatty acids are formed with the final product being acetyl

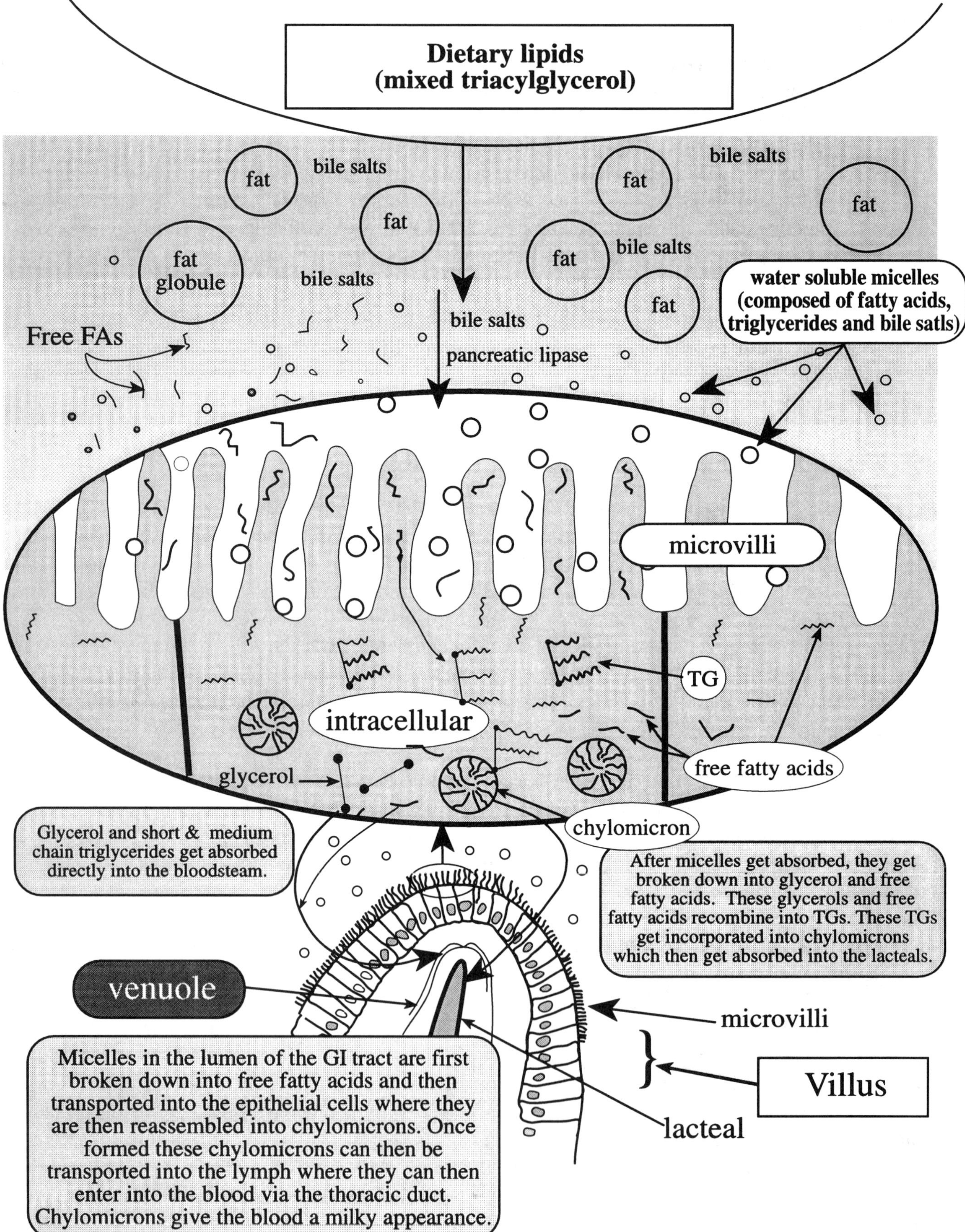
Dietary lipids
(mixed triacylglycerol)
fat
bile salts
fat
bile salts
fat
fat
globule
bile salts
fat
bile salts
fat
fat
water soluble micelles
(composed of fatty acids,
triglycerides and bile satls)
Free FAs
bile salts
pancreatic lipase
microvilli
TG
intracellular
free fatty acids
glycerol
chylomicron
Glycerol and short & medium
chain triglycerides get absorbed
directly into the bloodsteam.
After micelles get absorbed, they get
broken down into glycerol and free
fatty acids. These glycerols and free
fatty acids recombine into TGs. These TGs
get incorporated into chylomicrons
which then get absorbed into the lacteals.
venuole
microvilli
Villus
lacteal
Micelles in the lumen of the GI tract are first
broken down into free fatty acids and then
transported into the epithelial cells where they
are then reassembled into chylomicrons. Once
formed these chylomicrons can then be
transported into the lymph where they can then
enter into the blood via the thoracic duct.
Chylomicrons give the blood a milky appearance.

CoA. The rate limiting step in beta oxidation involves L-carnitine, an amino acid compound that is used in nutritional medicine to treat various cardiovascular disorders. The end result of beta oxidation leads to the formation of energy rich molecules which can be used for energy. Unoxidized fatty acids get stored throughout the body as subcutaneous fat which in turn can later be accessed and used as an energy source when needed.

Glycerol in the liver is either incorporated back into triglycerides or converted into glucose to be used as an energy source.

**Ketone Bodies**

Usually the liver produces more acetyl CoA than it can oxidize. The excess is condensed into two molecule units to form acetoacetic acid. This acetoacetic acid can diffuse from the liver into the circulation where it can be carried to the peripheral tissues to be converted into acetyl CoA and used for Beta oxidation. During periods of starvation, including very low carbohydrate diets, or in diabetes, the body relies mostly on fats for energy. Large quantities of fats from around the body get mobilized and transported to the liver where they are broken down into acetoacetic acid subunits. These subunits get converted into beta-hydroxybutyric acid and acetone. These 3 compounds are collectively known as *ketone bodies*. Skeletal muscle and the heart use these ketone bodies for producing energy. It is interesting that after several days of a low glucose availability, the brain starts using ketone bodies for its energy requirements and even prefers them over glucose.

The initial breakdown of the fatty acids into acetoacetic acid in the liver requires a supply of oxaloacetic acid, which is generated primarily from carbohydrate metabolism. Once oxaloacetic acid is produced, it can combine with acetoacetic acid to make citric acid. Citric acid is the beginning substrate for the Kreb cycle. In severe carbohydrate restriction or starvation, not enough oxaloacetic acid is present to combine with acetoacetic acid. The result is that ketone bodies start to build up in the tissues. This causes ketones to appear in the urine (ketonuria) and to be excreted in the breathe (acetone smell in the breath).

Excessive ketones in the liver must be removed from the body. They must be carried into the blood and excreted in the urine in combination with a neutralizing base. The available base in the blood, sodium ions, becomes used up. This results in the depletion of body stores of alkalinizing fluids which causes an overall acidification of the blood called *ketoacidosis.* Ketoacidosis can cause a number of deleterious effects including excessive excretion of calcium and, if severe enough, death.

**Hormonal Regulation of Lipid Metabolism**

A number of hormones in the body have a significant regulatory action on lipid metabolism. Below is a list of a few active hormones:

*Insulin* increases lipogenesis and inhibits lipolysis (fat breakdown and metabolism) by fat tissues. It also decreases the activity of hormone sensitive lipase (HSL). HSL is responsible for the enzymatic breakdown of triglycerides into free fatty acids stored in fat tissues.

*Thyroid hormones* increase cellular metabolism (particularly T3) and increases fat mobilization from fat cells.

*Glucocorticoids (ACTH and cortisol)* increases the rate of fat mobilization by increasing the activity of HSL and increasing the permeability of the fat cell membranes to fatty acids.

*Epinephrine, norepinephrine, adrenal* (medulla hormones) increase the activity of HSL and, therefore, indirectly increase the rate of fat mobilization.

*Growth hormone* has pronounced lipolytic effects.

## X. Lipid Transport and Storage

1) **White fat**–Most of our fat is stored as white fat. It is not very metabolically active.

2) **Brown Adipose Tissue (BAT or Brown Fat)**–We are born with a higher percentage of brown fat which is metabolically more active. As we age, brown fat slowly gets replaced with less active white fat. Evidence today indicates that we can actually change the type of fat in the body by the types of carbohydrate that we consume.

3) **Chylomicrons**–Once fatty acids and glycerol are absorbed into the epithelial cells, they recombine to form triglycerides. These triglycerides, inside the epithelial cells at the endoplasmic reticulum, then combine with cholesterol, phospholipid and protein to form chylomicrons. Once formed, they circulate in the lymphatic system where they eventually return to the blood via the thoracic duct. (See diagram concerning triacylglycerol digestion, absorption and metabolism)

4) **HDL**–High density lipoprotein is considered protective against heart disease. It is composed of more protein than fat and cholesterol and, thus, it is very dense. HDL transports fat and cholesterol from the peripheral circulation back to the liver to be metabolized. The higher the level of HDL in the blood, the lower the risk of heart disease. Some HDL ($HDL_3$) moieties are *not* considered protective.

5) **LDL**–Low density lipoprotein is considered to be atherogenic. It is composed of a higher percentage of cholesterol and fat than protein, thus, it tends to be lighter in density. LDL transports cholesterol from the liver to the peripheral circulation where it can accumulate in the blood vessel walls.

6) **Apolipoprotein A**–These are the beneficial lipoproteins found in the HDL cholesterol. They have been found to be inversely correlated to heart disease even more than HDL.

7) **Apolipoprotein B**–These are the apolipoproteins that have been found to be more highly correlated to heart disease than LDL cholesterol.

## XI. The Functions of Fats

1) **Energy**–Fats are the richest source of energy used by the body. They are relatively light weight and ideal for storing calories for future requirements.

2) **Protection**–Fat surrounding the organs makes an excellent protective pad. It also fills in spaces that would tend to allow the organs to slide downward due to gravity.

3) **Maintain body temperature**–Fat has excellent insulating properties and helps maintain proper body temperature for metabolic activities.

4) **Transport nutrients**–Dietary fats provide the stimuli for bile salt secretion from the gall bladder and are crucial for the absorption of fat soluble vitamins.

5) **Regulate stomach emptying**–Fat in the stomach is responsible for stimulating the enterogastric reflex which, in turn, keeps food in the stomach, thus allowing greater digestive action.

**6) Palatability & satiety**–Fat in foods tastes good and, without fats, food would be much less satisfying. In addition, since it keeps food in the stomach longer, fat allows satiety signals to reach the brain.

## XII. Eicosanoid Metabolism

Eicosanoids are 20 carbon chain fatty acids composed from essential fatty acids. Eicosanoid metabolism is complex and there are many things we do not know. From theoretical and clinical perspectives, we have learned a great deal about various pathways and some of the clinical effects of ingesting these oils. There are many ways to classify fats. One way is to classify them according to the series of prostaglandins to which they give rise. Below is the general scheme.

**Linoleic acid–18:2n-6(omega 6 fatty acid)**–This oil is found in many nuts and seeds including safflower, sunflower, sesame, soy bean, corn, cottonseed, and wheat germ (in approximate descending order). These oils eventually get converted into series 1 prostaglandins (PGE1). PGE1 relaxes smooth muscles; decreases platelet aggregation; prevents the release of arachidonic acid from cell membranes, thus decreasing the amount of inflammatory substrate available; enhances mucin production in the stomach for protection; inhibits tumor growth; decreases inflammation; stabilizes red blood cell membranes; and blocks the conversion of arachidonic acid into inflammatory eicosanoids.

**NOTE**–Because there has been a lot of misinformation concerning the conversion of one of linoleic acid's metabolites–dihomogamma linolenic acid (see diagram)–an important point needs to made. In most biochemistry text books, and in many less technical books and periodicals on the subject, it is stated that DHGLA gets converted to arachidonic acid via the enzyme delta 5 desaturase. This may be true in certain mammalian species such as rats and mice, but in humans this conversion is *very* slow. The activity of the enzyme delta 5 desaturase is minimal in humans, rabbits and guinea pigs. In addition, both DHGLA and GLA actually inhibit the action of delta 5 desaturase. It is sometimes mentioned that GLA supplements can be harmful because they increase the levels of arachidonic acid in the body which also increases inflammation. This is not true in humans. Only small amounts of arachidonic acid are produced and this small amount is blocked in its transformation into inflammatory mediators by delta 5 desaturase and DHGLA via its competition for cyclooxygenase.

**(Alpha) α linolenic acid–18:3n-3 (omega 3 fatty acid)**–Originally this fatty acid was thought to be a *non* essential fatty acid because it could be made from linoleic acid. Symptoms related to an essential fatty acid deficiency could for the most part be aleviated via the supplementation of linoleic acid. However it seems that there are some unique features

**PGE1**–Derived from omega 6 fatty acids–which are found in many nuts, seeds and grains as well as evening primrose, borage and blackcurrent oils–PGE1 has many effects. These include keeping blood pressure under control, regulating the secretion of the protective substances of the stomach, reducing inflammation and influencing mood and emotions. There are certain pathologies–such as diabetes, alcoholism, hypertension, and atopic dermatitis–that involve a decreased production of PGE1. The enzyme delta 6 desaturase is the rate limiting enzyme for the production of PGE1. A synthetic analog of PGE1, "Cytotek,® is sometimes prescribed for the prevention of stomach ulcers when NSAIDS are being used to treat inflammation. Certain nationalities such as Irish, Celtic, Scandinavian, Scottish, and American Indian have deficiencies of delta 6 desaturase and may require the more immediate precursor (GLA) to generate adequate levels of PGE1. It should also be noted that DHGLA may have properties of its own as it generates some unique metabolites that have not been studied much.

**PGE2**–Derived from arachidonic acid–20-4 omega-6 which come almost entirely from animal derived foods, PGE2 is responsible for generating the body's inflammatory response. This is vital for normal immune function. It acts to increase platelet aggregation, increase permeability, increase temperature, pain, and increase contraction of smooth muscle in the blood vessels. However, in many disease processes the reduction in these prostaglandins is very important in improving the condition. Most inflammatory conditions, as well as asthma and cardiovascular pathologies, benefit from a reduction of PGE2. Aspirin has been found to decrease production of PGE2. It is believed that this is the mechanism by which it exerts its anti-inflammatory effects by blocking the cyclooxygenase, the enzyme that is critical for converting arachidonic acid into PGE2.

**PGE3**–Derived from omega-3 fatty acids, this prostaglandin is responsible for anti-inflammatory action, decreasing platelet adhesiveness, decreasing serum triglycerides and improving the integrity of cell membranes. It has also been shown to have a regulatory effect on blood pressure similar to PGE1. Generally, it is in a balance with the other prostaglandins, especially PGE1. Currently, PGE3 levels in the U.S. are probably on the deficient side because the U.S. diet is very low in omega-3 fatty acids. Like PGE1, the rate limiting enzyme for PGE3 production is delta-6 desaturase which can be antagonized by a number of different factors such as coffee, insulin, trans-fatty acids, alcohol, and aging. It is believed that our diet as hunters and gatherers was much higher in omega 3 fatty acids; therefore our levels of PGE3 were considerably higher.

In some people there may be a problem converting alpha linolenic acid into eicosapentaenoic acid, 20:5 omega 3 (EPA) and docosahexaenoic acid, 22:6 omega 3(DHA). In such cases, it may be necessary to directly supply these in the diet either through foods or supplements. In infancy DHA is supplied directly through mother's milk. Infants not receiving this DHA (formula fed infants) have been found to develop their brain function and visual acuity more slowly.

References:


**Handbook of the Eicosanoids: Prostaglandins & Related Lipids. A.L. Willis, CRC Press, Incorp; August 1989. ISBN # 0-8493-3220-6. A.L. Willis is probably the foremost expert in the field of eicosanoid metabolism, prostaglandins and fats. He has been involved in much of the current research on eicosanoids.

STUDY–*GLA in diabetes: Results form the GLA Multicenter Trial Gruppl.* Diabetes Care. 16:8-15, 1993. ABSTRACT–In 111 pts with mild diabetic neuropathy, it was shown that GLA 480mg/day over the course of 1 year prevented further deterioration and in some cases was seen to actually get better.

STUDY– *Flax Oil and Prostaglandin Synthesis.* Nutrition 8:211-212, 1992. ABSTRACT–Alpha-linolenic acid was shown to decrease the levels of arachidonic acid. This suppression of arachidonic acid was found to be dependent upon the dose of alpha-linolenic acid unless linoleic acid intake was allowed to go up.

STUDY– *GLA in RA:Results form a double-blind study.* Annals of Internal Medicine. 119:867-873, 1993. ABSTRACT–1.4gms/day of GLA was given in form of borage oil while they were taking their NSAIDS. There was a significantly reduced number and severity of painful joints in 37 patients after 24 weeks.

STUDY– *Omega-3 oils in RA:Results form a long-term double-blind study.* Arthritis & Rheumatism, 37:824-9, 1994. ABSTRACT–90 patients with RA were treated with 2.5gms omega-3 oils from fish for 12 months. There was a significant clinical benefit from both subjective and objective evaluations.

# SUMMARY OF LIPID METABOLISM

## DIETARY LIPIDS
**Triacylglycerol**

**MOUTH**
**very mild mechanical digestion of all lipids via chewing and lingual lipase**

**STOMACH**
**lingual lipase & gastric lipase provide some enzymatic digestion**

**SMALL INTESTINE**
**bile salts from gall bladder emulsifys fats**
**pancreatic lipase digests TGs into glycerol, FAs, mono & diglycerides (MGs & DGs)**
**human milk lipase in infants acts like pancreatic lipase**

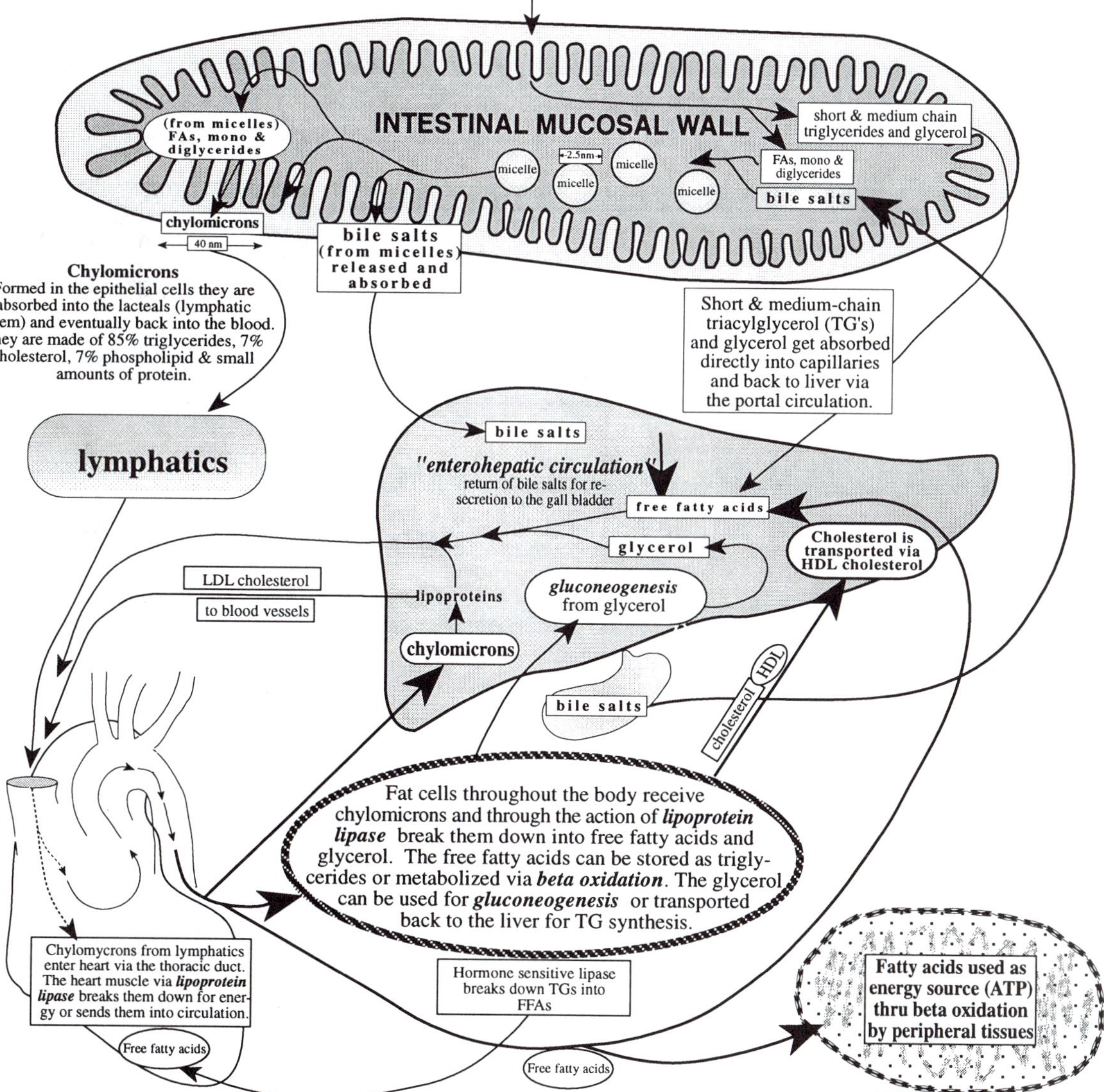

Fat content of selected foods with breakdown of polyunsaturated vs saturated fats

| Salad and cooking oils | Total Fat % | % Sat | % Monounsat | (Mostly linoleic acid) % Polyunsat | P/S ratio | P-M/S ratio |
|---|---|---|---|---|---|---|
| Safflower | 100 | 9 | 12 | 74 | 8.2 | 9.5 |
| Wheat germ | 100 | 19 | 15 | 62 | 3.3 | 4.1 |
| Corn | 100 | 13 | 24 | 59 | 4.5 | 6.4 |
| Soybean | 100 | 14 | 23 | 58 | 4.1 | 5.8 |
| Cottonseed | 100 | 26 | 18 | 52 | 2.0 | 2.7 |
| Sesame | 100 | 14 | 40 | 42 | 3.0 | 5.9 |
| Peanut | 100 | 17 | 46 | 32 | 1.9 | 4.6 |
| Rapeseed (canola) | 100 | 7 | 56 | 33 | 4.9 | 12.7 |
| Olive | 100 | 14 | 74 | 8 | 0.6 | 5.9 |
| Palm | 100 | 49 | 37 | 9 | 0.2 | 1.0 |
| Coconut | 100 | 87 | 6 | 2 | 0.02 | 0.09 |
| Palm kernel | 100 | 81 | 11 | 2 | 0.02 | 0.16 |
| Butter | 81 | 51 | 23 | 3 | 0.05 | 0.51 |
| Margarine, first ingredient on label | | | | | | |
| Safflower oil—tub | 80 | 9 | 23 | 44 | 4.9 | 7.4 |
| Corn oil (liquid)—tub | 80 | 14 | 32 | 31 | 2.2 | 4.5 |
| Soybean oil—stick | 80 | 17 | 39 | 21 | 1.2 | 3.5 |
| Corn oil—stick | 80 | 13 | 46 | 18 | 1.4 | 4.9 |
| Lard | 100 | 39 | 45 | 11 | 0.3 | 1.4 |
| Animal fats | | | | | | |
| Poultry | 100 | 30 | 37 | 20 | 0.7 | 1.9 |
| Beef, lamb, pork | 100 | 50 | 36 | 3 | 0.06 | 0.78 |
| Fish, raw | | | | | | |
| Salmon | 9 | 2 | 2 | 4 | 2.0 | 3 |
| Mackerel | 13 | 5 | 3 | 4 | 0.8 | 1.4 |
| Herring, Pacific | 13 | 4 | 2 | 2 | 0.5 | 1 |
| Tuna | 5 | 2 | 1 | 1 | 0.5 | 1 |
| Nut | | | | | | |
| Walnuts, English | 64 | 9 | 23 | 63 | 7.0 | 9.5 |
| Brazil | 67 | 13 | 32 | 17 | 1.3 | 3.8 |
| Peanuts or peanut butter | 51 | 17 | 46 | 32 | 1.9 | 5.6 |
| Pecan | 65 | 4-6 | 33-48 | 9-24 | — | — |
| Egg yolk | 33 | 10 | 12 | 4 | 0.4 | 1.6 |
| Avocado | 16 | 3 | 7 | 2 | 0.6 | 3 |

From USDA Handbook 8-4: Composition of fats and oils, 1979.
*Total is not expected to equal total fat.
†Polyunsaturated fatty acids: saturated fatty acids (excluding monounsaturated fatty acids).
‡Polyunsaturated fatty acids plus monounsaturated fatty acids: saturated fatty acids.

| Food | % of fat made of omega-3 | amt. of fat per serving |
|---|---|---|
| **Oils** | | grams per 2T or 1 ounce |
| Menhaden | 23 | 6.9 |
| Salmon | 22 | 6.6 |
| Cod liver | 20 | 6.0 |
| Canola | 10 | 3.0 |
| Soybean | 7 | 2.1 |
| Butter fat | 2 | 0.6 |
| Corn | 1 | 0.3 |
| **Fish** | | grams per 2T or 1 ounce |
| Cod | 42 | 0.3 |
| Shrimp | 38 | 0.5 |
| Tuna | 30 | 2.3 |
| Pink salmon | 29 | 1 |
| King crab | 20 | 0.6 |
| Mackerel | 17 | 1.8-2.6 |
| Herring | 6 | 1.0-2.0 |

| FAT CONTENT OF FOODS | | | |
|---|---|---|---|
| **FOOD ITEM** | **SERVING SIZE** | **CALORIES** | **% CALORIES FROM FAT** |
| **DAIRY PRODUCTS AND EGGS** | | | |
| Butter | 1 T | 102 | 99 |
| Cheese | | | |
| Cheddar | 3 oz | 342 | 72 |
| Cottage, 2% | .5 cup | 102 | 20 |
| Cream | 3 oz | 300 | 88 |
| Mozzarella, part skim | 3 oz | 215 | 55 |
| Parmesan | 3 T | 70 | 70 |
| Swiss | 3 oz | 321 | 70 |
| Cream, 1/2 & 1/2 | 3 T | 60 | 76 |
| Egg, 1 large | 80 | 62 | |
| Milk, cow | | | |
| Whole milk, 4% fat | 1 cup | 150 | 55 |
| Low fat, 1% fat | 1 cup | 144 | 21 |
| Milk, goat | 1 cup | 168 | 54 |
| Yogurt, whole milk, plain | 1 cup | 139 | 49 |
| **FRUITS** | | | |
| Apple | 1 medium | 81 | 5 |
| Apricots, dried | 6 halves | 50 | 8 |
| Avocado | 1 medium | 324 | 80 |
| Blackberries | 1 cup | 74 | 5 |
| Banana | 1 medium | 105 | 4 |
| Cantaloupe | half of 5 in. melon | 80 | 7 |
| Cherries | 20 whole | 97 | 11 |
| Grapes | 1 cup | 114 | 8 |
| Grapefruit | 1 medium | 80 | 3 |
| Kiwi | 2 whole | 92 | 6 |
| Orange | 1 medium | 62 | 1 |
| Papaya | 1 medium | 117 | 4 |
| Peach | 1 medium | 37 | 1 |
| Pear | 1 medium | 98 | 6 |
| Pinapple | 1 cup | 77 | 6 |
| Prunes, dried | 5 large | 117 | 2 |
| Strawberries | 1 cup | 45 | 5 |
| **MEAT** | | | |
| Bacon | 3 strips | 109 | 77 |
| Beef, bottom roast, no fat | 3 oz | 191 | 40 |
| Ground, lean | 3 oz | 231 | 61 |
| Hot dog | 1 medium | 142 | 82 |
| Ham, chopped | 3 oz | 195 | 68 |
| Lamb | 3 oz | 205 | 57 |
| Liver | 3 oz | 185 | 34 |
| Pork, spare ribs | 3 oz | 338 | 69 |
| Sausage | 3 oz | 274 | 72 |
| **SEAFOOD** | | | |
| Clams, raw | 3 oz | 65 | 14 |
| Fish stick | one | 70 | 38 |
| Flounder, baked, no fat | 3 oz | 80 | 11 |
| Oysters, raw | 1 cup | 160 | 20 |
| Salmon | 3 oz | 120 | 38 |
| Shrimp, canned, drained | 3 oz | 100 | 9 |
| Tuna | 3 oz | 108 | 6 |
| Tuna salad | 1 cup | 375 | 45 |

**FAT CONTENT OF FOODS**

| FOOD ITEM | SERVING SIZE | CALORIES | % CALORIES FROM FAT |
|---|---|---|---|
| **POULTRY** | | | |
| Chicken breast, roasted | 3 oz | 140 | 20 |
| Drumstick, roasted | 3 oz | 147 | 30 |
| Wing | 3 oz | 174 | 36 |
| Turkey leg, roasted | 3 oz | 135 | 21 |
| **SALAD DRESSING** | | | |
| Blue Cheese | 1 T | 75 | 96 |
| French | 1 T | 67 | 84 |
| Italian | 1 T | 69 | 91 |
| Thousand Island | 1 T | 60 | 90 |
| Oil and vinegar | 1 T | 70 | 100 |
| **VEGETABLES** | | | |
| Alfalfa sprouts | 1 cup | 10 | tr |
| Artichokes | 1 whole | 55 | tr |
| Asparagus | 1 cup | 45 | 1 |
| Beets | 1 cup | 55 | tr |
| Broccoli | 1 cup | 46 | 8 |
| Cabbage, cooked | 1 cup | 30 | tr |
| Carrots | 1 cup | 70 | 3 |
| Cauliflower, cooked | 1 cup | 30 | 6 |
| Eggplant, steamed | 1 cup | 25 | tr |
| Mushrooms, raw | 1 cup | 20 | tr |
| Onions, raw | .5 cup | 28 | 7 |
| Potatoes, baked w/skin | 1 medium | 220 | tr |
| French fries | 10 strips | 158 | 46 |
| Pumpkin, cooked, raw | 1 cup | 50 | tr |
| Squash, summer, cooked | 1 cup | 35 | 25 |
| Squash, winter, cooked | 1 cup | 80 | 11 |
| Tomatoes | 1 medium | 25 | tr |
| Tomato juice | 1 cup | 40 | tr |
| **GRAINS** | | | |
| Bread, whole wheat | 1 slice | 61 | 11 |
| Brown rice, cooked | 1 cup | 223 | 4 |
| Buckwheat, cooked | .5 cup | 104 | 7 |
| Corn | 1 ear | 85 | 10 |
| Corn, canned | 1 cup | 165 | 5 |
| Millet, cooked | .5 cup | 54 | 8 |
| Oats, rolled, cooked | .5 cup | 73 | 15 |
| Popcorn, plain | 1 cup | 23 | 12 |
| Quinoa, cooked | .5 cup | 118 | 13 |
| Wild rice, cooked | .5 cup | 92 | 2 |
| **NUTS & LEGUMES** | | | |
| Almonds | .25 cup | 209 | 74 |
| Cashews | 11 medium | 98 | 73 |
| Coconut, shredded | 1 cup | 493 | 90 |
| Peanuts | .25 cup | 207 | 73 |
| Peanut butter | 1 T | 94 | 75 |
| Pine nuts | 1 oz | 170 | 71 |
| Pistachios | 30 nuts | 105 | 80 |
| Pumpkin seeds | 2 T | 97 | 76 |
| Walnuts | .25 cup | 193 | 81 |
| Black beans | .5 cup | 85 | 4 |
| Kidney beans | .5 cup | 113 | 4 |
| Lima beans | .5 cup | 104 | 2 |
| Lentils, cooked | .5 cup | 99 | 4 |
| Peas, green | .5 cup | 67 | 2 |
| Soy milk | 1 cup | 73 | 40 |
| Tofu, 1" thick slice | 1 slice | 86 | 52 |
| Tempeh | 2 oz | 117 | 40 |

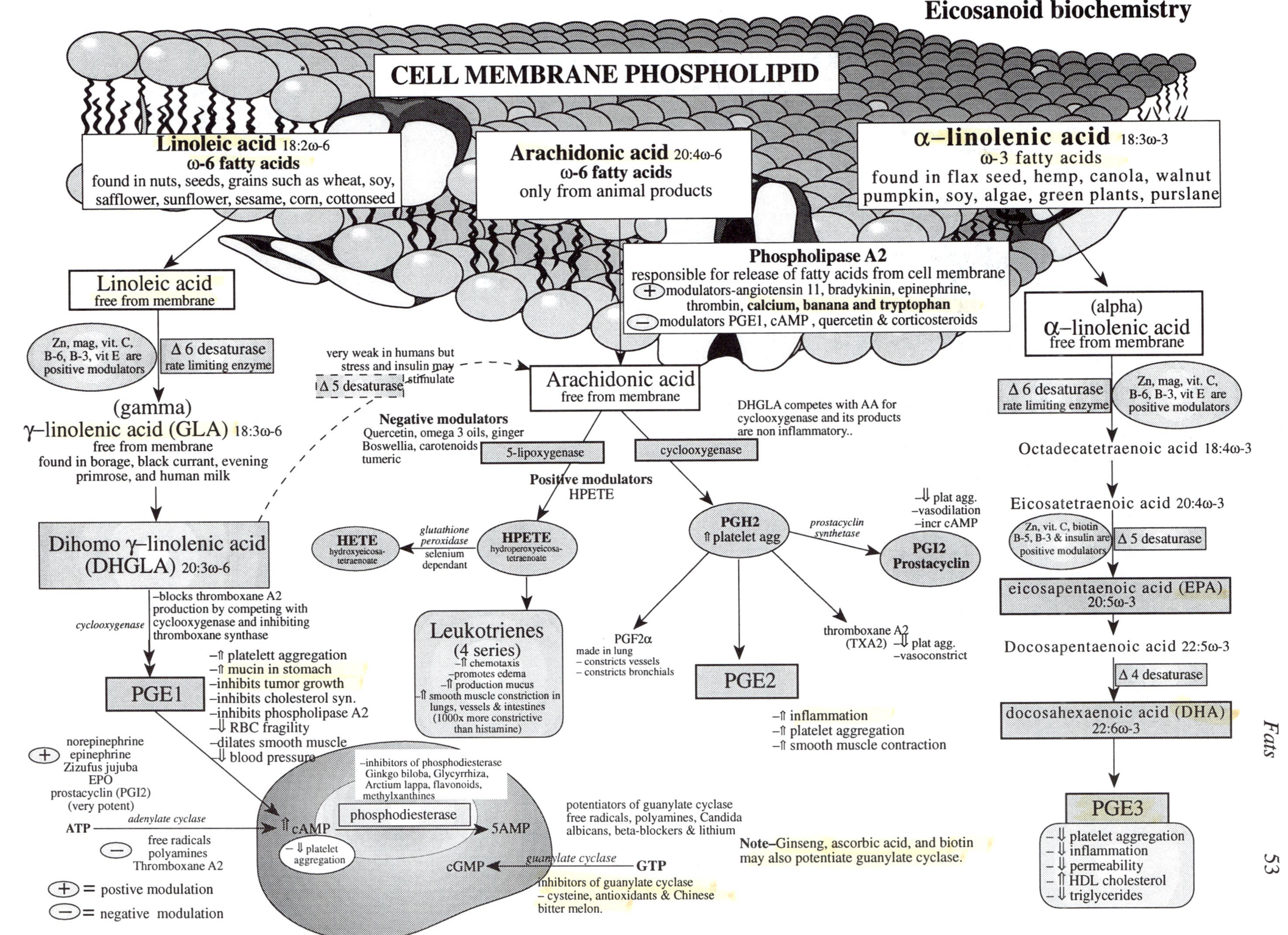
Eicosanoid biochemistry
CELL MEMBRANE PHOSPHOLIPID
Linoleic acid 18:2ω-6
ω-6 fatty acids
found in nuts, seeds, grains such as wheat, soy, safflower, sunflower, sesame, corn, cottonseed
Arachidonic acid 20:4ω-6
ω-6 fatty acids
only from animal products
α–linolenic acid 18:3ω-3
ω-3 fatty acids
found in flax seed, hemp, canola, walnut pumpkin, soy, algae, green plants, purslane
Phospholipase A2
responsible for release of fatty acids from cell membrane
+ modulators-angiotensin 11, bradykinin, epinephrine, thrombin, calcium, banana and tryptophan
− modulators PGE1, cAMP, quercetin & corticosteroids
Linoleic acid
free from membrane
Zn, mag, vit. C, B-6, B-3, vit E are positive modulators
Δ 6 desaturase
rate limiting enzyme
(gamma)
γ–linolenic acid (GLA) 18:3ω-6
free from membrane
found in borage, black currant, evening primrose, and human milk
very weak in humans but stress and insulin may stimulate
Δ 5 desaturase
Arachidonic acid
free from membrane
Negative modulators
Quercetin, omega 3 oils, ginger Boswellia, carotenoids tumeric
5-lipoxygenase
cyclooxygenase
DHGLA competes with AA for cyclooxygenase and its products are non inflammatory..
Positive modulators
HPETE
Dihomo γ–linolenic acid (DHGLA) 20:3ω-6
–blocks thromboxane A2 production by competing with cyclooxygenase and inhibiting thromboxane synthase
cyclooxygenase
PGE1
–⇑ platelett aggregation
–⇑ mucin in stomach
–inhibits tumor growth
–inhibits cholesterol syn.
–inhibits phospholipase A2
–⇓ RBC fragility
–dilates smooth muscle
–⇓ blood pressure
HETE
hydroxyeicosa-tetraenoate
glutathione peroxidase
selenium dependant
HPETE
hydroperoxyeicosa-tetraenoate
Leukotrienes
(4 series)
–⇑ chemotaxis
–promotes edema
–⇑ production mucus
–⇑ smooth muscle constriction in lungs, vessels & intestines (1000x more constrictive than histamine)
PGH2
⇑ platelet agg
prostacyclin synthetase
PGI2
Prostacyclin
–⇓ plat agg.
–vasodilation
–incr cAMP
PGF2α
made in lung
– constricts vessels
– constricts bronchials
PGE2
thromboxane A2 (TXA2)
–⇓ plat agg.
–vasoconstrict
–⇑ inflammation
–⇑ platelet aggregation
–⇑ smooth muscle contraction
norepinephrine
epinephrine
Zizufus jujuba
EPO
prostacyclin (PGI2)
(very potent)
adenylate cyclase
ATP
free radicals
polyamines
Thromboxane A2
–inhibitors of phosphodiesterase
Ginkgo biloba, Glycyrrhiza, Arctium lappa, flavonoids, methylxanthines
phosphodiesterase
⇑ cAMP
5AMP
– ⇓ platelet aggregation
cGMP
guanylate cyclase
GTP
potentiators of guanylate cyclase
free radicals, polyamines, Candida albicans, beta-blockers & lithium
inhibitors of guanylate cyclase
– cysteine, antioxidants & Chinese bitter melon.
Note–Ginseng, ascorbic acid, and biotin may also potentiate guanylate cyclase.
+ = postive modulation
− = negative modulation
(alpha)
α–linolenic acid
free from membrane
Δ 6 desaturase
rate limiting enzyme
Zn, mag, vit. C, B-6, B-3, vit E are positive modulators
Octadecatetraenoic acid 18:4ω-3
Eicosatetraenoic acid 20:4ω-3
Zn, vit. C, biotin B-5, B-3 & insulin are positive modulators
Δ 5 desaturase
eicosapentaenoic acid (EPA)
20:5ω-3
Docosapentaenoic acid 22:5ω-3
Δ 4 desaturase
docosahexaenoic acid (DHA)
22:6ω-3
PGE3
– ⇓ platelet aggregation
– ⇓ inflammation
– ⇓ permeability
– ⇑ HDL cholesterol
– ⇓ triglycerides

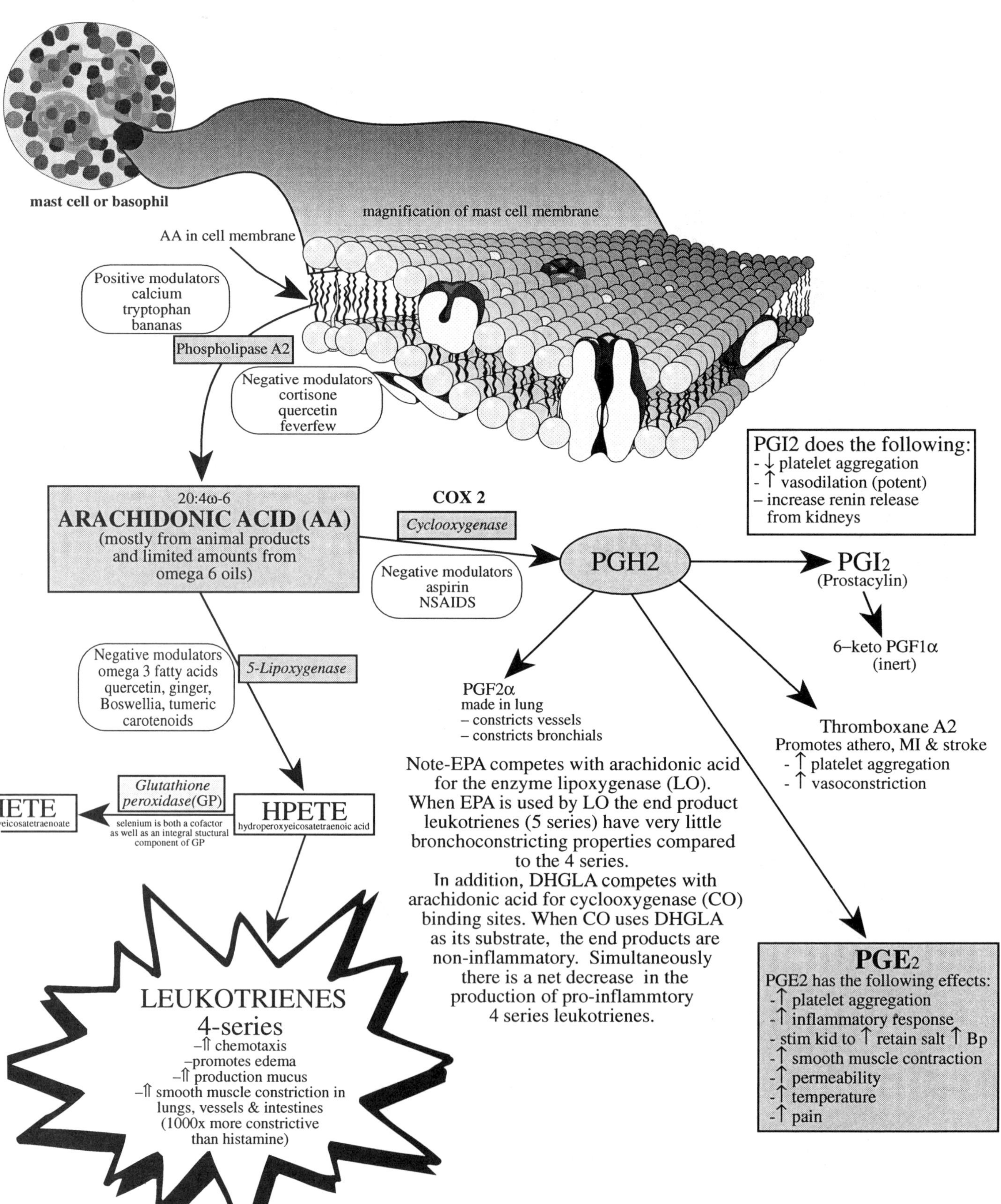

mast cell or basophil
magnification of mast cell membrane
AA in cell membrane
Positive modulators
calcium
tryptophan
bananas
Phospholipase A2
Negative modulators
cortisone
quercetin
feverfew
20:4ω-6
ARACHIDONIC ACID (AA)
(mostly from animal products
and limited amounts from
omega 6 oils)
COX 2
Cyclooxygenase
Negative modulators
aspirin
NSAIDS
PGH2
PGI2 does the following:
- ↓ platelet aggregation
- ↑ vasodilation (potent)
– increase renin release
from kidneys
PGI2
(Prostacylin)
6–keto PGF1α
(inert)
Negative modulators
omega 3 fatty acids
quercetin, ginger,
Boswellia, tumeric
carotenoids
5-Lipoxygenase
PGF2α
made in lung
– constricts vessels
– constricts bronchials
Thromboxane A2
Promotes athero, MI & stroke
- ↑ platelet aggregation
- ↑ vasoconstriction
Glutathione
peroxidase(GP)
IETE
eicosatetraenoate
selenium is both a cofactor
as well as an integral stuctural
component of GP
HPETE
hydroperoxyeicosatetraenoic acid
Note-EPA competes with arachidonic acid
for the enzyme lipoxygenase (LO).
When EPA is used by LO the end product
leukotrienes (5 series) have very little
bronchoconstricting properties compared
to the 4 series.
In addition, DHGLA competes with
arachidonic acid for cyclooxygenase (CO)
binding sites. When CO uses DHGLA
as its substrate, the end products are
non-inflammatory. Simultaneously
there is a net decrease in the
production of pro-inflammtory
4 series leukotrienes.
PGE2
PGE2 has the following effects:
-↑ platelet aggregation
-↑ inflammatory response
- stim kid to ↑ retain salt ↑ Bp
-↑ smooth muscle contraction
-↑ permeability
-↑ temperature
-↑ pain
LEUKOTRIENES
4-series
–⇑ chemotaxis
–promotes edema
–⇑ production mucus
–⇑ smooth muscle constriction in
lungs, vessels & intestines
(1000x more constrictive
than histamine)

# PROTEINS

- Protein was the first substance to be recognized as an essential component for living tissue. The name was derived from the Greek word meaning "of first importance." It is composed of carbon, hydrogen and oxygen. It also contains about 16% nitrogen, along with sulfur and, occasionally, other elements.
- Plants synthesize protein from nitrogen which they obtain from nitrates and ammonia in the soil. Some plants, like legumes, can extract nitrogen from bacteria that fix atmospheric nitrogen while growing on the root nodules. Animals obtain their nitrogen requirements by eating either plants or animals. Upon the death of the animal, the nitrogen goes back into the soil, resulting in the cyclic renewal of the nitrogen cycle.
- The average American consumes, on the average, about 101gms. **This is about twice the recommended dosage for the day.**

## I. Structure and Classification

The basic building blocks of proteins are amino acids. There are about 23 amino acids which have been recognized as constituents of most protein. All of the amino acids are alpha amino carboxylic acids in which the basic amino group and an acid carboxyl group are attached to the same carbon atom.

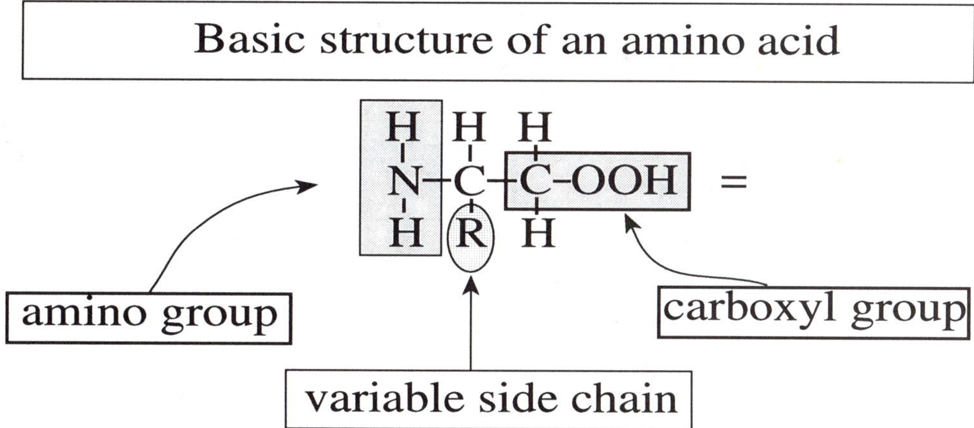


The R is the side chain which distinguishes the individual amino acid. Amino acids can combine by means of a peptide bond. Proteins vary in size from small (23 amino acids) to very complex (with thousands of amino acids). Polypeptides, which constitute the primary structure of proteins, may contain from a few to hundreds of amino acid subunits. Several polypeptide chains may be linked together in a helical or coiled form. This is called the secondary structure of a protein. More complex proteins feature a tertiary structure in which the polypeptide chain is wound upon itself into a globular form, with the whole structure held rigid by inter atomic forces such as hydrogen bonds. The structures that they may take are extremely varied and offer an infinite variety of compounds. Lastly, proteins can be found in quaternary structures similar to those found in hemoglobin. Four heme molecules, which are in the tertiary structure, are found in relationship with others in a quaternary pattern.

Proteins can be found in either fibrous or globular forms.

**Fibrous forms** occur mostly in connective tissue such as ligaments and tendons.

**Globular forms** occur as tissue fluids and include casein in milk, egg albumin and the albumins and globulins of blood, plasma, and hemoglobin.

Simple proteins yield only amino acids upon hydrolysis. They include albumins, globulins, glutelins, prolamins, and albuminoids. These proteins, such as albumins and globulins from animal fluids, may be soluble in water. Proteins such as myosin and muscle protein are less soluble.

Conjugated proteins are combinations in which a non protein substance is attached to a simple protein molecule as a prosthetic group, thus facilitating functions that neither could perform by themselves. They include RNA, and DNA, which combine simple proteins and nucleic acid; mucoproteins and glycoproteins, which combine proteins with variable quantities of complex polysaccharides, such as in mucin found in gastric secretions; and lipoproteins.

## II. The Functions of Proteins

1) **Anabolic proteins** are used to build connective tissue, bone, muscle, the lens of the eye, antibodies used to fight infections, enzymes used for digestion and various hormones such as insulin and gastrin. They are also involved in the synthesis of various other tissues which need repair and maintenance.

2) **Structural proteins** are used for various structural components. They are also said to be used during the process of anabolism.

3) **Energy source**–When proteins are deaminated, they can be used as a source of energy. The synthesis of carbohydrates from non-carbohydrate sources is known as gluconeogenesis.

4) **Transport**–Some proteins are used to transport other molecules across cell membranes, around the blood stream and also in tissues.

5) **Homeostasis** (old term)–This is a term used to describe proteins which are used for buffering the pH of the blood, and maintaining the correct oncotic pressure in the blood vessels. Albumin is the major protein in the blood involved with maintaining correct oncotic pressure.

## III. Protein Quality

Protein comes from various sources and in different forms. The degree to which the body is able to digest and absorb nitrogen from a food determines its quality. Currently the most commonly used measurements of protein quality in foods are *biological value* (BV), *net protein utilization* (NPU), *protein efficiency ratio* (PER), and chemical scores.

**Biological value of a food** is measured as the % of absorbed nitrogen that is retained in the body for growth or maintenance. It is determined by controlled animal feeding studies in which nitrogen is retained more fully when the essential amino acids are present in sufficient quantity. A food in which 70% of the absorbed nitrogen is retained is considered to be of good quality. It is capable of sustaining life.

**Net protein utilization** is another term that is used to describe the quality of a protein based on the ratio of weight gained by a person on a particular protein compared to the weight that person gains on casein, a known high quality protein. It is based upon the assumption that weight gain is proportional to the gain in body protein. This is a method to try to determine whether a protein has *all of the essential amino acids in correct ratios.* Protein sources that are poorly digested but yet have a high quality protein will yield a false low reading. **Eggs are considered to have the highest biological value or highest quality of protein (complete protein).** All other foods are compared to eggs because they have almost a perfect amino acid ratio for the body.

**Protein efficiency ratio** is the simplest measure of protein quality. It is based on weight gain per gram of protein ingested in young rats. It assumes that all weight gain is due to gain in body protein.

**Chemical scores** are based on methods which require information on the amino acid composition of the food or the diet. The chemical score is usually expressed as the ratio of amino acid mg per gram of protein in the food compared to the amino acid requirement per gram of protein for the age and sex of the group whose diet is being evaluated. Using this method, a particular amino acid has a different score for each age and sex group. ,For example wheat, which is low in the limiting amino acid, lysine, has a score of 54 for a 10 year old but exceeding 100 for an adult. This means that it could support the growth and repair of tissues in an adult but not in a child.

## IV. Protein Metabolism

Protein is mostly found in foods as polypeptides. These polypeptides must be broken down into amino acids before they can be absorbed. Physical breakdown of proteins starts in the mouth. Enzymatic digestion of protein starts in the stomach and continues into the small intestine. This process requires the breaking of the peptide bonds between amino acids. In the stomach HCL is an important mediator of protein digestion as it both breaks down proteins directly and activates certain enzymes which, in turn, break down the proteins. Final breakdown of smaller peptides occurs in the small intestine. Oligopeptides (smaller protein fragments) are broken down by enzymes contained in the brush border of the epithelial cells of the small intestine. Thus, substantial quantities of small peptides may get absorbed into the epithelial cells of the intestines, but only trace amounts actually end up appearing in the blood stream. These trace amounts get hydrolyzed by the liver and peripheral tissues. A substantial number of the amino acids which are absorbed actually get used by the enterocytes (epithelial cells of the small intestine) to synthesize their own protein requirements since these cells tend to be very metabolically active. Both glutamine and arginine are conditionally essential amino acids which are required in relatively large amounts by the enterocytes of the intestines.

> **Note**–Previously it was thought that whole proteins could not enter directly into the blood stream, but through radioactive labeling of certain proteins, such as bromelain, horse radish peroxidase, xanthene oxidase, it has been found that they do indeed enter into the blood stream as intact proteins. This has clinical significance because it means that administration of proteins that must be absorbed intact to have therapeutic efficacy, may indeed occur.

**Amino acid catabolism**–Amino acids are catabolized in the body through the process of oxidative deamination. This process takes place mostly in the liver and involves the removal of the amino group and formation of a keto acid. The carbon skeletons are converted into various intermediates which can eventually be used for energy. In times of abundant caloric intake this glucose gets stored in the body as adipose tissue. Small amounts get converted to glycogen in the liver and the muscles.

The amino group, removed during deamination, becomes ammonia which is then converted in the liver into urea. The ammonia that is formed is highly toxic and must be transported while conjugated to glutamic acid thus yielding the compound glutamine.

**Essential Amino Acids**–These amino acids must be eaten in the diet because they can not be manufactured in the body in sufficient amounts.

- histidine
- isoleucine
- leucine
- lysine
- methionine
- phenylalanine
- threonine
- tryptophan
- valine

**Conditionally essential amino acids**–These amino acids are sometimes considered essential in certain situations.

- arginine
- cysteine
- glutamine
- glycine
- proline
- serine
- taurine (preterm infants)
- tyrosine

## V. Protein Requirements

| AGE | grams per Kg weight | avg weight | approx total gms protein |
|---|---|---|---|
| 0-6 months | 2.2gms/kg | 6kg | 13gms of 90% NPU |
| 6-12 months | 1.4gms/kg | 9kg | 14gms or 70% NPU |
| 1-3yrs | 1.14gms/kg | 13kg | 16gms of 74% NPU |
| 4-6 | 1.03gms/kg | 20kg | 24gms of 90% NPU |
| 7-10 yrs | 1.00gms/kg | 28kg | 28gms of 90% NPU |
| males 11-14 | .98gms/kg | 45kg | 45gms of 90% NPU |
| 25-100yrs | .75gms/kg | 79kg | 63gms of 90% NPU |
| Females 11-14 | .94gms/kg | | of 90% NP |
| 19-100yrs | .75gms/kg | 47kg | 46gms of 90% NPU |
| Pregnancy 1st tri | | | +10 |
| Pregnancy 2nd tri | | | +10 |
| Pregnancy 3rd tri | | | +15 |
| lactation 1st 6mo | | | +15 |
| lactation 2nd 6mo | | | +12 |

**Note**–Animal protein has a higher qualitative value. Therefore, vegetarians need somewhat higher quantities of protein to allow for the lesser quality of vegetable protein (not having all of the essential amino acids in the correct ratio). It is also possible to combine vegetarian sources to get the correct balance of amino acids. An example of this is the combination of beans, which are deficient in lysine, and rice, which is ample in lysine but deficient in methionine.

Most people in the U.S. get more than sufficient protein in their diet. The table below which describes protein intake in this country shows that even vegans get at least 50% more protein than they require. Obviously we must ask the question, "What is the ideal amount of protein in the diet?" The answer to this question is probably very individualized. From amino acid studies (see RDA's) we know that there are very large variations in the requirements for individual amino acids. Epidemiological studies tell us that large amounts of protein may cause problems. It has been clearly shown that the higher the animal protein consumption in the diet, the greater the risk for heart disease. Other conditions that are associated with higher protein intakes include osteoporosis, gout, allergies, various digestive disorders, and certain forms of cancer. Most excess protein merely gets used to make glucose and if activity levels are not high enough to use it then it will get stored as fat in the body.

Some benefits of protein consumption are protein's stabilizing effect on blood glucose levels and the fact that protein does not promote the growth of Candida species in the gastrointestinal tract. Proteins are essential for maintaining body weight during periods of stress or trauma, especially trauma to the GI tract. In the past high fat and high protein diets, taking advantage of the high specific dynamic action of protein, were used to promote weight loss. The *specific dynamic action* of protein means that if calories come almost exclusively from protein, a significant amount of energy is required to catabolize the proteins. As a result, extra calories, which might otherwise cause a person to gain weight, are burned off. Unfortunately, people who tried these diets often went into ketosis, a condition which is not considered to be a healthy one.

Dr. James D'Adamo and his son Dr. Peter D'Adamo have written several books, the latest of which, *4 blood types and 4 diets*, 1997, tries to demonstrate that a person's blood type may determine the ideal amount of protein in his/her diet. There have also been other books which have advocated the use of high protein diets. It does seem that some people may be significantly healthier if they eat higher amounts of protein. We must ask, however, if a person feels better on a high protein diet because of the quantity of protein consumption or because he/she is avoiding the grains which had previously provoked an extremely allergic reaction. Recent evidence indicates that the incidence of celiac disease may be considerably higher than previously thought–especially those cases which are not full blown. People have only been eating grains for about 9,000 years, which is a very small amount of time from an evolutionary standpoint (see *Your Family Tree Connection* by Redding). Thus, when a person feels better on a high protein diet, it may well be that he/she is simply avoiding grain sensitivities.

In the meantime, it is probably wiser to consume a lower protein diet rather than to eat a gluttonous amount. From an ecological standpoint, it is clear that high protein diets are not healthy for our environment and that the planet can not possibly sustain the entire population if everyone ate these diets. In the future it may be possible to evaluate more clearly who needs to consume more protein. Blood typing may possibly be a tool that we can use to further evaluate a person's requirements.

| Amino acid | Nonvegetarians | Lacto-, ovovegetarians | Pure vegetarians |
|---|---|---|---|
| Isoleucine | 6.6 | 5.4 | 4.0 |
| Leucine | 10.1 | 8.2 | 6.0 |
| Lysine | 8.3 | 5.4 | 3.7 |
| Phenylalanine and tyrosine | 10.4 | 8.8 | 7.0 |
| Methionine and cysteine | 4.3 | 3.2 | 2.7 |
| Threonine | 5.0 | 3.8 | 2.9 |
| Tryptophan | 1.5 | 1.2 | 1.1 |
| Valine | 7.1 | 5.6 | 4.3 |
| Total protein intake | 121 | 97 | 82 |

Hardage MG, et.al. Consumption of Essential Amino Acids & Protein by Vegetarians in the U.S. J Am Dietetics 48:25, 1966.

**Synthesis of urea occurs through the ornithine cycle**

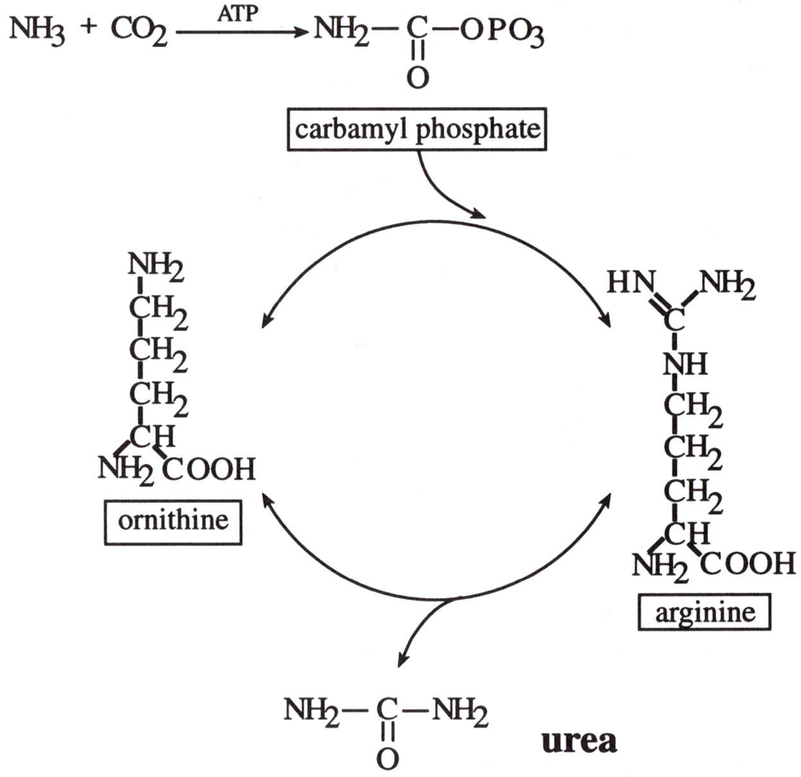

$$NH_3 + CO_2 \xrightarrow{ATP} NH_2-\underset{\underset{O}{\|}}{C}-OPO_3$$

carbamyl phosphate

$NH_2-CH_2-CH_2-CH_2-CH(NH_2)-COOH$

ornithine

$HN=C(NH_2)-NH-CH_2-CH_2-CH_2-CH(NH_2)-COOH$

arginine

$$NH_2-\underset{\underset{O}{\|}}{C}-NH_2$$

**urea**

## VI. Protein-Calorie Malnutrition (PCM)

Also known as Protein-Energy Malnutrition, it is found primarily in young children who live in poverty. The World Heath Organization estimates that 300 million children in the world have growth retardation as a result of malnutrition. In addition to feeling fatigued, many people with PCM have increased susceptibility to infections and an increased mortality from infections that normally can be handled by the immune system. Severe PCM can cause a mortality rate of nearly 50%.

- **Marasmus** refers to a lack of energy providing foods combined with a deficiency of protein. Marasmus is a Greek word which means "wasting." It results in growth retardation and a wasting away of tissues. It is caused by a lack of calories in the diet which requires the person to convert his/her protein supply into energy compounds. This results in a net deficiency.

- **Kwashiorkor**–First described in 1933 by Dr. Cicely Williams, who was a pediatrician working among the native children of the African Gold Coast in Ghana, this specifically refers to protein malnutrition. Kwashiorkor literally means *"the disease of the deposed baby when the next one is born."* It commonly affects the 1st born child between the ages of 1-4 years. It occurs because the child is weaned from his/her best source of protein and is forced to eat starchy vegetables which are high in fiber and carbohydrate. The lack of protein results in hypoalbuminemia, marked pitting edema, and an enlarged fatty liver.

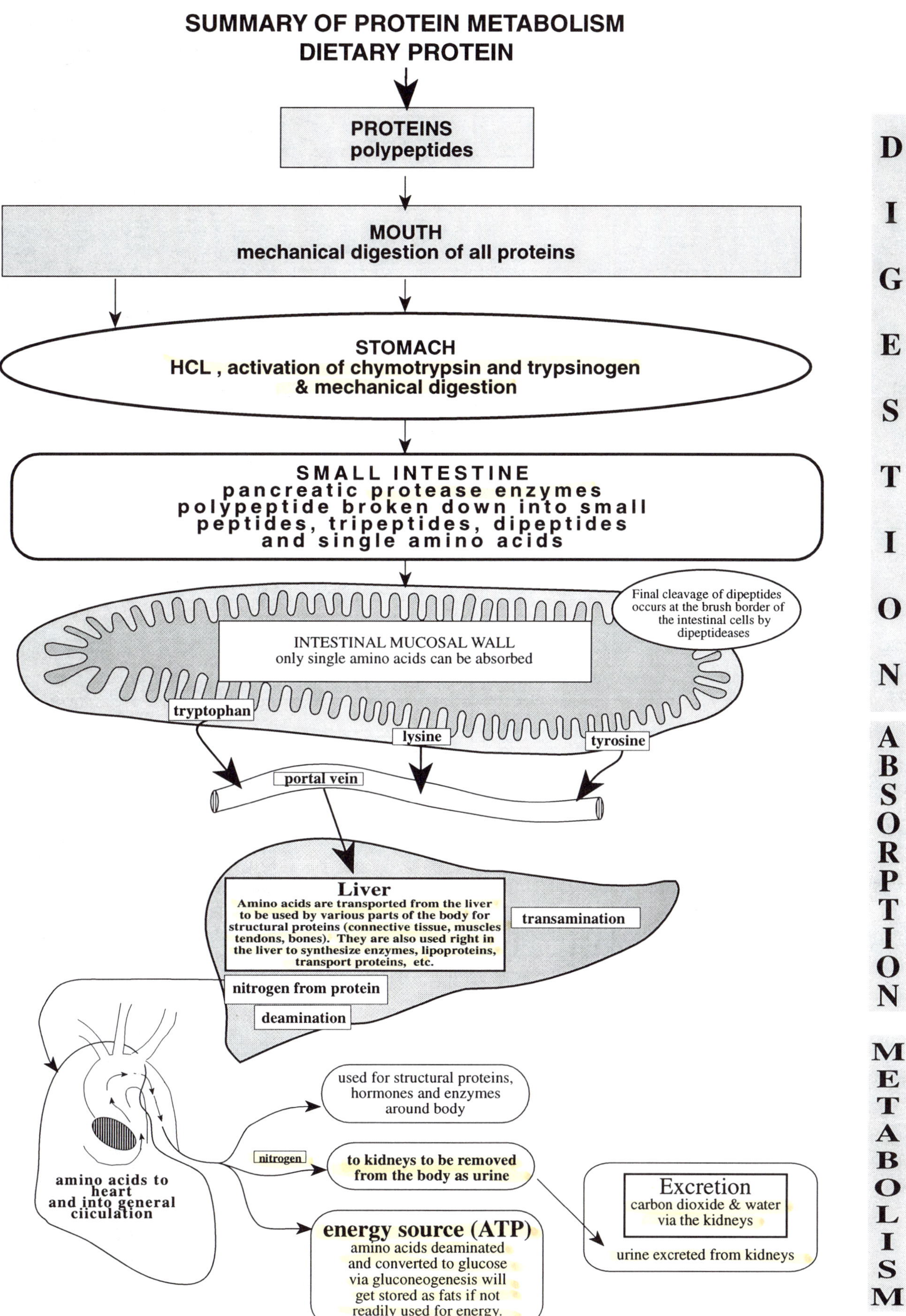
SUMMARY OF PROTEIN METABOLISM
DIETARY PROTEIN
PROTEINS
polypeptides
MOUTH
mechanical digestion of all proteins
STOMACH
HCL , activation of chymotrypsin and trypsinogen
& mechanical digestion
SMALL INTESTINE
pancreatic protease enzymes
polypeptide broken down into small
peptides, tripeptides, dipeptides
and single amino acids
Final cleavage of dipeptides occurs at the brush border of the intestinal cells by dipeptideases
INTESTINAL MUCOSAL WALL
only single amino acids can be absorbed
tryptophan
lysine
tyrosine
portal vein
Liver
Amino acids are transported from the liver to be used by various parts of the body for structural proteins (connective tissue, muscles tendons, bones). They are also used right in the liver to synthesize enzymes, lipoproteins, transport proteins, etc.
transamination
nitrogen from protein
deamination
amino acids to heart and into general ciiculation
used for structural proteins, hormones and enzymes around body
nitrogen
to kidneys to be removed from the body as urine
energy source (ATP)
amino acids deaminated and converted to glucose via gluconeogenesis will get stored as fats if not readily used for energy.
Excretion
carbon dioxide & water via the kidneys
urine excreted from kidneys

## Notes

# ENERGY

Energy expenditure is expended by the body in three ways:

- Resting energy expenditure
- Voluntary activity
- The thermal effect of food

## I. Basal Metabolic Rate (BMR)

When the body is totally at rest, the amount of energy the body expends carrying out activities necessary to sustain life–such as respiration and circulation, synthesis of organic constituents, pumping ions across membranes and maintaining body temperature–is called the *basal metabolic rate* (BMR). The BMR is measured in the morning after a person awakens, when he/she is in the post absorptive state (10-12 hrs. after eating).

Another measurement of energy expenditure is called the *resting metabolic rat*e (RMR). This measurement differs from the BMR in that the test it can be measured at any time in the day, usually 3-4 hrs. after a meal. Both the BMR and the RMR are measured in a neutral environment with a comfortable temperature. BMR may vary as much as 10% plus or minus in cold or hot temperature extremes.

- 50% of the energy expenditure is used for the nervous system.
- 27% is used by the liver (much of this is to synthesize glucose and ketone bodies as fuel for the brain).

**Factors affecting the metabolic rate**

Factors which affect the metabolic rate include body size and composition. While total body surface area is a determinant in energy expenditure, it appears that lean body mass is the most important factor regarding BMR & RMR. Women generally have a 5-10% lower BMR compared to males. This is because men tend to have leaner bodies. Typically women have 25% body fat while men have 15% body fat. Generally, adipose tissue has very little metabolic activity, but brown adipose tissue tends to have some heat producing metabolic activity because of the higher concentration of mitochondria.

**NOTE**–Thyroid status is perhaps the most important determining variant in BMR. Hyperthyroidism may cause up to a 50% increase in the metabolic rate while hypothyroidism may cause a 50% decrease.

Other factors affecting metabolic rate are:

- Sleep (decreases BMR by 10%)
- Fevers (every degree of temperature rise above 37 degrees C increases BMR 10%)
- Temperature extremes (tropical climate increases BMR 5-20%)
- Menstrual cycle (post ovulatory 150 kcal/day increase)
- Pregnancy
- Breast feeding

When figured over 24 hours BMR values for men and women are as follows:

- 1680 kcal for an average 70-kg man
- 1173 kcal for an average 58-kg woman

If a totally inactive 70kg man consumes a diet of 1680 calories, he will maintain his weight. If he consumes more than 1680 calories, he will start to gain weight.

While rapid fluctuations in weight are usually reflective of fluid retention or loss, true weight gain or loss is determined by a positive or negative calorie balance. The total energy required as determined by the BMR, calorie expenditure (physical activity) and specific dynamic action of food is subtracted by the total caloric intake.

**3500kcal is equivalent to 1 pound of body weight**

If a person's total expenditure for the day is 2500 kcal and he/she only eats 2000 kcal, there is a negative balance of 500 kcal. If this routine is repeated for 7 days, that person would have had a net negative balance of 3500kcal, or the equivalent of 1 pound of body weight loss. If this person went on a total fast for the week, we might expect that he/she would have a net kcal negative balance of 2500kcal per day or 17,500kcal for the week. However, when someone goes into a starvation mode such as a fast, the BMR drops drastically. This is the body's emergency response to conserve energy. Under this condition the person might only have a total requirement of 1500kcal. Hence, after one week the net loss would only be 10,500kcal, or the equivalent to 3 pounds of actual body weight.

## II. Thermic Effects of Food

Thermic effects of food (TEF) are measurements of the energy required to metabolize foods. This energy expenditure is also called diet-induced thermogenesis (DIT). Obligatory thermogenesis is the energy required to digest, absorb, and metabolize nutrients. The specific dynamic action of foods (SDA) is an antiquated term that is rarely used anymore.

Consumption of carbohydrates and fats generally increases the metabolic rate by about 5% of the total calories consumed. An all protein diet can increase the rate by 25%. A mixed diet adds an additional 10% onto total energy requirements. Both coffee and nicotine increase the TEF by approximately 10%.

## III. Energy Measurements

A *calorie* is the amount of heat energy required to raise the temperature of 1ml of water at a standard initial temperature by 1 degree C. In the metabolism of foods large amounts of energy are expended and the kilo calorie, which is equal to 1000 calories, is used. Popular use of the word "Calorie" with a capital letter is generally used to denote one kilo calorie.

In most countries other than the U.S. and Canada, the term *joule* is used. This is a measurement of energy in terms of mechanical work. In fact the joule is currently the preferred unit for measuring energy by international standards.

**One kilocalorie = 4.184 kilojoules.**

**Calorimetry** is the measurement of energy generated by the body. It can be measured both directly and indirectly. It's purpose is to evaluate a person's exact energy requirements.

**Direct calorimetry** requires monitoring the amount of heat produced by a subject placed inside a structure large enough to permit moderate movements. This method allows measurement of exactly how much heat is being generated, but not what type of fuel is being burned.

**Indirect calorimetry** measures the metabolic rate by using a spirometer. Both oxygen consumption and $CO_2$ production are measured over a set time period. The data can be used to calculate the *respiratory quotient (RQ).*

*RQ* = moles $CO_2$ expired/moles $O_2$ consumed

The RQ for different food nutrients are as follows:

| | |
|---|---|
| carbohydrate | 1.00 |
| protein | 0.82 |
| fat | 0.7 |

Generally a mixed diet will provide an RQ of 0.85.

## IV. Food Energy

The amount of energy available from a food can be measured by means of a bomb calorimeter. This is a closed combustible oven which burns the food completely and, as it is placed in a known volume of water, the exact amount of generated heat can be measured by the temperature rise in the water.

Not all of the energy of food is actually available to the cells of the body because the processes of digestion and absorption are not completely efficient. In addition, *the nitrogen moiety of proteins does not get oxidized, but rather gets excreted in the urine in the form of* ***urea***. The values that are biologically available have been calculated and rounded off to be used for practical application.

**CHO = 4.0 kcal/gm**
**Pro = 4.0 kcal/gm**
**Fat = 9 kcal/gm**
**ETOH = 7.0 kcal/gm**

For example, a food per serving may have the following breakdown:

**101 calories**
**8gms of CHO X 4kcal= 32 CHO calories = 32% CHO**
**6gms of Pro X 4kcal = 24 Pro calories= 24% Pro**
**5gms of fat X 9kcal= 45 fat calories=45% fat**

The nutritional label below has changed significantly in the last 10-20 years to include more useful information for the consumer. This label allows us to calculate the percentage of the calories which come from carbohydrates, proteins and fats. In addition, information about saturated and unsaturated fats can also be evaluated.

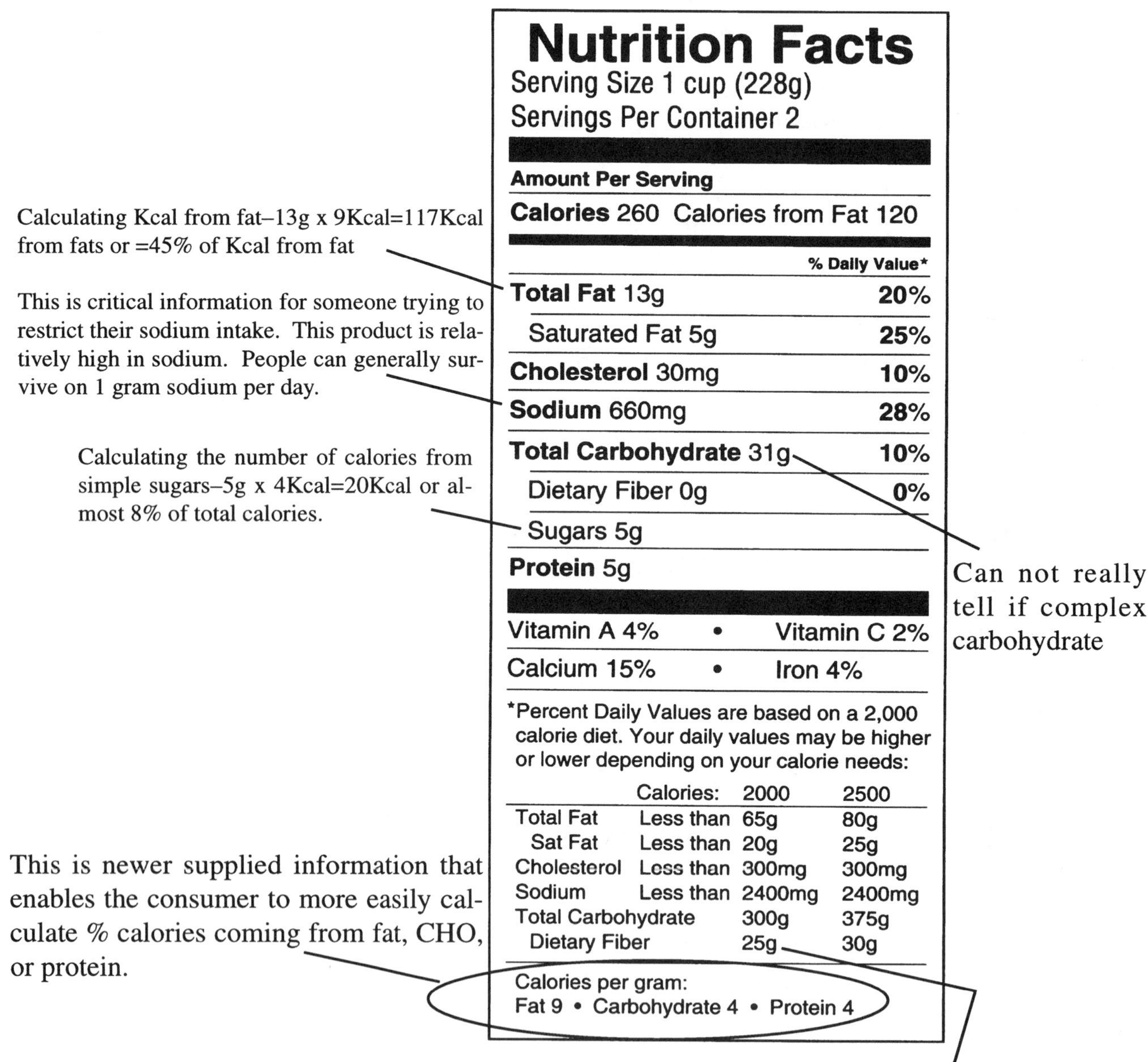


Ideal levels of fiber in the diet should be considerably higher than 25g but at least this gives the consumer an idea of how much they should be getting and how much the food that they are eating is adding to their ideal fiber intake. This particular food product has no fiber and therefore is adding calories but no fiber. Since one serving is supplying 260 calories, this means that they will have a more difficult time trying to reach their fiber goal.

| Activity | kcal/min |
|---|---|
| Sleeping | 1.2 |
| Resting in bed | 1.3 |
| Sitting, normally | 1.3 |
| Sitting, reading | 1.3 |
| Lying, quietly | 1.3 |
| Sitting, eating | 1.5 |
| Sitting, playing cards | 1.5 |
| Standing, normally | 1.5 |
| Classwork, lecture (listen to) | 1.7 |
| Conversing | 1.8 |
| Personal toilet | 2.0 |
| Sitting, writing | 2.6 |
| Standing, light activity | 2.6 |
| Washing and dressing | 2.6 |
| Washing and shaving | 2.6 |
| Driving a car | 2.8 |
| Washing clothes | 3.1 |
| Walking indoors | 3.1 |
| Shining shoes | 3.2 |
| Making bed | 3.4 |
| Dressing | 3.4 |
| Showering | 3.4 |
| Driving motorcycle | 3.4 |
| Metal working | 3.5 |
| House painting | 3.5 |
| Cleaning windows | 3.7 |
| Carpentry | 3.8 |
| Farming chores | 3.8 |
| Sweeping floors | 3.9 |
| Plastering walls | 4.1 |
| Truck and automobile repair | 4.2 |
| Ironing clothes | 4.2 |
| Farming, planting, hoeing, raking | 4.7 |
| Mixing cement | 4.7 |

Listed on this page are activities and the energy required to perform each activity. Each activity will thus burn the number of Calories listed. Obviously there are different levels you can perform each activity therefore different people will expend different levels of energy performing each task. Prolonged activities can burn off a tremendous amount of energy. E.g., bicycle touring with packs can burn up to 7,000 to 10,000 Calories over the course of a day. Similar activities such as Ironman events can also burn enormous amounts of energy.

| Activity | kcal/min |
|---|---|
| Mopping floors | 4.9 |
| Repaving roads | 5.0 |
| Gardening, weeding | 5.6 |
| Stacking lumber | 5.8 |
| Chain saw | 6.2 |
| Stone, masonry | 6.3 |
| Pick-and-shovel work | 6.7 |
| Farming, haying, plowing with horse | 6.7 |
| Shoveling (miners) | 6.8 |
| Walking downstairs | 7.1 |
| Chopping wood | 7.5 |
| Crosscut saw | 7.5–10.5 |
| Tree felling (axe) | 8.4–12.7 |
| Gardening, digging | 8.6 |
| Walking upstairs | 10.0–18.0 |
| Pool or billiards | 1.8 |
| Canoeing: 2.5 mph–4.0 mph | 3.0–7.0 |
| Volleyball: recreational—competitive | 3.5–8.0 |
| Golf: foursome—twosome | 3.7–5.0 |
| Horseshoes | 3.8 |
| Baseball (except pitcher) | 4.7 |
| Ping pong—table tennis | 4.9–7.0 |
| Calisthenics | 5.0 |
| Rowing: pleasure—vigorous | 5.0–15.0 |
| Cycling: 5–15 mph (10 speed) | 5.0–12.0 |
| Skating: recreation—vigorous | 5.0–15.0 |
| Archery | 5.2 |
| Badminton: recreational—competitive | 5.2–10.0 |
| Basketball: half—full court (more for fast break) | 6.0–9.0 |
| Bowling (while active) | 7.0 |
| Tennis: recreational—competitive | 7.0–11.0 |
| Water skiing | 8.0 |
| Soccer | 9.0 |
| Snowshoeing (2.5 mph) | 9.0 |

| Activity | kcal/min |
|---|---|
| Handball and squash | 10.0 |
| Mountain climbing | 10.0 |
| Skipping rope | 10.0–15.0 |
| Judo and karate | 13.0 |
| Football (while active) | 13.3 |
| Wrestling | 14.4 |
| Skiing: | |
| Moderate to steep | 8.0–12.0 |
| Downhill racing | 16.5 |
| Cross-country: 3–8 mph | 9.0–17.0 |
| Swimming: | |
| Pleasure | 6.0 |
| Crawl: 25–50 yd/min | 6.0–12.5 |
| Butterfly: 50 yd/min | 14.0 |
| Backstroke: 25–50 yd/min | 6.0–12.5 |
| Breaststroke: 25–50 yd/min | 6.0–12.5 |
| Sidestroke: 40 yd/min | 11.0 |
| Dancing: | |
| Modern: moderate—vigorous | 4.2–5.7 |
| Ballroom: waltz—rhumba | 5.7–7.0 |
| Square | 7.7 |
| Walking: | |
| Road—Field (3.5 mph) | 5.6–7.0 |
| Snow: hard—soft (3.5–2.5 mph) | 10.0–20.0 |
| Uphill: 5–10–15% (3.5 mph) | 8.0–11.0–15.0 |
| Downhill: 5–10% (2.5 mph) | 3.6–3.5 |
| 15–20% (2.5 mph) | 3.7–4.3 |
| Hiking: 40-lb pack (3.0 mph) | 6.8 |
| Running: | |
| 12-min mile (5 mph) | 10.0 |
| 8-min mile (7.5 mph) | 15.0 |
| 6-min mile (10 mph) | 20.0 |
| 5-min mile (12 mph) | 25.0 |

# AMINO ACIDS

Amino acids are classified as essential, conditionally essential or nonessential depending upon whether or not the body can synthesize adequate amounts to meet metabolic needs. Inadequate absorption or intake of any of the essential amino acids results in growth retardation, weight loss, and a wide array of clinical symptoms. There is a very wide divergence of requirement in the population. The conditionally essential amino acids are required only under certain circumstances, such as excessive stress and/or metabolic demands. For the most part amino acids must be taken in on a daily basis, i.e., they are not stored in the body to any appreciable level. They are required for the synthesis of: tissue protein, various enzymes, cellular components, transport proteins in the blood, blood proteins for maintaining acid-base & fluid balance, neurotransmitters in the brain, hormones, structural components, and as an energy source.

There has been much research concerning the therapeutic use of amino acids to treat disease and many therapeutic uses have been discovered. As of yet there are probably many uses yet to be found and the study of amino acid and protein therapy is still in its infancy. Often times single amino acids have much different functions than when given together with other amino acids. Even slight variations in structure can cause pronounces differences in pharmacological properties. While other amino acids undoubtedly have therapeutic value, I have chosen those with the most clinical significance at this time. The following selected amino acids are covered in this book:

# ARGININE

## I. Metabolism

Arginine is made in the body from glutamic acid in a series of reactions which form ornithine (an immediate precursor). Arginine is broken down so rapidly by arginase to form urea and ornithine that the body sometimes has a difficult time keeping up the supply. Furthermore, it is generally poorly absorbed from the gut. Thus, it is considered *a semi-essential amino acid.* It is required for the synthesis of guanidinoacetic acid, polyamines, and creatine. Its primary role, however, is involved in the urea cycle. Arginine stimulates the action of carbamyl phosphate synthetase which is the first step in the urea cycle. Approximately 50% of all the arginine present in the body is related to the urea cycle. Most of the urea is made in the liver and then sent to the kidneys to be removed as urine. The amino acids citrulline, aspartate and ornithine are also involved in the urea cycle and aid arginine in its function to rid the body of nitrogenous waste.

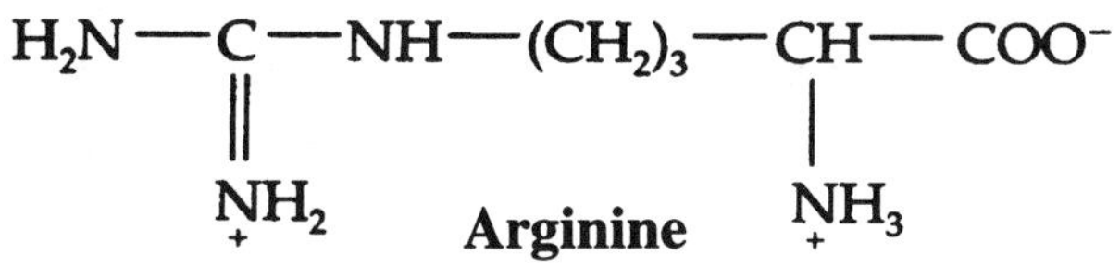

$$H_2N-\underset{\overset{\|}{\overset{+}{N}H_2}}{C}-NH-(CH_2)_3-\underset{\overset{|}{\overset{+}{N}H_3}}{CH}-COO^-$$

**Arginine**

**Genetic inborn errors in arginine metabolism**

- **Citrullinemia**–Argininosuccinate synthetase deficiency.
- **Arginino succinicaciduria**–Argininosuccinate lyase deficiency, with an incidence of 1 per 60,000 infants, causes infant retardation, seizures, ataxia and eventually death. Another peculiarity is marked by short, dry and brittle hair with minute nodes on the hair shaft. This defect can also occur in normal people who have suboptimal levels of arginine in their hair.
- **Arginemia**–arginase deficiency.

## II. Function

Arginine's primary function is the detoxification of urea. As mentioned above, the majority of arginine is used in urea metabolism. Arginine is involved with immunity and also in maintaining body weight during acute trauma. It is considered only semi-essential because it is made in the body from ornithine.

In animal studies the survival rate and bacterial containment within the gut are significantly improved during acute trauma when arginine is present in sufficient amounts. Concentrated in the muscles, it is responsible for the high energy compounds guanidophosphate, phosphoarginine and creatine which the muscles use. It also has a protective effect against certain liver toxins such as carbon tetrachloride, alcohol, and galactosamine-induced hepatitis.

## III. Requirements

**RDA**– only semi essential
**ESDDAI**-?/day
Average intake in the U.S.– 5g/day

## IV. Sources

Arginine is found in higher amounts in chocolate, peanuts, almonds, other nuts, and seeds.

**Best Sources of Arginine**

| Food | amount | mg | Food | amount | mg |
|---|---|---|---|---|---|
| Turkey (baked light meat w/o skin) | 3 oz | 1770 | Wheat germ, toasted | 1/4 c | 675 |
| Chicken (baked light meat w/o skin) | 3 oz | 1584 | Cashews, roasted | 1/4 c | 650 |
| Lamb, leg roasted | 3 oz | 1531 | Oats | 1 c | 600 |
| Pork | 3 oz | 1470 | Meat, luncheon | 3 oz | 592 |
| Tuna | 1/2 sm can | 1400 | Soybeans, cooked | 1/2 c | 540 |
| Beef, chuck | 3 oz | 1372 | Bacon | 3 med slices | 525 |
| Liver, beef | 3 oz | 1362 | Kidney beans, cooked | 1/2 c | 420 |
| Salmon | 3 oz | 1311 | Duck | 3 oz | 412 |
| Shrimp | 3 oz | 1166 | Egg | 1 med | 400 |
| Peanuts | 1/4 c (1.3oz) | 1080 | Sausage | 3 oz | 315 |
| Wild game | 1/4 c | 966 | Milk, whole | 1 c | 300 |
| Almonds, whole | 1/4 c | 910 | Chicken, white fried | 3 oz | 278 |
| Granola | 1 c | 900 | Bread, whole wheat | 2 slices | 255 |
| Cheese, ricotta | 1/2 c | 800 | Yogurt | 1 c | 250 |
| Walnuts | 1/4 c | 750 | Collards, cooked | 1/2 c | 240 |
| Cheese, cottage | 1/2 c | 700 | Rice, brown, cooked | 1 c (185g) | 183 |

From USDA: Composition of Foods. USDA handbook # 8 Washington DC, ARS, USDA, 1976-1986

## V. Deficiency

Usually related to overall protein malnutrition, an arginine deficiency can occur with excessive ammonia production, excess lysine, amino acid imbalances, rapid growth, pregnancy, trauma, protein or enzyme deficiency. Arginine deficiency is associated with rash, hair loss, poor wound healing, constipation, fatty liver, and cirrhosis.

## VI. Therapeutics

1) **Infertility from oligospermia**–4gms/day–There have been both positive and negative studies on arginine's effect on increasing sperm count and motility. It may work best in mild problems.

STUDY–Schachter, A., et al. *Treatment of oligospermia with the amino acid arginine.* J Urol. 110(3):311-313, 1973. ABSTRACT–178 men with mild to severe abnormalities in sperm count and motility received L-arginine 4gms/day for 3 months. 62% had a marked improvement, 12% had moderate improvement, and 26% had no improvement. 12% of men with sperm counts below 20 million per ejaculate increased their sperm count at least 100% compared to 36% of men with sperm counts of 20-50 million per ejaculate. No side effects were noted.

STUDY–Papp, G.Y., et al. *The importance of arginine content and arginase activity in fertility.* Andrologia 11:37, 1979.

STUDY–Papp, G., et al. *The role of basic amino acids of the seminal plasma in fertility.* Int Urol Nephrol. 15(2): 195-203, 1983. ABSTRACT–15.7% of 47 patients with pathospermia had mean seminal arginine concentrations which were significantly lower by 57% than normozoospermic patients while arginine values in the remaining pathospermia group were similar to those of the normozoospermic group. The mean seminal arginine concentrations of the azoospermic group were 28% lower than those of the normozoospermic group while the arginine concentrations of the oligozoospermic group corresponded to those of the normozoospermic group. Levels of arginine and ornithine in seminal plasma, if low, should be a strong indicator for supplementation of these 2 amino acids.

2) **Inflammatory bowel disease**–It has been found that arginine is especially useful in preventing secondary infections and weight loss during acute inflammatory bowel reactions.

STUDY–Barbul, A., et al. *Immunostimulatory effects of arginine in normal and injured rats,* J Surg Res 29:228-35, 1980.
STUDY–Barbul, A., et al. *Arginine: Thyrotrophic and wound healing promoting agent,* Surg Forum 28:101-102, 1977.

3) **Immunity enhancement**–30g/day–may enhance lymphocyte activity. It has been found that during acute trauma, an arginine deficiency greatly increases mortality and morbidity.

4) **Wound healing enhancement**–During acute trauma arginine is especially useful in maintaining epithelial integrity against bacterial translocation both on skin and in intestines.

5) **Trauma**–Arginine helps maintain weight, especially during acute traumas of various types.

6) **Increase lean body mass**–Studies show mild effects at large doses.

7) **Cancer Treatment**–In animals arginine has been shown to inhibit tumor growth by activating macrophage cytotoxic effects.

8) **Hypercholesterolemia**–Arginine inhibits fat absorption. The higher the levels of arginine, the lower the cholesterol levels found.

## VII. Toxicity

Herpes simplex (see table under lysine)–Arginine has been found to promote the growth of Herpes simplex, especially if lysine levels are low. In addition, excessive arginine (greater than 40gms per day) can cause diarrhea. Hyperkalemia and hyperphosphatemia can be induced by arginine in patients with severe hepatic disease and kidney problems. They can, in turn, increase ornithine and citrulline levels which can produce ataxia.

## Notes

---

# CARNITINE

## I. Metabolism

Carnitine is an amino acid derivative synthesized from the essential amino acids lysine and methionine. It has similarities to choline and resembles some of the B vitamins because of its amine group and properties. It is made in the liver, kidneys and brain. Iron, vitamin C, vitamin B-6, and niacin are required for the hydroxylation steps that are vital for the synthesis of carnitine.

It was originally isolated from meat extracts in 1905 and its structure was determined in 1932. In 1952 it was established as a growth factor of the mealworm, *Tenebrio molitor* and given the name vitamin $B_T$.

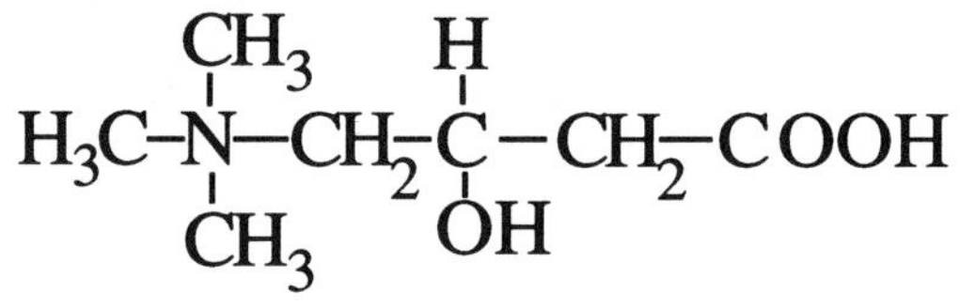

$$H_3C-N(CH_3)_2-CH_2-CH(OH)-CH_2-COOH$$

L-CARNITINE

Certain tissues, including the **heart**, skeletal muscles, epididymis, liver and kidneys, have specific transport proteins which actively concentrate carnitine into the tissue as high as 10x the rate found in the plasma. In the heart carnitine is particularly concentrated in the sarcoplasma reticulum. In semen carnitine is concentrated 5x higher than in the serum.

Carnitine synthesis in infants is limited. It has been found that both fetal and umbilical cord blood have higher levels of carnitine than maternal blood. This means that active transport is taking place, offsetting the fetus's inability to adequately synthesize carnitine.

Because carnitine is synthesized in the body, it is often not considered to be an essential nutrient. However, it is probably essential for preterm infants who can not make enough. It also may be considered conditionally essential in those with heart conditions which might require an additional supply.

## II. Function

Carnitine has been determined to be an essential substance in humans for the metabolism of fats. It is involved in the rate limiting step for beta oxidation which allows fats to be transported across mitochrondrial cell membranes. Fatty acids must be transferred from CoA to carnitine. Then the acyl-carnitine molecule can transport the fatty acid into the mitochondria to be oxidized.

Brown fat (which is metabolically more active than yellow fat) is highly dependent on carnitine to aid in the heat producing beta oxidation reaction.

Carnitine helps the body oxidize amino acids when necessary as in the case of a fast or low carbohydrate diet. It therefore helps the body metabolize ketones for energy utilization.

Carnitine also seems to be involved with prostaglandin production, especially in smooth and skeletal muscles, where it provides these cells with needed energy.

It is also involved in the conversion of certain amino acids–valine, leucine, and isoleucine–into energy products.

Finally, carnitine appears to decrease ketones in the body. Therefore, it may be useful for diabetics.

## III. Requirements

**RDA**–? (not considered essential)
Average intake in the U.S.–5-100mg/day
Lab–A muscle biopsy works best, however RBC will give approxi mate levels.

### Best Sources of Carnitine

| Food | amount | nmol |
|---|---|---|
| Beef, ground | 3oz | 640 |
| Beef, steak | 3oz | 540 |
| Bacon | 3oz | 135 |
| Milk, whole cows | 1c | 45 |
| Fish | 3oz | 30 |
| Chicken | 3oz | 30 |
| Milk formula based on milk | 1c | 25-50 |
| Milk, Human | 1c | 25 |
| Infant formula based on beef | 1c | up to 150 |
| Wheat whole bread | 2 slices | 2 |
| Soy based formula | 1c | 1 or less |

From USDA: Composition of Foods. USDA handbook # 8 Washington DC, ARS, USDA, 1976-1986

## IV. Sources

Carnitine is found only in animal products such as human milk, meat, poultry, and dairy products.

## V. Deficiency

Carnitine deficiency can occur in premature infants, people with total parenteral nutrition or on starvation diets, and those with liver damage. Symptoms may include muscle weakness, fatty deposits, impaired ketogenesis with hyperlipidemia, and impaired glucose control. Deficiencies have been found in cer
tain conditions such as Duchenne-type muscular dystrophy, and in people receiving dialysis.

Children at 21/2yrs of age synthesize carnitine at about 30% the rate of adults. Full synthesis does not occur until 15 yrs of age. Symptoms in children may resemble *Reye's syndrome* with acute brain swelling, hypoglycemia, and heart disturbances. Several fatal cases of acute carnitine deficiency have been reported.

## VI. Therapeutics

1) **Heart diseases including cardiomyopathy, arrhythmias, congestive heart failure, mitral valve prolapse**–1-4gms per day–It has been found that carnitine can increase HDL cholesterol while decreasing LDL and triglycerides. It works by providing energy to the heart muscle. There have been many positive studies concerning L-carnitine. With taurine and Coenzyme Q 10, carnitine may be an effective treatment for congestive heart failure.

STUDY–Pola, P., et al. *Statistical evaluation of long term L-carnitine therapy in hyperlipoproteinemias..* Drugs Exptl Clin Res 9:925-34, 1983. ABSTRACT–39 patients aged 50-60yrs of age with Fredrickson's type II, IV, or V hyperlipoproteinemia were studied. 1/3 of these patients were unresponsive to previous therapy with cholesterol lowering drugs. Patients were treated with 1gm per day and after 4 months serum cholesterol fell from 295 to 234 and HDL increased by 15%. TG's fell from 345 to 208 (40% reduction). In type IV patients and from 170 to 124 in type II patients. In 3 type V patients TG levels of 950 avg. fell rapidly to below 400. The L-carnitine eventually brought cholesterol levels down below 240 in 90% of the patients, and 66% of them occurred in 4 months.

STUDY–Davini, P., et al. *Controlled study on L-carnitine therapeutic efficacy in most MI patients.* Drugs Exptl Clin Res 18:355-65, 1992. ABSTRACT–160 patients following MI's were randomly assigned to receive either 4g/day of carnitine in addition to standard treatment or standard treatment alone. During the follow up period the next year, the carnitine group had significant reductions in blood pressure, fewer anginal attacks and a significant reduction in cholesterol levels. The mortality rate in the carnitine group was 1.2% compared to 12.5% in the control group (p=0.005)

2) **Enhanced Athletic Performance and Peripheral Vascular Circulation**–1-4gms per day–may especially enhance endurance capacity.

STUDY–Leibovitz, B. *Carnitine the Vitamin BT Phenomenon* New York: Dell Pub Co. Inc, 1984

STUDY–Annon *Role of carnitine in branched chain ketoacid metabolism* Nutrition Reviews 39(11):406-7, 1981.

3) **Angina pectoris**–In double blind controlled trials it has been shown that carnitine gives significant benefits to angina patients by improving circulation to peripheral tissues.

STUDY–Cherchi, A., et al. *Effects of L-carnitine on exercise tolerance in chronic stable angina: a multicenter, double blind randomized placebo controlled crossover study.* J Clin Pharm Ther Toxicol 23:569-572, 1985. ABSTRACT–1g bid of carnitine or placebo was used to treat 44 males with chronic stable effort induced angina. The trial lasted for 4 weeks and then the patients switched. Carnitine significantly increased the amounts of work required to induce the angina. EKG showed ST segment depression was significantly worse on placebo compared to the carnitine.

STUDY–Orlando, G., Rusconi, C. *L-carnitine in the treatment of chronic cardiac ischemia in elderly patients.* Clin Trials J 23:338-44, 1986. ABSTRACT–30 patients experiencing symptoms such as palpitations, asthenia, and precordial pain were treated with 2gms carnitine tid for 2 months. Via the NYHA functional class evaluation, 4 of these patients improved significantly. In 30% of the patients EKG and echocardiographic evidence showed improvement. Most of the patients showed significant improvement in their symptoms.

4) **Cirrhosis of the liver**–Carnitine may prevent or reduce fatty infiltration of the liver. It may also reduce toxicity to various toxic agents.

5) **Diabetes mellitus**–Carnitine can have significant effects on circulation and improve cardiovascular parameters.

6) **Trauma**–Carnitine helps maintain weight when there is a limited intake of nutrients, especially in total parenteral nutrition and during acute trauma.

7) **Infant formula, especially premature infants or soy milk fed infants or vegetarian babies**–Carnitine only occurs in animal foods and strictly fed vegetarian infants may develop a deficiency. It is wise to supplement 250-500mg per day as a prevention. It may be of value in prevention of *Reye's syndrome* in children. Preterm infants may require additional carnitine because of a decrease ability to store and synthesize carnitine. It may enhance weight gain and growth.

8) **Intermittent claudication**–Just as it can improve problems with angina, carnitine can reduce intermittent claudication by improving oxygenation of the peripheral tissues.

9) **Infertility**–It has been found that carnitine is concentrated in semen 5x that of serum.

STUDY–Costa, M., et al. *L-carnitine in idiopathic asthenozoospermia: a multicenter study.* Andrologia 26:155-59, 1994. ABSTRACT–100 infertile men with poor sperm motility were given L-carnitine 3gms/day for 4 months. There was a significant increase in sperm motility which was especially apparent with the men with the lowest sperm motility.

STUDY–Vitali, G., et al. *L-carnitine supplementation in human idiopathic asthenospermia: clinical results.* Drugs Exptl Clin Res 21:157-59, 1995. ABSTRACT–47 infertile males of at least 2 years duration who had failed to respond to previous therapy and who had at least 10 million sperm per ml were given 1gm tid L-carnitine for 3 months. 79% of the patients responded. Of those who responded, the mean sperm count increased from 88 million to 159 million per ml and the mean number of motile sperms increased from 27 to 54 million per ml.

10) **Alzheimer's disease or related conditions**–The L-acetylcarnitine form may significantly improve the symptoms of depression and memory problems. L-acetylcarnitine is a major neurotransmitter in the brain. There have been numerous studies to date which have shown benefits in mental function, particularly in enhancing memory and constructional thinking.

Because Down Syndrome shares many of the characteristic brain abnormalities that Alzheimer's disease does and its efficacy hs been studied. There have been some favorable studies using L-acetylcarnitine.

STUDY–Cipolli, C., & Chiari, G. *Effects of L-acetylcarnitine on mental deterioration in the aged: Initial results* Clin Ther 132, 479-510, 1990 ABSTRACT–236 elderly patients with mild mental deterioration in a double blinded clinical trial who received 1500mg L-acetylcarnitine per day showed significant improvement in memory and other mental functions.

STUDY–Cipolli, C., & Chiari, G. *Effects of L-acetylcarnitine on mental deterioration in the aged: Initial results* Clin Ther 132, 479-510, 1990 ABSTRACT–Down syndrome was studied comparing mental deficiency related to Down Syndrome and mental deficiency related to other causes. It was found that L-acetylcarnitine was statistically significant in terms of improving visual memory and attention span only in the Down Syndrome subjects.

11) **AIDS**–Carnitine may improve symptoms of fatigue and muscle wasting. In addition it may enhance lymphocyte function as involved in immunity. L-carnitine may protect the liver against the deleterious effects of AZT which can damage the mitochondria.

12) **Miscellaneous inborn errors in metabolism**–Glutaric aciduria, isovaleric acidemia, propionic acidemia and methylmalonic aciduria may all respond to carnitine therapy.

13) **COPD and other chronic lung conditions** which involve difficulty breathing–Carnitine may improve intercostal muscle strength.

## VII. Toxicity

L-Carnitine is very safe, producing few side effects even at high doses.

The D,L-carnitine has produced side effects, including muscle pain and decreased exercise tolerance in compromised patients, and can deplete levels of L-carnitine in the heart and skeletal muscles. These effects were reversed when the D,L form was discontinued.

Some people who are taking carnitine may experience a fishy smell from bacterial amines that are produced. Heartburn can sometimes occur.

In addition, some people may experience diarrhea if they begin supplementation with a too high dose.

Use with caution in patients with kidney problems.

## VIII. Interactions

L-carnitine has synergistic activity with other nutrients such as taurine, coenzyme Q 10 and pantetheine.

Valproic acid, Pivampicillin, emetine, sulfadiazine, Adriamycin, Lovestatin and pyrimethamine may deplete carnitine supplies. Beta blockers may also deplete carnitine stores.

### Notes

---

# CYSTEINE/GLUTATHIONE

- Cysteine is a water soluble amino acid containing the sulfur containing thiol group. Thiol is in the common antibacterial agent, merthiolate.
- The Greeks used garlic and the element sulfur to treat a variety of ailments–such as psoriasis, rheumatoid arthritis and psychosis.
- As glutathione, it is an antioxidant necessary for the protection of proteins. It is used by the liver to detoxify formaldehyde, acetaminophen, benzpyrene and many other compounds.
- Selenium is required to keep glutathione in its reduced form so it acts as an antioxidant.
- Several tests have been devised using 24 hour urine collection of D-glucaric acid and or mercapturic acid to evaluate toxicity in the body.

## I. Metabolism

Cysteine is one of the sulfur containing amino acids used for the synthesis of glutathione, which is very critical in detoxification. The *thiol* group is the active part of the molecule which serves as a reducing agent to prevent oxidation of tissues. Glutathione is synthesized from glutamate and glycine as well.

Glutathione acts as one of the major detoxifiers in the body, but it must be in the reduced form to work properly. Sometimes glutathione will be listed on the label of a product, however it won't be specifically listed as being reduced. The unreduced form is much cheaper and isn't metabolically active. Riboflavin, niacinamide and glutathione reductase are all essential cofactors for generating reduced glutathione. Once the cysteine moieties become oxidized, they combine to form cystine. Cystine taken by itself is poorly absorbed. Forms include reduced glutathione, N-acetyl cysteine, and cysteine.

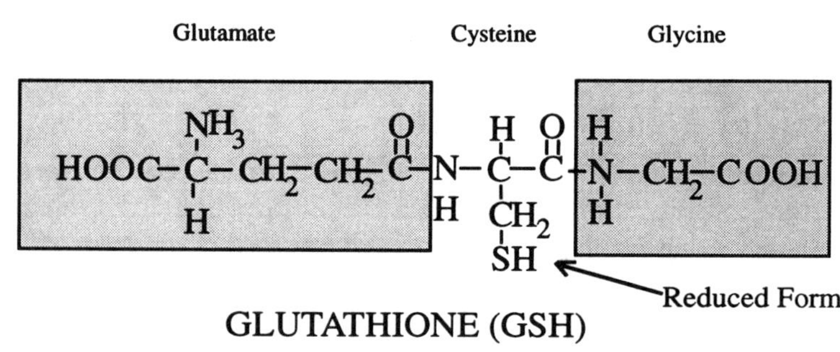

GLUTATHIONE (GSH)

An inborn error in metabolism, **cystinuria**, occurs in 7 out of every 10,000 births. The excessive excretion of cystine results in low levels of cysteine in the brain and causes mental retardation. In addition, excessive accumulation of cystine in the kidneys can result in the formation of cystine crystals which can damage the kidneys. Low cystine levels have been found in allergy, asthma, depression, psychosis, rheumatoid arthritis and hypertension.

thiol sulfur group

$H_3N-CH-COOH$, $CH_2$, $SH$

Cysteine

Glutathione, which is synthesized from cysteine and selenium, is found in almost all living cells. The liver, spleen, kidneys, pancreas, and the lens and cornea, have the highest concentrations in the body. Glutathione levels decrease with age. It is believed to be an essential antioxidant factor in slowing down the aging process. Glutathione peroxidase is another compound which is involved in detoxification against peroxides and other xenobiotics. It is synthesized from selenium and cysteine.

## II. Function

1) **Protection of proteins**–As *glutathione*, it is necessary as an antioxidant. Selenium is required to keep glutathione in its reduced form so it can act as an antioxidant.

2) **Liver detoxification** of formaldehyde, acetaminophen, benzpyrene. Several tests have been devised using 24 hour urine collection of D-glucaric acid and or mercapturic acid. It also helps remove heavy metals from the body.

3) **Transport across cell membranes**–It is part of amino acid transport across cell membranes.

4) **Cell membrane integrity**–this includes RBCs and mucosal cells.

5) **Cancer prevention**

6) **Synthesis of fatty acids**

7) **Taurine precursor and bile acid conjugator**

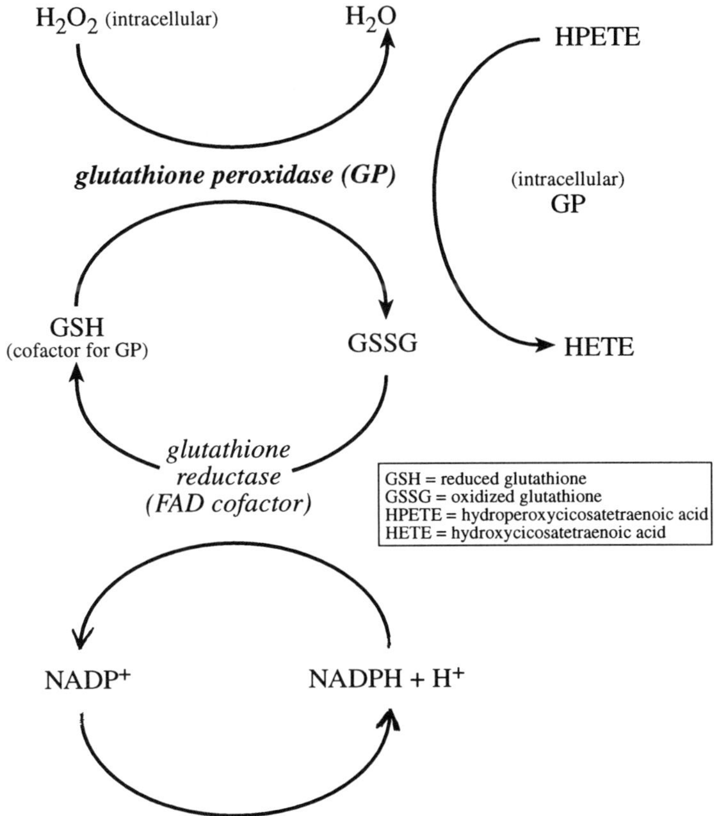


## III. Requirements

**RDA**–nonessential
Average intake in the U.S.– 5-100mg/day
*Optimal daily intake*– depends on exposure to toxins

## IV. Sources

BEST SOURCES OF CYSTINE
(Cysteine is very difficult to measure)

| Food | amount | mg | Food | amount | mg |
|---|---|---|---|---|---|
| Yogurt | 1 cup | 930 | Turkey | 3 oz | 94 |
| Granola | 1 cup | 300 | Cheese | 3 oz | 90 |
| Duck | 3oz | 225 | Chicken | 3 oz | 75 |
| Oatmeal flakes | 1 cup | 200 | Egg | 1 med | 70 |
| Wheat germ toasted | 1/4 cup | 180 | Wild game | 1/4 cup | 67 |
| Cheese, cottage | 1/2 cup | 150 | Sausage | 3 pz | 66 |
| Cheese, ricotta | 1/2 cup | 120 | Meat, luncheon | 3 oz | 54 |
| Pork | 3 oz | 120 | Milk, whole | 1 cup | 33 |

From USDA: Composition of Foods. USDA handbook # 8 Washington DC, ARS, USDA, 1976-1986

## V. Deficiency

A lack of cysteine results in a deficiency of glutathione which may result in mental retardation. A deficiency of glutathione results in diminished macrophage activity, increased fragility of RBCs, increased susceptibility to cancer and other toxins. A reduced level can be found in people who are protein deficient or who are fasting.

## VI. Therapeutics

**CYSTEINE** [Dosages should start low (500mg) and work up to 4-5 grams per day. Excess cysteine can cause an increase in cystine which can be nephrotoxic.]

1) **Detoxification and heavy metal toxicity**–Cysteine has been shown to be effective against molybdenum and cobalt toxicity. It has been shown to protect against liver toxins. One study showed that the ability of the body to make cysteine from N-acetyl cysteine makes it critical in its effectiveness in preventing chemotherapy damage. Other common toxins that glutathione may help protect against are car exhaust, cigarette smoke, aspirin and alcohol (check environmental toxicities via 24 hr urine collection of D-glucaric acid and or mercapturic acid).

2) **Bronchitis and/or asthma (COPD, cystic fibrosis, emphysema etc.)**–1-3gms/day–N-acetyl cysteine has been found to have mucolytic activity as well as immune enhancing properties. Chronic smokers may benefit from cysteine supplementation. It may be used in an aerosol form.

3) **Immune enhancement**–1-3gms/day–This is especially effective against clostridium in the GI. It helps prevent translocation.

4) **Cancer**–N-acetyl cysteine form 1-3gms/day–as an adjunct treatment for cancer and for people receiving chemotherapy treatments. NAC has been shown to mitigate the toxicity of acetaminophen, doxorubicin, cyclophophamide, ifosfamide, and radiation.

5) **Psoriasis**

6) **Hair loss**–1-5gms/day–The hair and fingernails are composed of keratin which is 12% cysteine. Certain types of baldness may respond to cysteine.

7) **AIDS**–In vitro studies have shown N-acetyl cysteine inhibits HIV.

8) **Diabetes mellitus**–Especially in ketosis as DM patients will generally excrete increased amounts of sulfur containing amino acids.

9) **Liver disease including cirrhosis and fatty liver disease caused by alcohol**–Studies show mild effects at large doses.

10) **Ulcers intestinal or stomach**–In patients with stomach ulcers, low levels of GSH have been found.

**GLUTATHIONE**

Most therapeutics for glutathione can use cysteine, which is considerably less expensive. There are some inborn errors in metabolism that may require glutathione directly. Supplementation of glutathione does not necessarily raise tissue levels of glutathione in all cases however. Other supplements such as vitamin C, selenium and N-acetyl cysteine may have a more significant effect at actually raising glutathione levels in the liver and other tissues. Certain labs such as Metametrix, Antibody Assay Labs, Great Smokies, and Diagnostechs may be able to assess glutathione status directly or indirectly. Since glutathione is involved in various liver detoxification processes, various cytochrome systems may not be working at their optimal capacity. This can be evaluated through certain tests such as caffeine clearance and glucuronic acid.

## VII. Toxicity

**Toxins Requiring Glutathione**

| | |
|---|---|
| 1) Halogenonitrobenzenes and congeners (fungicides) | 13) Other eposice intermediates (solvents) |
| 2) 2-Chloro-S-triazines and congeners (herbicides) | 14) Arylamines, arylhydroxylamines, carbamates, and related compds (phenols) |
| 3) Aryl Nitrocompounds (nitrates, nitrosamines) | 15) Steroids |
| 4) Phenoltetrabromphthaleins (dyes) | 16) Quinones and catechols (meds) |
| 5) Aryl and alkyl haldies (solvents) | 17) Isothiocyantes (methylisocyanate) |
| 6) Aryl and alkyl ester (solvents and flavorings) | 18) Trichloromethylsufenyls (pesticides) |
| 7) Alkene halides (plastics, vinyl chloride) | 19) Theocaramatess (pesticides) |
| 8) Allyl compunds (intermediates) | 20) Heavy metals including lead, mercury, arsenic, cadnium |
| 9) Alkyl methanesulfonates (dyes and detergents) | 21) Bacterial toxins (Clostridia difficile) |
| 10) Organophosphorus compounds (insecticides) | 22) Automobile exhaust and cigarette smoke |
| 11) Arylhydrocarbon epoxides or arene oxides (solvents) | 23) Pharmaceuticals (very long list that need to be detoxified by the liver) |
| 12) Arylhalide epoxides (solvents) | |

Cysteine has very little toxicity. No toxicity has been reported even at 10gms per day taken orally. Cystine however has been shown to have toxic effects as in Fanconi's syndrome and cystinosis. Fanconi's syndrome causes kidney damage resulting from the accumulation of cystine crystals. Cystinosis results in kidney damage as well. Both conditions may be treated with D-penicillamine 1.5-2.0gms per day. D-penicillamine is dimethyl cysteine and seems to inhibit the cystine formation but does not effect cysteine. Large IV doses of cysteine have resulted in increased accumulation of cystine in the kidneys and resultant damage.

# GLUTAMINE

## I. Metabolism

Glutamine is considered a conditionally essential amino acid since it is essential during periods of excessive stress (injury, septicemia, acute burns, inflammatory bowel disease, etc.). It is the most abundant amino acid in the skeleton, muscle and blood. Glutamine is 10-15x more concentrated in the brain than in the blood. It is synthesized from glutamic acid.

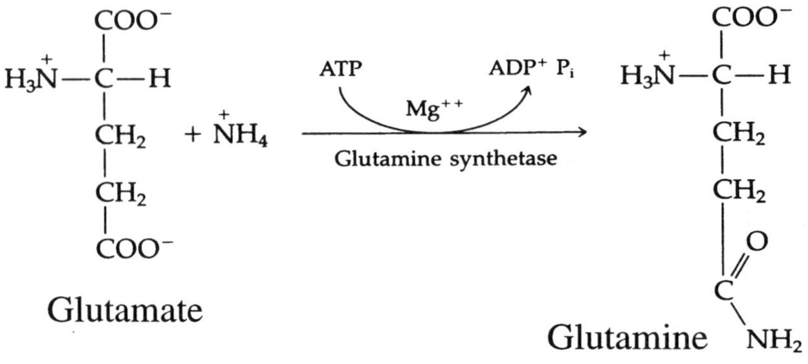

$$\underset{\text{Glutamate}}{{}^{-}OOC-CH_2-CH_2-CH(\overset{+}{N}H_3)-COO^-} + \overset{+}{N}H_4 \xrightarrow[\text{Glutamine synthetase}]{ATP \rightarrow ADP^+ \; P_i,\; Mg^{++}} \underset{\text{Glutamine}}{H_2N-C(=O)-CH_2-CH_2-CH(\overset{+}{N}H_3)-COO^-}$$

Synthesis of glutamine from glutamate and ammonium ion

## II. Function

- Glutamine is essential and is the preferred source of energy for enterocytes of the GI tract. With alanine, it provides over 75% of the fuel for enterocytes during acute stress. It is also a preferred source of energy for the brain. It is involved as a neurotransmitter in the brain.
- In athletes who overtrain, glutamine can become depleted. This results in increased infections, especially respiratory type infections.
- Other cells which rapidly divide–including lymphocytes, macrophages, thymocytes–rely on glutamine as well. It is also involved with acid base balance in the body.
- In the intestines it is critical for repair of tissue, especially in returning the tissue's normal permeability characteristic.
- Glutamine is essential for the synthesis of vitamin B-3, and is a cofactor in the metabolism of benzoates. It is essential in the metabolism of uric acid and arginine.

### Best Sources of Glutamic Acid

| Food | amount | mg | Food | amount | mg |
|---|---|---|---|---|---|
| Cheese | 3 oz | 4800 | Meat, luncheon | 3 oz | 1875 |
| Cheese, cottage | 1/2 c | 3400 | Milk, whole | 1 c | 1700 |
| Cheese, ricotta | 1/2 c | 3000 | Oatmeal flakes | 1 c | 1400 |
| Granola | 1 c | 2600 | Wheat germ, toasted | 1/4 c | 1400 |
| Pork | 3 oz | 2438 | Turkey | 3 oz | 1125 |
| Yogurt | 1 c | 2300 | Chicken | 3 oz | 844 |
| Wild game | 3 oz | 2250 | Duck | 3 oz | 844 |
| Sausage | 3 oz | 1875 | Egg | 1 med | 800 |

From USDA: Composition of Foods. USDA handbook # 8 Washington DC, ARS, USDA, 1976-1986

## III. Requirements

**RDA**–Glutamine is considered only conditionally essential
Average intake in the U.S.–2–3gm /day

## IV. Sources

**See previous page**

## V. Deficiency

Glutamine is considered a conditionally essential amino acid because it can be synthesized from glutamic acid. There are certain conditions where the body's demand for glutamine exceeds its ability to synthesize it. Such conditions as acute bowel inflammation or acute trauma require greatly increased amounts. Under such conditions the body takes its supply from muscle tissue. This can be an obvious problem when its comes to maintaining lean body mass. In such situations large oral doses of glutamine may spare muscle tissue from becoming catabolized.

## VI. Therapeutics

1) **Inflammatory bowel disease especially in extreme weight loss**–6-12gms per day. Ideally, it can be added as a powder to drinks to help maintain weight and heal the gut mucosa.

2) **Peptic ulcers**

3) **Alcoholism**–It has been used for years in the treatment of alcoholism. It may decrease cravings for alcohol.

STUDY–Rogers, L.L., et al. Quar. J of Studies on Alcohol 18:4: 581-7, 1957. ABSTRACT–In a double blind crossover trial 7 men and 3 women with long histories of excess drinking took 5 caps/day divided through day of lactose placebo or 200mg of glutamine. After 6 wks on L-glutamine 9 of 10 subjects, as well as friends and relatives, stated that the glutamine diminished the desire to drink and decreased anxiety and improved sleep. 2 or 3 subjects continued to do well after placebo substitution, but no subjects responded to placebo unless they had first responded to glutamine.

4) **Total Parenteral Nutrition treatment or starvation diet to prevent villus atrophy in the small intestine.**

5) **Enhancement of mental function in Alzheimer's patients**

6) **Cancer**–Glutamine may be an essential respiratory fuel for tumor cells. A drug glutaminase which breaks down glutamine is used to treat acute leukemia and lymphocytic malignant cells. Vegetarian diets have sometimes worked in the treatment of some cancers since glutamine is usually on the low side for vegetarian foods.

## VII. Toxicity

Glutamine has very little toxicity.

# L-LYSINE

## I. Metabolism

Lysine is one of the essential amino acids. It is found highest in muscles–only glutamic acid and aspartic acid being higher. Lysine is degraded to acetyl CoA, a critical intermediate in the Krebs cycle. Enzymes involved with acetyl CoA have been found in decreasing order in the liver, kidneys, heart, adrenal glands, thymus gland, brain and skin. Lysine is the precursor to carnitine and citrulline. Minor amounts of lysine can be made into pipecolic acid, a neurotransmitter in the brain, and it works with the help of niacin. Arginine and ornithine are antagonistic to lysine and if given in large amounts can lead to a deficiency of lysine.

There are some inborn errors in metabolism which can lead to an elevation of lysine. High amounts of lysine can result in mental retardation along with a host of different physical abnormalities including delayed sex development, facial bone abnormalities, enlarged liver and obesity. Lysine is metabolized with the help of vitamins B-2 and B-3.

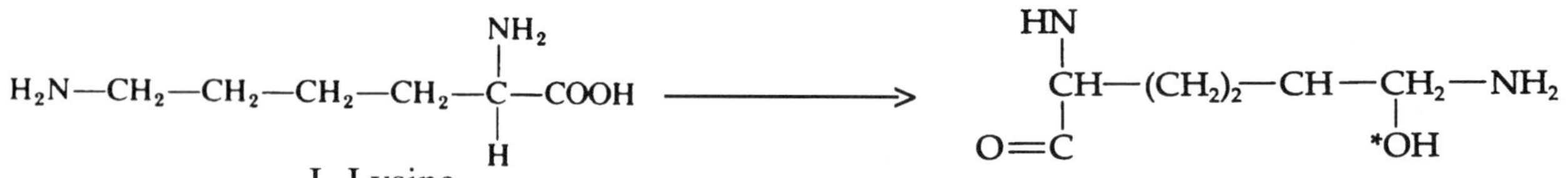

$$H_2N-CH_2-CH_2-CH_2-CH_2-\underset{H}{\overset{NH_2}{C}}-COOH \longrightarrow \underset{O=C}{\overset{HN}{CH}}-(CH_2)_2-CH-\underset{*OH}{CH_2}-NH_2$$

L-Lysine

**Hydroxylysine**

(involved with collagen synthesis)

**SPECIAL NOTE**–(see special note on next page).

## II. Function

Lysine is involved with the synthesis of connective tissue, brain neurotransmitters and carbohydrate metabolism through its role as a precursor to acetyl CoA.

## III. Requirements

**RDA**–Adults–840mg/day or 12mg/kg body weight
Children below twelve–44mg/kg
Infants–97mg/kg per day
Average intake in the U.S.–70mg to 80mg/day
Therapeutic range–.5-4gms/day

## IV. Deficiency

Certain vegetarian foods can be found to be deficient in lysine. Refined grains, corn, sunflower seeds, peanuts, and vegetables are generally low in lysine. In vegetarian diets, legumes are used to supply the needed lysine. Deficiency symptoms usually show a decreased immune function as well as decreased growth.

**SPECIAL NOTE**–Lysine is involved in a reaction in foods called ***Caramelization.*** This reaction is also called the ***Mailliard Reaction*** or ***Browning Reaction***. It takes place in foods such as pastries, doughnuts, cookies, puffed and flaked cereals which contain lysine and simple sugars. When, during preparation, these foods are heated, a sugar hooks onto the lysine moiety of the protein chain. The body is unable to hydrolyze the protein chain that contains this caramelized lysine molecule. Absorption of this peptide can trigger immune responses or allergies.

In addition, if a person already has borderline lysine levels, these foods can cause a deficiency in lysine. In fact, a study done in the 70's by Dr. Constance Kies of the University of Nebraska and Dr. William Caster of the University of Georgia examined 38 cereals and their effect on the growth of rats. The cereal was their sole source of nutrition. 20 of the cereals failed to keep the rats alive, while another 12 provided little or no growth. The only cereals that did well were fortified with soy protein which made up for the deficiency of lysine that occurred because of the Maillard reaction. Others, such as wheat germ, which do not have any sugars, did not cause a lysine deficiency. There may also be a connection with lysine deficiency and kidney stones (calcium oxalate) as well.

## V. Sources

### Best Sources of Lysine together with Arginine

| Food | amount | mg lysine | mg arginine | Ratio Arg to Lys | | Food | amount | mg lysine | mg arginine | Ratio Arg to Lys |
|---|---|---|---|---|---|---|---|---|---|---|
| Tuna 3 oz | 1/2 can | 2400 | 1450 | .6 | | Beans, red canned | 1/2 cup | 630 | 510 | .8 |
| Turkey (baked light meat) | 3 oz | 2400 | 1770 | .74 | | Oatmeal flakes | 1 cup | 600 | 600 | 1.0 |
| Halibut, baked | 3oz | 2083 | 1357 | .65 | | Carrot juice | 12 cup | 600 | | .8 |
| Salmon | 3 oz | 2014 | 1311 | .65 | | Granola | 1 cup | 500 | 900 | 1.85 |
| Liver, beef | 3 oz | 1671 | 1363 | .82 | | Wheat germ, toasted | 1/4 cup | 500 | 675 | 1.3 |
| Cheese | 3 oz | 1650 | 600 | .4 | | Bacon | 3 slices | 500 | 525 | .9 |
| Cheese, ricotta | 1/2 cup | 1600 | 800 | .5 | | Duck | 3 oz | 480 | 407 | .85 |
| Pork | 3 oz | 1586 | 1470 | .83 | | Sausage | 3 oz | 420 | 315 | .8 |
| Cheese, cheddar | 3  0z | 1497 | 729 | .49 | | Egg | 1 med | 400 | 400 | 1.0 |
| Wild game | 3 oz | 1300 | 962 | .75 | | Chicken (baked light meat) | 3 oz | 2232 | 1584 | .71 |
| Cheese, cottage | 1/2 cup | 1200 | 700 | .6 | | Peanuts | 1/4 cup | 363 | 1080 | 3.0 |
| Sardines, canned in oil | 3 med | 814 | 531 | .65 | | Avocado | 1 med | 200 | 100 | .5 |
| Meat, luncheon | 3 oz | 740 | 592 | .8 | | Cashews | 10 nuts | 185 | 490 | 2.6 |
| Yogurt | 1 cup | 700 | 250 | .35 | | Almonds | 18 nuts | 145 | 683 | 4.7 |
| Milk, whole | 1 cup | 650 | 300 | .45 | | | | | | |

From USDA: Composition of Foods. USDA handbook # 8 Washington DC, ARS, USDA, 1976-1986

## VI. Therapeutics

1) **Herpes Simplex–3-9gms per day in divided doses for acute conditions.** For prevention 500-1500mg per day–Lysine is a well known inhibitor of the herpes virus.

2) **Osteoporosis**–Lysine may effect calcium metabolism by increasing absorption and decreasing excretion. In animal studies lysine deficiency results in an increased excretion of calcium.

3) **Aphthous ulcers**–In rare cases lysine may have dramatic effects.

## VII. Toxicity

In mice and chicks high intakes of lysine can cause increased cholesterol levels. In humans lysine has very little toxicity, even at high doses. Doses up to 8gms per day seem to be innocuous.

## VIII. Interactions

Lysine is an antagonist to arginine and could result in an arginine deficiency if taken in high amounts with borderline intakes of arginine.

As mentioned previously, lysine in cereals and other carbohydrate foods can interact and actually cause a lysine deficiency. Too many cereals, especially if they contain significant quantities of simple sugars can cause a lysine imbalance.

### Notes

---

# METHIONINE

## I. Metabolism (see diagram p.89)

One of the sulfur containing amino acids, methionine is *essential* because we cannot synthesize it from aspartic acid. However, there have been reports of people surviving on only potatoes which are deficient in methionine. This may be because bacteria in the gut can synthesize significant amounts.

Methionine is converted into **S-adenosyl methionine** (SAM), which is considered to be the *activated* form of methionine. This happens in the first step of the metabolism of methionine. This step requires energy in the form of ATP. In this activation of methionine, an adenosyl moiety is transferred from the ATP molecule.

SAM is an important biological methylating agent. Its methyl group, which is attached in a sulfonium linkage with high-energy characteristics, may be donated to any of a large number of methyl-group acceptors in the presence of the appropriate enzyme (Biochemistry Lehninger, 1975).

SAM was first discovered by G. Cantoni and colleagues in 1952 in Italy. Interestingly enough, when high doses of methionine are given orally, levels of SAM do not go up correspondingly as one would expect. SAM is an extremely potent methyl donor.

## II. Function

It performs as a sulfur donor, a methyl donor, as a precursor for other sulfur amino acids as well as a metabolizer of polyamines. Decreased levels are associated with an increase in polyamines (see eczema).

1) S-adenosyl methionine synthesis is one of the most potent methyl donors and is involved in many methylation reactions. It is intimately involved in the synthesis of brain chemicals and also in detoxification reactions. This compound has pronounced analgesic properties and is currently being investigated in Italy. It has been commercially available in Europe since 1975, but, currently, it is not available in the U.S.

2) As a methyl donor, SAM is involved in the following:
- a) Breakdown of estrogens
- b) Carnitine synthesis
- c) Choline synthesis
- d) Creatine synthesis
- e) Epinephrine synthesis
- f) Melatonin synthesis
- g) Nucleic acid synthesis
- h) Degradation of histamine

$$H_3C{-}S{-}CH_2{-}CH_2{-}\overset{\displaystyle NH_2}{\underset{\displaystyle H}{C}}{-}COOH$$

**Methionine**

3) Glutathione synthesis– increases levels of glutathione

4) Antioxidant functions–especially the sulfur component

5) Maintains cartilage health

## III. Requirements

**RDAs**–22mg/kg for children and 10mg/day/kg or 1.5 gms per day for adults.
WHO recommends 9g/day
Homocysteine in the diet can eliminate the requirement for methionine
Average intake in the U.S.–2.7 to 5g/day

| Intake of cysteine and methionine: | Omnivores– | 4.3 |
|---|---|---|
| | Lacto-ovo-vegetarian | 3.2 |
| | Vegans– | 2.7gm |

## IV. Sources

Sunflower seeds are a good source of methionine, but generally animal products are the best source. Soybeans are a poor source and soy-based infant formulas are generally low in methionine. Egg yolks are particularly high in sulfur. Methionine and cysteine make up 91% of the sulfur in the yolk.

**Best Sources of Methionine**

| Food | amount | mg | Food | amount | mg |
|---|---|---|---|---|---|
| Tuna | 3 oz | 733 | Turkey | 1 oz | 167 |
| Cheese, Cheddar | 3 oz | 555 | Sausage | 3 oz | 166 |
| Salmon | 3oz | 505 | Almonds | 1/2 c | 160 |
| Wild game | 3 oz | 444 | Wheat germ, toasted | 1/4 cup | 158 |
| Shrimp, mixed cooked | 3 oz | 400 | Duck | 3 oz | 157 |
| Cheese, Ricotta | 1/2 cup | 350 | Chicken | 3 oz | 120 |
| Pork | 3 oz | 333 | Filberts | 1/2 c (70gm) | 120 |
| Meat, luncheon | 3 oz | 241 | Cheese, cottage | 1/2 cup | 100 |
| Granola | 1 cup | 200 | Sesame seed butter | 2T(30gm) | 100 |
| Egg | 1 med | 200 | Peanut Butter | 2 T | 94 |
| Milk, whole | 1 cup | 200 | Potato, baked | 1 med | 73 |
| Chocolate | 1 cup | 200 | Sweet potato | 1 med | 48 |
| Cashews | 1/2 c | 188 | Avocado | 1/2 med | 25 |
| Walnuts | 1/2 c | 170 | Mushrooms, Shitake | 8 med | 36 |

From USDA: Composition of Foods. USDA handbook # 8 Washington DC, ARS, USDA, 1976-1986

## V. Deficiency

Methionine deficiency is usually related to overall protein malnutrition. Experimentally, a methionine deficiency causes premature atherosclerosis in monkeys, especially if they are also deficient in vitamin B-6. Methionine deficiency can also cause a folate deficiency since a deficiency causes 5-methyl-tetrahydrofolate to accumulate in the liver.

Deficiencies of B-12, folate and methionine can cause a deficiency of SAM.

## VI. Therapeutics

1) **Depression**–SAM 400mg qid–Methionine is readily absorbed into the brain and gets converted into SAM where it increases the effects of norepinephrine likethe neurotransmitters. SAM is one of the most effective natural anti-depressant remedies, comparing more favorably than MAO inhibitors and some tricyclics such as Tofranil and Elavil! SAM may be superior to methionine for the treatment of depression. It may be especially useful in treating postpartum depression and depression associated with drug withdrawal.

STUDY–Kagan, B.L., et al. *Oral SAM in depression: A randomized , double blind placebo-controlled trial.* Am J Psychiatry 147:591-95, 1990.

STUDY–Rosenbaum, J.F., et al. *An open label pilot study of oral SAM in major depression.* Psychopharmacol Bull 24:189-94, 1988.

STUDY–Salmaggi, P., et al. *Double blind, placebo-controlled study of SAM in depressed postmenopausal women.* Psychotherapy Psychosom 59:905-13, 1993.

2) **Osteoarthritis**–SAM 400mg tid (reduce dose after a few weeks)–SAM has proven in a number of large studies to be as or more effective than many of the standard medications (NSAIDS) without any of their side effects.

STUDY–Muller-Fassbender, H. *Double blind, clinical trial of SAM versus ibuprofen in the treatment of osteoarthritis* Am J Med 83 (suppl. 5A), 81-3, 1987.

STUDY–Glorioso, S., et al. *Double blind, multicenter study of the activity of SAM in hip and knee osteoarthritis.* Int J Clin Pharmacol Res 5, 39-49, 1985.

STUDY–Marcolongo, R., et al. *Double blind, multicenter study of the activity of SAM in hip and knee osteoarthritis.* Current Ther Res 37:82-94, 1985.

STUDY–Caruso, I. and Pietrogrande, V. (Italian) *Double blind, multicenter study comparing SAM, naproxen, and placebo in the treatment of degenerative joint disease.* Am J Med 83:(suppl 5A), 66-71, 1987.

STUDY–Burger, R., and Nowak, H. *A new medical approach to the treatment of osteoarthritis: Report of an open phase IV study with ademetionin (Gumbaral) SAM.* Am J Med 83:(suppl 5A), 84-88, 1987. ABSTRACT–Over 20,000 patients with osteoarthritis of the knees, hip, spine and fingers were studied over an 8 week period. Patients received 400mg tid for first week, then 400mg bid for second week and 200mg bid from the third week on. No added treatment was permitted. The results revealed 71% of the patients had very good or good response which is comparable to NSAIDS but without the side effects.

3) **Pain control**

4) **Fibromyalgia**–SAM

5) **Schizophrenia**–SAM may increase levels of dopamine in the brain and may be an effective adjunct therapy with L-dopa.

STUDY–Bidard, J.N. et al. *Effect de la SAM sur le catabolisme de la dopamine.* J Pharmacol. (Paris)8, I:83-93, 1977.

6) **Detoxification and allergies**–SAM may be helpful in withdrawal symptoms of barbiturates or amphetamines. It may protect the body against radiation. In addition, it may be effective in the treatment of various liver disorders such as elevated liver enzymes due to alcohol, Gilberts syndrome, Gauchers, cholestasis, cirrhosis, hepatitis, and other liver toxins. SAM has been found to increase levels of glutathione.

7) **Wilson's disease**–SAM can lower levels of copper in the body.

8) **Parkinson's**–SAM may stimulate the production of L-dopa in the brain.

9) **Migraine headaches–** may require long term treatment to be effective.

10) **Acrodermatitis enteropathica**–a condition similar to pronounced atopic dermatitis and related to a genetic defect in zinc absorption. Methionine can reduce polyamines which may exacerbate the symptoms.

## VII. Toxicity

Although it rarely occurs, nausea and GI irritation are signs of methionine toxicity. Use caution if someone has bipolar depression because SAM may precipitate the manic phase of the disorder. It is unclear if SAM has the same problems with elevated levels of homocysteine as methionine does. In cases of strong family history of CHD, it is wise to check homocysteine levels before and during treatment.

# Notes

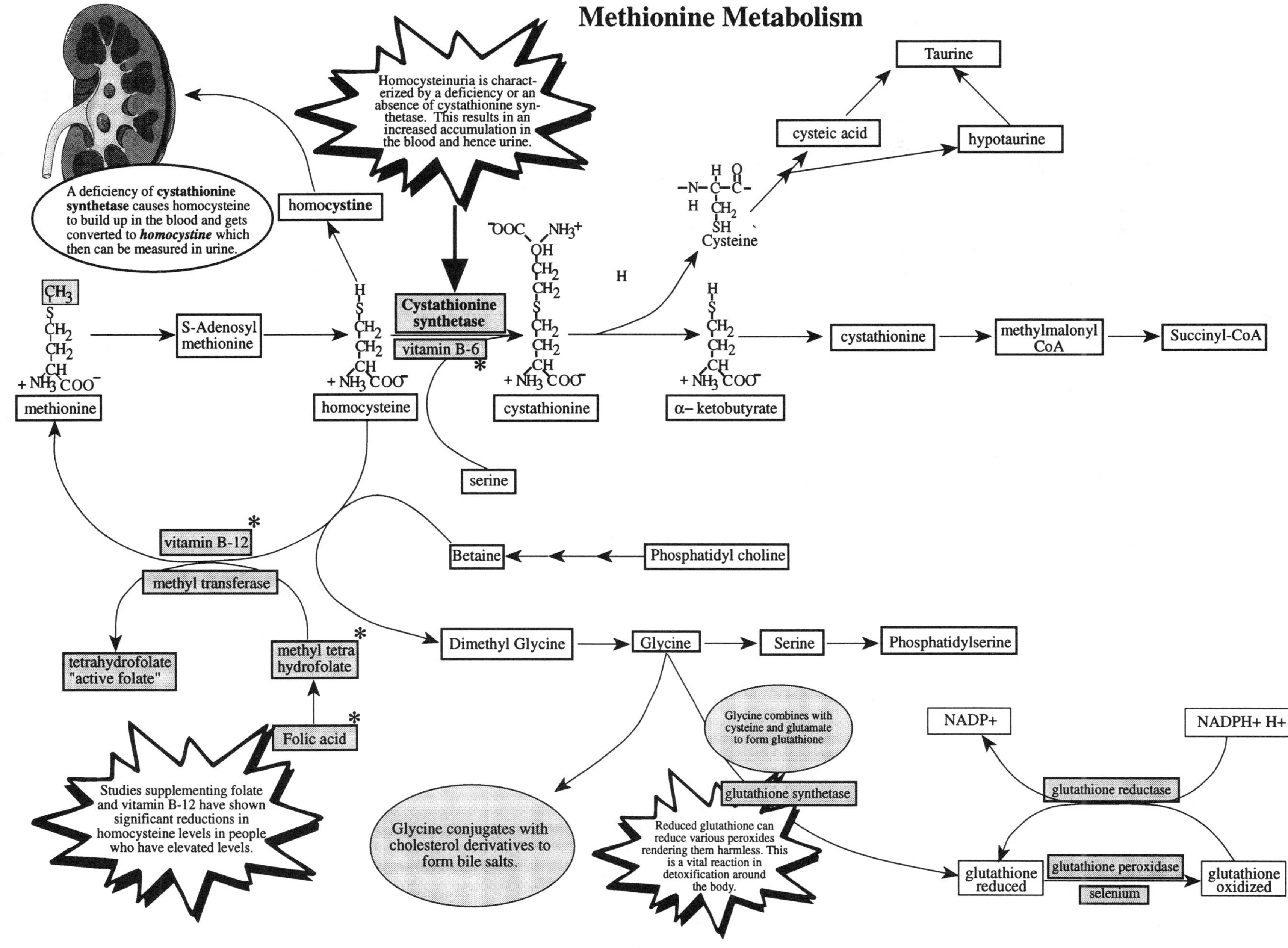
Methionine Metabolism
Homocysteinuria is characterized by a deficiency or an absence of cystathionine synthetase. This results in an increased accumulation in the blood and hence urine.
A deficiency of **cystathionine synthetase** causes homocysteine to build up in the blood and gets converted to ***homocystine*** which then can be measured in urine.
homocystine
methionine
S-Adenosyl methionine
homocysteine
Cystathionine synthetase
vitamin B-6
cystathionine
α– ketobutyrate
Cysteine
cysteic acid
hypotaurine
Taurine
cystathionine
methylmalonyl CoA
Succinyl-CoA
serine
vitamin B-12
methyl transferase
tetrahydrofolate "active folate"
methyl tetra hydrofolate
Folic acid
Betaine
Phosphatidyl choline
Dimethyl Glycine
Glycine
Serine
Phosphatidylserine
Studies supplementing folate and vitamin B-12 have shown significant reductions in homocysteine levels in people who have elevated levels.
Glycine conjugates with cholesterol derivatives to form bile salts.
Glycine combines with cysteine and glutamate to form glutathione
glutathione synthetase
Reduced glutathione can reduce various peroxides rendering them harmless. This is a vital reaction in detoxification around the body.
NADP+
NADPH+ H+
glutathione reductase
glutathione reduced
glutathione peroxidase
selenium
glutathione oxidized

# D,L-PHENYLALANINE (DLPA)

## I. Metabolism

Phenylalanine is the precursor for tyrosine. Many of the conditions that tyrosine is used for may also respond to phenylalanine. DLPA is considered to be one of the essential amino acids. It is also one of the aromatic amino acids. Phenylalanine is metabolized primarily by the liver through the action of phenylalanine hydroxylase. This enzyme directly metabolizes DLPA into tyrosine except in PKU and also in the synthesis of a metabolite tyramine. It is considerably better absorbed than tyrosine.

**NOTE**–DLPA follows a slightly different metabolic pathway than tyrosine as it forms an important brain neurotransmitter, ***phenylethylamine*** (PEA). PEA is a compound that has amphetamine like actions in the brain. Chocolate contains significant amounts of it.

DLPA is normally found free in the blood stream. But in the brain it is found to be part of other important brain proteins, peptides and neurotransmitters.

One defect in DLPA metabolism is **Phenylketonuria** (PKU) which was first identified in 1934. It was then discovered that 1% of the institutionalized retarded population was high in phenylpyruvic acid. From 1965-70 states adopted newborn screening programs to detect phenylketonuria. *Occurrence is 1 in 5,000 births with the heterozygous condition occurring in as high as 1% of the population.* 97% of cases show a deficiency of **phenylalanine hydroxylase**, the enzyme that converts DLPA into tyrosine. Children who are not treated with a restricted diet may become severely retarded. Treatment should begin as early as possible. Certain forms of PKU may be resistant to restriction of the diet. These cases have responded favorably to large amounts of folate supplementation.

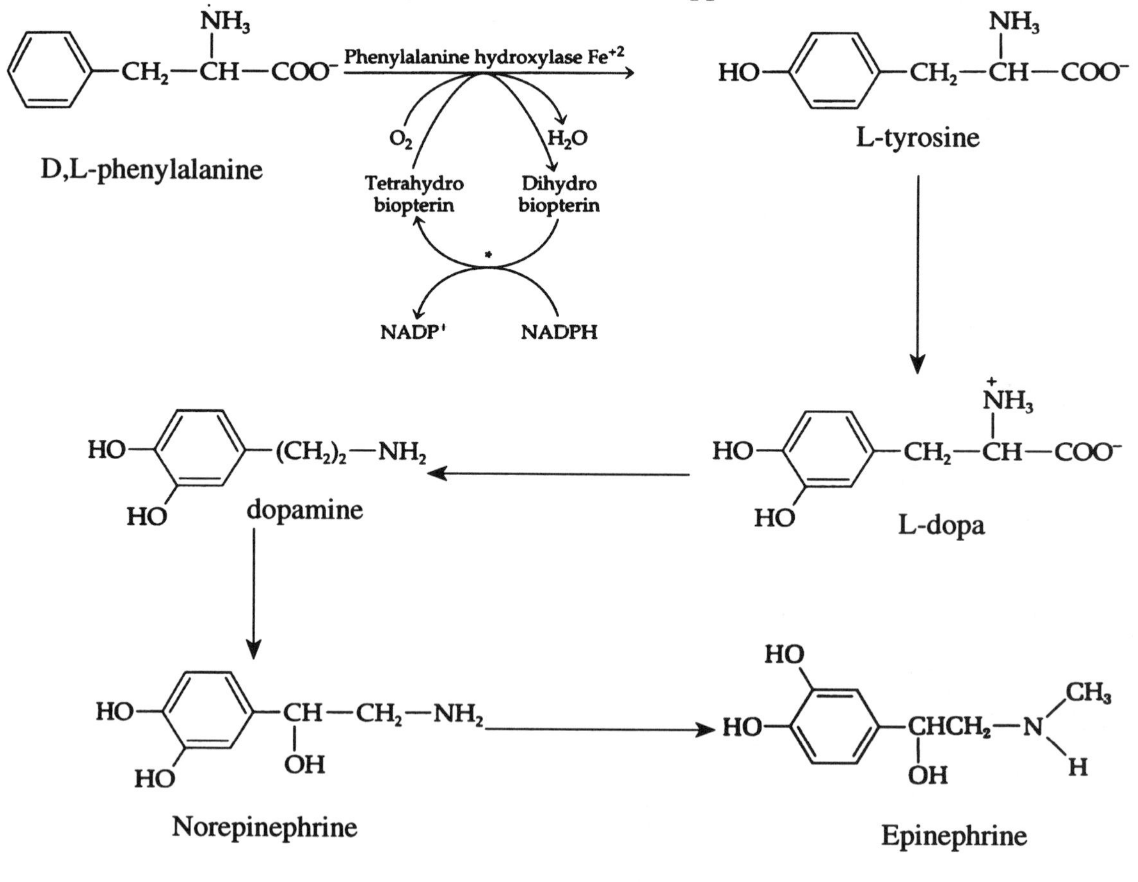

$NH_3$ — $CH_2$—CH—$COO^-$ → Phenylalanine hydroxylase $Fe^{+2}$ → HO— —$CH_2$—CH—$COO^-$ ($NH_3$)

$O_2$   $H_2O$

D,L-phenylalanine   Tetrahydro biopterin   Dihydro biopterin   L-tyrosine

NADP'   NADPH

HO— HO —$(CH_2)_2$—$NH_2$ ← HO— HO —$CH_2$—CH—$COO^-$ ($\overset{+}{N}H_3$)

dopamine   L-dopa

HO— HO —CH—$CH_2$—$NH_2$ (OH) → HO— HO —$CHCH_2$—N ($CH_3$, H) (OH)

Norepinephrine   Epinephrine

## II. Function

DLPA is involved with neurotransmitters in the brain and so is chiefly involved with brain chemistry.

## III. Requirements

**RDA**–1gm /day
Average intake in the U.S.–4-5g/day
Therapeutic range–1.0-8gms/day

**NOTE**–Children with PKU should be restricted to 60mg phenylalanine/kg/day.

## IV. Sources

### Best Sources of Phenylalanine

| Food | amount | mg | Food | amount | mg |
|---|---|---|---|---|---|
| Cheese, cottage 2% fat | 1 cup | 1700 | Milk, whole | 1 cup | 400 |
| Chicken | 3 oz | 1100 | Chocolate | 1 cup | 400 |
| Cheese, cheddar | 3 oz | 1116 | Yogurt | 1 cup | 400 |
| Turkey | 3 oz | 950 | Meat, luncheon | 3 oz | 390 |
| Tuna | 3 oz | 776 | Wheat germ toasted | 1/4 cup | 350 |
| Cod, Atlantic cooked | 3 oz | 776 | Egg | 1 med | 350 |
| Salmon, Chinook | 3 oz | 666 | Bread, whole wheat | 2 slices | 285 |
| Granola | 1 cup | 650 | Walnuts | 10 whole | 265 |
| Wild game | 3 oz | 600 | Cashews | 10 nuts | 250 |
| Pork | 3 oz | 540 | Duck | 3 oz | 240 |
| Oatmeal flakes | 1 cup | 500 | Sausage | 3 oz | 185 |
| Soybeans | 1/2 c cooked | 480 | Avocado | 1/2 med | 75 |

## V. Deficiency

A deficiency of DLPA may lead to depression and diminished growth.

## VI. Therapeutics

1) **Depression**–1-6gms per day. Certain types of depression may respond favorably to DLPA. There have been a significant number of controlled trials which showed improvement comparable to many of the common antidepressants that are used. It may be more effective than tyrosine in the treatment of depression because of its ability to make PEA which is often deficient in depressed people.

2) **Pain, chronic**–DLPA may block certain enzymes such as enkephalinase, which normally breaks down enkephalines, and endorphins which have morphine like activity in the body. The endorphins and enkephalines have mild mood enhancing effects, but stronger analgesic effects. Such conditions as OA, PA, low back pain, menstrual cramps, and migraine headaches may respond to DLPA.

3) **Parkinson's disease**–750mg/3x/day–DLPA may help with symptoms of rigidity and depression but not the tremors.

## VII. Toxicity

DLPA may cause symptoms of anxiety, jitteriness and hyperactivity in children. Sufferers of phenylketonuria must avoid DLPA. Children with attention deficit disorder or hyperactivity may need to avoid foods containing aspartamine (Nutrasweet). It may also cause problems with migraine headaches and hypertension due to tyramine sensitivity because phenylalanine may lead to an increase in tyramine levels.

## VIII. Interactions

Tyramine containing foods may potentiate the effects of DLPA. People taking significant amounts of DLPA and eating tyramine containing foods may possibly have an increase in blood pressure. Caution must also be used with patients who are taking monoamine oxidase inhibitor type antidepressant medications since phenylalanine can precipitate a hypertensive crisis and there have been reports of cerebral hemorrhaging.

**Tyramine Containing Foods**

| **Foods very high in tyramine** | **Moderately high in tyramine** | **Medium levels of tyramine** |
|---|---|---|
| Yeast extracts & breads made with yeast | Cheeses | Broad beans (fava, Chinese pea pods, lima, lentils& snow peas) |
| Cheeses | Blue | Caffeine (in large amounts) |
| Boursalt | Brick, natural | Chocolate (in large amounts) |
| Camembert | Brie | Liver (Chicken or beef) |
| Chedder | Gruyere | Pineapple |
| Stilton | Mozzarella | Plums |
| **Foods highs in tyramine** | Parmesan | Prunes |
| Bologna | Romano | Raisins |
| Herring, dried, salted, pickled | Roquefort | Soy sauce |
| Cod, dried, salted or pickled | Chianti wine | |
| Pepproni | Meat tenderizers | |
| Salami | | |
| **Foods low in tyramine** | | **Tyramine, unknown amounts** |
| Ale | Figs | Legumes |
| Beer | Sherry | Nuts |
| Cheeses | Wine, white | Soy sauce |
| American, processed | Sour cream | Vanilla |
| Cottage | Avocados | Monosodium glutamate (MSG) |
| Cream | bananas | Chinese foods with MSG |
| Ricotta | | |

# TAURINE

## I. Metabolism

Taurine is one of the sulfur containing amino acids along with cystine, cysteine and methionine. It is a nonessential amino acid. Preterm infants and term infants have very small amounts of taurine and need to get their taurine from breast milk or formula. As infants mature, they quickly gain the ability to synthesize their own taurine. Under certain conditions–such as hypertension, heart disease, and seizure disorders–the taurine requirement goes up considerably. Taurine tends to be well absorbed and tissue levels can go up rapidly after oral administration.

$$NH_2CH_2{-}CH_2{-}SO_3^-$$

L-Taurine

## II. Function

Taurine modulates the production and activity of cAMP. It is intimately involved with the contractility of the heart. It may decrease cholesterol levels by increasing excretion through the action of taurocholate, a substance found in bile salts. It is involved in gall bladder function through the synthesis of this taurocholate. It concentrated in the eyes especially the retina.

## III. Requirements

**RDA**–Taurine is a nonessential amino acid.
Average intake in the U.S.–40-400mg/day.
Therapeutic range–1.5-3gms/day

## IV. Sources

Taurine is concentrated in animal and fish protein. Organ meats, particularly brains, are very high in taurine.

## V. Deficiency

In animals like cats,who don't synthesize much taurine, a deficiency can cause blindness. Inborn errors in taurine metabolism, in which there are decreased levels of taurine, result in depression, fatigue, insomnia, weight loss, and vision disturbances. In another inborn error in metabolism, there are decreased levels in the heart muscle which result in mitral valve prolapse, and rapidly progressing cardiomyopathy. Taurine may be deficient in preterm infants. It is especially important in seizure disorders in newborns.

**Best Sources of Taurine**

| Food | amount | mg |
|---|---|---|
| Cheese, cottage | 1 cup | 1700 |
| Cheese | 3 oz | 1000 |
| Granola | 1 cup | 650 |
| Wild game | 3 oz | 600 |
| Pork | 3 oz | 540 |
| Oatmeal flakes | 1 cup | 500 |
| Milk, whole | 1 cup | 400 |
| Chocolate | 1 cup | 400 |
| Yogurt | 1 cup | 400 |
| Meat, luncheon | 1 cup | 390 |
| Wheat germ, toasted | 1/4 cup | 350 |
| Egg | 1 med | 350 |
| Turkey | 3 oz | 240 |
| Duck | 3 oz | 240 |
| Chicken | 3 oz | 185 |
| Sausage | 3 oz | 185 |
| Avocado | 1/2 med | 75 |

From USDA: Composition of Foods. USDA handbook # 8 Washington DC, ARS, USDA, 1976-1986

## VI. Therapeutics

1) **Cardiovascular disease**–Taurine has been found to be particularly concentrated in the heart with its levels exceeding the combined total of all other amino acids. During active stress the levels of taurine go up in the heart. Levels go down after an MI or ischemic attack. In Japan Taurine is widely used to treat various types of heart disease.

2) **Seizure disorders**–Serum levels may actually be elevated in certain seizure disorders.

3) **Congestive heart disease, arrhythmias–may require IV administration for certain types of arrythmias.**

4) **Macular degeneration**–Taurine has been found in very high concentrations in the eyes. It is the most abundant amino acid in the retina. People suffering from the condition, retinitis pigmentosa, have been found to have abnormally low levels of taurine. Taurine may have a protective effect on the delicate tissues of the retina. When animals have been put on a taurine deficient diet, they suffer blindness that is reversible upon taurine supplementation.

5) **Diabetes mellitus**–Low serum taurine has been found in diabetics. It may help with the release of insulin from the pancreas.

## VII. Toxicity

May cause stomach ulcers in susceptible individuals. Taurine should not be given to people who are taking aspirin.

### Notes

---

# TRYPTOPHAN

## I. Metabolism

Tryptophan is found in the serum, both free in small amounts, and bound to albumin in much larger amounts. Availability to the brain depends on a number of factors. It is actively transported into the brain and competes with other amino acids for active transport systems. Tyrosine, phenylalanine, valine, leucine and isoleucine all compete with tryptophan for transport into the brain. In depressed and suicidal patients, abnormalities in tryptophan binding have been found.

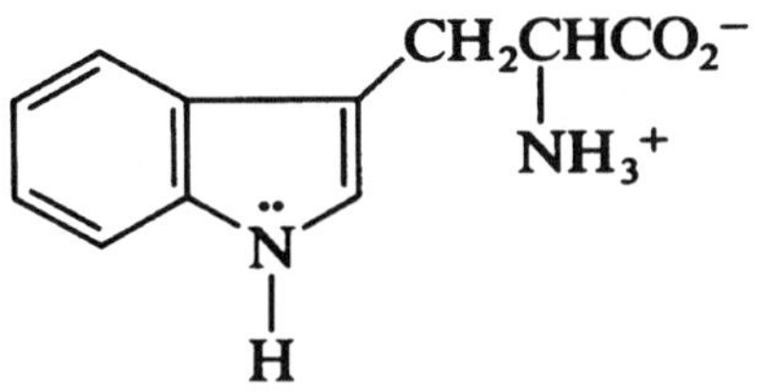

$CH_2CHCO_2^-$, $NH_3^+$, N, H

L-Tryptophan

Measurement in the blood vary greatly when measured by different labs. Tryptophan can be measured via fluorometric and high performance liquid chromatography techniques. Some experts believe chromatography may be the most accurate. Other indirect methods can also be employed, such as the *tryptophan load test.* This test involves measuring a metabolite of tryptophan, xanthurenic acid, in the urine after a standard 2 gram dose is given. The more xanthurenic acid found in the urine, the greater the need for either vitamin B-6 or tryptophan (see tryptophan load test in the chapter on pyridoxine).

When tryptophan is therapeutically administered, it is usually given with vitamin B-6 away from meals with a small amount of carbohydrate to facilitate uptake by the brain. Tryptophan gets metabolized into niacin, melatonin and serotonin. If enough tryptophan is present in the diet, niacin is not required.

### DISORDERS OF TRYPTOPHAN METABOLISM

**Carcinoid syndrome**–Certain tumors of the intestines, stomach, lung, pancreas, thyroid, ovary and testicles can make increased amounts of serotonin. Tryptophan may actually become deficient in the presence of these cancers because of the increased turnover of tryptophan. Symptoms may include diarrhea, flushing, cardiovascular disease, bronchoconstriction and vasodilation. In addition niacin frequently becomes deficient when these tumors are present because of its increased metabolism to form tryptophan.

**Hartnup's disease**–This is a congenital disease that is characterized by ineffective absorption of tryptophan from the intestine. Because tryptophan gets broken down in the gut by bacteria, symptoms similar to pellagra–such as dementia and ataxia–frequently develop (see niacinamide and pellagra).

## II. Functions

1) Niacin synthesis
2) Serotonin precursor
3) Melatonin precursor
4) Proper brain function

## III. Requirements

**RDA's**–200mg/day
Average daily intake–1-1 1/2gms per day
Therapeutic range–.5-4gms/day

## IV. Sources

Tryptophan is the least abundant amino acid in foods. It tends to be deficient in most dietary proteins and has a rather odd distribution. Corn is particularly low in tryptophan, but if treated with lime, the small amount is made more available.

### Best Sources of Tryptophan

| Food | amount | mg | Food | amount | mg |
|---|---|---|---|---|---|
| Cheese, cottage 2% fat | 1 cup | 400 | Cheese | 3 oz | 180 |
| Liver, beef | 3 oz | 334 | Milk, whole | 1 cup | 110 |
| Peanuts | 3 oz | 291 | chocolate | 1 cup | 110 |
| Turkey | 3 oz | 283 | Wheat germ, toasted | 1/4 cup | 110 |
| Lamb, leg roast | 3 oz | 283 | Egg | 1 med | 100 |
| Tuna, 1/2 reg can | 3 oz | 270 | Meat, luncheon | 3 oz | 100 |
| Beef, chuck | 3 oz | 260 | Collards, boiled | 1 cup | 100 |
| Salmon | 3 oz | 231 | Duck | 3 oz | 80 |
| Wild game | 3 oz | 230 | Bacon | 3 slices | 80 |
| Cashews | 20 whole | 215 | Bread, whole wheat | 2 slices | 70 |
| Halibut | 3 oz | 214 | Sausage | 3 oz | 61 |
| Shrimp | 3 oz | 210 | Raisins | 7 T | 60 |
| Granola | 1 cup | 200 | Chicken | 3 oz | 56 |
| Oatmeal flakes | 1 cup | 200 | Yogurt | 1 cup | 50 |
| Pork | 3 oz | 200 | Sweet potato | 1 small | 50 |
| Avocado | 1/2 med | 200 | Spinach | 2 cup raw | 50 |

From USDA: Composition of Foods. USDA handbook # 8 Washington DC, ARS, USDA, 1976-1986

## V. Deficiency

A deficiency of tryptophan may lead to pellagra, depression, insomnia, suicidal thoughts.

## VI. Therapeutics

Relative to other amino acids, small amounts are required to have a therapeutic effect.

1) **Insomnia**–1-3 gms has been used very successfully to treat insomnia although studies have been mixed. Tryptophan has been shown to increase both melatonin and serotonin levels in the brain.

2) **Depression**–1-3gms can be used to treat a variety of depression syndromes. It is especially effective when treating depression which is accompanied by insomnia. Depression associated with menstrual cycles and postpartum depression sometimes respond very well to tryptophan supplementation. Postpartum women usually have high estrogen levels and it has been found that high estrogens increase the conversion of tryptophan to niacin. Progesterone and hydrocortisone decrease its conversion. Women on birth control pills, when given vitamin B-6 and tryptophan, generally tend to metabolize tryptophan more normally.

3) **Mental disorders including mania, psychosis, suicidal tendencies**–Many patients suffering from mental disorders have been found to have low tryptophan levels.

4) **Pain syndromes**

5) **Schizophrenia**–Tryptophan may be more useful when used in conjunction with other nutrients such as niacin and vitamin B-6. Studies show mixed results with tryptophan supplementation. When histamine levels are low, tryptophan supplementation seems to be more effective. Certain tryptophan metabolites, N-methylated tryptamines, have been found to have hallucinogenic properties. These have been found in increased amounts in certain cases of schizophrenia. While these compounds are also formed in normal brains, it seems likely that schizophrenics abnormally metabolize tryptophan.

6) **Anorexia and bulimia**–Low serum tryptophan levels are found in anorexic patients but this may be a result of a generally low intake of all amino acids. One study showed tryptophan together with 50mg/day of pyridoxine helped moods and eating behavior.

7) **Appetite suppression**–Tryptophan has been shown to increase growth hormone and prolactin which seems to inhibit appetite.

8) **Hartnup's disease**–Supplementation may be necessary because of the malabsorption of tryptophan.

9) **Carcinoid syndrome**–Supplementation may be necessary because of the increased metabolism of tryptophan.

10) **Premenstrual Syndrome**

11) **Migraine headaches**–500mg 4-6x/day–may be useful occasionally.

## VII. Toxicity

L-tryptophan has low toxicity. Studies in humans have shown that 100mg/kg/day of tryptophan corresponding to 7 gms per 150lbs, can cause gastric irritation, vomiting and head twitching. In some animals the equivalent of 8gms/day was found to be teratogenic. Therefore caution should be used in pregnancy. In women it has been found that the downline metabolite form of tryptophan, 5 hydroxytryptophan, has fewer side effects. Foods containing tryptophan have been found to be extremely carcinogenic, especially to breast and bladder tissues, when they have been charbroiled or heated to high temperatures .

In 1989 L-tryptophan supplements were found to have caused a number of deaths (35) and severe allergic reactions called eosinophilia myalgia. These symptoms were found to occur more often in the elderly. L-tryptophan was taken off the market following this connection. It was subsequently found that one manufacturer from Japan had used a new bacterial strain to synthesize tryptophan and the bacteria produced some toxic by-products. The FDA decided, for some little known reason, to keep tryptophan off the market indefinitely. It was an interesting coincidence that in March of 1990 a front page story came out in TIME magazine extolling the miracle benefits of Prosac. Prosac sales were more than 3/4 billion dollars per year at that time. Today, sales of prosac gross well over 2.5 billion dollars. Many people who had been taking tryptophan for depression switched to the Prosac medication. During the FDA's ban on tryptophan, it had to allow tryptophan in many products including infant formulas, elemental formulas, and other parenteral formulas. The reason is simply because humans can not live without tryptophan, it is an essential amino acid.

## VIII. Interactions

Long-term supplementation of tryptophan increases plasma levels of other amino acids and this may have many side benefits. Caution should be used when taking antidepressant medications like Prozac since its effects could be amplified. Tyrosine, phenylalanine, valine, leucine and isoleucine all compete with tryptophan for transport into the brain. Tryptophan should not be used by people with asthma, because it stimulates phospholipase $A_2$ which increases the release of arachidonic acid and may exacerbate the condition.

### Notes

---

# TYROSINE

## I. Metabolism

Tyrosine is involved with the synthesis of neurotransmitters in the brain. It is a precursor to dopamine, norepinephrine and epinephrine. Brain concentrations of these neurotransmitters are dependent upon intake of tyrosine. Tyrosine requires biopterin (a folate derivative), NADPH and NADH (forms of niacin), copper and vitamin C.

L-dopa is an amino acid which is synthesized from tyrosine.

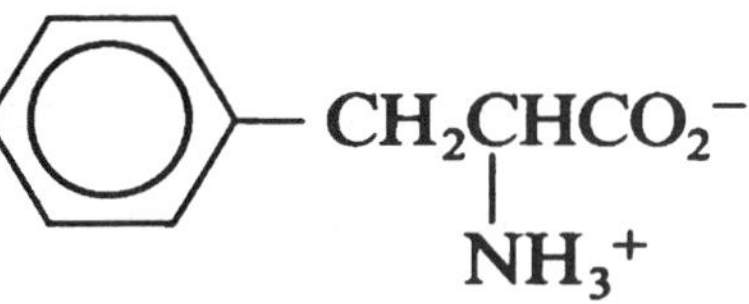

**L-tyrosine**

**Inborn errors in tyrosine metabolism:**

**Tyrosinemia**–Extremely high levels of tyrosine accumulate. Symptoms include mild mental retardation, neurological damage, abnormal pigmentation, migraine headaches and other effects. Premature infants who have an elevation of tyrosine usually show decreased motor activity, lethargy and poor feeding. In addition, infection and intellectual deficiencies may occur. This increased level of tyrosine can be reduced to normal levels with the supplementation of vitamin C. Treatment also involves decreasing intake of protein and tyrosine. It is interesting that vitamin C may decrease the incidence of SIDS, which may have a connection to tyrosine excess.

**Methionemia**

## II. Function

Tyrosine is a precursor to thyroid hormones and catecholestrogens (compounds that have estrogen and catecholamine like effects). Tyrosine is also involved with the synthesis of enkephalins, substances which have pain relieving effects in the body, and melanin, a pigment in the body.

## III. Requirements

**RDA–7.3mg/pound** body wt. /day ~ 1gm per day
Average intake in the U.S.–3.5-5gms/day
Therapeutic range 1-10gms/day

## IV. Sources

**Best Sources of Tyrosine**

| Food | amount | mg | Food | amount | mg |
|---|---|---|---|---|---|
| Cheese, cottage | 1 cup | 1700 | Turkey | 3 oz | 260 |
| Cheese | 3 oz | 900 | Wheat germ, toasted | 1/4 cup | 250 |
| Wild game | 3 oz | 600 | Egg | 1 med | 250 |
| Pork | 3 oz | 500 | Duck | 3 oz | 220 |
| Granola | 1 cup | 400 | Chicken | 3 oz | 160 |
| Milk, whole | 1 cup | 400 | Avocado | 1/2 med | 50 |
| Chocolate | 1 cup | 400 | Meat, luncheon | 3 oz | 20 |
| Yogurt | 1 cup | 400 | Sausage | 3 oz | 10 |
| Oatmeal flakes | 1 cup | 350 | | | |

From USDA: Composition of Foods. USDA handbook # 8 Washington DC, ARS, USDA, 1976-1986

## V. Deficiency

Since tyrosine is a precursor to thyroid hormones and catecholamines, a deficiency leads to hypothyroidism and low adrenal function. It is also a precursor to melanin, the pigment that gives skin its color. A lack of melanin due to a tyrosine deficiency could predispose a person to cancer.

## VI. Therapeutics

1) **Depression**–1-6gms/day can increase tyrosine metabolites such as thyroid hormones and catecholamines.

2) **Narcolepsy**–3-4g/day for 6months may help.

3) **Physical performance enhancement**–Because of its role in catecholamine and thyroid hormone synthesis and stress, tyrosine may benefit athletes who have been training excessively.

4) **Cardiovascular disease**–There have been reports that tyrosine can increase or decrease blood pressure depending upon conditions. In addition, some reports show that tyrosine can decrease PVC's in dogs.

5) **Increased sex drive**–Combined with yohimbine, which can prolong the effects of tyrosine, increased sex drive may occur through the increased stimulation of the beta receptors and increased production of catecholamines.

6) **Decreased appetite**–Large doses, up to 6 gms per day, may decrease appetite through the enhanced production of catecholamines.

7) **Stress conditions**

8) **Addictions**–There have been reports that tyrosine can help with cocaine and nicotine addiction.

9) **Parkinson's disease**–Increased excretion of tyrosine may require supplementation.

## VII. Toxicity

L-Tyrosine has very low toxicity. There have been very few reports of toxicity.

## VIII. Interactions

Caution should be used when using tyrosine with MAOI antidepressant drugs. Theoretically, a hypertensive crisis could occur.

## Notes

# Minerals

Minerals are components in the body that have many essential roles. They occur in both food and water in various forms and amounts. In the body minerals are usually found in the ionic form. Many of them in the body are found as components of bodily fluids and tissues as salts such as sodium chloride but also as components of organic compounds such as phospholipid and hydroxyapatite. When minerals occur in large amounts in the body, such as calcium, they are referred to as macrominerals and when they occur in very small amounts such as selenium, they are called trace minerals or microminerals. The quantity that minerals exist in the body has no bearing on their relative importance in the body. In the last 10-15 years, thanks to more sophisticated techniques in analysis and measurements, there have been many new discoveries concerning the roles of trace minerals in human nutrition and health. Minerals play many roles in the body including the regulation of many enzymes by acting as cofactors, maintaining acid-base balance, osmotic pressure, facilitating transfer of essential compounds across membranes, maintaining proper nerve and muscle conduction and contraction, regulating growth of tissues, and making up critical components of structural tissue. Much of the information that has been found out about trace minerals has occurred because of people being put on long term parenteral nutrition and developing deficiency symptoms. It seems likely that there are as yet many undiscovered functions of trace minerals and that over the next 10-20 years many more discoveries will be made regarding their function.

It appears as though many of the current diseases of today may stem from the depletion of trace minerals from our diet. Trace minerals are found in whole unprocessed foods and are generally dependant upon the health of the soil for their mineral content. When the soil becomes depleted in certain trace minerals the result is food that is also devoid of trace minerals. With our current farming practices here in the U.S., most soils are quite deficient in many trace minerals and the deficiency is only growing worse. Enrichment of grains does nothing to put back trace minerals that are lost during processing of foods. It is almost essential to take trace mineral supplements if we are to achieve optimal nutrition. Unfortunately many multivitamins themselves are deficient in trace minerals although there have been great improvements in the quality of supplements offered today.

# MAGNESIUM

- Magnesium is the second most abundant cation after potassium.
- 60% is found in the bone, 25% in muscle and the remainder in soft tissues and fluids (especially gastric juice).
- In the muscle tissue the majority of magnesium is found in the mitochondria, the organelles that are responsible for oxidative phosphorylation and producing ATP.
- Magnesium intake has gone down dramatically in the last 100 years. In areas where drinking water tends to be hard, having higher levels of magnesium, the incidence of coronary heart disease is lower.

## I. Chemistry

Serum magnesium is a very poor indicator of how much magnesium is actually in the tissues. For example, magnesium concentrates in the heart muscle at almost 20x higher level than in the serum. Measuring white blood cell magnesium is a more sensitive indicator of tissue levels, but ionic magnesium measurement, pioneered by Drs. Burton and Bella Altura at Down-State University of New York in Brooklyn (718) 270-2194, appears to be a considerably more accurate indicator of tissue levels of magnesium than either WBC or RBC measurements, especially in correlating to symptomatology. Dr. Burton Silver in San Jose, California has developed a elemental X-ray analysis technique that uses a bucal smear. An X-ray beam is passed through the cells and different minerals fluoresce at different wavelengths (available through IntraCellular Diagnostics Inc. (800) 874-4804). These newer techniques I believe are critical for evaluating true magnesium tissue levels.

## II. Metabolism

The rate of magnesium absorption varies from as low as 24% to as high as 85%. While absorption occurs mostly in the jejunum via facilitated and simple diffusion, significant amounts are also absorbed in the ileum and large intestine. Many factors regulate magnesium absorption. As the level of calcium intake goes down, the level of magnesium absorption goes up. A significant amount goes to the stomach for HCL production. Magnesium is very involved with ATP production via the Krebs cycle. Glycolysis, adenyl cyclase and other reactions involving nerve impulse transmission also require high quantities of magnesium. High intakes of calcium, protein, vitamin D and alcohol all function to increase the magnesium requirement. In the blood magnesium is found bound to proteins, complexed to small anion ligands and finally as free ionized magnesium. Most labs measure total magnesium which consists of all 3 fractions.

STUDY–Lakshman FL, Rao RB, Kim WW. *Magnesium intakes, balances, and blood levels of adults consuming self selected diets.* AJCN 40(suppl 6): 138 0-89, 1984. Abstract–Men and Women were studied periodically over the course of one year. They were allowed to eat ad lib. It was found that men and women consumed 323mg and 234mg magnesium respectively. (This represents only 84% of the RDA.) Absorption rates were 21% and 27% respectively.

STUDY–Altura BM & Altura BT. *Magnesium and cardiovascular biology: an important link between cardiovascular risk factors and atherogenesis.* Cellular and Molecular Biology Research 41(5): 347-59, 1995.

STUDY–Altura BM & Altura BT. *Role of magnesium in patho-physiological processes and the clinical utility of magnesium ion selective electrodes.* Scand H Clin Lab Invest 56, Suppl 224: 211-234, 1996. Abstract–In this review article ionic magnesium appears to show the best correlation to depleted tissue stores of magnesium. Patients with cardiovascular disease including CHD, MI and hypertension have been found to have low levels of ionic magnesium but normal total serum magnesium levels.

## III. Function

- Magnesium regulates the absorption of calcium and is involved in the structural integrity of bones and teeth. If it is deficient in the bones, the bones may be dense but have poor trabecular integrity, and thus may be brittle. In both Finland and the Netherlands, there is a high ratio of calcium to magnesium intake (4 to 1); the rates of osteoporosis in these countries are the highest in the world.

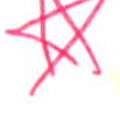

- Magnesium regulates the contractility of the heart muscle. It is concentrated around 20x greater in the heart muscle than in the bloodstream. A decreased magnesium level in the heart muscle may predispose a person to coronary spasms. In areas where the water is harder (mainly due to magnesium), there is a much lower rate of heart disease.
- Magnesium has a relaxing effect on smooth muscle. It may be helpful in relaxing the smooth muscle of the bronchioles (improving asthma) and the arterioles (lowering blood pressure). It relaxes uterine smooth muscle tissue (decreasing the cramping of dysmenorrhea) and is useful in the treatment of angina, myocardial infarction and stroke.
- Magnesium decreases coagulation and acts as a calcium channel blocker. Thus, it helps the heart to pump more effectively, to regulate blood pressure, and to control bleeding after a stroke.
- It is also one of the cofactors for delta 6 desaturase which is involved in the production of PGE1. It works synergistically with pyridoxine in this and many other reactions.
- Magnesium is necessary for the actions of PTH and 1,25 DHCC in bone calcium mobilization.

## IV. Requirements

The average intake of magnesium by so called healthy adults in the U.S. and Western Europe ranges between 143-266mg/day. *In 1985 the average adult American man consumed 329mg/day and woman 207mg/day.* Paleolithic diets probably contained 600-800 mg of magnesium per day. High intakes of calcium, vitamin D, and protein increase the requirement for magnesium. Vitamin D, lactose and HCL all act to enhance absorption.

**RDA** males–350mg/day

**RDA** females–280mg/day; pregnancy and lactation 350mg/day

*Optimal daily intake* – 600-800mg/day

**Progressive decline in dietary intake in the USA of magnesium over the past century**

From Magnesium deficiency in the pathogenesis of disease, New York: Plenum Press, 1980

| Years | Magnesium intake (mg per day) |
|---|---|
| 1900-1908 | 475-500 |
| 1909-1913 | 415-435 |
| 1915-1929 | 385-398 |
| 1935-1939 | 360-375 |
| 1947-1949 | 358-370 |
| 1957-1959 | 340-360 |
| 1965-1976 | 300-340 |
| 1978-1985 | 225-318 |
| 1987-1992 | 175-248 |

## V. Sources

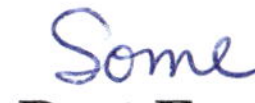

**Best Food Sources for Magnesium**

| Food | amount | mg | Food | amount | mg |
|---|---|---|---|---|---|
| Soybean flour | 1 c | 310 | Mendocino Sparkling Water | 2 c | 56 |
| Buckwheat flour | 1 c | 246 | Avocado | 1/2 med | 56 |
| Cereal, raisin bran | 3 oz | 144 | Baked potato w/skin | 1 med | 55 |
| Soybeans, dried | 1/4 c | 138 | Oat bran | 1/4 c (25g) | 55 |
| Whole wheat flour | 1 c | 136 | Navy beans, cooked | 1/2 c | 54 |
| Tofu, firm | 1/2 c | 118 | Watermelon 1"x10" diameter | 1 slice | 53 |
| Cherrios | 3 oz | 117 | Acorn squash, baked | 1/2 c | 53 |
| Rye | 1 c | 102 | Millet, cooked | 1/2 c | 53 |
| Figs, dried | 5 med | 100 | Bread, whole wheat | 2 slices | 52 |
| Black-eyed peas, cooked | 1/4 c | 98 | Cocoa powder | 2 T | 52 |
| Chard, Swiss | 1 c | 96 | Molasses, black strap | 1 T | 52 |
| Almonds, whole | 1/4 c | 96 | Sweet potato w/skin | 1 med | 50 |
| Cashews, roasted | 1/4 c | 89 | Oatmeal | 1 c | 50 |
| Rice, brown cooked | 1 c | 84 | Wheat bran | 2 T (10g) | 49 |
| Kidney beans, dried | 1/4 c | 82 | Tomato sauce | 1 c | 47 |
| Filberts | 1/4 c | 82 | Okra, cooked | 1/2 c | 47 |
| Lima beans, dried raw | 1/4 c | 81 | Kiwi fruit | 2 med | 46 |
| Halibut, baked | 3 oz | 78 | Spinach, fresh | 1 c | 44 |
| Brazil nuts | 1/4 c | 78 | Beans, garbanzo | 1/2 c | 40 |
| Pecans | 1/4 c | 77 | Potato, baked w/o skin | 1 med | 39 |
| Kelp | 2 T (10g) | 76 | Peas, green | 3/4 c | 35 |
| Peanuts | 1/4 c | 67 | Squash, winter | 1 c | 34 |
| Shredded wheat | 1/2 c | 67 | Milk, 2% | 1 c | 33 |
| Walnuts, chopped | 1/4 c | 60 | Collards, cooked | 1/2 c | 33 |
| Chocolate chips, semi-sweet | 1/4 cup | 58 | Grapefruit juice | 1 c | 30 |
| Banana | 1 med | 58 | Brewer's yeast | 2 T | 23 |
| Beet greens, raw, chopped | 1 c | 58 | | | |

From USDA: Composition of Foods. USDA handbook # 8 Washington DC, ARS, USDA, 1976-1986

## VI. Deficiency

Magnesium deficiency is very common in the West, since magnesium is found predominantly in whole unprocessed foods. Deficiency symptoms include fatigue, irritability, weakness, muscle tightness or spasms, dysmenorrhea, high blood pressure, cardiomyopathy, nerve conduction problems, anorexia, insomnia, sugar cravings, poor nail growth, anxiety.

Magnesium deficiency may be caused by any condition which increases loss or shifts the electrolyte balance, (such as renal disease) or diuretic therapy (such as antihypertensive medications). A magnesium deficiency has been found to lower cellular potassium and a depletion of potassium reduces cellular magnesium both in bone and muscles. Malabsorption, hyperthyroidism, pancreatitis, kwashiorkor, diabetes, parathyroid gland disorders, poor intake, and diarrhea may also cause a deficiency.

## VII. Therapeutics

1) **Constipation**–400mg-800mg (higher dosages can be used for significant pathologies such as megacolon or MS)

2) **Muscle cramping**–1 gm IM 2x per week for 2-3 weeks–is effective for both skeletal and smooth muscle cramping. This also works for esophageal spasms.

3) **Torticollis**–for acute conditions use IV (IM may work but not as effectively as IV). If the condition is chronic, use orally. Bowel tolerance is the rate limiting factor.

4) **Acute angina or after a myocardial infarction**– Dr. Mildred Selig has reviewed the most efficacious protocols for the treatment of MI with magnesium(see magnesium under cardiovascular disease). For further information, contact: *Dr. Mildred Selig; 1076-F North Jamestown Dr.; Decatur, GA 30033 (404) 329-1916.*

STUDY–Morten & Rasmussen, et al. *Magnesium in the treatment of MI.* Drugs *46:347-59, 1993.* ABSTRACT–Magnesium needs to be given IV immediately during an MI to work effectively. In 76 patients with MI there was a decrease mortality rate of 55% of the patients treated with magnesium IV.

STUDY–Rasmussen, H.S., et al. *Intravenous magnesium in acute myocardial infarction.* Lancet 1:234, 1986. ABSTRACT–In a double blind placebo-controlled study, 273 patients with suspected acute MI's were randomized to receive either magnesium chloride (MgCl) intravenously or placebo, immediately on admission to the hospital. The Mg group was given 50 mmol of elemental Mg (as Mg chloride) during the first 24 hours and an additional 12 mmol during the second 24 hours. Of the 130 patients with proven MI, 56 received Mg and 74 received placebo. During the first 4 weeks after treatment, mortality was 7% in the Mg group and 19% in the placebo group. This represents a 63.2% reduction in mortality in the Mg gp. In the Mg group, 21% of the patients had arrhythmias that required treatment, compared to 47% in the placebo group. There were no side effects attributable to Mg therapy.

5) **Stroke-**Perfusion of magnesium into the brain may prevent tissue damage by preventing small vessel spasm (Bella & Burton Altura, see tape).

6) **Asthma**–give orally as a prophylactic or, in acute situations, administer IV. Some studies have shown that the trabecular bone structure depends upon magnesium. Thus, even if the bone density looks good on a bone scan, the trabecular structure may be deficient if there is a magnesium deficiency.

7) **Kidney stone prevention**–especially effective when taken along with vitamin B-6.

8) **Dysmenorrhea**–give orally as a prophylactic, or in acute situations administer IV.

9) **Premenstrual syndrome**–70% of women with PMS are deficient in magnesium. It decreases sugar and chocolate cravings.

10) **Acute gastrointestinal spasms or cramping**–must give IV

11) **Eclampsia**–give 2gms magnesium sulfate IV along with 50mg of pyridoxine

12) **Heart disease, especially cardiomyopathy**–Sudden Death Ischemic Heart Disease may be particularly sensitive to magnesium deficiency, especially when excessive stress may be depleting magnesium levels. It has been found that the incidence of CVD rises in areas with softer drinking water (implying magnesium levels are low). Magnesium raises HDL levels.

13) **Diabetes mellitus**–especially IV to enhance delivery of nutrients to starved tissues

14) **Nocturnal muscle cramping**

15) **Mitral valve prolapse**–magnesium may improve the symptoms.

16) **Toxemia of pregnancy**–1-2 grams along with B-6 (may need to give IV).

17) **Panniculofibrositis or fibromyalgia**–give orally or IV along with other nutrients.

**18 Migraine headache**–it works best when given IV while the migraine is occurring, but can be used orally to prevent migraines. Can use up to 2 to 4 grams with caution.

**19) Lead toxicity**–magnesium inhibits the uptake of lead.

**20) Fatigue**–try especially if no reason for the fatigue can be found. Magnesium is concentrated in the mitochondria which generate ATP. Lead poisoning may retard mitochondria function.

**Miscellaneous treatments**–Magnesium tends to inhibit cravings for chocolate, may enhance athletic performance, protect against spasms, and mitigate anxiety and irritability.

## VIII. Interactions/Miscellaneous

- Thiazide diuretics increase urinary excretion of magnesium, however potassium spar ing diuretics also spare magnesium.
- Calcium generally competes with magnesium for absorption across the mucosa membrane, although smaller amounts enhance absorption.
- Other medications that may induce magnesium deficiency are:
  Antibiotics such as gentamicin, cargenicillin and amphotericin B;
  Chemotherapeutic drugs (cis platinum, vinblastine, and bleomycin);
  Cyclosporin used to prevent organ transplant rejection;
  Corticosteroids such as cortisone;
  Asthmatic medications;
  Alcohol;
  Laxatives, especially if they are used for a long time and cause loose stools.
- Magnesium is synergistic when given with vitamin B-6. It may be helpful in the prevention of kidney stones.
- Aspirin may work in part by increasing magnesium retention.
- There are slow release magnesium formulas, Slo-mag® and Omni Mag-Lo-Plex® (Omnivite Nutrition), that may be helpful in elevating the intracellular levels of magnesium. People with kidney failure must be cautious about magnesium supplementation since they may experience toxicity symptoms.

## IX. Toxicity

The biggest problem with magnesium is diarrhea. Too much magnesium can actually lead to a magnesium deficiency if it causes chronic diarrhea. Magnesium also competes with calcium and can induce a calcium deficiency if calcium intake levels are already low. About 800mg of elemental magnesium will generally cause loose stools, although some people may be able to tolerate much higher doses. Different forms of magnesium, such as magnesium glycinate, may be tolerated differently as well.

Intravenous magnesium, because of its effect on smooth muscles, may cause hypotension along with dizziness and fainting. It may also cause respiratory depression or depletion of potassium.

Intramuscular injections can often be painful and may cause a persistent lump if injection does not go deep enough to reach the muscle tissue. After the magnesium is loaded into the syringe a small amount of 2% lidocaine can be drawn into the tip of the syringe to ease the reaction.

# PHOSPHORUS

Phosphorus is the second most abundant mineral in the body after calcium. 80% of our bodily phosphorus resides in calcium phosphate crystals in the bone and teeth. Serum levels of phosphorus are closely maintained by parathyroid activity.

## I. Chemistry

Phosphorus is involved with many different reactions in the body, specifically the Kreb's cycle and glycolysis in the oxidative phosphorylation reactions, which generate energy molecules in the form of ATP.

## II. Metabolism

A 1:1 intake ratio between calcium and phosphorus is ideal for the maximum absorption of calcium. In older children and adults, the absorption rate is 50-80%. Infants absorb more than 85% from breast milk, and somewhat lower amounts from cow's milk. Most people maintain phosphorus levels in the serum within a very tight range. The adult absorption range is between 50-75%. Stimulation of adrenals, PTH, cortisone, and estrogen inhibits the function of phosphorus.

## III. Function

- Besides its structural role in the teeth and bony skeleton, phosphorus has numerous functions in the body.
- It is an essential component of nucleic acids and phospholipids, which are key components in the formation of cell membranes.
- Phosphorus is used in the body during glycolysis and oxidative phosphorylation to synthesize ATP, which is the major energy compound used by the body.
- Cyclic AMP is another intermediary compound, which is a cornerstone for the regulation of many metabolic processes in the body.
- Phosphorus is part of some conjugated proteins, such as casein in human milk. It is also part of the phosphate buffering system inside cells.

## IV. Requirements

Ideally, phosphorus should be ingested at a one to one ratio with calcium. The average intake in the U.S. is around 1600 mg per day. Food additives may contribute as much as 30% of total phosphorus intake per day. Generally, we consume twice as much phosphorus as we really need. Carbonated beverages, which make up as much as 20% of the total phosphorus intake, should be excluded. Vitamin supplements which contain phosphorus should also be excluded.

*Optimal daily intake* – 1000mg/day

## V. Sources

**Best Food Sources of Phosphorus**

Meat, poultry, fish and eggs rank at the top of the list.

From USDA: Composition of Foods. USDA handbook # 8 Washington DC, ARS, USDA, 1976-1986

| Food | Amount | mg | Food | Amount | mg |
|---|---|---|---|---|---|
| Cheese, Swiss | 3 oz | 650 | Tofu | 1/2 cup | 239 |
| Cheese, American | 3 oz | 635 | Milk, 2% | 1 cup | 232 |
| Ham | 6 oz | 630 | Pizza | 1 med slice | 216 |
| Grilled cheese sandwich | med | 531 | Split pea soup | 1 cup | 213 |
| Cheese, cheddar | 3 oz | 445 | Ice milk, soft serve | 1 cup | 202 |
| Macaroni & cheese | 1 cup | 322 | Almonds, raw | 1/4 cup | 184 |
| Milkshake, vanilla | 10 oz | 289 | Oatmeal | 1 cup | 178 |
| Sole, baked | 3 oz | 248 | Lentils, cooked | 1/2 cup | 178 |
| Tostada, beans & beef | 1 med | 247 | Cheese, cottage 2% | 1/2 cup | 170 |

## VI. Deficiency

Phosphorus is so ubiquitous in our food supply that there is little possibility of it becoming deficient in the diet. Deficiency may occur due to total parenteral nutrition, excess use of antacids (which bind phosphates), hyperparathyroidism, alcoholism or during the treatment of diabetic acidosis.

## VII. Treatment

There are a number of supplements containing phosphorus, such as phosphatidyl choline or phosphoserine, that have been used for various treatments. But, unless hypophosphatemia is present, phosphorus, by itself, is rarely indicated for the treatment of anything.

## VIII. Toxicity

Excessive phosphorus can inhibit calcium absorption and lead to problems such as osteoporosis or other related conditions related to calcium deficiency.

### Notes

---

# CALCIUM

- Calcium makes up 1.5%-2% of total body weight. 99% of this is in the bone and teeth. It is the most abundant mineral in the body.
- Increased levels of calcium in the blood increase calcitonin. This, in turn, increases calcium deposition in the bone and decreases calcium absorption.
- Decreased levels of calcium in the blood increase PTH. This causes increased calcium absorption from the gut and increases calcium resorption from bone.
- Vitamin D is intimately involved with calcium metabolism, regulating absorption, excretion and retention in the bone.

## I. Chemistry

Calcium absorption is regulated by a number of factors. Certain substances, such as oxalates and phytates, can interfere with its absorption. Oxalates are found in dark green leafy vegetables such as spinach and rhubarb. Fewer oxalates are found in other green leafy vegetables.

Phytates are found in whole grains, seeds, nuts and legumes. Phytase is an enzyme naturally found in these foods that breaks down phytates rendering them harmless. Sprouting, leavening, or gentle heating activates the phytase enzymes and allows them to break down phytates. Soaking the grains will also naturally aid in the activation of the phytase enzyme. Phytic acid may have a beneficial effect in preventing dental caries.

## II. Metabolism

Calcium is mainly absorbed in the duodenum. The more acidic the pH, the greater the absorption. At best, 30% of calcium is absorbed and sometimes as little as 4%, especially if a person is in an achlorhydria or hypochlorhydria state. Among people over 60 years of age it is estimated that 1/3 of the population is achlorhydric! This means that the majority of people over 60, who are at the greatest risk for osteoporosis, at least, have a deficiency of HCL. Almost half of post-menopausal women are achlorhydric. This means that most women should be taking some form of solubilized calcium. If they can be shown to have normal levels of HCL, they can get by with some of the cheaper forms of calcium such as calcium carbonate.

### Factors affecting calcium absorption

The form of the calcium, both in ingredients (lactose, citrate carbonate) and how it is taken (tablet or capsule, liquid or powder) has an effect on how well it is absorbed.

Decreased HCL, oxalates, phytates, excess magnesium, and malabsorption are all factors which may decrease the absorption of calcium.

### Forms of calcium

Calcium is found as citrate malate, citrate, aspartate, ascorbate, carbonate, gluconate, dolomite, bone meal, amino acid chelates, lactate etc. Different forms of calcium are absorbed at different rates. The pH of the stomach will determine how well they will be absorbed. The ionized forms of calcium, such as citrate and citrate malate, tend to be more soluble and have a greater absorption rate–especially in people who are deficient in HCL. From another prospective, it should be noted that different calcium compounds may be made up of varying % elemental calcium. For example, calcium citrate is composed of 16% calcium whereas calcium carbonate is made up of 40% elemental calcium. In terms of patient compliance in reaching recommended amounts, it may be most prudent to take in mixed forms of calcium so long as they are not contaminated with lead.

**Regulation of calcium in the body**

The body regulates calcium levels in the serum very carefully. Vitamin D is an essential factor which has different forms, depending upon what the brain is reading as levels of serum calcium. The level of calcium in the blood determines which of 2 hormones gets released.

- **PTH**–in response to low levels of calcium in the blood, PTH is released to stimulate the hydroxylation of 25 hydroxycholecalciferol into the 1,25 DHCC form. This causes an increased absorption from the gut and an increase in bone resorption.
- **Calcitonin**–stimulates hydroxylation of 25 HCC into the 24 position producing 24,25 DHCC which in turn decreases absorption from the gut and increases bone deposition.

## III. Function

- Calcium is intimately involved in the structures of bone and teeth where 99% of it is stored. Calcium ions add hardness to the bone matrix.
- Calcium aids transport across cell membranes. Muscles require calcium to function in their contractility. Without calcium, the muscles tend to stay contracted. Calcium also regulates membrane stabilization. Certain cells (mast cells) tend to rupture when calcium ions are depleted. In addition, neurotransmitters at synaptic junctions are regulated by calcium. This may have an effect on such states as anxiety, insomnia and other stress conditions.
- Like striated muscle throughout the body, the heart requires calcium for proper contractility. An increase in serum calcium can cause tetany, leading to cardiac or respiratory failure.
- Ionized calcium initiates the formation of blood clotting by stimulating the release of thromboplastin from the platelets. It is also a cofactor in the conversion of prothrombin to thrombin, which aids in the polymerization of fibrinogen to fibrin.
- As previously mentioned, calcium is responsible for maintaining proper contractility of smooth and skeletal muscles.

## IV. Requirements

**RDA**–800mg/day (adults 25-50); 1200mg (males & females 11-24); 400mg (0-1/2 infants); 600-800mg (children 1/2-10) Recently (1998) the National Acad of Science has recommended that people age 19-51 should consume 1000mg per day and people over 60 should take in 1200mg.

**Pregnant and lactating females**–1200mg/day

**LAB**–Calcium in the serum is not a good indicator of intracellular levels of calcium. Hair analysis may offer a general idea but has not been shown to be consistent or accurate.

*Optimal daily intake*–500mg-1500mg. This depends on the total intake of minerals, protein, phosphorus, magnesium, phytates, oxalates, and level of exercise, among other factors. Paleolithic diets probably contained 1500 - 2000ms/day.

**NOTE**–It has been found that the people in Gambia and Jamaica consume calcium at less than half of the RDA. Yet, their relative risk for osteoporosis is much less than many areas in the world where calcium intake is much higher.

STUDY–Hegsted J. of Nut. 116:2316, 1986 This study found ↑ protein intake ↑ osteoporosis.

## V. Sources

### Best Food Sources of Calcium

| Food | amount | mg Ca | mg Phos | Food | amount | mg Ca | mg Phos |
|---|---|---|---|---|---|---|---|
| Cheese, Gruyere | 3 oz | 860 | 450 | Edensoy, extra fortified | 1 cup | 167 | 120 |
| Cheese, mozzarella | 3 oz | 621 | 405 | Cheese, cottage 2% | 1 cup | 155 | 525 |
| Cheese, cheddar | 3 oz | 612 | 405 | Dandelion, greens cooked | 1/2 cup | 147 | 44 |
| Cheese, American | 3 oz | 525 | 405 | Swiss chard | 1 cup | 138 | 40 |
| Turnip greens, cooked | 1 cup | 492 | 100 | Molasses, blackstrap | 1 T | 137 | 15 |
| Torula yeast | 1 oz | 490 | 2000 | Soy flour, full fat | 1/2 cup | 132 | 280 |
| Lambs quarters, cooked | 1 cup | 400 | 100 | Rice Drink, Pacific, fortified | 1 cup | 120 | 80 |
| Sardines, with bones | 3 oz | 372 | 424 | Mustard greens, cooked | 1 cup | 104 | 60 |
| Collard greens, cooked | 1 cup | 357 | 50 | Almonds | 1/4 cup | 92 | 250 |
| Rhubarb, cooked | 1 cup | 348 | 55 | Beans, baked | 1/2 cup | 64 | 180 |
| Yogurt | 1 cup | 345 | 99 | Filberts | 1/4 cup | 60 | 90 |
| Milk, skim & 2% | 1 cup | 300 | 240 | Orange | 1 med | 52 | 25 |
| Spinach, cooked | 1 cup | 276 | 65 | Halibut | 3 oz | 51 | 200 |
| Oatmeal, fortified | 1 cup | 208 | 178 | Kale, cooked | 1 cup | 47 | 18 |
| Rice Drink, Westbrae, fort. | 1 cup | 200 | 80 | Spinach, fresh | 1 cup | 44 | 15 |
| Salmon, canned w/bones | 3 1/2 oz | 185 | 400 | Tahini, toasted sesame paste | 2T=15gms | 42 | 240 |
| Tofu, firm (about 2/3 cup) | 6.1oz | 190 | 170 | Garbonzo beans, chick peas | 1/2 c cook | 40 | 138 |
| Broccoli, cooked | 1 cup | 180 | 120 | Sesame seeds (varies) | 3T=24gms | 33 | 160 |
| Ice cream, vanilla | 1 cup | 176 | 125 | | | | |

From USDA: Composition of Foods. USDA handbook # 8 Washington DC, ARS, USDA, 1976-1986

**NOTE**–Calcium supplements may contain significant quantities of lead. Years ago it was found that dolomite and bone meal had high levels of lead. More recent studies have found that other sources, such as carbonate and other chelated forms, may also contain lead. The more refined forms tend to eliminate lead during processing.

## VI. Deficiency

A lack of calcium may cause osteoporosis and/or osteomalacia. Other symptoms related to a deficiency are tetany or other muscle spasms. These usually occur in the legs. However, they may also occur in the blood vessels and may lead to hypertension.

Periodontal disease, hyperactivity, anxiety, insomnia, and lead toxicity may also be associated with a calcium deficiency. *Pica*, a craving for nonfood items such as clay, ice, dirt, paint, paste which sometimes occurs in women and children, is a sign of calcium deficiency. However, it can also occur due to a zinc deficiency. In children who are deficient in vitamin D, rickets may occur. In adults, this condition is called *osteomalacia*.

Decreased intake, blood loss (both internal and external), menorrhagia, lead toxicity, and malabsorption are all factors that can lead to calcium deficiency.

## VII. Therapeutics

1) **Osteoporosis**–1-2gms/day–From a practical standpoint, using a combination of calcium citrate, citrate malate, aspartate, and carbonate works best. Citrate and citrate malate forms of calcium have shown promise of greater absorption in some studies, but they are only 18-20% calcium by weight (so you need to take a lot of capsules or tablets to get significant amounts). The dose depends upon how much protein, phosphorus, and acidic foods a person ingests. It also depends upon how much HCL is being secreted from the stomach. Generally, it is a good idea to take at least half as much magnesium with the calcium. Some believe equal amounts of magnesium and calcium may be best because of the lack of magnesium in most diets. Calcium reduces aluminum absorption which may cause osteomalacia. The ideal dose depends on many factors including: total intake of protein, trace minerals, vitamin K, magnesium, acid and basic ash foods, and numerous other nutritional and hormonal factors.

2) **Hypercholesterolemia**–1-2gms/day–It may take several months before any effect is seen. The literature shows very little to support this, but one study came up with fairly good results.

3) **Hypertension**–1-2gms/day–Evidence here is well supported. It may take 6-8 weeks to take effect. This effect has been shown in pregnancy, children, and in both male and female adults. The most significant effect is on people who are salt-sensitive hypertensive.

4) **Blood clotting**–Problems with blood clotting may arise in people who are very deficient in calcium. This is especially a problem for people undergoing renal dialysis.

5) **Periodontal disease**–This condition is one of the signs of low calcium levels in the tissues.

6) **Insomnia**–500-1000mg taken at bedtime.

7) **Smooth & skeletal muscle relaxant**
   - Dysmenorrhea along with PMS
   - Restless leg syndrome
   - Arthritis

8) **Anxiety**–1-2gms/day

9) **Hyperactivity**–1-2gms/day

10) **Depression, especially post menopausal**

11) **Lead toxicity**–Calcium has been shown to inhibit lead toxicity by competing with lead for binding sites in the bones; thus, higher levels of calcium intake inhibit bone uptake of lead.

12) **Prevention of calcium oxalate stones**–Use the calcium citrate form. Citrate reduces urinary saturation of calcium oxalate and calcium phosphate which, in turn, reduces the precipitation of calcium, the cause of calcium oxalate stones.

13) **Prevention of colon cancer** by binding onto endotoxins.

## VIII. Toxicity

**CI–Asthma** potentiates phospholipase $A_2$, which breaks down cell membranes and releases arachidonic acid. This eventually converts into leukotrienes of the 4 series, which have tremendous bronchoconstriction effects.

**Kidney stones**–There may be a concern if very high levels are ingested. Citrate forms of calcium actually inhibit stone formation.

## IX. Interactions

**Thyroid**–Excess thyroid hormones, specifically $T_4$, have been shown to cause bone loss, if given inappropriately, by causing excessive excretion of calcium.

**Digoxin**–if given without magnesium, may exacerbate digoxin toxicity.

**Tetracyclines** inhibit calcium absorption and vice versa.

**Corticosteroids** are well known to cause osteoporosis and calcium loss.

Calcium may be a factor in magnesium, iron, and zinc deficiency, if given in high doses. It may also interfere with other minerals such as manganese.

### Notes

---

# IRON

- Iron was first recognized as a body constituent in 1713 and as a dietary essential in the 1860's.
- Approximately 3-5gms are present in the body with about 1/3 found in storage form in the liver, spleen and bone marrow.
- The other 2/3 is found in functional forms, primarily as hemoglobin and, to a small extent, in myoglobin.

## I. Chemistry

Iron is transported in the bloodstream bound to a protein called *transferrin*. *Ferritin*, another iron containing substance, is also found in the bloodstream as well as in tissues such as the bone, liver, spleen and muscle. Ferritin levels parallel the storage of iron in the body. It is used as an indirect measurement of tissue supplies of iron. The degree of saturation of transferrin is also used as a measurement of body stores of iron.

**Ferric vs. ferrous iron**–reduced iron or ferrous iron is much more effectively absorbed.

**Heme vs. non-heme**–Absorption of heme iron is about 10x that of non-heme iron depending on whether body stores are replete.

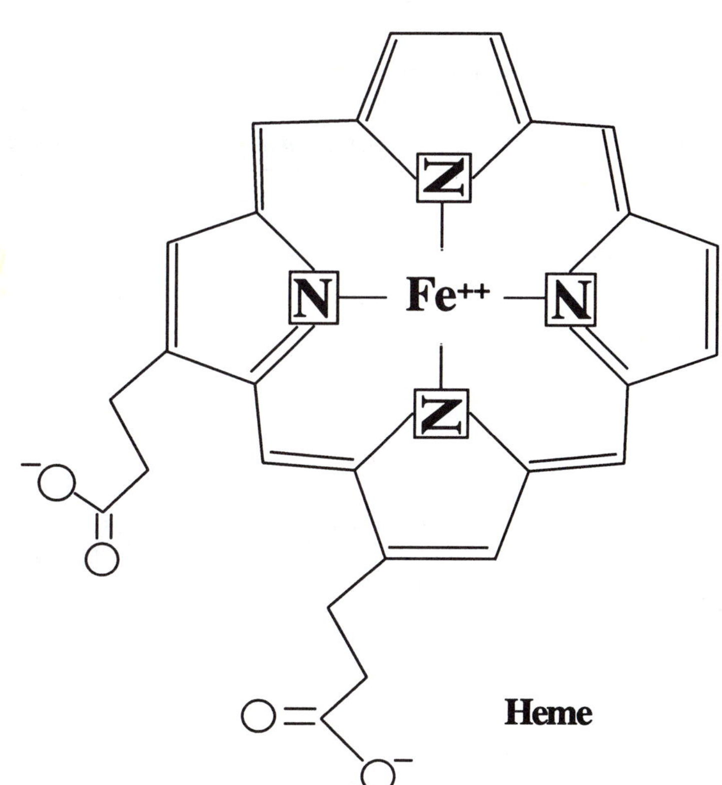


## II. Metabolism

Iron is absorbed from the intestines in different forms. When iron is found in meat, it is in the heme form. When the source of iron is from plants or from animal products such as milk, eggs and cheese, it is referred to as non-heme iron. In the heme form, once it is cleaved from the food, iron is directly absorbed intact into the blood.

In the non-heme form, iron must be cleaved from its food source, then reduced from the ferric to the ferrous form before it can be absorbed. This chemical change takes place with the help of HCL from the stomach or from vitamin C found in foods. Absorption takes place mostly in the upper part of the small intestine. The reduced iron or ferrous form must then be *chelated* to an amino acid so that it can be readily absorbed across the intestinal mucosa.

Iron is transported within the mucosal cell by transferrin. Transferrin is usually saturated to about 1/3 of its total iron binding capacity (TIBC). If no iron is needed, then transferrin remains saturated and less is absorbed from the intestinal mucosal cells. The transferrin that remains in the cells eventually gets sloughed away with the mucosal cells at the end of their 2-3 day life cycle. If iron is needed, the transferrin is less saturated when it reaches the intestinal mucosal cells and more iron passes from the mucosal cell to the transferrin.

Excretion of iron takes place through bleeding. It may also be excreted via the feces, sweat, and normal exfoliation of hair, skin and nails in very small amounts, usually between 0.9mg-1.2mg/day. Most iron expelled in the feces is lost through non-absorbed iron from the diet.

In menstruating women, however, iron losses are considerably greater, and vary widely from individual to individual.

| Factors that enhance Fe absorption | Factors that inhibit absorption of Fe |
|---|---|
| Vitamin C | Oxalates |
| Fructose | Tannins |
| Citric acid & fumarate | Phytates |
| Protein | Carbonate |
| Lysine | Phosphate |
| Histadine | Fiber (but not cellulose) |
| Cysteine &/or methionine | Hypo or achlorhydria |
| MFP (meat, fish and poultry) factor | Protein deficiency |
| EDTA & NTA | High iron stores |
| Natural chelation such as amino acids & heme | Infection or inflammation |
| Enhanced RBC synthesis associated with hypoxia & hemolysis, hemorrhage, androgens, cobalt salts, low iron stores, genetic effects as in hemochromatosis | Excess metal ions $Co^{+2}$, $Cu^{+2}$, $Zn^{+2}$, $Cd^{+2}$, $Mn^{+2}$, $Pb^{+2}$ |

## III. Function

- Iron is metabolized.
- Iron makes up heme which is a component of hemoglobin, an essential compound which transports oxygen.

## IV. Requirements

**RDAs**–18mg per day for females; males need 10mg/day
Infants require 1mg/kg body weight
6 months-3yrs need 10mg/day

**ODI**–0-60mg/day; is extremely variable depending on the individual
The age, sex, hormonal balance and genetic factors all play a role in determining the optimal levels. *It should be remembered that as many as one person in twelve may be heterozygous for hemochromatosis.*

## V. Sources

**Best Food Sources of Iron**

| Food item | amount | mg Fe | % absorb | Food item | amount | mg Fe | % absorb |
|---|---|---|---|---|---|---|---|
| Beef liver | 3 oz | 7.5 | 30.0 | Cocoa powder | 2 T | 1.5 | |
| Tofu | 1/2 c | 6.7 | | Peas cooked | 1/2 c | 1.5 | |
| Black strap molasses | 1 T | 5.0 | | Collard greens | 1 c cook | 1.5 | |
| Amaranth, cooked | 1 oz=2/3 c | 4.0 | | Beet greens | 1/2 c | 1.4 | |
| Oysters | 1 oz | 3.8 | | Brewers yeast | 1 T | 1.4 | |
| Lentils, cooked | 1/2 c | 3.3 | | Quinoa, cooked | 1 oz=2/3 c | 1.3 | |
| Swiss chard | 1 c | 3.2 | | Teff, cooked | 1 oz=2/3 c | 1.3 | |
| Ground beef | 3 oz | 3.0 | | Figs | 1/4 c | 1.3 | |
| Roast beef | 3 oz | 3.0 | | Sunflower seeds | 1/8 c | 1.3 | |
| Dulse, dried | 1/16 c=2 gm | 3.0 | | Raisins | 1/4 c | 1.3 | |
| Lima beans | 1/2 c | 2.9 | | Beans, green cook | 1/2 c | 1.2 | |
| Iron fortified formula | 8 oz | 2.9 | | Millet, cooked | 1oz=2/3 c | 1.2 | |
| Beef ground | 3 oz | 2.8 | | Shredded wheat | 1 biscuit | 1.2 | |
| Potato, baked | 1 med | 2.8 | | Whole wheat bread | 1 slice | 1.2 | 7.5 |
| Mustard greens | 1 c | 2.7 | | Lambs quarters | 1/2 c | 1.2 | |
| Wheat germ toasted | 1/4 c | 2.5 | | Prunes | 1/4 c | 1.1 | |
| Soy beans | 1/2 c | 2.5 | 5.2 | Endive or Escarole | 1 c | 1.0 | |
| Garbonzo beans, cook | 1/2 c | 2.4 | | Cod | 3 oz | 1.0 | |
| Rice white enriched | 1 c | 2.3 | 1.0 | Turkey white | 3 oz | 1.0 | |
| Pinto Beans, cooked | 1/2 c | 2.2 | | Egg | 1 large | 1.0 | |
| Kidney beans | 1/2 c dried | 2.2 | | Parsley, chopped | 1/4 c | 0.9 | |
| Turkey dark meat | 3 oz | 2.0 | 30.0 | Rye, cooked flakes | 1 oz=2/3 c | 0.9 | |
| Leeks | 1 c cooked | 2.0 | | Kelp, dried | 1/16 c=2 gm | 0.8 | |
| Dandelion greens | 1 c cooked | 1.9 | | Oats, cooked | 1 oz=2/3 c | 0.8 | |
| Apricots | 1/4 c | 1.8 | | Corn | 1/2 c 4 oz | 0.8 | 2.5 |
| Cornflakes | 1 c | 1.8 | | Frankfurter | 1 lg | 0.8 | |
| Kale | 1 c cook | 1.8 | | Peanuts | 1/4 c | 0.8 | |
| Pumpkin or squash | 2T seeds | 1.8 | | Cashew butter | 1 T | 0.8 | |
| Black beans | 1/2 c | 1.7 | 3.6 | Buckwheat, cooked | 1 oz=2/3 c | 0.7 | |
| Infant cereal | 1 T | 1.7 | | Rice | 1 oz dry | 0.7 | |
| Infant cereal rice | 1 T | 1.7 | | Pork chop | 1 med | 0.7 | |
| Spinach raw chopped | 1 c | 1.7 | 3.5 | Leaf lettuce | 1 c loose | 0.6 | 7.8 |
| Broccoli raw | 1 stalk 1/2 c | 1.7 | | Almond butter | 1 T | 0.6 | |
| Almonds chopped | 1/4 c | 1.6 | | Blueberries | 1/2 c | 0.5 | |
| Tuna | 3 oz | 1.6 | | Banana | 1 med | 0.4 | |
| Pumpkin canned | 1/2 c | 1.6 | | Raspberries | 1/2 c | 0.4 | |

USDA Handbook #8 Series Washington, DC, ARS, USDA, 1976-1986.

**NOTE**–A significant amount of iron can come from cast iron pots and pans

## VI. Deficiency

Anemia is a common result of iron deficiency. Fatigue, although popularly thought to be an early symptom of iron deficiency, has not been correlated with decreased HgB levels. Fatigue, weakness, anorexia and pica may be due to tissue depletion of iron containing enzymes and not to decreased levels of blood hemoglobin.

Iron deficiency may be the cause of symptoms such as sore tongue (glossitis), nail spooning (koilonychia), increased susceptibility to infection, brittle nails, and canker sores.

Other symptoms of iron deficiency may include hair loss, decreased endurance, impaired mental ability.

**Factors**–(See above) HCL, decreased intake, blood loss–both internal and external as in menorrhagia. Forms of calcium, both ingredient bound and in tablet or capsule form, may lead to iron deficiency.

**LAB**–Measure total iron binding capacity (TIBC), % transferrin saturation, and ferritin.

## VII. Therapeutics

1) **Anemia**–The best way to treat the anemia is slowly while monitoring the serum ferritin and % transferrin saturation. The first parameter to change will be the RBC count. This usually takes 1-3 weeks. The next change will be in the hemoglobin levels and, lastly, the ferritin. The correct ferritin level depends upon the individual. Continue supplementing or at least eating foods high in iron until the anemia is corrected.

2) **Menorrhagia**–Low levels of ferritin can actually cause the menses to be greater as a resul, it is important to build up the ferritin levels in the treatment of menorrhagia.

3) **Decreased immune function**–Low levels of iron or associated anemia can also cause problems similar to thyroid deficiency.

4) **Restless leg syndrome**

5) **Canker sores-**in cases of chronic canker sores check out ferritin levels.

6) **Glossitis-**a deficiency of iron as well as B-1 and, folate may cause glossitis.

**NOTE CONCERNING THERAPEUTICS**

Even though iron deficiency anemia is quite common in the U.S., I feel quite strongly that iron should never be prescribed unless there is a proven low ferritin level. No one, especially males who are at risk for heart disease, should take iron supplements unless lab values truly show deficient iron stores. If MCV is low normal (below 83) and ferritin in males is below 30mg/dl, then iron supplementation is indicated. Iron is indicated for females if ferritin levels are below 40 or below 60 during pregnancy. Low normal levels of ferritin (below the mean on the reference range) indicate that iron can be given safely, although this doesn't mean that supplementation is necessary. It is better to err on the side of caution by not giving iron to patients if you do not know the ferritin levels or the percentage of saturation. This is true even if hemoglobin or hematocrit levels are borderline low, especially if the patient has a normal or high MCV. If there is an inflammatory process possibly going on, a SED rate can differentiate between truly high ferritin or an acute phase reaction elevation of ferritin.

## VIII. Toxicity

10% of the population is heterozygous for hemochromatosis. Hemochromatosis is characterized by deposits of iron-containing pigments in many tissues. This results in tissue damage.

Hemosiderosis is characterized by excessive iron deposits in hemosiderin, the normal iron-storage protein. Vitamin C can potentiate this problem, so look at ferritin levels and check vitamin C intake as a possible precipitating cause.

## IX. Interactions

**Tricyclic antidepressants**–Iron deficiency induced by tricyclic antidepressants may increase symptoms of jitteriness.

**Thyroxine** can deplete iron stores.

**Ciprofloxacin**

**Neuroleptic drugs** may relieve some of the symptoms of akathisia.

# SUMMARY OF IRON ABSORPTION AND METABOLISM

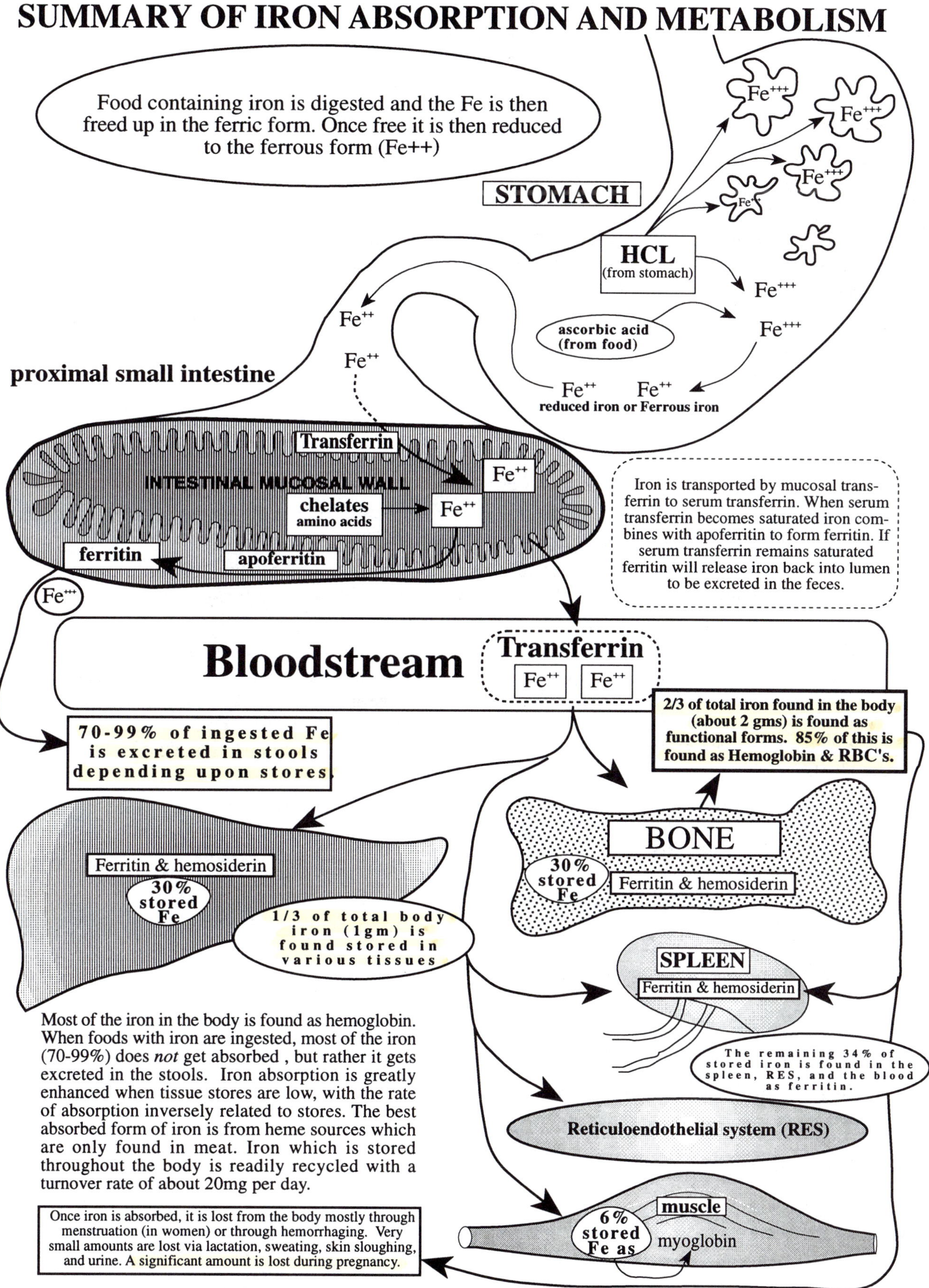


Most of the iron in the body is found as hemoglobin. When foods with iron are ingested, most of the iron (70-99%) does *not* get absorbed , but rather it gets excreted in the stools. Iron absorption is greatly enhanced when tissue stores are low, with the rate of absorption inversely related to stores. The best absorbed form of iron is from heme sources which are only found in meat. Iron which is stored throughout the body is readily recycled with a turnover rate of about 20mg per day.

Once iron is absorbed, it is lost from the body mostly through menstruation (in women) or through hemorrhaging. Very small amounts are lost via lactation, sweating, skin sloughing, and urine. A significant amount is lost during pregnancy.

# ZINC

## I. Chemistry

Zinc forms picolinate, citrate aspartate, gluconate, and oxide.

## II. Metabolism

Actively transported, zinc is regulated, in part, by sulfur containing amino acids.

Zinc absorption is enhanced by soy protein, red wine, glucose, and lactose. It is inhibited by iron, copper, and phytates.

Zinc is stored in muscle, spleen, bone marrow and liver. Both RBC'S and WBC's have high concentrations of zinc. Other tissues with high zinc concentrations are the skin, prostate, and retina (especially the macula).

## III. Function

- Zinc is involved in the synthesis of cholesterol, protein, and fats. In addition, it regulates the release of vitamin A from the liver.
- Zinc affects cell growth, especially the epithelial tissue.
- Prostate reproductive health require zinc. Zinc inhibits the activity of 5-alpha-reductase, the enzyme that irreversibly converts testosterone to dihydrotestosterone, a form of testosterone that binds most strongly to prostate tissue causing hypertrophy.

STUDY–Irving Bush and assoc. Cook County Hospital, Chicago. *Zinc and the prostate*. Presented at the annual meeting of the AMA, Chicago, 1974. ABSTRACT–19 patients took zinc sulfate–150mg (34mg elemental zinc) daily. All patients reported symptomatic improvement and 14/19 had shrinkage of the prostate, as determined by rectal palpation, X-ray and endoscopy. The supplemented group had higher levels of zinc in the semen.

STUDY–Fahim M.S., et al. *Zinc treatment for the reduction of hyperplasia of the prostate*. Fed Proc 35:361, 1976 ABSTRACT–Supplementation of zinc reduced symptoms as well as the size of BPH.

- Zinc is required for vision.
- Zinc is also needed as:
  - an antioxidant cofactor for SOD;
  - a cofactor for alcohol metabolism;
  - a cofactor for delta 6 desaturase—> PGE1 synthesis.
- Insulin function requires zinc.
- The immune system uses zinc.
- Zinc is crucial for taste perception.
- Zinc provides protection against heavy metal toxicity, such as cadmium and lead, as well as copper toxicity as in Wilson's Disease.

## IV. Requirements

**RDA**–15mg/day
**ODI**– 30-50mg/day
Average Daily Intake in the U.S.–10mg.

**Lab**–WBC levels appear to be the most accurate method of evaluating zinc status. Hair may show extreme deficiencies or excesses, but generally, like the serum, is not a very reliable indicator of zinc status. The Zinc TasteTest appears to be of some value in determining general zinc status.

## V. Sources

### Best Sources of Zinc

| Food | amount | mg | Food | amount | mg |
|---|---|---|---|---|---|
| Oysters, eastern | 1/2 c | 113 | Kidney beans | 1/2c dried | 2.2 |
| Oysters, pacific | 1/2 c | 21.0 | Ginger root | 1 oz | 2.2 |
| Beef, roast | 3 oz | 5.3 | Wild rice, cooked | 1 c | 2.2 |
| Wheat germ, toasted | 1/4 c | 4.7 | Peas, dried | 1 c | 2.2 |
| Turkey, dark meat | 3oz | 3.8 | Leeks | 1 c cook | 2.0 |
| Cheese, cheddar | 3oz | 3.3 | Lentils | 1 c | 2.0 |
| Cheese, Swiss | 3 oz | 3.3 | Cashews | 1/4th c | 2.0 |
| Swiss chard | 1 c | 3.2 | Sunflower seeds | 1/4 c | 2.0 |
| Ground beef | 3oz | 3.0 | Beans, lima | 1/2 c | 1.7 |
| Roast beef | 3oz | 3.0 | Pecans | 1/4 c | 1.6 |
| Lima beans | 1/2c | 2.9 | Tahini (sesame butter) | 1 T | 1.6 |
| Potato, baked | 1 med | 2.8 | Crab, canned | 1/4 c | 1.3 |
| Oats, rolled | 1 c | 2.8 | Peanuts | 1/4th c | 1.4 |
| Mustard greens | 1 c | 2.7 | Filberts | 1/4 c | 1.0 |
| Pumpkin seeds | 1/4 c | 2.6 | Whole wheat bread | 1 slice | 0.5 |
| Soybeans | 1/2 c/2.9 oz | 2.5 | White bread | 1 slice | 0.2 |
| Tuna | 3 oz | 2.5 | Milk, human (varies) | 1 c | .35 to 1 |
| Rice, white enriched | 1 c | 2.3 | Colostrum | 1 c | 5mg |

From USDCA Composition of Foods USDA handbook # 8 Washington DC ARS USDA 1976-1986

Food processing removes a large amount of zinc as well as other trace elements. For example, whole brown rice has more than 4x the zinc of polished white rice. Molasses has 42x more zinc than an equal amount of white sugar. Per weight, the germ part of wheat has 15x more zinc than can be found in white flour.

## VI. Deficiency

Deficiency symptoms include growth retardation (as related to protein metabolism), delayed sexual development, mild anemia, decreased taste sensation (hypogeusia), decreased or loss of sense of smell (hyposmia or anosmia), delayed wound healing, alopecia, glossitis, angular stomatitis, and diverse forms of skin lesions (including eczema, psoriasis, acne). Night blindness, associated with an inability to mobilize retinol from the liver, may also be caused by zinc deficiency.

Another classic condition that can develop, *Acrodermatitis enteropathica,* an autosomal recessive disease, is characterized by zinc malabsorption which results in eczematoid skin lesions, alopecia, diarrhea, and concurrent bacterial and yeast infections. GI malabsorption can lead to deficiency. About 25% of people who have an impairment in taste and/or smell are suffering from outright zinc deficiency.

Other symptoms that may be associated with decreased zinc include hang nails, inflammation of nail cuticles, white spots on finger nails, Beau's lines (transverse lines) and poor nail growth; impaired glucose tolerance; dandruff; arthritis; and alcoholism.

## VII. Therapeutics

**1) Rheumatoid arthritis**–Zinc is involved as an antioxidant through the enzyme superoxide dismutase. Zinc levels in patients with RA are usually reduced.

STUDY–Simkin, P.A.; *Oral zinc suphate in rheumatoid arthritis.* Lancet 2:539-42, 1976. ABSTRACT–Double blind. 12/24 patients with chronic RA received 50mg elemental zinc from sulfate 3x daily with meals for 12 weeks while the rest received placebo. Following this, all 24 patients received zinc for 12 more weeks. There were significant improvements in joint swelling, morning stiffness, walking time and subjective symptoms during the first part of the study with continued improvement in the second 12 weeks.

STUDY–Clemmensen ,O.J. *Psoriatic arthritis treated with Oral zinc suphate.* British Journal of Derm. :103:411-15, 1980. ABSTRACT–Double blind 24 patients with negative tests for rheumatoid factors, LE cells and ANA experienced reduction in signs and symptoms of RA following supplementation with zinc sulfate 220mg 3x per day for 6 weeks. At the end of this period of time serum immunoglobulins decreased and serum albumin increased. Joint pains were significantly reduced following the initial study. In a subsequent 24 week trial morning stiffness and improvement in overall condition was significant. The psoriatic lesions did not change.

**2) Immune enhancing, increase T cell function**–Low levels of zinc are associated with a drop in T cell functions. It has also been found that when the elderly are given low dose zinc sulfate supplements–20mg/day–they show an enhancement of thymus gland activity as demonstrated by an increase in levels of thymulin.

### Skin Damage

**3) Eczema**–30-90mg zinc picolinate. Zinc is involved as a cofactor with delta 6-desaturase in the production of PGE1. It can be used both orally and topically (zinc oxide ointment), especially in infants who have advanced inflammation of the skin.

**4) Acne**–Adolescent males have been found to have lower zinc levels than any other age group. In females it is often used with vitamin B-6.

**5) Skin damage**–Use topically or orally to enhance wound healing. Zinc may also be effective for the treatment of herpes, psoriasis, boils, furuncles, burns, etc. Burn victims can frequently become zinc deficient due to their increased requirements.

**6) Intestinal damage**–Both Crohn's disease and ulcerative colitis respond well to zinc. It may also be effective in repairing damage from parasites, c eliac disease, peptic ulcers, esophagitis, canker sores, periodontal disease etc. It can be used topically or systemically.

**7) Cervical dysplasia**–The rapidly dividing cells of the cervix are composed of epithelial cells that require zinc for their replication. When cervix tissue has depleted zinc levels, there are corresponding abnormalities in the cells.

**8) Anosmia or lack of taste sensation-**the zinc tally taste test (Metagenics or Thorne may be used to as both diagnostic test and treatment. technique

**9) Pharyngitis**–Local application in throat–Zinc lozenges have been found to be effective when locally applied to pharyngitis. It is better to use lower dosages of zinc locally to avoid nausea. Lozenges containing less than 10mg of zinc, with more frequent application are best.

STUDY–Eby, G.A., et al *Reduction in duration of common colds by zinc gluconate lozenges in a double blind study.* Antimicrob Agents Chemother 25, 20-24, 1984 ABSTRACT–23 mg of zinc gluconate lozenges were taken every 2 hours after an initial double dose. After 7 days 86% of the zinc treated patients were symptom free compared to 46% of the 28 placebo treated patients.

### Reproductive problems

**10) Prostate**–Zinc has been found to inhibit the activity of 5-alpha reductase, the enzyme that irreversibly converts testosterone to dihydrotestosterone, a form which binds more avidly to the prostrate and stimulates greater growth. It also decreases prolactin secretion by the pituitary gland, thus decreasing its binding to the prostate, both of which prevent prostatic hypertrophy.

**11) Infertility**–Zinc has been found to increase both sperm count and motility.

STUDY–Netter, A., et al. *Effect of zinc administration on plasma testosterone, dihydrotestosterone and sperm count..* Arch Androl 7, 69-73, 1981 ABSTRACT–37 men with infertility of greater than 5 years whose sperm counts were less than 25 million per ML had low blood testosterone levels. The men received 60mg of zinc sulfate per day for 45-50 days. In the 22 patients with initially low testosterone levels, their mean sperm count increased significantly from 8 to 20 million. Testosterone levels also increased and 9 out of the 22 wives became pregnant during the study. In the 15 men who had normal testosterone levels there was no further increase in testosterone levels and no pregnancies occurred even though there was an increase in sperm count.

### Toxicity exposure

**12) Lead and Cadmium toxicity**–Zinc inhibits the uptake of lead and cadmium by various tissues in the body.

**13) Copper toxicity**–Zinc is a well known antagonist to copper and can be used to treat Wilson's Disease.

**14) Cataracts**–The link between zinc deficiency and cataracts is weak. There have not been many human studies to support this claim.

STUDY–Heinity, M., et al. *Clinical and biochemical aspects of the prophylaxis and therapy of senile cataract with zinc aspartate.* Klin Monatsbl Augenheilkd 172 (5):778-83, 1978. ABSTRACT–Senile cataract glucose utilization is disturbed due to loss of activity of some key zinc dependent enzymes in the lens. Zinc supplementation improves the impaired glucose metabolism occurring in old age and prolonged administration of zinc aspartate is indicated for the prevention and treatment of senile cataracts. In the presence of magnesium deficiency magnesium should also be given.

**15) Macular degeneration**–90-120 mg zinc picolinate. Oral administration of zinc has shown improvement in vision. Intravenous administration along with selenium have demonstrated benefits in the treatment of macula degeneration. Zinc given in a lower dose in combination with *vaccinium myrtilus* might show even greater improvement .

STUDY–Newsome, D.A., et al, *Oral zinc in macular degeneration* Arch Ophthalmol 106, 192-98, 1988 ABSTRACT–This was a double blinded, placebo controlled study in which 151 elderly patients with macular degeneration were treated with either 100mg zinc or placebo. The zinc treated group had significantly more improvement than placebo over the course of 2 years. In some of the zinc taking group patients experienced loss of vision, but less loss than the placebo group.

**16) Anorexia nervosa**–There is evidence that some people with anorexia nervosa may have a zinc deficiency which may cause abnormalities in taste sensation which may lead to this eating disorder. Studies show there may be a subset population that is particularly sensitive to a deficiency. Alexander Schauss, author of *Diet Crime and Delinquency*, is one of the strong proponents of this theory.

**Miscellaneous**–Certain conditions may be related to a decrease in thyroid hormone or vitamin A. Zinc has been shown to be essential for sensitizing the tissues of the body to thyroid hormone and also responsible for releasing vitamin A from storage from the liver.

## VIII. Toxicity

Zinc at doses of 20 mg and above often causes stomach upset and/or nausea. Thus, it should always be taken with food.

Long term zinc supplementation above 50mg/day has shown to decrease HDL cholesterol and increase total cholesterol. This may be due to an induced copper deficiency. In addition copper deficiency anemia can occur as well. Zinc should always be taken with copper in a 10 to 1 through 30 to 1 zinc to copper ratio. Large doses of zinc may also promote folate deficiency.

## IX. Interactions

Copper, calcium and iron taken in large doses can interfere with zinc absorption and induce a deficiency, especially in pregnant women. People who take large doses of iron to correct anemia when they are already borderline zinc deficient can easily create a true zinc deficiency.

### Notes

---

# COPPER

- Copper was first found as a normal constituent of serum in 1875.
- It is found in highest concentrations in the brain, liver, heart, bones, teeth, and kidneys.
- Although muscle has a lower concentration, because of the large mass, the muscular system stores 40% of the copper.
- About 90% of copper in the blood is found as ceruloplasmin and the rest is bound to albumin and amino acids.

## I. Chemistry

Copper is a divalent cation. Its absorption can be inhibited by fructose and sucrose.

## II. Metabolism

Some copper can be absorbed from the stomach, but the majority is absorbed from the small intestine. It is both actively and passively transported across the intestinal mucosa. Normally about 30-50% of ingested copper gets absorbed. Fiber doesn't have the same ability to bind onto copper as zinc. Most copper is excreted via the bile.

## III. Function

- **Copper acts as a cofactor for the following enzymes:**

  **1) Cytochromic oxidase** is involved electron transport and energy production.
  **2) Dopamine β monooxygenase(previously β hydroxylase)** is involved with catecholamine synthesis in both the brain and adrenals.

**dopamine**—Dopamine β monooxygenase—**>norepinephrine**————**>epinephrine**

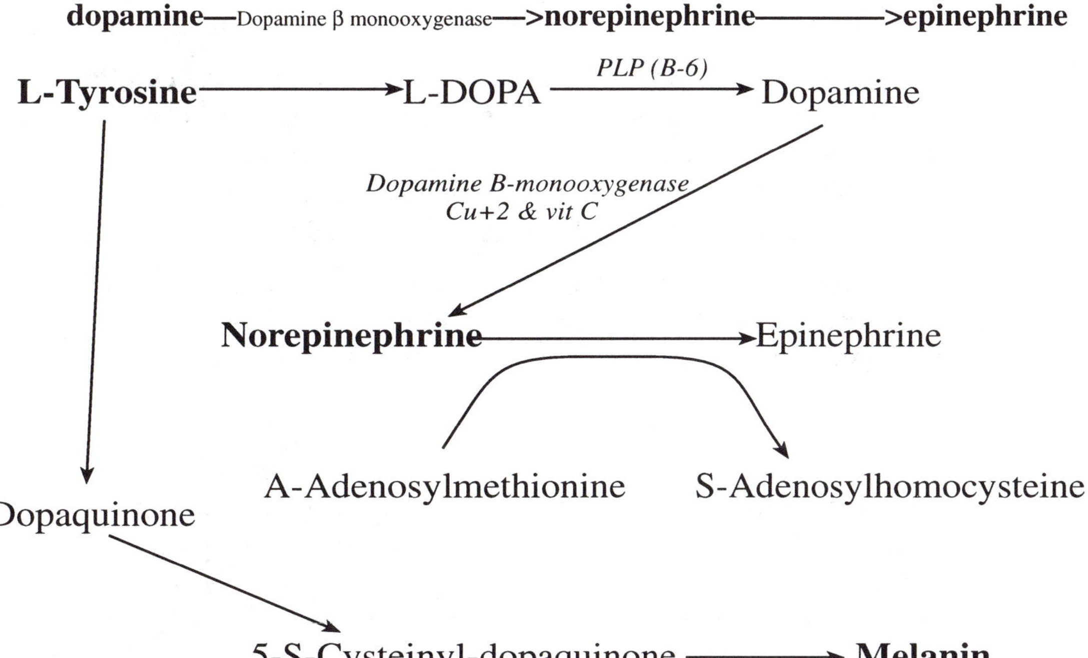

3) **Tyrosinase** is involved in melanin synthesis in the skin.
Vitamin C can potentiate problems, so control the intake of vitamin C.

**Tyrosine———————————————>melanin**

4) **Ceruloplasmin** is a broad-specificity oxidase and its main function is as an extracellular scavenger of superoxide and other oxygen radicals in copper transport and in antioxidant defense. Thus, it is intimately involved in detoxification. As a cofactor it reduces iron into the ferrous form, making it much more absorbable. It also facilitates iron availability from the liver.

**Other Functions**

- **Collagen cross linking**–Lysyl oxidase is a copper containing enzyme secreted by connective tissue cells that aid in the cross linking of elastin and collagen. This role makes copper indispensable for connective tissue repair.
- **Estrogen breakdown**–Copper is involved in the catabolism of estrogenic hormones.
- **Anti inflammatory**–During inflammatory conditions copper is increased in the serum by 20-30%. Through the action of ceruloplasmin, which acts as a radical scavenger, and superoxide dismutase (SOD), copper plays a pivotal role in decreasing inflammation. There are also copper containing amino acid chelates that have SOD activity.
- **Copper salicylate**–This compound has pronounced anti-inflammatory activity and, furthermore, was found to be healing to the stomach mucosa. The FDA took this compound off the market around 1989, but is available today through compounding pharmacists.
- **SOD**–Copper, along with zinc, is found in cytostolic superoxide dismutase enzymes that are involved with disposing of superoxide anions and ceruloplasmin. Ceruloplasmin is a weak broad specificity oxidase whose main function is to carry copper around. It is also an extracellular scavenger of superoxide and other oxygen radicals.
- **Myelin synthesis**–It is essential for the formation of the myelin surrounding the nerves.
- **Cancer inhibition–In various types of cancer serum copper and ceruloplasmin are increased. It has been shown in lab animals that dietary copper and certain copper chelates significantly inhibit chemical carcinogenesis A low copper/zinc ratio may be associated with a higher incidence of stomach cancer in humans. Linder theorizes that copper chelating agents may cause chromosomal damage in fast growing tumor cells.**
- **Cholesterol reduction**–The mechanism is unclear as to why it lowers cholesterol. If excessive zinc is ingested, cholesterol will go up. Supplementation of copper will decrease the elevated levels caused by the high zinc supplementation.

## IV. Requirements

There is no RDA for copper but the estimated safe and adequate daily dietary intake (ESADDI) for copper is from 1 to 3 mg/day. The average American gets about 1.2-1.7mg per day of copper.

**Lab**-Serum and hair levels are not very reliable. It is best to check WBC intracellular levels
Optimal daily intake-2-4 mg per day depending upon environmental exposure to copper

## V. Sources

**Best Food Sources of Copper**

| Food | Amount | mg | Food | Amount | mg |
|---|---|---|---|---|---|
| Beef liver | 3 oz | 2.4 | Millet flour | 1/2c | 0.47 |
| Rye | 1/2 cup | 0.9 | Cocoa powder | 2 T | 0.4 |
| Beans, dried | 1/2 cup | 0.9 | Prunes | 10 dried | 0.4 |
| Brazil nuts | 1/4 cup | 0.82 | Barley, raw | 1/4 cup | 0.4 |
| Cashews | 1/4 cup | 0.8 | Chicken, light meat | 3 oz | 0.4 |
| Peas, dried, cooked | 1/2 cup | 0.7 | Pecans | 1/4 cup | 0.37 |
| Molassas, black strap | 2 T | 0.6 | Banana | 1 med | 0.35 |
| Sunflower seeds | 1/4 cup | 0.6 | Peanuts | 1/4 cup | 0.22 |
| Mushrooms, raw | 1/2 cup | 0.6 | Halibut | 3 oz | 0.21 |
| Tofu, firm | 1/2 cup | 0.5 | Wheat germ | 1 T | 0.15 |
| Beans, refried | 1/2 cup | 0.5 | Apricots, dried | 1/4 cup | 0.15 |
| Almonds | 1/4 cup | 0.5 | Sesame seeds, unhulled 25 | 1 T | 0.13 |
| Wheat flour, whole | 1/2 cup | 0.47 | | | |

From USDA Composition of Foods USDA handbook # 8 Washington DC, ARS, USDA, 1976-1986

## VI. Deficiency

A deficiency of copper is not uncommon. Symptoms include hemolysis with liver and brain damage, anemia, neutropenia, degeneration of vasculature, depigmentation of skin, kinky hair, hypotonia, and hypothermia.

Copper deficiency can come from an inborn error in metabolism Known as **Menkes'**, an X-linked defect, this condition is characterized by a lack of absorption of copper from the intestine and a lack of uptake in the liver. Copper especially accumulates in the intestinal cells. All of the classic symptoms of copper deficiency, such as hemolysis with liver and brain damage, anemia, neutropenia, degeneration of vasculature, depigmentation of skin, kinky hair, hypotonia, and hypothermia, are seen with this disorder. Infants usually die due to this condition, rarely surviving to age 3.

**Anemia**–Copper is essential for the mobilization of iron from the liver. A deficiency of copper results in microcytic anemia.

## VII. Therapeutics

1) **Anemia**–microcytic anemia secondary to lack of iron absorption and mobilization from the liver. This is due to a lack of ceruloplasmin from decreased copper availability due to decreased absorption or decreased intake.

2) **Enhance Immunity**–A deficiency may cause problems with neutropenia.

3) **Vitiligo**–This inborn pigmentation problem may be a result of an increased requirement for copper which is a cofactor for *tyrosinase*, the enzyme responsible for the synthesis of melanin.

4) **Skin cancers**–Since copper is the cofactor for the enzyme tyrosinase, copper, tyrosine and vitamin B-6 may be helpful in preventing skin cancers.

5) **Prevention of Aneurysms & CVD**–Decreased copper increases the risk for heart disease. In people who have a genetic predisposition to aneurysms of the aorta, a moderate daily dose of copper may be a good idea. Copper is a cofactor for lysyl oxidase, an enzyme that is responsible for the connective tissue integrity surrounding the aorta.

6) **Stomach cancer prevention**–When the zinc/copper ratio becomes high and there is a relative copper deficiency, the rate of stomach cancer increases. Certain copper chelates may induce chromosomal damage in tumor cells, resulting in their death. In addition, it may be that chelating agents of copper help to inhibit certain cancers. Effects have also been noted on cell mediated immunity. Other observed phenomena in cancers is that the rate of copper turnover is significantly less and that ceruloplasmin actually can stimulate tumor growth. It has been found that when cancers go into remission, the levels of ceruloplasmin go back down to normal levels.

7) **PVC's**

## VIII. Toxicity

Some people have experienced nausea and vomiting with supplementation of copper which is similar to zinc toxicity. Long term supplementation may cause cirrhosis of the liver. Large doses of vitamin C may lower serum copper levels.

Copper overload may come from copper pots and pans and water that has been stored in copper pipes. The acidity or softness of the water determines how much copper goes into the water.

**Poor memory, depression, insomnia, and joint pain** are signs and symptoms of copper toxicity.

**Wilson's disease**, a copper accumulation in the liver, brain and eyes, usually manifests itself in late adolescence. Reduced excretion of copper from the body begins to cause a toxic accumulation in the liver, kidney, cornea, and CNS. A neuropsychiatric syndrome may develop from copper overload.

**Migraine headaches**–Catechol synthesis may be inhibited by copper excess and cause migraines to develop.

## IX. Interactions

### Zinc/Copper

A strong relationship exists between zinc and copper. Deficiency symptoms may manifest each way. Too much copper can cause zinc deficiency and too much zinc can lead to a copper deficiency. **Iron** can interfere with copper absorption.

### Pharmaceuticals

Non-steroidal anti-inflammatory drugs and penicillamine may cause copper deficiency. Chronic corticosteroid intake, which weakens connective tissue, may also cause a copper deficiency. Copper salicylate has good anti-inflammatory properties and is actually been found to be protective against stomach ulcers.

# POTASSIUM/SODIUM

- Sodium and potassium make up the majority of electrolytes in the body. They are the main substances responsible for maintaining fluid balance in the tissues. They also regulate transport mechanisms along cell membranes, and are responsible for maintaining membrane potential and membrane charge of mammalian cells.
- The largest dietary source of sodium comes from table salt or NaCl. Reading about salt and sodium is often confusing because the terms are often interchanged, though they really aren't the same. Sodium naturally occurs in many foods, and is often added to foods during processing and cooking.
- For millennia, salt has been our primary food seasoning and preservative; thus, it has played an important role in our history. Many wars have been fought to satisfy this need for salt. For ages, the only source of salt throughout the world was from the evaporation of sea water. This was usually done in small amounts at home.
- It wasn't until 1937 that salt was discovered to be a dietary essential.

## I. Chemistry

Both potassium and sodium are actively transported into and out of the cells of the body. They are both cations. They are very water soluble and, hence, tend to dissolve easily in cooking water. Foods cooked this way tend to be much lower in nutritional value.

## II. Metabolism

Normally 90-98% of ingested sodium is absorbed, mostly in the small intestine. Aldosterone increases the excretion of potassium. Also many diuretics increase excretion of potassium along with other minerals. Measuring sodium intake can be evaluated by measuring how much sodium is excreted in the urine in 24 hours. Normally, the amount of sodium that is required per day is around 200mg; however, losses on the average of 2200mg per day are typical in hot climates. 200mg of sodium per liter of perspiration is typical, but may vary with intake. During periods of intense sweating, when sodium levels start to decline in the blood, the kidneys will begin to retain more sodium in response to greater levels of aldosterone secreted by the adrenals. Aldosterone simultaneously increases the excretion of potassium.

## III. Function

- **Acid base balance**–Both potassium and sodium are intimately involved with acid base balance. If there is an imbalance, the heart may beat irregularly.
- **Electrical activity for nerve and muscle cell function including the heart**–Both a deficiency and an excess of potassium can cause electrical disturbances in the heart, which can lead to arrhythmias and other problems. Potassium deficiency in muscles can cause cramping and spasms in the muscles. In addition, because potassium is essential for the storage of glycogen in muscles, a deficiency can cause muscles to become fatigued and weak.

- **Water balance**–Sodium is pumped out of cells while potassium is pumped into cells. Without this active pumping of sodium out of cells, swelling of the cells occurs.
- **Kidney and adrenal function**–Sodium is intimately involved in the proper functioning of adrenals.

## IV. Requirements

**RDA:** Sodium: .5–2gms/day
Potassium: .8–5gms/day (potassium is only available at a maximum dose of 99mg)

Currently, the average American gets 3–7gms/day of sodium to only 2gms/day of potassium. This is equivalent to 12gms of NaCl of which 3gms are naturally found in food, 4gms in processed foods, and 5gms added.

**ODI**: Sodium: .5–2gms depending upon activity level.
Potassium: .5–10gms per day from food sources.

**Salt, Sodium, and Potassium Conversions**

| | |
|---|---|
| Sodium into salt (NaCl) equivalent | mg $Na^+$ x 2.5= mg of salt |
| Salt into sodium | mg of salt x .40 = mg of $Na^+$ |
| To convert mEq sodium into mg of sodium | mEq of sodium x 23 = mg of sodium |
| To convert millimoles of sodium or potassium into mg | multiply the millimoles x gm molecule wt. of $Na^+$ or $K^+$ (23 or 39) |
| $Na^+$ in mg converted to sodium in milliequivalents (dietary prescriptions are often given as milliequivalents or mEq) | mg $Na^+$ into 23 (atomic wt of sodium) = mEq $Na^+$mEq $Na^+$ x 23 = mg $Na^+$ e.g., 100mEq = 2.3gms $Na^+$ |
| 1 teaspoon salt (5gms) | 2gms sodium (salt is 40% $Na^+$) |
| To convert mEq potassium into mg | mEq potassium x 39= mg $K^+$ e.g. 10 mEq $K^+$ x 39= 390mg |

## V. Deficiency

A potassium deficiency leads to muscle weakness, fatigue, mental confusion, irritability, heart disturbances, muscle cramps, abdominal bloating and nerve conduction abnormalities.

Minimum requirements for adults
Sodium–500mg /day
Potassium–2000mg/day (this is not optimal)
(Replacement is required only in extreme sweating.)

> **NOTE**–The average intake of potassium today is about 1-3gms per day. This intake is only about 25% of what hunter/gatherers took in thousands of years ago. This means that the average ratio of sodium to potassium is 5 to 2. Ideally, this should be a 5 to 1, or even 10 to 1 ratio of potassium to sodium. Thus people should be ingesting a much higher amount of potassium in their diets, similar to what hunter/gatherers consumed.

**Lab:** Potassium RBC is the best indication of true intracellular levels. One can also do a 24 hour urine collection for both sodium and potassium to get an idea of what people are consuming.

Serum levels are a fair indicator.

# VI. Sources

### Best Sources of Potassium (along with sodium levels)

It should be noted that when potassium salts are supplemented orally symptoms of nausea, vomiting, diarrhea, and ulcers can occur. Consuming naturally occurring potassium in foods doesn't seem to cause the same side effects.

| Food | Amount | (mg) $K^+$ | (mg) $Na^+$ | Food | Amount | (mg) $K^+$ | (mg) $Na^+$ |
|---|---|---|---|---|---|---|---|
| Avocado | 1 med | 1360 | 10 | Kidney beans | 1 cup | 330 | 10-200 |
| Tomato Sauce | 1 cup | 909 | 10-1500 | Liver, beef | 3 oz | 323 | 90 |
| Apricots, dried | 1/2 cup | 896 | 18 | Artichoke | 1 med | 316 | 79 |
| Potato | 1 med | 782 | 6 | Prunes | 5 med | 315 | 1 |
| Cantaloupe | 1/2 med | 782 | 6 | Peach | 1 med | 308 | 2 |
| Papaya | 1 med | 781 | 9 | Beef, round steak | 3 oz | 298 | 46 |
| Prune Juice | 1 cup | 707 | 10 | Haddock | 3 oz | 297 | 150 |
| Figs, dried | 5 med | 666 | 10 | Spinach, cooked | 1/2 cup | 292 | 45 |
| Lima beans | 1/2 cup | 582 | 2 | Nectarine | 1 med | 288 | 0 |
| Parsnips | 1 cup | 573 | 16 | Pork | 3 oz | 283 | 48 |
| Pumpkin, cooked | 1 cup | 564 | 2 | Mustard greens | 1 cup | 283 | 22 |
| Watermelon 1"x10" dia. | 1 slice | 559 | 10 | Blackberries | 1 cup | 282 | 0 |
| Raisins | 1/2 cup | 545 | 9 | Lamb, leg of | 3 oz | 274 | 53 |
| Kiwi fruit | 2 med | 504 | 8 | Turkey, white meat | 3 oz | 259 | 54 |
| Sardines | 3 oz | 501 | 425 | Mushrooms | 1 cup | 259 | 3 |
| Flounder | 3 oz | 498 | 201 | Strawberries | 1 cup | 247 | 1 |
| Orange juice | 1 cup | 496 | 2 | Cherries | 1 cup | 239 | 17 |
| Soy beans | 1/2 cup | 496 | 2 | Orange | 1 med | 237 | 0 |
| Squash, winter | 1/2 cup | 473 | 11 | Celery | 2 stalks | 228 | 70 |
| Broccoli | 3.5 oz | 464 | 13 | Tuna | 3 oz | 225 | 70 |
| Tomato | 1 med | 444 | 13 | Peanut butter | 2 T | 220 | 150 |
| Pinto beans | 1/2 cup | 441 | 2 | Papaya | 3.5 | 211 | 3 |
| Banana | 1 med | 440 | 1 | Chicken, white meat | 3 oz<br>1 med | 201 | 54 |
| Milk, skim | 8 oz | 406 | 126 | Cashews | 1/4 cup | 194 | 4 |
| Pomegranate | 1 med | 400 | 5 | Asparagus | 4 spears | 186 | 2 |
| Eggplant | 1 cup | 397 | 5 | Rasberries | 1 cup | 186 | 0 |
| Sweet potato | 1 med | 397 | 11 | Apple | 1 med | 182 | 2 |
| Salmon | 3 pz | 378 | 99 | Cauliflower | 1/2 cup | 178 | 8 |
| Beans, great northern | 1/2 cup | 374 | 7 | Grapefruit | 1 med | 157 | 0 |
| Potato chips | 14 chips | 362 | usually 200 | Green beans | 3.5 oz | 54 | 4 |
| Cod, baked | 3 oz | 345 | 93 | | | | |

## Highest Sources of Sodium

| Food | Amount | mg | Food | Amount | mg |
|---|---|---|---|---|---|
| Lox (smoked salmon) | 3 oz | 2132 | Pork, bacon | 3 pieces | 303 |
| Anchovy paste | 1 T | 1540 | Crab | 3 oz | 280 |
| Soy sauce | 1 T | 1540 | Cherrios | 1 cup | 249 |
| Cheese, American | 3 pz | 1215 | Mustard | 1 T | 189 |
| McDonald's 1/4 w/cheese | 1 | 1209 | Saltines | 4 crackers | 156 |
| Baking soda | 1 t | 1123 | Bread, regular | 1 slice | 150 |
| Bologna | 3 slices | 1107 | Cheese, cottage | 1/4 cup | 130 |
| Corn chips | 6 oz | 1060 | Milk | 8 oz | 120 |
| Feta | 3 oz | 945 | Scallops | 1/2 cup | 111 |
| Egg McMuffin | one | 914 | Water, softened | 1/2 cup | 100 |
| Tortilla chips | 6 oz | 900 | Egg | 1 med | 70 |
| Corned beef | 3 oz | 720 | Halibut | 3 oz | 65 |
| Fried chicken | 2 legs | 792 | Salmon | 3 oz | 65 |
| Ham | 3 oz | 720 | Chicken, white meat | 3 oz | 60 |
| Bacon, Canadian | 1 slice | 537 | Turkey, white meat | 3 oz | 54 |
| Cheese, cheddar | 3 oz | 528 | Celery | 1 stalk | 50 |
| Grape Nuts | 1/2 cup | 396 | Mayonnaise | 1 T | 40 |
| Tuna | 3 oz | 384 | Venison (deer meat) | 3 oz | 40 |
| Raisin bran | 1 cup | 365 | Water, naturally hard | 1 cup | 5 |
| Baking powder | 1 t | 349 | Orange juice | 1 cup | 2 |
| Rice Crispies | 1 cup | 348 | Banana | 1 med | 1 |
| Cake, coffee | 1 slice 72g | 303 | Vegetables, most types | 1 serving | under 20 |

### Food Labeling

| | |
|---|---|
| **Sodium free** | Less than 5mg per standard serving and no sodium chloride. |
| **Very low sodium** | 35mg or less per serving. |
| **Low sodium** | 140mg or less per serving. |
| **Reduced sodium** | At least 25% less sodium than the regular food per the standard serving. |
| **Light in sodium** | 50% less sodium per standard serving than in the regular food. |
| **Unsalted** | No added salt during processing when the product it resembles is normally processed with salt. |
| **Lightly salted** | 50% less added sodium than is normally added; product must state that it is not a low sodium food if that criteria is not met. |

## VII. Etiology of Potassium Deficiency

1) **Diarrhea and/or vomiting**–GI disturbances caused by disease, parasites or food reactions can deplete potassium significantly.
2) **Diuretics**–Medications, especially anti-hypertensive medications, can deplete large amounts of $K^+$.
3) **COPD & Diabetes mellitus acidosis**–Excess loss of glucose will cause solute loss, especially in the form of $K^+$. The body, in attempt to buffer the hyperacidity, will lose $K^+$.
4) **Glucocorticoids**–Many medications, including adrenal steroid hormones, can disturb potassium levels in the body.
5) **Perspiration**–Up to 3 gms of potassium can be lost in one day from sweating. More may be lost in extreme cases–e.g. *ironman/woman* events.

## VIII. Therapeutics

**1) Hypertension**–There seems to be a significant correlation of hypertension with potassium deficiency and high sodium consumption in the diet. Since the average American has a high sodium diet, the issue is whether someone is getting enough potassium from their diet. This means that the average ratio of $Na^+$ to potassium is 15 to 2. Other cultures, such as the Chinese, Japanese, and Tibetan, have a particularly high prevalence of hypertension and stroke. This may be because they consume a diet low in potassium and somewhat high in sodium. Obesity also has the effect of making people more sensitive to $Na^+$.

STUDY–Patki, P.S., et al. *Efficacy of potassium and magnesium in essential hypertension: A double-blind, placebo-controlled, crossover study.* Br J Med 301, 521-23,1990 ABSTRACT–37 mild hypertensive adults were given 60mml/day K or placebo for 32 weeks. At the end of this period there was a significant drop in blood pressure attributed to the K. Added magnesium had no additional effect.

**2) Cancer**–Max Gerson developed a therapy which involves using large amounts of potassium-containing foods in the form of juices.

**3) Arrhythmias**–Be aware, specifically if $K^+$ is deficient or excess.

**4) Atherosclerosis**

**5) Glaucoma**–Give in the form of sodium ascorbate to bowel tolerance. This may have a significant effect. A synergistic effect of Na on the effect of Vitamin C on glaucoma has been shown.

## IX. Toxicity

### Potassium

Nausea, vomiting, and diarrhea with ulcers have been reported with high doses of supplemental $K^+$. This does not seem to occur when even very high levels are consumed through dietary means. Arrhythmias may also occur.

**Magnesium** is critical for maintaining intracellular levels of $K^+$ because it regulates the sodium/potassium ATP pump. However, if excessive supplemental intake occurs, an increased excretion of potassium can occur via the fecal route.

*The following increase the excretion, and therefore the requirement, of* $K^+$*:*

**Diuretics**–Many antihypertensive medications cause increased excretion of potassium and must therefore be supplemented with $K^+$.

**Caffeine**–Coffee and other caffeine compounds cause an increased excretion of potassium and should be limited to small amounts, especially in people with hypertension. One of the mechanisms by which caffeine may increase blood pressure, aside from increasing catecholamine release, is by decreasing the potassium to $Na^+$ ratio which is already very unbalanced.

### Sodium

Excessive sodium increases the requirement for potassium. It may cause problems with hypertension, promote renal stones, osteoporosis and congestive heart failure. Currently, essential hypertension affects 20% of adults over 40 years or age.

**Lithium** may cause an increased excretion of $Na^+$. Low sodium diets are contraindicated in people who are on lithium.

# CHROMIUM

- Walter Mertz first discovered that chromium was a trace nutrient in 1955.
- Chromium was determined to be essential for animals in 1959 by Schwarz and Mertz.

## I. Metabolism

Chromium, in its trivalent form, Cr+3, is about 10-25% absorbed. Only 1% of inorganic chromium is absorbed. Absorption comes from active transport. Amino acids keep chromium from precipitating in the small intestine where the pH is alkaline. The more acidic the milieu, the more soluble chromium becomes. Amino acids, oxalates and niacin may enhance absorption. Chromium is actively transported from the small intestine. Then it is transported via transferrin to the liver. In hemochromatosis, when transferrin is saturated, the rate of chromium excreted from the urine goes up since it can no longer bind to the transferrin.

During a carbohydrate meal, levels of chromium increase as much as 5 times in the blood. Increased intake of simple sugars, strenuous exercise, or physical trauma all elevate urinary excretion of chromium.

## II. Function

- Glucose tolerance–Chromium is involved in the production of glucose tolerance factor (GTF). This compound helps insulin bind to its proper receptors, thereby stabilizing blood glucose levels.
- Fat and cholesterol metabolism can use fairly high levels of chromium, in the range of 200-2000mcg per day. Chromium may have some synergistic effects with niacin.

## III. Requirements

**ESADDI**–50-200mcg/day
**ODI**–300-900mcg/day
*Average intake in the U.S. is estimated to be around 30mcg per day.*

## IV. Sources

Measuring chromium in both tissues and foods has been a problem because of contamination. In the past (prior to 1980) measurements of chromium have been artificially high and it is estimated that values are actually about 8 times lower than what was previously reported.

Brewer's yeast, oysters, liver, and potatoes are fairly high in chromium. Seafood, whole grains, cheeses, chicken, meats, bran, fresh fruits and vegetables are intermediate in levels. Unfortunately actual values for many foods is scant. Below is a partial list of foods containing chromium.

**Best Sources of Chromium**

| Food | Amount | µg | Food | Amount | µg |
|---|---|---|---|---|---|
| Liver, calf's | 2 oz | 55 | Cornmeal | 1 cup | 10 |
| Potato with skin, 1 med. | 200g | 48 | Brewer's yeast | 1T (8g) | 9 |
| Bread, whole grain | 2 slices 57g | 24 | Banana | 1 med | 9 |
| Pepper, green | 1 med | 23 | Spinach, cooked | 1 cup | 6 |
| Rye bread, whole grain | 2 slices | 18 | Cabbage, cooked | 1 cup | 6 |
| Carrot | 1 med | 12 | Orange | 1 med | 4 |
| Apple | 1 med | 10 | Blueberries | 1 cup | 3 |

## V. Deficiency

Chromium deficiency was first recognized in parenterally fed long term patients. Long term deficiency results in glucose intolerance, elevated cholesterol and triglycerides.

## VI. Therapeutics

### 1) Hyperglycemia

STUDY–Mertz, W. *Chromium in human nutrition: A review.* J Nutr 123, 626-33, 1993. ABSTRACT–This review article has over 15 controlled studies showing how chromium can enhance the body's ability to metabolize glucose if it is impaired.

STUDY–Canfile, W. *Chromium in nutrition and metabolism.* Shapcott D, Hubert J, eds, New York: Elsevier, p145123, 626-33, 1993. ABSTRACT–11 elderly glucose intolerant men were supplemented with GTF-chromium for 1-2 months. Average fasting glucose levels went from 106 to 99mg/dl and one hour rises went from 201mg/dl to 162 mg/dl. At 2 hours the unsupplemented group was still at 162 and the supplemented group was at 132gm/dl. Furthermore, 2 hour mean insulin levels in the unsupplemented group were at 118 whereas the supplemented group was at 83. In younger diabetic patients (n=38) average glucose levels before supplementation was at 923 and afterward went down to 817.

**2) Hypoglycemia**–Empirically chromium seems to have a stabilizing effect on blood glucose. It also seems to decrease cravings for sweets.

**3) Hypercholesterolemia**–One study found chromium to have a synergistic effect with niacin in lowering cholesterol. Much less niacin may be required to lower cholesterol.

**4) Increasing lean body mass**–There have been several studies showing that chromium picolinate increased muscle mass over a period of 21/2 months.

STUDY–Katts, G.R., Ficher, J.A., and Blum, K. *The effects of chromium picolinate supplementation on body compostition in different age groups.* Age 14 138 abstract 40, 1991. ABSTRACT–400mcg per day was found to significantly increase lean body mass in 15 patients compared to placebo and a group that was supplemented with 200mcg per day.

**5) Acne**–May be effective when acne is related to blood glucose levels Consider using chromium with *Gymnema sylvestra*.

## VII. Toxicity

Very little toxicity to chromium has been shown. Large amounts of refined sugar increases the requirement for chromium. One double blind study showed increased dream activity with diminished sleep requirements. There has been one study in animals that has shown very high doses of chromium picolinate caused some chromosomal damage.

## Notes

# SELENIUM

- Initially, selenium was thought to be a toxic element due to diseases which appeared in animals who grazed on land that had high selenium levels. "Blind staggers" and "alkali disease" can occur in cattle and sheep.
- Scattered findings of selenium deficiencies in humans and animals were reported as far back as 1295 by Marco Polo.
- Prior to 1957 symptoms of selenium deficiency were thought to be caused by a vitamin E deficiency.

## I. Metabolism

Selenium is absorbed fairly easily in the upper GI. Plant sources of selenium may be more bioavailable compared to animal sources. There is some controversy over which form of selenium is more bioavailable. Currently the literature shows that the organic and inorganic forms may have different properties.

Organic forms include selenomethionine, selenocysteine, amino acid chelates, yeast, and kelp bound selenium.

Inorganic forms include sodium selenite and sodium selenate. Some rat studies have shown that the selenite form of selenium raised tissue levels of glutathione peroxidase the most and the organic selenium from tuna was the worst. It seems that certain plant forms of selenium may be the best sources.

Stephen Levine, author of *Antioxidant Adaptation: It's role in Free Radical Pathology,* recommends using incrementally increasing doses of sodium selenite especially for decreasing sensitivity to environmental toxins. Some people can not tolerate high doses of selenium and this method may allow someone to slowly acclimate to high doses of selenium.

Selenocysteine is the form in which selenium is incorporated into the glutathione peroxidase molecule. There is a specific genetic code that requires insertion of selenocysteine into certain proteins used in the synthesis of glutathione peroxidase. Selenium may thus regulate the transcription of glutathione peroxidase. It is known that selenium supplementation will increase glutathione levels in the liver of a person who is deficient in selenium.

## II. Function

- Selenium is involved in the synthesis of the enzyme **glutathione peroxidase (GP)**. GP consists of a 4 subunit enzyme with one selenium per subunit in the form of selenocysteine. This enzyme is responsible for detoxification in the body. Selenium, both makes up the active site and induces its activity. This enzyme is responsible for detoxifying hydrogen peroxide intracellulary.
- Converts **HPETE** (hydroperoxyeicosatetraenoic acid) into **HETE** (hydroxyeicosatetraenoic acid) extracellulary, thereby reducing leukotriene 4 series and inflammation.

**HPETE** ———→ *glutathione peroxidase* ———→ **HETE**

- Selenium may be an important inhibitor of various types of cancer.
- The enzyme type 1 iodothyronine 5'– diodinase is a selenium-containing protein molecule that is responsible for converting thyroxine (Ty) into triiodothyronine ($T_3$).

## III. Requirements

**RDA**–55-70mcg/day
Average intake in the U.S.–100mcg/day
*Optimal daily requirement*–200-300mcg/day depending upon toxin exposure

## IV. Sources

**Best Sources of Selenium**

| Food | Amount | µg | Food | Amount | µg |
|---|---|---|---|---|---|
| Brazil nuts | 1/4 cup | 380 | Sunflower seeds | 25 | 25 |
| Snapper, baked | 3 oz | 148 | Granola | 1 cup | 23 |
| Halibut, baked | 3 oz | 113 | Ground beef | 3 oz | 22 |
| Salmon | 3 oz | 70 | Bread, whole wheat | 1 slice | 20 |
| Scallops, steamed | 3 oz | 70 | Rice, brown | 1 cup | 20 |
| Swiss chard, cooked | 1 cup | 57 | Turnips, cooked | 1 cup | 18 |
| Clams, steamed | 20 | 52 | Chicken breast, baked | 3 oz | 17 |
| Oats | 3 oz | 50 | Egg | 1 med | 12 |
| Orange juice | 1 cup | 50 | Barley, uncooked | 1 cup | 12 |
| Oysters | 1/4 cup | 35 | Milk, 2% | 1 cup | 6 |
| Wheat germ | 1/4 cup | 35 | Garlic | 3 cloves | 2.5 |
| Molasses, blackstrap | 2 T | 25 | Yeast | good but variable | |

It should be noted that selenium quantities vary in foods depending upon the levels in the soil. Many agricultural areas are extremely deficient in selenium. Generally grains are a fairly good source. Garlic and mushrooms are sometimes quite high in selenium. Asparagus is a good source of selenium, but other fruits and vegetables are poor sources.

## V. Deficiency

**Keshan disease**–Cardiomyopathy develops in children and young women in a certain area of China where soil selenium is deficient. This condition is reversible upon selenium supplementation. It has been postulated that this condition might be due to a viral condition that only manifests itself when there is a deficiency of selenium.

**Kashin-Beck disease**–This is an arthritis condition that also develops where there are low levels of selenium in the soil.

**Duchennes muscular dystrophy** is also associated with increased selenium excretion.

There are other diseases in which ceroid pigment granules accumulate in nervous tissue. Other symptoms may include anemia, growth retardation, and painful muscles. In Finland, there has been shown to be an extreme selenium deficiency in the soil. This may be a link to the high incidence of cardiovascular disease. A double-blinded trial of vitamin E and selenium in Finland was found to improve mental, emotional, and physical parameters of well-being.

## VI. Therapeutics

1) **Cancer prevention**–200-800mcg/day. Selenium acts to detoxify many bodily toxins via the enzyme glutathione peroxidase. Low levels of soil selenium have been linked to increases in various forms of cancer in the U.S. and Finland. Selenium seems to exert its highest protection against lung and intestinal cancers. Selenium may be used as an adjunct therapy in the treatment of cancer.

2) **Allergies, detoxification and immunity**–200-800mcg/day. Steven Levine from the Allergy Research Group has a protocol for allergy desensitization. Some studies have shown selenium supplementation of 200mcg may increase levels of white blood cells and thymus activity.

3) **Cystic fibrosis**–Joel Wallach has pioneered the use of selenium and vitamin E in the treatment of this condition with reported success.

4) **Cardiovascular disease**–Like cancer, there is an association with higher incidence of heart disease where there are lower levels of selenium in the soil, although the relationship is not quite as strong. Selenium acts by protecting endothelial cells of the arteries against oxidative damage.

5) **Arthritis and other inflammatory conditions** require increased amounts of antioxidant nutrients. Selenium is a major antioxidant. Glutathione peroxidase is low in most inflammatory conditions such as: RA, eczema, and psoriasis.

6) **Osgood Slaughter and growing pains** respond to 200-400mcg selenium and 400-800iu of vitamin E.

7) **Chemotherapy protection**–Along with other antioxidant nutrients, selenium is a critical nutrient for the protection of cells thoughout the body.

8) **Heavy metal toxicity**–Selenium, being involved with glutathione peroxidase, is critical for the protection of the liver.

9) **Cataracts and macular degeneration**–Studies using both IV or oral selenium supplementation have shown it then to be helpful in the treatment of these conditions.

STUDY–Swanson, A. and Truesdale, A. *Elemental analysis in normal and cataract human lens tissue.* Biochem Biophys Res Comm 45, 1488-96, 1971 ABSTRACT–It was found that people who had developed cataracts had 85% less selenium than controls concentrated in the lens.

STUDY–Karakucuk, S., et al. *Selenium concentrations. in serum, lens, and aqueous humour of patients with senile cataract.* Archiv Ophthamolgy Scand 73, 329-32, 1995 ABSTRACT–It was found that there was a 25 times greater concentration of hydrogen peroxide levels compared to normals.

10) **SIDS**–It has been found that selenium levels become depleted at the end of pregnancy. This may explain why there is a problem with toxemia toward the end of pregnancy. Low selenium levels in newborns have been linked to Sudden Infant Death Syndrome (SIDS). SIDS is highest in areas of the world where selenium in the soil is lowest. Heart failure is common in SIDS, a problem found in Keshan Disease.

11) **Myotonic dystrophy and other forms of dystrophy.**

12) **Prevention and treatment of viral illness especially retroviruses.**

STUDY–Hou, J.C., et al. *Inhibitory effect of selenium on complement activation and its clinical significance.* Chung-Hua-I-Hsueh-Tsa-Chih 73, (11) a645-6, 699, 1993 ABSTRACT–Sodium selenite inhibited hemolysis induced by complement activation in-vivo in mice. 80 patients with epidemic hemorrhagic fever received multiple dosages of 2 mg selenite per day during the 1st 9 days of hospitalization. In fulminant cases mortality fell from 100% in the untreated patients to 36% in those receiving selenium. In severe cases mortality fell from 22% in untreated cases to zero in those receiving selenium.

## VII. Toxicity

900-1000mcg/day is probably the highest long-term daily dose that can be taken without the development of toxicity in most people. There are variations in the toxic dose, as with other nutrients, but selenium must be used with caution. Estimates from cattle and other animals show that the toxic long-term dose is probably closer to 2.4-3mg per day. This would lead to symptoms such as liver, skeletal and cardiac muscle damage.

**Selenium has a narrow margin of safety.**

Toxic signs may also include garlic breath and sweat, metallic taste in mouth, depression, nervousness, emotional instability, nausea, vomiting, weight loss, brittle hair & nails, hair loss, fingernail damage, and GI irritation.

## VIII. Interactions

Selenium generally has a synergistic relationship with the other antioxidant nutrients. It appears to lose some of its normal function when exposed to lead, mercury, cadmium, and arsenic. Chronic exposure to environmental toxins, including chemotherapeutic drugs, radiation and other toxic medications, increases its requirement, since selenium is used in the generation of glutathione peroxidase, an enzyme used in the detoxification process.

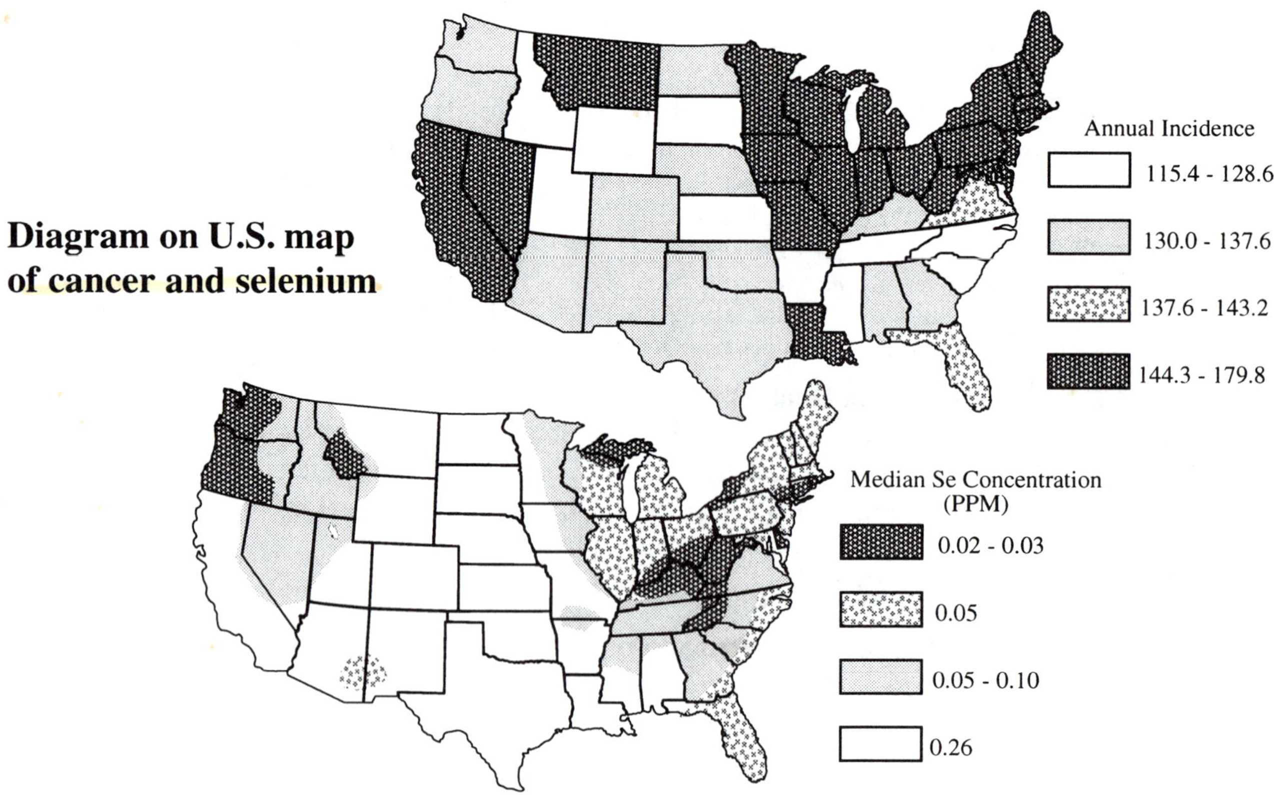


**Diagram on U.S. map of cancer and selenium**

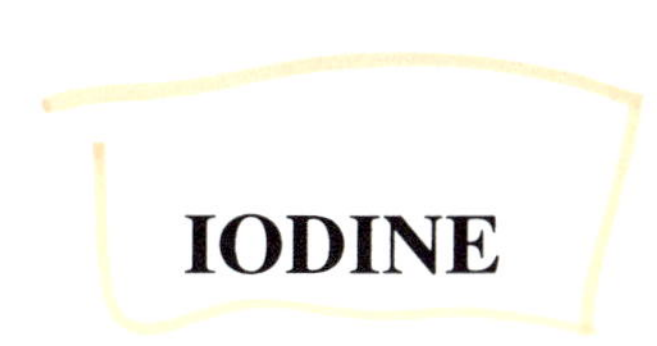

# IODINE

- The body contains 20-30mg of iodine with more than 75% found in the thyroid gland.

## I. Metabolism

Iodine is easily absorbed from the intestines. It is found in serum both in a free state and bound to protein. Stored in the thyroid gland, it is used to synthesize thyroid hormones. Iodine tends to be more involved metabolically with the regulation of estrogen actions on breast tissue. Breast tissue does not have the necessary enzymes to oxidize iodide to iodine, thus it requires the free form of iodine.

*Iodine* should be used to describe free iodine. *Iodide* is the term used to describe iodine that is bound to another compound such as potassium. Iodide tends to be more involved with thyroid function. Organic forms of iodine may be preferred to the inorganic iodides such as potassium iodide.

STUDY–Ghent, W.R., et al. *Iodine replacement in fibrocystic breast disease.* Canadian J Surg 36, 453-6, 1993 ABSTRACT– It was determined that breast tissue responds better to iodine. 70% of patients had positive effects while iodine produced fewer side effects compared to the iodide forms (such as acne, altered thyroid function).

## II. Function

- Iodine is specifically involved with thyroid hormone synthesis.
- No other known functions have been discovered, however, gastric mucosa, salivary glands, choroid plexus, and lactating mammary glands seem to concentrate iodine as well.

## III. Requirements

**RDA**–150 μg/day adults; 175μg/day in pregnancy; 200μg/day lactation
*Average adult intake is between 200μg/day-600μg/day*
The high daily intake of iodine is primarily due to excessive consumption of iodinated salt.

## IV. Sources

Iodine levels are extremely variable in foods and drinking water. The amount of iodine in a food depends on the type of fertilizer, quality of soil used to grow it and the way the food has been processed. Seafoods are generally quite high in iodine with saltwater fish containing between 300-3000 μg/kg of flesh. Freshwater fish contains 20-40μg/kg. Iodinized salt contains 76μg/gram of iodine in the U.S. and Canada. In certain areas where people have a high incidence of goiters, it may be necessary to add iodine to the food supply.

**Best Sources of Iodine**

| Food | Amount | μg | Food | Amount | μg |
|---|---|---|---|---|---|
| Kombu, dried strip | 2 gms | 6,000 | Cod | 3 oz | 341 |
| Arame, dried 1/16 c | 2 gms | 6,000 | Shrimp | 3 oz | 79 |
| Kelp | 1 t | 3,400 | Halibut | 3 oz | 56 |
| Dulce, dried 1/16 c | 2 gms | 3,000 | Herring | 3 oz | 56 |
| Haddock | 3 oz | 341 | Sardines | 3 oz | 30 |

## V. Deficiency

**Goiter**–Low iodine intakes result in the development of goiter, an enlargement of the thyroid gland. WHO estimates that approximately 200 million people in the world have goiters. Some estimates report that endemic goiter exists in at least 12 European countries, including countries that require iodine supplementation. In the U.S. approximately 1/470 people have goiter with the rate being higher in women.

Goitrogens are naturally occurring substances found in foods which block absorption or utilization of iodine. Goitrogenic foods include cabbage, turnips, rapeseeds, peanuts, cassava, and soybeans. Cooking these foods inactivates their goitrogenic substances. Some studies suggest that certain waters may contain goitrogenic substances from rock origin or possibly from E. coli.

**Cretinism**

**Hypothyroidism**

## V. Therapeutics

**Forms of iodine** include SSKI (saturated solution of potassium iodine), Lugol's Solution (sodium iodide)–these 2 forms supply about 40-45 mg of iodide per drop–caseinated iodine (iodaminol), aqueous iodine, elemental diatomic or molecular iodine.

Dosage range:

15 drops per day and 1-8 drops per day for chronic conditions.

1) **Goiter**–If the goiter is very chronic, it may require thyroid hormones to reduce the size of the thyroid gland. Less chronic goiter may be treated with 300-600µg/day of iodine.

2) **Fibrocystic Breast Disease/Syndrome**–It has been found that using iodine intravaginally or orally may help. It may be that the iodine makes the breast tissue less sensitive to the effects of estrogen. In addition, it may work by enhancing the effect of thyroid hormones. The thyroid hormones are known to help with FBD. Dr. Meyer, who pioneered this treatment, insisted that magnesium must be given IV or IM immediately after iodine application.

3) **Hyperthyroidism** may require 300-900mg/day iodine.

4) **Atherosclerosis**–Iodine is a great solvent of cholesterol, at least in vitro.

5) **Asthma and bronchitis**–Iodine can be used as an expectorant and as a mucolytic agent.

6) **Lymphatic stasis** (chronic lymphadenopathy), **Sebaceous Cysts**–Iodine used both orally and topically can be used to soften the tissues.

7) **Salivary duct stone dissolution**–Use SSKI 7-10 drops tid for 1-2 weeks.

8) **Keloid, Dupuytren's contracture, Peyronie's disease** can all be treated with topical iodine. This can be applied with arnica oil and DMSO.

9) **Antiviral, antifungal, anti-bacterial**–In patients with depleted immune function, use iodine over an extended period of time to enhance immunity.

10) **Sarcoidosis**

11) **Estrogen metabolism**–Iodine can be used to reduce the estrogen quotient converting

estrone and estradiol to estriol in the liver. This may be useful in preventing breast cancer and also in the treatment of PMS.

**NOTE–**A tape by Dr. Richard Kunin which describes the many uses of iodine in the treatment of disease may be obtained by calling (415) 346-2500.

## VI. Toxicity

Iodine may cause rashes, nausea, headaches, excess secretions or other allergic reactions.

Iodine has a wide margin of safety. Very high intakes have been found to inhibit the thyroid gland. Long term intakes of 20-30mg/day may inhibit thyroid function. This may result in thyroid goiter. Some clinicians believe it takes much higher levels, up to 300mg/day, to inhibit thyroid function.

## Notes

---

# MANGANESE

- Found particularly in mitochondria, manganese is a component of several enzymes, including glutamine synthetase, pyruvate carboxylase, and mitochondrial superoxide dismutase (SOD).

## I. Metabolism

Manganese is poorly absorbed. Less than 1% of dietary intake is used by the body. Citrate enhances absorption.

## II. Function

- Manganese is needed for connective tissue and bone function, including skin integrity, tendon & ligament strength, skeletal development, and ear otolith development.
- **Bone remodeling**–Manganese may work with vitamin K by enhancing alpha c carboxylation of glutamate side chains. These are vital for the binding of calcium ions in the bone.
- Pancreatic and brain function. Diabetics only have only half the levels of manganese compared to normals and there are reports of improved glucose tolerance with 5mg/day supplementation.
- In mitochondria, manganese may protect the membranes from oxidative damage by acting as part of and stimulating SOD activity.

## III. Requirements

**ESADDI** (1989)–2-5mg/day.
Average daily intake in the U.S.–3mg day
*Optimal daily intake* – 10-20mg/day

## IV. Sources

Rich food sources include nuts and whole grains, especially those high in the germ moiety. Meat poultry, fish, and dairy are generally poor sources.

**Best Sources of Manganese**

| Food | amount | mg | | Food | amount | mg |
|---|---|---|---|---|---|---|
| Four, whole wheat | 1/2 cup | 2.6 | | Beans, dried | 1/2 cup | 0.7 |
| Peas, dried, cooked | 1/2 cup | 2.0 | | Lettuce, shredded | 1 cup | 0.68 |
| Rice, brown, raw | 1/4 cup | 1.9 | | Oats, dry | 1 c (80g) | 0.6 |
| Barley | 1 cup | 1.8 | | Sweet potato | 1 med | 0.6 |
| Rye, whole, uncooked | 1 c (100g) | 1.3 | | Corn | 1/2 cup | 0.56 |
| Buckwheat, dry | 1 cup | 1.3 | | Beets, diced | 3 oz | 0.41 |
| Banana | 1 med | 1.1 | | Spinach, raw | 1 cup | 0.41 |
| Pecans | 1/4 cup | 1.0 | | Liver | 3 oz | 0.41 |
| Brazil nuts | 1/4 cup | 0.8 | | Kale | 1/2 cup | 0.33 |
| Spinach, cooked | 1/2 cup | 0.75 | | Walnuts | 1/4 cup | 0.2 |
| Almonds | 1/4 cup | 0.7 | | Peanuts | 1/4 cup | 0.2 |
| Rhubarb | 1 cup | 0.7 | | Raisins | 1/4 cup | 0.1 |

## V. Deficiency

Manganese is not commonly deficient. Magnesium can substitute for many manganese functions. Symptoms of deficiency include sterility, skeletal abnormalities, glucose intolerance, and ataxia. Other symptoms noted are temporary inflammations of the skin, nausea and vomiting.

Decreased serum levels have been found in diabetics, epileptics, people with osteoporosis, and in people with pancreatic insufficiency.

## VI. Therapeutics

1) **Arthritis**

2) **Connective tissue damage**

3) **Bone repair**–Certain non-healing fractures may respond to the supplementation of manganese. Bill Walton, the famous center for the Portland Trailblazers, had chronic stress fractures in his feet. He retired from basketball for a while. It was then found that he had a hereditary decrease in his body stores of manganese. After supplementation with manganese, he was able to return to playing professional basketball for a few more years.

4) **Epilepsy**–Animal studies show a deficiency of manganese results in seizures.

## VII. Toxicity

Parkinson's like neurological symptoms can develop if manganese is inhaled. Other symptoms associated with manganese inhalation include psychiatric symptoms such as hallucinations and violent actions.

There are few toxic symptoms associated with large ingested intakes of manganese. Over 100mg/day may cause nausea

## VIII. Interactions

Manganese may interfere with the absorption of iron, copper, and zinc. Conversely, high doses of magnesium, calcium, iron, copper, and zinc may inhibit the absorption of manganese.

### Notes

---

# BORON

- Not previously known to be essential, boron is now being studied as a mineral needed for numerous bodily functions.

## I. Metabolism

Boron is very readily absorbed yet its concentration remains quite low in the serum. It appears to be concentrated in the thyroid gland.

## II. Function

- For a long time boron has been a known essential for plants and various diseases have been shown to result from boron deficiency.
- In humans boron is responsible for the hydroxylation of various substances in the body.
- It may enhance the production of various hormones such as testosterone, estrogen, DHEA, and 1,25 dihydroxycholecalciferol.

## III. Requirements

No requirements have been set as of 1996. Estimates are that between 1-2mg/day may be required. Average intake in the U.S. has been estimated at between 1.7-4.3mg/day, although 3 U.S. reference diet composites estimated an intake of about 1mg/day.

## IV. Sources

Boron is found in legumes, fruits, and nuts. Food levels vary widely depending upon the soil in which the food was grown. Generally, vegetables contain much higher quantities of boron than animal sources.

**Best Sources of Boron**

| Food | Amount | Mg | Food | Amount | Mg |
|---|---|---|---|---|---|
| Tomato | 1 oz | 3.5* | Peanuts | 1 oz | 0.5 |
| Pear | 1 oz | 2.9* | Almonds | 1 oz | 0.5 |
| Apple | 1 oz | 2.0* | Dates | 1 oz | 0.3 |
| Wine | 4 oz | 1.0 | Honey | 1 oz | 0.2 |
| Soymeal | 1 oz | 0.8 | Filberts | 1 oz | 0.3 |
| Prunes | 1 oz | 0.7 | Seafood | 3 oz | 0.4 |
| Raisins | 1 oz | 0.7 | Thyroid, sheep | 60mg | 0.45mcg |

*Values are from a single report and may be falsely elevated.

## V. Deficiency

There has been very little research to date on the effects of boron deficiency in humans. Studies done with rats in the 1940's showed no signs of deficiency. Recently, however, there is evidence that boron deficiency is involved with bone metabolism problems and arthritis.

## VI. Therapeutics

1) **Osteoporosis–**1-3mg/day–Recently it has been shown that osteoporotic people have lowered levels of boron and that supplementary boron can increase endogenous estrogen levels and markedly reduce calcium excretion levels.

STUDY–Nielsen, F.H., Hunt, C.D., Mullen, L.M., Hunt, J.R. *Effect of dietary boron mineral, estrogen, and testosterone metabolism in postmenopausal women.* FASEBJ 1:394-397, 1987. ABSTRACT–Postmenopausal women were fed a standard diet for 119 days consisting of 0.25mg boron. Supplementation of this diet with 3mg boron reduced urinary calcium excretion by 44% and markedly increased serum concentration of the estrogenic hormone, 17ß-estradiol. The increased levels of 17ß-estradiol were the same as in women receiving estrogen therapy.

2) **Osteoarthritis** (OA)–recent studies have shown that 3mg/day of boron may reduce OA pain. The synovial fluid of rheumatoid arthritis joints have been found to have lower levels of boron.

## VII. Toxicity

Very little toxicity has been associated with high intakes of boron, which may be as high as 40mg/day in some parts of the world.

### Notes

---

# SILICON

- Silicon has recently been added to the list of essential trace minerals.

## I. Metabolism

Different forms of silicon are absorbed at varying rates. It is estimated that 30-50% of ingested silicon is absorbed. Aluminosilicates are very poorly absorbed while organic forms are easily absorbed.

## II. Function

- Silicon is necessary for the proper formation of glycosaminoglycans and collagen as well as for the formation of matrix and ground substance of bones. It thus provides the organic matrix for the proper mineralization of bones and teeth.
- Silicon accumulates during the early phases of bone mineralization (found to be especially high in the epiphyseal plates).
- It is also necessary for the formation of elastin and maintains the integrity of elastic tissues such as blood vessels.

## III. Requirements

The basic requirement is approximately 20-50mg/day.
No RDA has been established.
Average intake in the U.S.–21-46mg/day.

## IV. Sources

Silicon is generally found in high fiber foods, especially in the husks of grains. Beer is especially high in silicon. During refining of foods, most silicon is lost. Meats, fish, and dairy products are poor sources of silicon.

**Best Sources of Silicon**

| Food | Amount | Mg |
|---|---|---|
| Oats, raw | 1 cup | 368 |
| Beets, cooked | 1/2 cup | 170 |
| Barley | 1 cup | 170 |
| Soybeans, cooked | 1/2 cup | 170 |
| Rice, brown | 1 cup | 70 |
| Wheat bran | 2 T | 30 |
| Turnips, cooked | 1 cup | 19 |
| Rice, white | 1 cup | 14 |
| Raisins | 1/2 cup | 11 |
| Beans, green string | 1/2 cup | 6 |

## VI. Deficiency

A deficiency of silicon in animals results in growth retardation and bone deformities.

## VII. Therapeutics

1) **Osteoporosis**–Silicon is found in high concentrations in connective tissue including bone. Botanical–Horsetail Equisetum

2) **Atherosclerosis**–It has been found that there is an inverse relationship of silicon content of the intima of blood vessel walls and the degree of atheromatous lesions. Normal arterial walls contain extremely high concentrations of silicon. With age the silicon

content goes down. Hard water, which has significantly more silicon, has been associated with lowered heart disease.

## VIII. Toxicity

Very low toxicity

## Notes

---

# VANADIUM

- Vanadium is named after the Scandinavian goddess of beauty, youth, and luster.
- It was established as an essential mineral after studies on 2 different species.

## I. Metabolism

Very little is known, but absorption may be very low, around 1% of the total ingested. It concentrates in the dentin of teeth and also in the bone. It appears to be involved with bone mineralization by promoting osteoblastic activity. After being absorbed from the GI tract it becomes bound to transferrin in the blood. 80-90% of vanadium is lost from the body via the urine. It appears as though vanadyl or vanadate may be the most biologically active forms.

## II. Function

Glucose, cholesterol and bone metabolism may require vanadium. Vanadium may act independently from insulin in lowering glucose levels. It has also been found to suppress cholesterol synthesis in the liver of younger humans who have high cholesterol levels. Trials in adults with higher cholesterol failed to reduce levels. Some studies have shown promise in vanadium's effect at decreasing dental carries by enhancing the integrity of tooth enamel. In addition it may have effects on the thyroid.

## III. Requirements

**ESADDI**–100-300µg/day
Average intake in the U.S.–10-60µ/day

## IV. Sources

The best sources of vanadium occur in certain spices such as dill seeds, parsley, black pepper, mushrooms, and shellfish. Grains have fairly high levels with lesser amounts in meat, fish and poultry.

**Best Sources of Vanadium**

| Food | Amount | µg | Food | Amount | µg |
|---|---|---|---|---|---|
| Buckwheat groats | 1 cup | 100 | Sunflower oil | 1 T | 6 |
| Corn, whole | 1 cup | 30 | Olive oil | 1 T | 4 |
| Oats, raw | 1 cup | 28 | Wheat, whole | 1 cup | 4 |
| Safflower oil | 1 T | 9 | Sunflower seeds | 1 oz | 4 |
| Tomato | 1 med | 8 | Apples | 1 med | 4 |
| Parsley | 10 sprigs | 8 | Peanut oil | 1 T | 2 |
| Carrot | 1 med | 7 | | | |

## V. Deficiency

The average intake in the U.S. is variable, but can be quite low. Very little is known about the possible effects of vanadium deficiencies.

## VI. Therapeutics

**1) Diabetes mellitus**–Vanadium may enhance glucose tolerance since it shows an insulin-like activity, especially on adiposites. It has been shown in some studies to actually decrease insulin requirements and may even have effect without insulin present. High doses of vanadate sulfate may be necessary for this effect.

STUDY–Cohen, N., et al. *Oral vanadly sulfate improves insulin sensitivity in NIDDM but not in obese nondiabetic subjects.* Diabetes 45(5):659-66, 1996 ABSTRACT–100mg/day of oral vandyl sulfate was used in moderately obese NIDDM and nondiabetic subjects. Both fasting plasma glucose and HgbA1c were reduced in the NIDDM subjects but not in the non diabetic group.

STUDY–Cohen, N., et al. *Oral vanadyl sulfate improves epatic and peripheral insulin sensitivity in patients with non-insulin dependant diabetes mellitus.* J Clin Invest 95(6):2501-9, 1995. ABSTRACT–6 NIDDM patients were treated with placebo or vandyl sulfate 100mg/day for 3 wks. Fasting plasma glucose average was 210mg/dl and HgbA1c 9.6 and improve after treatment to 181mg/dl and 8.8. The effects continued for 2 wks after the treatment was discontinued.

## VII. Toxicity

Little is known. 12 human subjects were fed 13.5mg daily for 2 wks followed by 22.5mg daily for 5 months. 5 patients experienced cramps and diarrhea at the high dose level. In patients with NIDDM no side effects were noted at doses of 100mg per day. Excessive vanadium may trigger mania as patients with mania have been found to have high levels in hair samples. Both iron and vitamin C can reduce vanadium toxicity in animal studies. High dose vanadium may deplete vitamin C.

## VIII. Interactions

Lithium

**Notes**

---

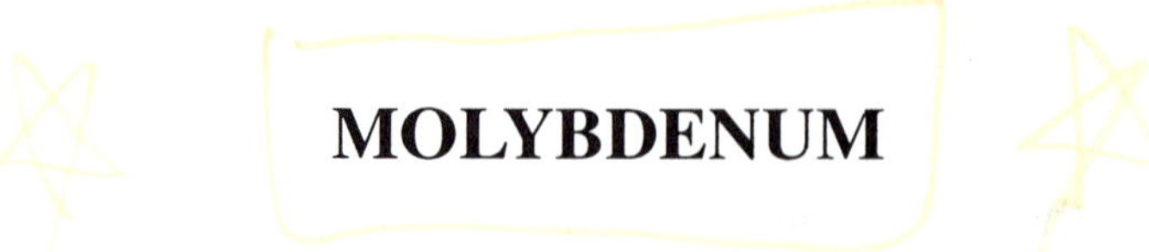

# MOLYBDENUM

## I. Metabolism

Molybdenum is readily absorbed (90%) in the stomach and also the small intestine from dietary sources.

## II. Function

- Involved with iron, copper and sulfur in the body, molybdenum functions as a co-factor for oxidation-reduction reactions. The enzymes involved are xanthine oxidase, aldehyde dehydrogenase, and sulfite oxidase.
- **Sulfite oxidase** is an important enzyme for the degradation of amino acids cysteine and methionine. A genetic disorder involving a deficiency of sulfite oxidase is a fatal disorder of cysteine metabolism which results in severe brain damage, mental retardation, dislocation of ocular lenses and increased urinary output of sulfate. It is also responsible for the inactivation of sulfite ions which may be involved with asthma.
- **Xanthine oxidase** is an enzyme found in several tissues including the liver, intestine, spleen, kidney and others. It is also found in milk. It is responsible for the terminal oxidation of purines so that they may be excreted as uric acid.

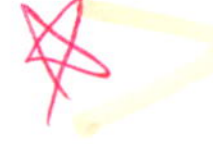

- **Aldehyde oxidase** is found in the liver. It can substitute for many of the same substrates as xanthine oxidase. This enzyme is responsible for the detoxification of alcohol.

## III. Requirements

**ESADDI**–75-250μg/day
Average intake in the U.S.–75-110μg/day

## IV. Sources

Molybdenum is found in the germ of grains and legumes.

**Best Sources of Molybdenum**

| Food | Amount | μg | Food | Amount | μg |
|---|---|---|---|---|---|
| Lentils, cooked | 1 cup | 310 | Corn | 1/2 cup | 36 |
| Split peas, cooked | 1 cup | 260 | Rye bread | 2 slices | 25 |
| Green peas | 1 cup | 170 | Wheat bread, whole | 2 slices | 25 |
| Rice, brown | 1 cup | 150 | Apricots | 3 raw | 15 |
| Spinach | 1/2 cup | 90 | Brewer's yeast | 1 T | 10 |
| Potato | 1 med | 60 | Wheat germ | 1 T | 10 |
| Oats, raw | 1 cup | 43 | Garlic | 2 cloves | 8 |
| Cantaloupe | 1/2 med | 43 | Molasses | 2 T | 8 |
| Wheat, whole | 1 cup | 36 | Raisins | 1/2 cup | 8 |

## V. Deficiency

Molybdenum deficiency is very rare and may be related to a genetic defect such as sulfite oxidase deficiency. It has also been known to become deficient during long-term TPN (Total Parenteral Nutrition or Totally Poor Nutrition).

## VI. Therapeutics

Molybdenum may be useful in the treatment of certain cardiovascular conditions, asthma, allergies and mercury toxicity. Because of its involvement with sulfur, it may be warranted to use in asthma associated with sulfite sensitivity. It may be wise to balance molybdenum intake with copper supplements.

1) **Asthma**–50-500µg per day orally or 250-500µg IV–This is especially effective for sulfite sensitivity. Sulfites in foods can trigger many allergic reactions. They were finally banned for use on produce in 1986. At that time the FDA also required other beverages containing sulfites, such as wine, beer and dried fruit to have warning labels.

2) **Rheumatism**–Molybdenum may help with various types of muscle neuralgia.

3) **Hypouricemia**

4) **Wilson's syndrome**–Etrathiomolybdate is the form used to bring down copper levels. This should be taken in conjunction with zinc.

5) **Dental caries prevention**–In several population studies it has been found that areas that have the highest molybenum intake have the lowest rate of tooth decay. By the same token, areas where molybenum intake is the lowest have the highest rate of tooth decay. One study has shown that when molybdenum was added to a fluoride treatment, the treatment was more effective than fluoride alone.

6) **Cancer prevention**–It has been found that areas with the lowest levels of molybdenum have the highest rate of cancer, especially esophageal cancer. In China esophageal cancer was also linked to lowest levels of molybenum.

## VII. Toxicity

500µg/day may result in impaired copper status because molybdenum increases excretion of copper. Thus it may be important to give copper supplements. High levels–10-15mg/day–may precipitate gout by raising uric acid levels.

## Notes

# FLUORINE

## I. Metabolism

Fluorine is one of three halogens essential for health and reproduction in humans. It is as abundant as iron in the body and it is found mostly in bone tissue. As part of bone, it is complexed with calcium or hydroxyapatite to form fluoroapatite. Plasma fluorine levels are related to dietary intake. Industrial exposure may also play a role in plasma levels. It should be noted that only very small amounts pass from the placenta to fetus. Fluoride is readily absorbable in the small intestine. It is lost mainly through the urine.

## II. Function

- Fluorine, found complexed with calcium and hydroxyapatite, plays an important role in making bones and tooth enamel hard (harder and more resistant to decay compared to hydroxypatite). It provides nucleation sites for bone mineral crystallization. It is also responsible for giving bone its density.
- In rats and mice low fluorine diets have resulted in growth retardation, increased infertility and anemia. Addition of fluorine corrects these problems.

## III. Requirements

**ESADDI**–1.5-4.0mg/day
Average intake in the U.S.–2.7mg/day (1.5mg from food & 1.3 from water)

**Note**–An 8oz glass of fluoridated water (1ppm or 1 mg/l) provides about 0.2 mg of fluoride.

One study showed that in areas where water contained more than 0.7 ppm of fluoride, the mean dietary intake for:

6 month old infants–0.418 mg/day
1 year old toddler–0.621 mg/day

When drinking water contained less than the 0.7 ppm, intake was significantly less with the highest intakes not exceeding 0.08m/kg/day.

## IV. Sources

Most fluoride comes from drinking water but food can contribute nearly as much. Black tea and seafood contain very high amounts. 1 cup of tea may have up to 1mg of fluoride. Soups made in societies that use fish and meat bones may provide considerable amounts of fluoride. In China, plants, rather than water, have very high fluoride content. Beef liver is also high in fluoride and significant amounts of fluoride can be taken in from Teflon pans, especially if they are heated to higher temperatures or scraped.

**Best Sources of Fluoride**

| Food | Amount | Mg | Food | Amount | Mg |
|---|---|---|---|---|---|
| Wine | liter | 6.3 | Grapefruit | 1/2 | 0.07 |
| Mackerel | 100g | 2.70 | Egg | 1 large | 0.062 |
| Sardines | 3.5 oz | 1.14 | Oatmeal | 1 cup | 0.06 |
| Cod | 3.5 oz | 0.7 | Corn | 1/2 cup | 0.05 |
| Salmon | 3.5 oz | 0.66 | Onions | 100g | 0.05 |
| Tea | 100g | 0.47 | Beef | 3.5 oz | 0.03-0.2 |
| Shrimp | 3.5 oz | 0.4 | Wheat germ, toasted | 1/4 cup | 0.02-0.1 |
| Coffee | 100g | 0.25 | Spinach | 1/2 cup | 0.02-.16 |
| Buckwheat | 100g | 0.17 | Soybeans | 100g | 0.02 |
| Chicken | 3.5 oz | 0.145 | Potato | 1 med | 0.01-1.0 |
| Milk, whole | 1 cup | 0.12 | Lettuce | 100g | 0.01 |
| Kale, cooked | 1/2 cup | 0.08-0.2 | Apple | 1 med | 0.008-0.2 |
| Rice | 100g | 0.07 | | | |

USDA Handbook #8 Series Washington, DC, ARS, USDA, 1976-1986

## V. Deficiency

Symptoms of fluoride deficiency include growth retardation, dental caries, anemia, and weakened bones.

## VI. Therapeutics

1) **Dental caries prevention**–It has been well documented that fluoride intake positively correlates with a decreased incidence of dental caries in children. Areas that have less fluoride in their drinking water have more dental caries and less bone density. At least one study has shown that molybdenum has synergistic effects with fluoride and, if supplemented together, less fluoride can be used.

don't agree!

STUDY–Riggs, B., et al. *A four year controlled trial of fluoride suppementation of women with osteroporosis does not change fracture rate.* N Engl J Med, 332:802, 1990 ABSTRACT–Fluoride supplementation in women with osteoporosis did not change the hip fracture rate.

## VII. Toxicity

Fluorine has very high levels of toxicity. Chronic ingestion of 2.5ppm or more in children will strengthen their teeth and bones but will also cause permanent mottling of teeth. At 3-5 ppm, toxic effects have been shown to occur in cattle with symptoms of weakness, loss of appetite, and gastroenteritis. At higher intakes in humans, gastroenteritis has been documented. Other long term exposure symptoms–from ingestion of 8 ppm over 35 years–include skeletal abnormalities such as osteoporosis and/or osteomalacia; calcification of tendons, ligaments and interosseous membranes; and development of bone spurs. These toxic effects have become quite common in certain areas in India and China where fluoride levels are high in water and soil.

**NOTE**–Carbon block filters only remove about 30% of fluoride from drinking water.

STUDY–National Center for Toxicological Research, US Food and Drug Administration–noted in FDA Consumer May, 1991. The risk for developing osteosarcoma may go up.

STUDY–Tsutsui, T., et al. *Induction of unscheduled DNA synthesis in cultured human oral keratinocytes by Sodium Fluoride*. Mutation Res 140:43-48, 1984. ABSTRACT–45-135 ppm fluoride, given as sodium fluoride, caused unexpected DNA synthesis in human oral keratinocytes within 4 hours.

## Notes

---

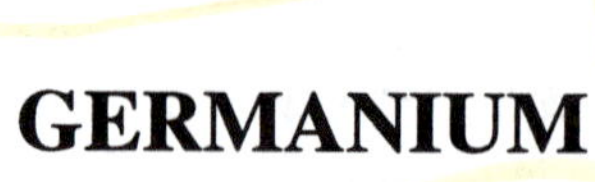

# GERMANIUM

## I. Metabolism

The total amount of germanium in the body is about 20mg. It is mainly concentrated in the thyroid gland. It has been found to be associated with T3 and T4 bound in the plasma. The absorption rate seems to be excellent. Most excretion takes place in the urine.

## II. Function

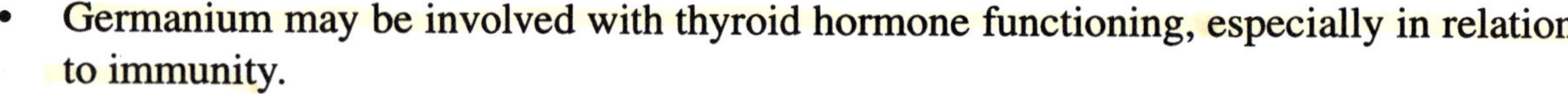

- Germanium may be involved with thyroid hormone functioning, especially in relation to immunity.

## III. Requirements

**ESADDI**–probably about 500μg/day
Average intake in the U.S.–?/day

## IV. Sources

Wheat bran, vegetables and leguminous seeds.

## V. Deficiency

In rats a germanium deficiency may cause altered bone and liver mineral composition and decreased tibial DNA.

## VI. Therapeutics

Germanium may have some immune stimulating properties. In addition it may reverse changes in rats caused by a silicon deficiency. Some organic germanium compounds have antitumor activity.

STUDY–Sato, I., Yuan, B.D., et al. *Inhibition of tumor growth and metastasis in association with modification of immune response by novel organic germanium compounds.* J Biol Response Mod 4; 159-68, 1985.

STUDY–Suzuki, F., Brutkiewicz, R.R., et al. *Cooperation of lymphokines and macrophages in expression of antitumor activity of carboyethlgermanium sesquioxide.* .Anticancer Res 6:177-82, 1986.

STUDY–Jacobs, M.M., & Griffin, A.C. *Inhibition of tumor induction and development.* Zedeck, M.S., Lipkin, M. eds. NewYork: Plenum, 1981.

## VII. Toxicity

More than a few mg/day may result loose stools and skin irritations. There have been several reports concerning kidney failure in patients taking large doses of contaminated germanium.

# TIN

- Tin was first found to be an essential growth factor in rats who were made deficient on an ultra clean chemical diet in the early 1970's.
- Its highest concentrations are found in the liver and spleen. People living in cities have a higher concentration in their tissues.
- Little or no tin is found in fetuses or newborns. It accummulates progressively after birth.

## I. Metabolism

Tin is very poorly absorbed, depending upon the intake. At low intakes as much as 50% may be absorbed and at higher intakes less than 3% gets absorbed. It is excreted in the bile and in small amounts in the urine.

## II. Function

Little is known about the function of tin in the body, but it may be involved in electron transport systems and in protein binding.

## III. Requirements

ESADDI–none
Average intake in the U.S.–3-4mg/day
Intakes may be up to 38mg/day for people eating a lot of canned foods.

## IV. Sources

Most tin comes from the consumption of canned foods. Tomato, pineapple and orange juices are often placed in unlacquered tin cans, therefore they may contain as high as 50mg of tin per container.

## V. Deficiency

A deficiency in rats results in stunted growth and anemia.

## VI. Therapeutics

None known

## VII. Toxicity

Oral tin has very low toxicity. A 50mg/day tin intake may have a negative effect on zinc balance. Decreased hematocrits, hemoglobin and serum iron in rats fed equivalent of 170mg/day tin has also been noted. Organo-tin compounds tend to much more toxic because they may be absorbed more efficiently. In humans inhalation of tin has been associated with a mild benign pneumoconiosis.

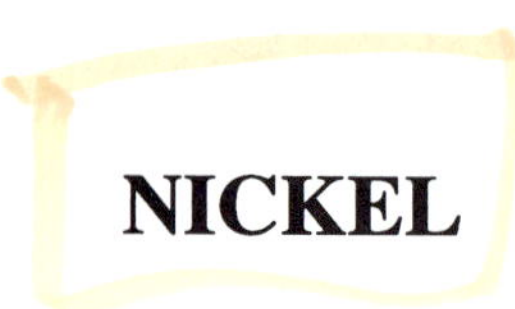

# NICKEL

## I. Metabolism

- About 10 mg of nickel are found in the body, mostly in the skin and bone marrow. The largest amount (18%) is found in the skin.
- The liver and the muscle tissues are the most responsive to the dietary intake of nickel.
- Average absorption is about 3-10%. It is enhanced during pregnancy. Absorption increases with dose and appears to share the same receptors as cobalt and iron.
- Following absorption and distribution, 60% is lost in the urine with smaller amounts found in the bile and the sweat. Excretion varies depending upon intake with the higher intakes resulting in greater excretion.

## II. Function

Found to be essential in 1973 for chicks, rats, mini pigs and goats, nickel is present in RNA and DNA. It may help stabilize the tertiary structure of the nucleic acids and proteins or function as a cofactor for certain enzymes, especially liver dehydrogenases. It may be involved with iron or vitamin metabolism to some extent. Levels of nickel rise during trauma as from MI, stroke and labor.

## III. Requirements

**ESADDI**–/day
Average intake in the U.S.–300µg-600µg/day

## IV. Sources

Nickel is found primarily in plants, nuts and fruits. Wheat contains 40µg per 100gms; nuts, 100µg-500µg per 100gms; legumes, 40-160µg per 100gms; fruits contain lesser amounts.

**Best Sources of Nickel**

| Food | Amount | Mg | Food | Amount | Mg |
|---|---|---|---|---|---|
| Beet greens, cooked | 1/2 cup | .14 | Spinach, raw | .02 | 0.4 |
| Cider | 1 cup | .14 | Peanuts | 1/4 cup | 0.2 |
| Kindney beans, dried | 1/4 cup | .12 | Raisins | 1/4 cup | 0.2 |
| Peas, split, dried | 1/4 cup | 0.08 | Rhubarb | 1 cup | 0.7 |
| navy beans, dried | 1/4 cup | 0.08 | Pear | 1 med | 0.04 |
| Lentils, dried | 1/4 cup | 0.08 | Broccoli | 1/2 cup | 0.026 |
| Clams, uncooked | 3 oz | 0.07 | Peas | 1/2 cup | 0.024 |
| Kale, cooked | 1/2 cup | 0.06 | Bread, whole wheat | 1 slice | 0.021 |
| Banana | 1 med | 0.06 | Celery, chopped | 1/2 cup | 0.022 |
| Swiss chard, cooked | 1/2 cup | 0.05 | | | |

## V. Deficiency

Nickel deficiency results in decreased levels of glucose 6-phosphate which is involved in the production of NADPH via the pentose phosphate shunt pathway. In animals a nickel deficiency may result in decreased levels of iron. It may also be related to problems with decreases in pancreatic amylase production. Chiefly, its effects occur with regard to mitochondria and hepatocytes.

## VI. Therapeutics

Nickel bromide 30mg per day may be helpful in the treatment of psoriasis.

## VII. Toxicity

Nickel has a very low toxicity level, usually related to the inhalation of certain forms, such as nickel carbonyl, which has been shown to cause lung cancer in several animal species. In animals chronic excessive intake or exposure causes degeneration of the myocardium, brain, lung, liver, and kidney.

**Notes**

---

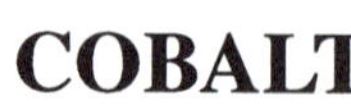

# COBALT

## I. Metabolism

Cobalt in an intrinsic part of vitamin B-12. However most cobalt is absorbed through sources other than vitamin B-12. In the body only 10% of cobalt is found as vitamin B-12. Iron deficiency increases absorption of cobalamin. Where cyanocobalamin is mainly stored in the liver, cobalt is initially deposited in the liver and kidneys and later in the bone, spleen, pancreas, intestine, and other tissues.

## II. Function

Involved as a constituent of cyanocobalamin, cobalt is essential to the normal function of cells–particularly the bone marrow, the nervous system, and the gastrointestinal tract.

In addition, cobalt has been found to function independently from B-12 in the form of glycylglycine dipeptidase.

## III. Requirements

**ESADDI**–2µg/day

Average intake in the U.S.–5-20 µg/day

Dietary cobalt comes primarily from vegetables and whole grains which contain no vitamin B-12.

## IV. Sources

See Vitamin B-12. Vitamin B-12 usually comes from animal products, although it may also be found in some bacterially contaminated foods.

## V. Deficiency

Cobalt deficiency is rare but cyanocobalamin is not uncommon in vegans or in people with malabsorption syndromes, pernicious anemia, or in surgically treated persons who have had their distal ileum or stomach removed.

In certain areas of the Soviet Union, the incidence of goiter is related to deficient levels of cobalt in food and drink. In rats cobalt may be necessary for the formation of thyroxine. Excess levels of inorganic cobalt have been found to cause goiters.

Wild animals have 2-6 times more cobalt in their tissues than Westerners.

## VI. Therapeutics

1) **Hypertension**–50mg/day for 10-65 days caused vasodilation, release of bradykinin and lowered Blood pressure in 8 of 9 subjects. No side effects were noted.

STUDY–Perry & Schroeder 1954. See Maria Linder, p.260.
STUDY–LaGoff, J.M. J Qual. 38:, 1940.

## VII. Toxicity

At high oral doses cobalt can cause goiter, and proliferation of bone marrow erythropoietic cells. This response may occur in people who are given frequent IM cobalt and/or who have excessive exposure other than through the diet. Injections of cobalt oxides or sulfides has been shown to produce proliferation of otherwise normal cells and to form cancer in both animals and humans at the injection site in muscle or thyroid tissue. This only occurs if the cobalt is injected. Children tend to be much more sensitive to oral cobalt. Doses of greater than 1mg/kg body weight will cause cardiotoxic reactions.

In years past beer was treated with cobalt salts to enhance the foaming. Heavy beer drinkers would sometimes die of cardiac damage. Administration of methionine and cysteine protect against this effect.

## Notes

---

# LITHIUM

## I. Metabolism

Lithium is one of the most abundant elements in nature. Plant and tissue concentrations appear to be low and it is estimated that less than 1mg exists in total body stores. Lithium tends to be stored in ovaries, thyroid, adrenal and pituitary glands. Its levels are maintained even if diet sources are low.

## II. Function

Goats and rats placed on low lithium diets were less fertile. The growth and survival rates of goats were also lower. Lithium has profound pharmacologic effects on manic depressive psychosis or bipolar disorder. It may effect the production or turnover of cAMP. By speeding up metabolism it may ↓ in cAMP and make psoriasis, eczema, or asthma worse. It may also activate glucocorticosteroid receptors (inhibiting the effects of glucocorticosteroids) which may exacerbate the symptoms of manic depression.

## III. Requirements

**ESADDI**–Not yet determined

Average intake in the U.S.–100 µg/day

This level is highly variable depending upon soil and water concentrations. Hard water is a significant source of lithium. Recent estimates, not including water sources, show an average intake of 10-25µg per day. Some hard water has as much as 80µg lithium per liter.

## IV. Sources

| Food | amount | mg |
|---|---|---|
| Yeast | 1 T | 8 |
| Grains | 1 cup | 5 |
| Leafy vegetables, cooked | 1/2 cup | 3-9 |
| Liver, beef | 3 oz | 3 |
| Seafoods | 3 oz | 1-3 |
| Legumes | 1/2 cup | 1 |

**Best Sources of Lithium**

## V. Deficiency

Lithium deficiency is very rare. It may be related to a genetic defect.

## VI. Therapeutics

Lithium concentration has been inversely related to atherosclerosis and, in some areas, homicides.

STUDY–Dawson, E.B., Moore, T.D., et al. Disease Nerv Syst 33:546, 1972.

**Nutritional therapy** (dose range 5-10mg/day)

**1) Depression**–5-10 mg/day elemental lithium–has been shown to be effective in the treatment of depression in recovering alcoholics and their relatives who may have a genetic tendency toward depression. If hair levels are low and there is fx of depression strong indications for its use according to Jonathan Wright.

**2) Idiopathic neutropenia** and neutropenia induced by cancer chemotherapy. Lithium may also increase platelet and RBC counts.

**3) Premenstrual syndrome**–J. Wright.

**Pharmacological therapy**

**4) Alcohol recidivism**

**5) Hyperthyroidism–**300mg lithium carbonate 3x/day or monitor serum levels. Hans Neiper says lithiam orotate–20x more potent even though it won't show up as higher in RBC's or serum.

**6) Asthma**–J. Wright

**7) Gout**–J. Wright

**8) Kidney stones (uric acid)**–J. Wright

**9) Headaches, cluster acute attack**

**10) Skin–seborrheic dermatitis**–lithium succinate - 8% solution compounding pharmacists.

## VII. Toxicity

Lithium toxicity is closely related to serum levels. Nutritionally therapeutic levels of 5-10mg/day rarely produces toxicity. Cardiovascular or renal disease is a significant problem with lithium. Polyurea, tremors, dehydration, sodium depletion, and hypothyroidism may also be induced by lithium toxicity. These toxic effects may be alleviated with supplementation of essential fatty acids–either omega 3 or 6. Lithium aspartate, 100mg per day may significantly reduce glucose levels in diabetics according to Dr. Alan Gaby.

Lithium should not be given in pregnancy or lactating women.

## VIII. Interactions

See a pharmacology text for more details. NSAIDS, diuretics and calcium channel blockers could cause problems.

**Notes**

---

# Vitamins

Vitamins are organic compounds that are found in the body in small amounts. They are essential for survival and must be taken in by the foods that we eat. They can not be synthesized in the body in significant quantities to be considered nonessential, with the exception of vitamin D, which is considered by some to be a hormone. A minimal exposure to ultra violet light can stimulate the synthesis of vitamin D in adequate amounts. Other B vitamins, such as folate, biotin, folate, cobalamin, and one fat soluble vitamin, vitamin K, can be synthesized by microorganisms in the gastrointestinal tract in significant quantities to minimize their requirement.

The term *"vitamine"* was first coined in 1912 by Casimir Funk to designate the *vital amine* compounds that were found necessary to sustain life. The vitamins got their names original in the order in which they were discovered or from the source where they were discovered, or after the description of their function. Vitamins are classified according to their solubility whether they are more soluble in water or fat. Generally the fat soluble vitamins do not need to be consumed in foods on a daily basis because they are stored in the body in significant amounts. The water soluble vitamins are generally not stored in the body, with the exception of vitamin B-12, and need to be consumed on a daily basis for optimal health and survival.

The use of vitamins to treat disease is sometimes referred to as orthomolecular medicine or megavitamin therapy when they are used to treat conditions that are not the classic deficiency conditions such as pellagra, scurvy or beriberi. There are many uses for vitamins therapeutically and like minerals and amino acids we are constantly finding more therapies for the use of vitamins. Often times vitamins have synergistic activity with each other and they often have side benefits when used in a broad treatment plan.

| **FAT SOLUBLE VITAMINS** | | ***Rating of toxicity** |
|---|---|---|
| Vitamin A (Retinol & ß-carotene) | 168-174 | "8" (retinol) |
| Vitamin D (Cholecalciferol, Dihyroxy Cholecalciferol) | 175-180 | "4" |
| Vitamin E (Tocopheryl) | 181-187 | "4" |
| Vitamin K (Menadione, phytonadione, aquamephyton) | 188-191 | "4" |
| **WATER SOLUBLE VITAMINS** | | |
| Vitamin B-1 (Thiamin) | 192-196 | "1" |
| Vitamin B-2 (Riboflavin) | 197-199 | "1" |
| Vitamin B-3 (Niacinamide, niacin) | 200-205 | "9" (niacin) |
| Vitamin B-5 (Pantothenic acid) | 206-210 | "1" |
| Vitamin B-6 (Pyridoxine, pyridoxal 5-phosphate) | 211-219 | "3" |
| Vitamin B-12 (cyanocobalamin, hydroxycobalamin) | 220-225 | "1" |
| Folate (Tetrahydrofolate, folic acid, folacin) | 226-230 | "1" |
| Biotin | 231-324 | "1" |
| Vitamin C (Ascorbic acid) | 235-241 | "2" |

***Rating of toxicity** is a relative toxicity that is based on a 1-10 scale with "10" being the most toxic. It is a toxicity scale comparing the relative toxicity of the vitamins with themselves. Compared with prescription drugs, they are relatively low in toxicity with the highest being perhaps a "4" rating overall.

# VITAMIN A

Vitamin A was discovered almost simultaneously in 1913 by McCollum and Davis at the University of Wisconsin, and Osborne and Mendel at Yale University. Both teams observed that rats developed inflamed, infected eyes and failed to grow when they were fed diets lacking in natural fats. It was found that butterfat or cod liver oil could quickly remedy the problem. Vitamin A was then isolated from rat intestines. In 1928, a yellow pigment of plants was discovered to be a precursor to vitamin A. The term, "vitamin A," is used to refer to the alcohol, aldehyde and acid forms of vitamin A, all of which are biologically active.

retinol–alcohol

retinal–aldehyde

retinoic acid–acid

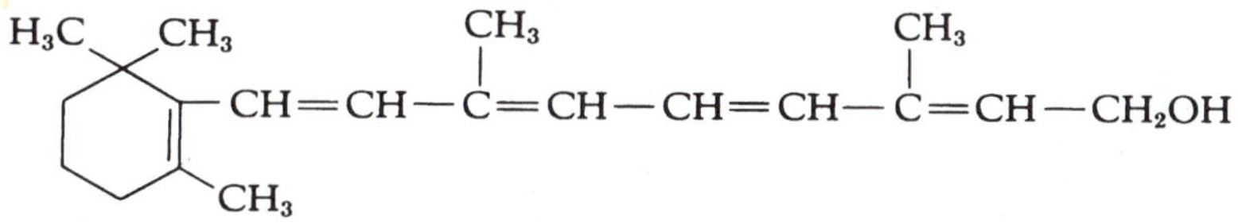

$H_3C$ $CH_3$ $CH_3$ $CH_3$

$-CH{=}CH{-}C{=}CH{-}CH{=}CH{-}C{=}CH{-}CH_2OH$

$CH_3$

*Retinol*

## I. Chemistry and Properties

**Water miscible preparations of retinol usually lead to greater concentrations in the plasma, whereas oil-soluble preparations lead to a greater storage of retinol in the liver.**

**Carotenoids** alpha, gamma, and beta are **converted to** vitamin A primarily in the **intestinal mucosa.** Theoretically, ß carotene should be twice as active as the alpha and gamma carotenoids because it is composed of 2 molecules of retinol while the others contain only one molecule of retinol. However, only 1/3 of the available retinal molecules found in Beta carotene from foods actually get converted to retinol (the % is higher for synthetic beta carotene) and only 1/3 of ß carotene gets absorbed. As the intake of carotene goes above 5,000 IU/day the % absorption rate goes down proportionally. **Thus, ß carotene is considered to be significantly less biologically active** (approximately 1/6) **than pure retinol.**

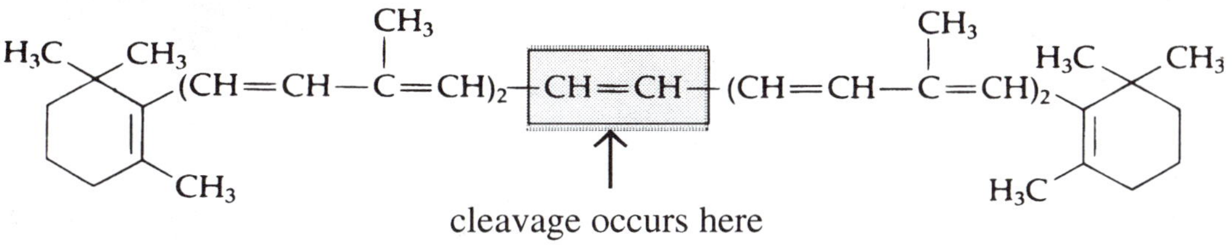

$H_3C$ $CH_3$ $CH_3$ $CH_3$ $H_3C$ $CH_3$

$(CH{=}CH{-}C{=}CH)_2{-}CH{=}CH{-}(CH{=}CH{-}C{=}CH)_2$

$CH_3$ $H_3C$

cleavage occurs here

*ß carotene*

**Blood carotene levels reflect dietary carotene and not the storage of vitamin A.** Therefore, with decreased intake, a rather rapid drop in serum carotene occurs. Vitamin A is stable to heat and light and is thus resistant to most processing and cooking.

Until 1974 the U.S. used international units (IU) to describe the potency of the different forms of vitamin A. IUs represent equivalent potencies of preformed vitamin A (or its precursor, carotene) which cause a specific growth response in rats whose reserves of vitamin A have been depleted. The unit of measure was changed to retinol equivalents (RE). The advantage of the term, retinol equivalents, is that it takes into consideration the variation in absorption and conversion of different precursors into vitamin A.

| | | |
|---|---|---|
| 1 RE | =1mcg of retinol | =3.33 IU retinol or 10 IU ß-carotene |
| | =6mcg of ß-carotene | =3.33 IU retinol or 10 IU ß-carotene |
| | =12mcg of other carotenoids | |
| 1000 RE | =1mg of retinol | =3,333 IU retinol or 5,000 IU of a mixture of retinol & ß-carotene |

**1mg of Beta carotene = 1670 IU Beta carotene**

## II. Metabolism

More than 90% of all dietary retinol is in the form of esters, usually retinyl palmitate. These esters must be hydrolyzed in the intestinal lumen by pancreatic enzymes and within the brush border of the intestinal epithelial cells before absorption. Retinol is transported across intestinal epithelial cells by a carrier mediated mechanism which involves a protein called "cellular retinol-binding protein." In average doses, retinol is almost entirely absorbed. Peak concentrations are reached in 4 hours. When large amounts are taken, some is excreted in the feces. Absorption is reduced in patients with pancreatic, hepatic or intestinal pathologies. Retinol is absorbed 2-4x more efficiently than ß carotene. **Only 1/3 of ingested ß carotene is absorbed.** Of that which is taken up by the intestinal mucosa, only 1/3-2/3 is converted into retinyl esters. Presumably, as retinol stores get built up to saturation levels in the liver, the intestinal mucosa stops converting ß carotene into retinyl esters and drastically reduces absorption. The remainder stays as ß carotene. Carotenes rely on fats in the diet and on bile salts for absorption to a *much greater* extent than retinol does.

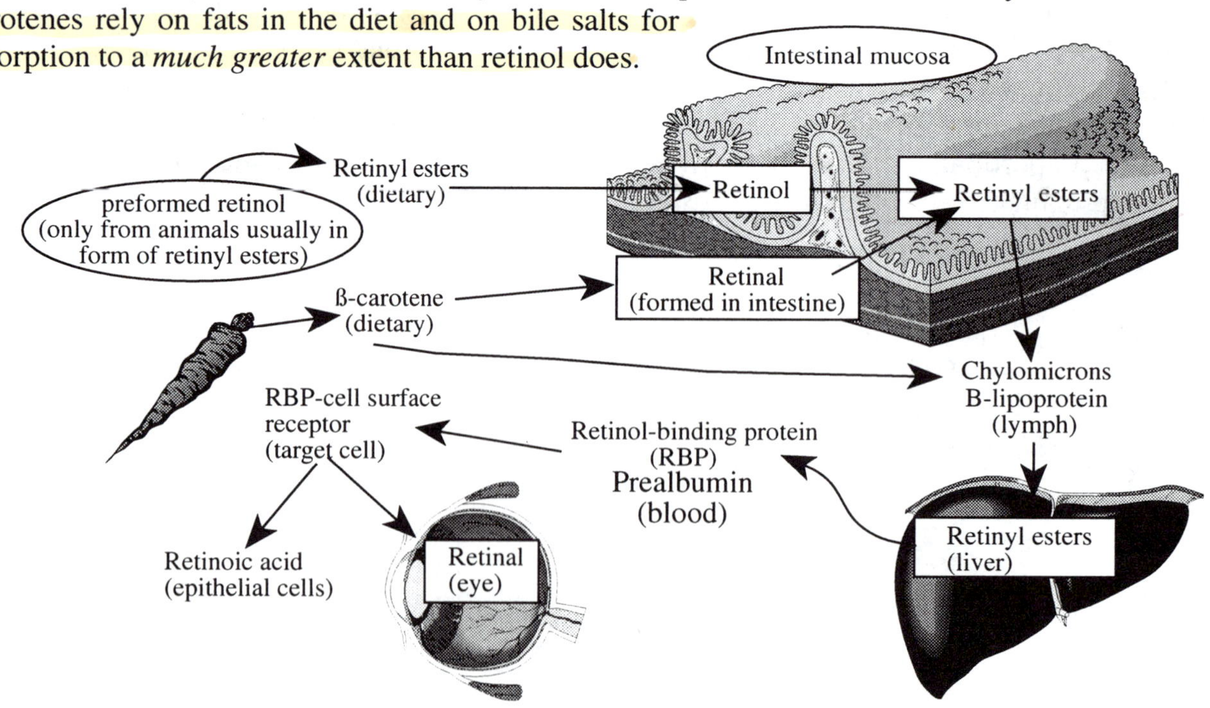


*Pathway by which preformed dietary vitamin A and ß carotene reaches target cells of an organ.*

**ß carotene is stored in fat deposits and in the adrenals** rather than in the liver. Serum levels of ß carotene directly reflect daily consumption, not storage. Both thyroxine and vitamin E enhance the conversion of carotene to retinol. **Most ingested retinol is stored in the liver.** Retinol storage has a half life of 50-100 days. Minor amounts of ß-carotene get converted to retinol in the liver and the lungs. Zinc, thyroid hormones, and proteins are responsible for proper metabolism. There are over 50 carotenoids such as lutein and zeaxanthin, (see *Encyclopedia of Nutritional Supplements*, Michael Murray) all which have different activities in the body; not all of them have been found to have vitamin A activity.

## III. Function

**1) Vision**–Both retinyl esters and ß carotene from the diet are converted to retinal (11 cis isomer). Retinal is combined with the protein opsin to form rhodopsin in the rods of the retina and iodopsin in the cones. Light hitting the retina causes visual excitation and changes the cis configuration into the all trans form of retinaldehyde. The rods are particularly sensitive to a vitamin A deficiency. When it is in low supply, the *all trans form* that is generated during the light reaction cannot be converted back to the active rhodopsin.

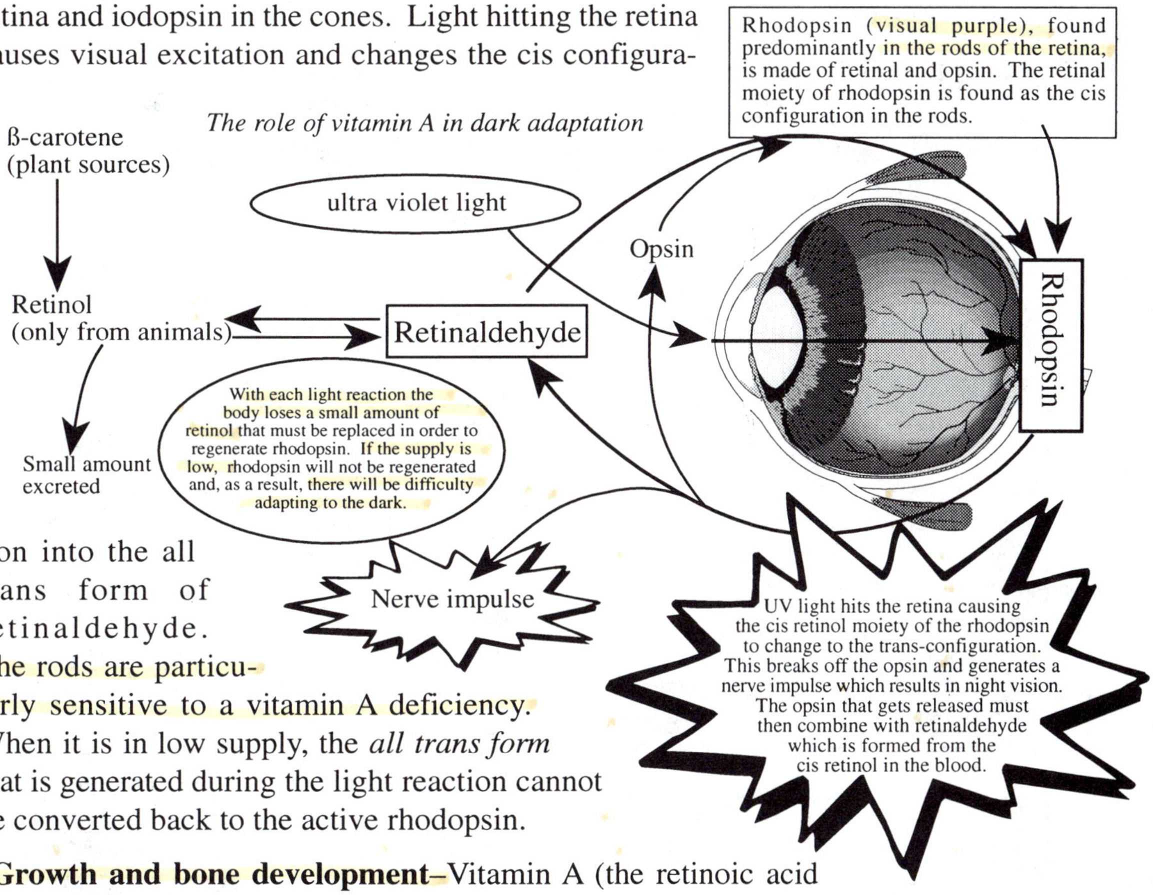

Rhodopsin (visual purple), found predominantly in the rods of the retina, is made of retinal and opsin. The retinal moiety of rhodopsin is found as the cis configuration in the rods.

*The role of vitamin A in dark adaptation*

ß-carotene
(plant sources)
ultra violet light
Opsin
Retinol
(only from animals)
Retinaldehyde
Rhodopsin
With each light reaction the body loses a small amount of retinol that must be replaced in order to regenerate rhodopsin. If the supply is low, rhodopsin will not be regenerated and, as a result, there will be difficulty adapting to the dark.
Small amount
excreted
Nerve impulse
UV light hits the retina causing the cis retinol moiety of the rhodopsin to change to the trans-configuration. This breaks off the opsin and generates a nerve impulse which results in night vision. The opsin that gets released must then combine with retinaldehyde which is formed from the cis retinol in the blood.

**2) Growth and bone development**–Vitamin A (the retinoic acid form) is necessary for growth and development of skeletal and soft tissues through its effect upon protein synthesis. It has an essential role in the differentiation of bone cells. Normal enamel-forming epithelial cells also require vitamin A to develop. A deficiency of vitamin A in the first 5 years of life results in a deficient enamel layer on teeth.

**3) Epithelial tissue development and maintenance**–Retinoic acid is needed for the differentiation of basal cells into mucus epithelial cells. A deficiency results in keratinization (drying and hardening) of mucus membranes that line the respiratory tract, intestines, urinary tract, and epithelium of the eye. A loss of cilia, which is critical to the removal of mucus, also occurs. This decreases the protective barrier role played by these membranes, resulting in an increased number of infections and other pathologies.

4) **Immunity**–As previously mentioned, vitamin A maintains the integrity of the mucus membranes and, thus, is vital for protecting the body against bacterial, viral or parasitic infections. This has led vitamin A to be called "*the anti-infective vitamin.*" It is also involved in humoral and cell-mediated immunity. The number of T lymphocytes, as well as their response to mitogens, is reduced in vitamin A deficiency.

5) **Reproduction**–Vitamin A is involved in steroid hormone synthesis and cell differentiation. It is critical for healthy growth, normal reproduction and lactation.

6) **Anti-cancer function**–Numerous studies have shown that retinoid deficiency enhances susceptibility to carcinogenesis both in experimental animals and in humans. Analogues of vitamin A, or retinoids, are being used in humans to treat cancers (particularly skin, lung, bladder, cervical or breast) which involve epithelial tissues.

## IV. Requirements

**RDA**–1,000 RE men (5,000 IU)        800 RE women (4,000 IU)
pregnancy–1,000 RE        lactation–1,200 RE
The 5,000 IU assumes a mixed diet of 2/3 vegetable and 1/3 animal sources of vitamin A.

**Lab**–Plasma retinol and plasma ß carotene 20-80µg & 50-250µg/dl

*Optimal daily intake*–15,000 IU Retinol (with caution periconceptionally)
25,000 IU ß carotene & mixed carotenoids (depending upon family history and exposure to environmental toxins)

## V. Sources

**Best Food Sources of Vitamin A or Beta Carotene**

| Food | Amount | Beta Carotene (IU) or Retinol (IU) if * | Food | Amount | Beta Carotene (IU) or Retinol (IU) if * |
|---|---|---|---|---|---|
| Liver, Polar Bear | 3 oz | extremely high * | Broccoli | 1 med stalk | 4,500 |
| Dunaliella salina | 1 t (3gms) | 250,000 | Pepper, mature red | 1 med (100g) | 4,500 |
| Carrot juice | 1 cup | 120,000 | Winter squash | 1/2 cup | 4,300 |
| Liver, beef | 3 oz | 45,000* | Mustard greens | 1/2 cup | 4,000 |
| Liver, chicken | 3 oz | 27,000* | Mango | 1/2 med | 4,000 |
| Spirulina | 1 T (7.5g) | 21,293 (50,000mix) | Chicory greens, steamed | 1/2 cup | 4,000 |
| Dandelion leaf, cooked | 1/2 cup | 14,000 | Watermelon | 1"x10" slice | 2,500 |
| Cod liver oil | 1 T | 14,000 | Nectarine | 1 med | 1,650 |
| Burdock/yellow dock | 1c steamed | 12,900 | Endive | 1c packed | 1,600 |
| Liver, pork | 3 oz | 12,000* | Edensoy, extra fortified | 1 cup | 1,500 |
| Sweet potato | 1 med | 12,000 | Cheese, cheddar | 3 oz | 1,290 |
| Carrot | 1 med | 11,000 | Leaf lettuce | 1 c packed | 1,000 |
| Mango | 1 med | 8,000 | Tangerine/Guava | 1 med | 780/710 |
| Pumpkin, cooked | 1/2 cup | 8,000 | Margarine (maybe carotene) | 1 T | 700*/460 |
| Spinach, steamed | 1/2 cup | 7,300 | Plums/Prunes | 3 med | 650/420 |
| Pepper, hot chili | 1 med (30g) | 7,000 | Egg, whole/yolk | 1 med | 590/580* |
| Papaya | 1 med | 6,100 | Asparagus | 4 spears | 540 |
| Apricots (med size) | 10 halves | 6,000 | Butter | 1 T | 535* |
| Wild blue-green algae | 1 T (7.5g) | 5,962 (12,700 mix) | Pacific Rice Drink | 1 cup | 500* |
| Chives, steamed | 1/2 cup | 5,800 | Pepper, green | 1 med (100g) | 430 |
| Wheat/Barley grass | 1 T (7.5g) | 5,621 (12,400 mix) | Peas | 1/2 cup | 430 |
| Collard greens/Kale | 1/2 cup | 5,400/4,600 | Milk, whole/nonfat | 1 cup | 390/10* |
| Cantaloupe | 1/2 melon | 5160 | Green beans | 1/2 cup | 340 |
| Chlorella (dried) | 1 T (7.5g) | 4,685 (11,200 mix) | Yellow corn | 1/2 cup | 330 |

USDA Handbook #8 Series, Washington, DC, ARS, USDA, 1976-1986. The Secrets of Spirulina, Hills, 1981.
* indicates preformed retinol

9 carrots = 99,000 Beta Carotene (IU)

## VI. Deficiency

Symptoms may result from low intake, problems with absorption and/or storage, or from interference with the conversion of ß carotene to retinol. In addition, a deficiency of protein or zinc can reduce the amount of vitamin A released from the liver. Symptoms include night blindness, dry eyes, keratinization, opacity and sloughing of the epithelial cells of the cornea.

**Bitot's spots ——————→ xerosis conjunctiva ——————→ xeropthalmia**

*Bitot's spots are triangular gray spots appearing on conjunctiva.*

Other symptoms include respiratory infections, follicular hyperkeratosis (commonly seen on the anterior thighs and posterior arms due to keratinization of the hair follicles), reduced immunity, diarrhea, loss of tooth enamel, loss of bone mass, and the loss of both taste and smell.

## VII. Therapeutics

1) **Enhance immunity**–vitamin A 100,000-150,000 IU for 5-7 days then cut back to 25,000-50,000 IU

**NOTE**–Use vitamin A for any acute infectious condition. Usually it's best to begin with a high dose for a short (5-7days) time, then cut back. Vitamin A can be used in the treatment of AIDS and other related infectious conditions. Recent studies have shown beta carotene may also be beneficial.

STUDY–Coutsoudis, Hons, Kiepiela, Coovadia, Broughton. *Vitamin A supplementation enhances specific IgG antibody levels and total lymphocyte numbers while improving morbidity in measles.* The Pediatric Infectious Disease Journal Vol 11, #3 p.203-9, 1992. ABSTRACT–In a randomized double blind trial, 31 African children, aged 4-24 months, infected with measles, were given either 100,000 IU of retinyl palmitate (if under 12 months of age), 200,000 IU retinyl palmitate (if over 12 mo.), or placebo. The supplemented group had a significant reduction in morbidity during the acute (Day 8, P=0.006) and chronic (Day 42, P=0.02; 6 months, P=0.002) phases. In the treated group there was an increase in total number lymphocytes P=0.05 and measles IgG antibody concentrations (Day 8 P=.02), both of which have been shown to correlate more closely with outcome in measles than other immunologic factors.

STUDY–Alexander, M., et al. *Oral Beta carotene can increase the number of OK4+ cells in human blood.* Immunol. Letters 9, 221-25, 1994. ABSTRACT–Daily supplementation of 300,000 IU beta carotene/day for 7 days increased the frequency of OK4+(helper inducer T cells) by about 30% and after 14 days increased all T cells.

STUDY–Brevard, P.B. *Beta carotene affects WBCs in human peripheral blood.* Nutr Rep Internat .40,139-15, 1989. ABSTRACT–126 healthy college students were randomly assigned to 3 groups, a placebo, synthetic beta carotene 15,000 IU and an equivalent of 15,000 IU of beta carotene from foods. The synthetic beta carotene group had the greatest increase in WBC count and function.

2) **Cancer**–Vitamin A can be used to both treat (adjunctive therapy) and prevent cancers (see toxicity). There have been a number of studies showing beta carotene's cancer protective effects. More recently, carotene compounds called lycopenes, which are found in high amounts in tomatoes, have been shown to protect against prostate cancer. Several studies have shown that males consuming regular amounts of tomato sauce experience cancer protective effects. Watermelon, guava and pink grapefruit have significant amounts as well.

**Epithelial pathologies:**

**3) Acne**–200,000 IU-500,000 IU/day for 3 -5 months. Vitamin A may regulate prostaglandins that control the secretion of sebaceous glands in the skin. Vitamin E may enhance the effectiveness of vitamin A. One study used tetracyclin 1x/day after vitamin A treatment and was very effective and prevented the reoccurance of the acne.

STUDY–Kligman, A.M., et al. *Oral vitamin A in acne vulgaris.* Int. J. Dermatol. 20:278, 1981. ABSTRACT–123 cases of acne were treated. Most subjects responded favorably, but doses under 300,000 IU were ineffective. After 5 months of treatment, there were no serious cases of toxicity. Only 1 patient had a transient elevation of liver function tests and 1 or 2 patients had transient headaches.

STUDY–Ayres, S. Jr., Mihan R. *Acne vulgaris and lipid peroxidation: New concepts in pathogenesis and treatment.* Int. J. Dermatol. 17:305, 1978. ABSTRACT–Over 100 patients with acne were successfully treated with average daily doses of 100,000 IU vitamin A and 800 IU of vitamin E. Most responded within weeks and maintenance of control was obtained with lower doses.

**4) Menorrhagia**–Vitamin A 50,000 IU-75,000 IU

STUDY–Lithgow, D.M., Politzer, Wm. *Vitamin A in the treatment of menorrhagia.* S. Afr. Med. J. 51:191-3, 1977. ABSTRACT–71 women with menorrhagia were found to have significantly lower serum vitamin A levels than healthy controls. 40 of these women were treated with vitamin A 25,000 IU 2x daily for 15 days. Menstruation returned to normal in 57.5% and diminished in an additional 35%.

**5) Wound healing** (stomach ulcers, colitis, burns, respiratory tract injury as in emphysema etc.)–Vitamin A is involved in the formation and regeneration of epithelial cells. In animal and human studies increased stress may increase cortisol levels which increase the incidence of stomach ulcers. Vitamin A has been shown to significantly decrease ulcer formation.

**6) Cervical dysplasia**–60,000 IU-100,000 IU/day of vitamin A (not ß carotene). It has been found in a few studies that women who consume less than average vitamin A and ß carotene were 3x more likely to have dysplastic changes or carcinoma in situ. Both ß carotene and vitamin A can be used topically.

**7) Lupus**–Vitamin A is indicated especially regarding the epithelial skin damage.

**8) Psoriasis**–Vitamin A inhibits ornithine decarboxylase, the rate-limiting step in endogenous polyamine synthesis (see psoriasis). Polyamines are endogenous endotoxins which exacerbate any dermatological pathology.

**9) Seborrheic keratosis or Senile keratosis**–100,000 IU/day for 1-2 years (monitor toxicity)

**10) Ichthyosis**–100,000 IU/day for a few months

**11) Prevention of sunburn**–give both 150,000 IU β carotene and 100,000 IU vitamin A a few days before exposure to sun. Give along with 500mg calcium carbonate.

**12) Follicular hyperkeratosis (Keratosis pilaris)**–25,000-75,000 IU day / 4-6 wks. Follicular hyperkeratosis is a classic sign of vitamin A deficiency (keratosis is a thickening and hardening of the cells); EFA, folic acid, or zinc deficiency; and hypothyroidism. The typical presentation is a gooseflesh appearance of the skin which begins on the posterior arms, anterior thighs, and buttocks.

13) **Photosensitivity disorders including erythropoietic protoporphyria (EPP)**–age 1-4, 60-80mg/day; adults 180mg/day–In EPP, elevated levels of porphyrins get deposited in various tissues, including the skin. Ultra Violet light reacts with the porphyrins causing free radicals and extensive damage to the skin. Redness, burning, swelling, itching and general inflammation typically occur. Topical sunscreens apparently have little protective effect. Beta carotene has been found to be highly effective in preventing damage to the skin. A long term study, from 1969-75, of 133 patients showed 84% had a 3 times greater tolerance to sunlight with β carotene supplementation.

**Ophthamological conditions:**

14) **Night blindness**–5,000-20,000 IU/day–This is the classic sign of vitamin A deficiency. It readily responds to vitamin A or beta carotene therapy.

15) **Dry eyes (Sicca syndrome)**–Vitamin A drops 1-2 drops tid or as needed [Viva Eyedrops; available from Vision Pharmaceuticals (800)442-6789]. For eye irritation due to allergies, use vitamin A and C eyedrops. Also consider Sodium Cromolyn drops (Apothecure or Pfizer) and Similasan eye drops #2 [(800)426-1644]. For eye irritation due to viral conjunctivitis also try vitamin A and C drops, Rue fennel drops (Herb Pharm), Similasan #1 eye drops and Succus Cineraria maritima (Luyties Pharm Co.).

16) **Chalazion**–50,000-100,000 IU/day for several weeks. Use with poultice of French Green Clay, potato, carrot. Consider iodine therapy as well.

17) **Macular degeneration**–Lutein and zeaxanthin may offer significant protective effects.

## VIII. Drug Interactions

Vitamin A has been shown to diminish the decreased wound healing and immunosuppressive effects of corticosteroids.

## IX. Toxicity

### Vitamin A (retinol)

Toxicity to vitamin A varies greatly with the individual. Sketchy reports of toxicity have been reported in subjects supplementing as low as 20,000 IU/day. Alleged toxicity at this lower dose has occurred in persons with liver dysfunction caused by drugs, viral hepatitis, aging, or protein calorie malnutrition. Most cases of toxicity in nonpregnant females result from more than 200,000 IU/day supplementation for at least 6-8 months. The synthetic water soluble form of retinol produces the most toxicity. Reports of side effects have been caused by 20,000 IU/day supplementation for 4-6 months. However, doses as high as 500,000 IU-1,000,000 IU/day extending over several years have not caused any adverse effects in many people.

Typical symptoms, especially in children, include drowsiness, fatigue, irritability, vomiting and bulging of the fontanelle. In adults, bone pain, headaches, dry scaly skin, brittle nails, alopecia, gingivitis, cheilosis, hepatosplenomegaly, and visual disturbances have been reported. Generally, discontinuation of supplemental vitamin A causes symptoms to disappear within a few days with no permanent repercussions.

***The greatest concern about toxicity occurs during early pregnancy***. A report in the NEJM in 1995 reported doses of vitamin A greater than 10,000 IU/day during the first 7 wks of conception increased birth defects significantly. Another study in Lancet actually showed a decreased incidence of birth defects with doses over 10,000 IU/day when taken with a multivitamin supplement. It seems highly unlikely that such low doses could increase the risk of birth defects. If this were true, we would see a much higher incidence of birth defects in cultures like the Eskimos where people normally consume larger amounts of vitamin A from foods. Furthermore, there are many women in the U.S. who consume more than 10,000 IU of vitamin A from both dietary sources and supplements and we don't see any increase in birth defects.

STUDY-Rothman KF, et al. –*Teratogenicity of high vitamin A intake* NEJM 333:1369-73, 1995. ABSTRACT-22,748 pregnancies were studied looking at intake of vitamin A and incidence of birth defects. It was found that the number of total birth defects was 339 and the number of neural crest defects was 121. When the amount of vitamin A from supplements alone was studied in these 121 birth defects it was found that the relative risk was 4.8x in women taking greater than 10,000IU per day.

STUDY-Shaw GM, et al.High maternal vitamin A intake and risk of anomalies of structures with a cranial neural crest cell contribution Lancet 347:899-900, 1996. ABSTRACT-A study of 552,601 deliveries found a 45% lower risk of cleft lip or palate in women who took vitamin A supplements along with a multivitamin supplement compared to women who took no supplements.

STUDY–Diet and health NRC-p.516. NY State Dept of Health studied 16 out of 492 women who took between 15,000 IU to 50,000 IU per day with no side effects and no birth defects. Intakes in excess of 50,000 IU may lead to increased risk of birth defects according to animal studies. To date there is at least one anecdotal study that involves a woman ingesting 150,000 IU/day for 2 months before and 3 months after conception. Her pregnancy had to be terminated because of fetal malformations at 23 weeks.

STUDY–Von Lennep, E., et al. Prenatal Diag. 5:35-40, 1985.

STUDY–Hathcock, J., et al. *Evaluation of vitamin A toxicity*. AJCN, 52:183-202, 1990.

STUDY–Bernhardt, I. & Dorsey, D. *Hypervitaminosis A and congenital renal anomalies in a human infant.* Obster. Gynecol. 43, 750-55, 1974.

## Beta Carotene

The ingestion of ß carotene and the rest of the carotenoids in very high amounts may result in hypercarotenemia and reversible yellow discoloration of the skin. This can be distinguished from jaundice by the absence of scleral pigmentation. Beta carotene may have antagonistic effects on vitamin E status. Thus, it is a good idea to supplement vitamin E if large doses of beta carotene are given for prolonged periods. For that matter, it is wise to give all the fat soluble nutrients to someone who is taking large doses of beta carotene for prolonged periods of time. There have been some reports of women who consume large amounts of carotenoids from foods becoming amenorrheic.

In the NEJM 330, 1029-35, 1994, there was a study of 29,000 men in Finland who smoked and drank alcohol. These men were divided into several groups. It was found that the group that consumed only beta carotene had an 18% increase in lung cancer. The group that also took vitamin E had no such increase and even saw a significant decrease in prostate cancer. In another large trial in the U.S., the CARET study (Carotene and Retinol Efficacy Trial Cancer Research 54, 2038S-43S, 1994), over 18,000 men and women who were smokers and/or asbestos workers showed, after 4 years of 50,000 IU/day, a 28% increase in lung cancer and a 17% increase in cancer mortality. That study was discontinued prematurely because of this finding. Dr. Gaby has theorized that beta carotene may decrease levels of other carotenes such as lycopene and lutein in the body. In smokers and people exposed to asbestos these carotene levels may already be low. Surely it would make sense to do a trial with multiple carotenes as well as vitamin E and with vitamin E alone in order to differentiate the effects of these nutrients which should prove beneficial.

# VITAMIN D

Vitamin D is known as the "sunshine vitamin" or "rickets-preventive factor." In 1918, Mellanby, a British nutritionist, presented the first evidence of this fat soluble vitamin and its anti-rachitic properties. It had been known for over a century that cod liver oil could prevent rickets. In 1924, Steenbock and Hess discovered independently that ultraviolet light would give antirachitic properties to certain foods.

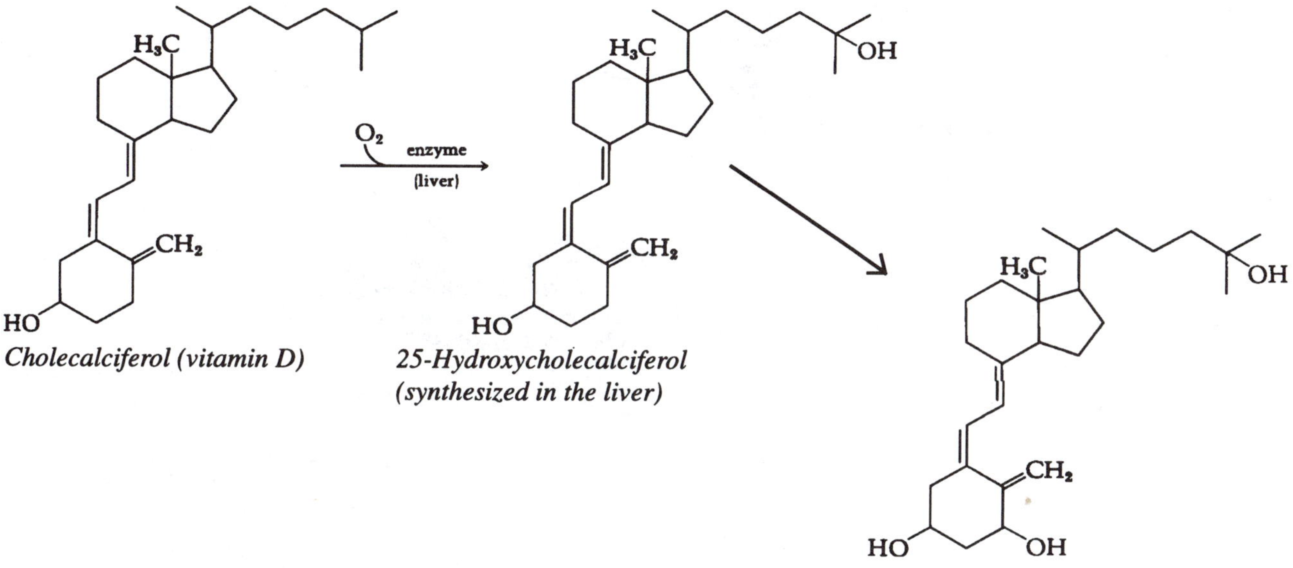

$O_2$ enzyme (liver)

*Cholecalciferol (vitamin D)*

*25-Hydroxycholecalciferol (synthesized in the liver)*

**1, 25 dihydroxycholecalciferol (most active form of vtiamin D)**

## I. Chemistry and Properties

Vitamin D (cholecalciferol) is stable to heat, light, and storage.
Vitamin D2 (ergocalciferol) is obtained from plants.
Vitamin D3 is cholecalciferol derived from animal products.

Relative potencies of vitamin D analogs:

| | | |
|---|---|---|
| 1x | cholecalciferol (1mcg = 40iu) | 1iu = .025mcg |
| 5x | 25 hydroxycholecalciferol | |
| 10x | 1,25 dihydroxycholecalciferol | |

**NOTE**–Calcitriol is the name of a drug which is the active (1,25 dihydroxycholecalciferol) form of vitamin D.

## II. Metabolism

Vitamin D can be synthesized in the skin with the aid of ultraviolet light. It is estimated that the RDA can be achieved with the exposure of 30% of a person's skin surface for 30 minutes at moderate latitudes.

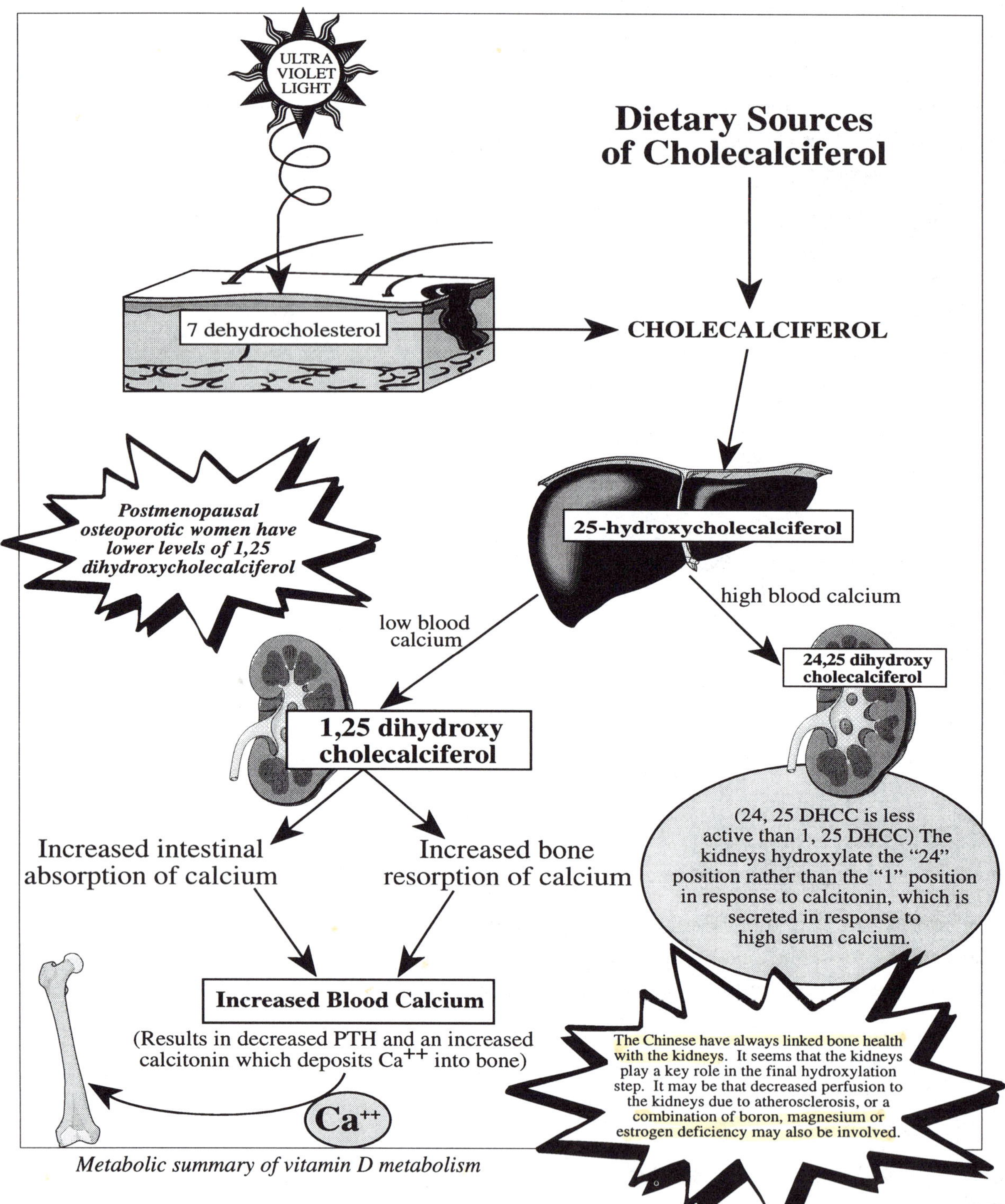


*Metabolic summary of vitamin D metabolism*

Vitamin D is absorbed from the small intestine in the presence of bile and is transported into the circulation via the lymph in chylomicrons (similar to vitamin A transport).

Vitamin D is stored in the liver, bone, brain, and skin.

**NOTE**–Osteoporotic women have normal 25 HCC but low levels of 1,25 DHCC. Diagnostic tools should include active vitamin D levels and treatment should be geared to enhance the function of the kidneys. Medications that effect kidney function should be re-evaluated.

## III. Function

**1,25 DHCC is the most active form of vitamin D. It functions to:**

- increase the absorption of calcium from the intestines by stimulating the synthesis of calcium-binding protein. This occurs in the brush border of the intestinal mucosa.
- increase the resorption of calcium from bone.
- increase serum calcium levels. Once this occurs calcium can then be stored in the bones. Thus, even though it initially causes bone resorption, the net effect is to increase calcium deposition in the bone.

## IV. Requirements

**RDA**–200IU for adults
400IU for children, adolescents and pregnant or lactating women
**LAB**– cholecalciferol 10-80ng/ml and 1,25 DHCC 21-45pg/ml
*Optimal daily intake*– depends upon sun exposure, latitude, time of year, pollution, clouds, skin color, family history, and vitamin D antagonists; could be from 0–800IU.

Requirements depend upon the exposure of a person's skin to ultraviolet (UV) radiation. Exposure is a function of the intensity of UV light and is determined by many factors, such as the latitude and altitude where one lives as well as the level of pollution and cloud cover in the environment. These are key factors in determining the amount of time one needs to be exposed to the sun in order to meet their requirement for vitamin D. Skin color is another factor which affects a person's ability to produce vitamin D. The darker the skin the less vitamin D will be produced, with as much as 95% blockage of UV light in people with very dark skin. However, even with the darkest skin color, sufficient levels of vitamin D are produced with long enough UV exposure and intensity. It should be noted that ordinary glass blocks almost all UV light. The sunscreens and sunblocks used on the skin to prevent sunburn also prevents formation of vitamin D. Any screen with a sun protection factor (SPF) of 8 or greater starts to block vitamin D synthesis.

## V. Sources

- **Sunshine**–With exposure to ultraviolet light the skin synthesizes vitamin D. It is estimated that 20 minutes, with face and arms exposed, will stimulate about 200 IU per day. A moderate sunburn can produce 10,000 IU per day. Significant amounts of vitamin D can be synthesized and stored to carry one through the winter.
- **Foods**–Vitamin D is found primarily in foods of animal origin, unless they are fortified (usually with ergocalciferol). Mushrooms are a significant non-animal source of vitamin D.

**Vitamin D Content in Unfortified Foods**

| Food | IUs per 100g | Food | IUs per 100g |
|---|---|---|---|
| Halibut liver oil (1T) | 16,800 | Mushrooms, morel (1 cup) | 87 |
| Sardines | 1150-1570 | Mushrooms, shitake (1 cup) | 70 |
| Codliver oil (1T) | 1200 | Mushrooms, chanterelle (1c) | 60 |
| Mackerel | 820-1100 | Pork | 45 |
| Herring | 320-840 | Halibut | 44 |
| Tuna | 252 | Egg yolk | 25 |
| Salmon | 150 -550 | Lamb | 20 |
| Shrimp | 150 | Beef | 9-42 |
| Human milk | | | |

**Vitamin D Content in Fortified Foods**

| Food | IUs per serving | Food | IUs per serving |
|---|---|---|---|
| Milk | 1 cup - 100 | Cherrios 3oz | 48 |
| *Pacific Rice Drink (plain) | 1 cup - 60 | Corn Flakes 3oz | 48 |
| *Rice Dream Beverage (enriched) Imagine Foods | 1 cup - 50 | Most all commercial cereals fortified 1 cup 30- 40gms | 36-48 |
| *Westbrae Westsoy (plus) | 1 cup - 50 | *Edensoy Extra (plain) | 1 cup - 20 |
| *Westbrae Rice Bev (enrich) | 1 cup - 50 | Cheese | 12-20 |
| Margarine (USA) 1pat-14g | 8.4 - 62 | Butter 1 T=14gms | 8 - 35 |

Milk used to make cheese or yogurt is usually not vitamin D fortified. Human milk contains the 25 hydroxycholecalciferol form of D probably because the liver in infants is relatively nonfunctional for the first hydroxylation of cholecalciferol. The vitamin D in human milk varies with sun exposure and vitamin D intake.

- **Tanning lamps**–it is possible to stimulate vitamin D synthesis with the UV light from tanning lamps and tanning booths. However, caution should be used with these lamps as they can ↑ risk of skin cancer.

## VI. Deficiency

In children a deficiency of vitamin D causes "**rickets,**" a malformation of the bones due to decreased deposition of calcium phosphate (hydroxyapatite). The signs and symptoms of this disease in young infants are restlessness, poor sleep and reduced mineralization of the skull away from the sutures. In older infants, sitting and crawling are delayed; bossing of the skull and costochondral beading (rachitic rosary) occur. There is also enlargement of epiphyseal growth plates, especially noted in the radius and ulna. Failure of the fontanelles to close results in a large head with delayed teeth eruption, stunted growth, bow legs, or "knock knees."

Deficiency of vitamin D in adults causes **"osteomalacia,"** a skeletal demineralization especially in the spine, pelvis, and lower extremities. Signs and symptoms of osteomalacia are burning mouth and throat, nervousness, diarrhea, and insomnia.

**Lab**–shows increased alkaline phosphatase, and decreased 25 HCC, and serum phosphorus. Serum calcium may be low or normal. Bone densiometry is very helpful in determining the density of the bone and this test is widely available now.

–1,25 DHCC (Meridian Labs)
–hair analysis to monitor progression of mineral absorption

**Etiology**–poor exposure to sun; dark skin; malabsorption (as in celiac disease); intestinal surgery; Ulcerative Colitis; Crohn's disease; decreased consumption of vitamin D; kidney or liver disease; vitamin D-resistant rickets; Cushing's disease; hypothyroidism; and anticonvulsive drug therapy.

## VII. Therapeutics

1) **Rickets**–1000 to 5000 IU/day vitamin D along with 1gm Calcium. Vitamin D-resistant rickets may require 50,000 IU to 500,000 IU per day or ***Calcitriol*** ®.
   This therapy may take up to two months before the symptoms are alleviated. If it is due to a malabsorption syndrome, the underlying etiology must be corrected. Bile salts may need supplementation. If there is a liver or kidney problem, or if it is vitamin D-resistant rickets, then use the 1,25 DHCC form ***Calcitriol*®.**

2) **Fractures** (especially in the elderly)–1000-3000 IU/day along with calcium and vitamin K. The activated form, 1,25 DHCC, may be indicated.

3) **Osteoporosis**–consider 1000 to 3000 IU vitamin D. Monitor 1,25 DHCC. The activated form, 1,25 DHCC, may be indicated. It appears that the best way for the elderly to get their daily dose of vitamin D is to get some natural sunlight so that they can synthesize cholecalciferol in the skin.

STUDY–Lancet ABSTRACT–Biopsies of 134 patients with femur fractures were shown to have osteomalacia. The largest number of fractures occurred from February to June.

STUDY–AJCN, Aug, 1981 ABSTRACT–The highest levels of 25 HCC were reached in November even though the strongest "ultraviolet exposure" was in July.

STUDY–Israeli J Med Sci. Jan 1981 ABSTRACT–82 elderly patients were compared to 30 young control subjects. 15 (19%) of the elderly had outright deficiency and 28 more had borderline levels. Even the elderly farm workers who got plenty of sunshine were significantly lower than controls. It is postulated by others that there is an impairment in the conversion to the active forms of vitamin D in the elderly.

**4) Cancer prophylaxis–200-400 IU/day**

Vitamin D has been shown to be protective against colon cancer. It may also be effective in the treatment of breast cancer.

STUDY–Garland, C. et al. *Serum Vitamin D and the risk of colorectal cancer.* Lancet, Nov.18, 1989. ABSTRACT–People with serum levels of at least 20mg/ml had a 70% reduction in colon cancer risk compared to those with lower vitamin D levels.

**5) Psoriasis**–Topical treatment with 1,25DHCC (Dovonex®)

STUDY–Kragballe, Knud. *Treatment of Psoriasis by the topical application of the Novel Cholecalciferol analogue Calcipotriol.* (MC 903) Arch Dermatol Vol 125; 1647-52, Dec 1989. ABSTRACT–A double-blind study of 50 patients with psoriasis vulgaris were treated topically (right and left sides) with different concentrations. Patients were treated 2x daily for 8 weeks. Marked improvement was seen in 40% of the patients treated with the 25 mcg/g concentration of Calcipotriol and in 88% treated with 100mcg/g concentration. No patient treated with the placebo had more than slight improvement.

## VIII. Toxicity

**Children**–Vitamin D intakes of 2,000 IU to 3,000 IU/day may cause toxicity symptoms in some children. Also, some hypersensitive infants have developed toxicity symptoms at 1,000 IU/day Most cases of toxicity involve the intake of 25,000-60,000 IU/day for 1-4 months. Children taking 10,000 IU/day for 4 months can develop the following **toxicity symptoms**: headaches, weakness, nausea & vomiting, constipation, polyuria, polydipsia, diarrhea, and calcification of soft tissues such as kidneys, lungs, tympanic membrane or ears.

**NOTE**–Large doses of vitamin A given concurrently with vitamin D tend to reduce the toxic effects of vitamin D.

STUDY–Kummerow, Cho, Huang, Imai, Kamio, Deutsch, Hooper. *Additive risk factors in atherosclerosis.* AJCN 2:579-584,1976. In pigs it was noted that supplementing 12.5x that which is recommended produced atherosclerotic lesions after 3 months. This would be the equivalent of an adult supplementing about 5,000 IU/day of vitamin D. The author, Kummerow, notes that the average per capita intake per day from vitamin D-enriched foods is about 2,435 IU Most of the foods that contain significant amounts of vitamin D are from animal sources such as meat and dairy.

STUDY–Kamio, A., Kummerow, F., and Imai, H. *Degeneration of aortic smooth muscle cells in swine fed excess vitamin D3.* Arch Pathol Lab Med 101: 378, 1977.

**Editorial**–There has been extensive talk about the development of arteriosclerosis due to excessive intake of vitamin D. Kummerow seems to be the biggest proponent, allegedly linking vitamin D to premature calcification of soft tissues especially concerning arteriosclerosis. After reviewing these studies and talking to numerous experts in the field, I have concluded that the problem seems to have been blown out of proportion. It appears that most people will benefit from a small amount of additional vitamin D (200-400 IU/day). Even daily consumption of 1,000 IU/day is probably innocuous.

## Notes

# VITAMIN E

Discovered as a dietary essential in 1922 by Evans and Bishop, Vitamin E became known as the "antisterility vitamin" because it was found to be necessary for normal reproduction in animals. Tocopherol (Gk."to bear offspring") was the name given to the isolate of wheat germ oil which contains Vitamin E.

HO, $H_3C$, $CH_3$, $CH_3$, $CH_3$, 5, 7, 8, O — $CH_2CH_2CH_2CH(CH_3)CH_2CH_2CH_2CH(CH_3)CH_2CH_2CH_2CH(CH_3)_2$

*d-α-Tocopherol (vitamin E)*
*RRR-a-tocopherol*

The position of the methyl groups on either the phenyl ring or side chain distinguishes the different forms of tocopherol.

## I. Chemistry

Tocopherols are oily yellow liquids, water insoluble, heat and acid stable, that deteriorate with exposure to alkali, light, oxygen, and on contact with iron and lead. Frying and freezing of foods also decreases the potency of Vitamin E. However, tocopherol esters, which are most commonly found in foods, tend to be fairly resistant to both frying and freezing.

There are 8 tocopherols. Of these, 4 occur naturally in foods, (alpha, beta, gamma, and delta or α, β, γ and δ ). d-alpha tocopherol accounts for 80% of the activity of the vitamin, however it may exhibit lower *in-vivo* or *in-vitro* antioxidant activity when compared to the other *less biologically* active tocopherols. **d,l -alpha tocopherol** (SRR a-tocopherol) is the name given to synthetic derivatives which are composed of equal amounts of all the stereoisomers.

**NOTE**–When you see mixed tocopherols on vitamin labels, it indicates that 80% of the natural "d-alpha" variety is present with the remaining 20% being a mixture of β, γ and δ. An important distinction should be made regarding the different forms. The **d-alpha tocopherol** has the "*most biological activity*" of all the forms (currently this stereoisomer is now referred to as RRR-α-tocopherol where the Rs refer to the stereoisomers of tocopherol). This means that it will prevent deficiency symptoms in laboratory animals (chicks and rats) more efficiently than any of the other form. However, there is a question as to whether animal assays are appropriate for evaluation of human requirements. In addition, merely preventing deficiency symptoms may not be the best way to assess the function of tocopherol or, for that matter, other nutrients as well. Where one tocopherol form may prevent deficiency symptoms, another, with less "biological activity" may be better at preventing oxidation of LDL cholesterol or lipid membranes, and at lowering serum cholesterol, which is the case of γ tocopherol. The tocotrienols, which are less distributed in nature than the tocopherols, have not been well studied probably because they have so-called less biological activity. However, one study reported that they have greater antitumor effects than the most biologically active tocopherol.

STUDY– Komiyama, K, et. al., *Studies on the biological activity of tocotrienols.* Chem Pharm Bull 37, 1369-81, 1989.

## II. Metabolism

Vitamin E requires the presence of bile for absorption. At normal levels of intake only 20-30% of dietary vitamin E is absorbed. This percentage decreases with increased dosage. Vitamin E is stored in high amounts in the pituitary gland and the adrenals. There is no correlation between serum levels and Vitamin E stores. A serum peroxide value can give an indirect status.

## III. Function

**Anti-oxidant**–Vitamin E protects cell membranes, especially in the lungs and red blood cells. It particularly protects fatty acids against oxidative damage caused by various pollutants, peroxides, and free radicals formed during metabolic processes. It aids in the prevention of lipofuscin, an oxidized fat that has been implicated in the aging process. If insufficient vitamin E is present, PUFAs may become oxidized in the body. This causes various toxins to be formed. These toxins may lead to chromosomal damage and the formation of cancers. Evidence has been presented that supplemental vitamin E along with vitamin C may greatly inhibit the formation of mutagens in the feces, thus preventing the formation of polyps and cancer. Vitamin E may protect the liver and the rest of the body against environmental pollutants such as ozone and other constituents of smog. People receiving chemotherapy or radiation can also be protected with additional vitamin E supplementation.

**_The antioxidant function of tocopheral_**

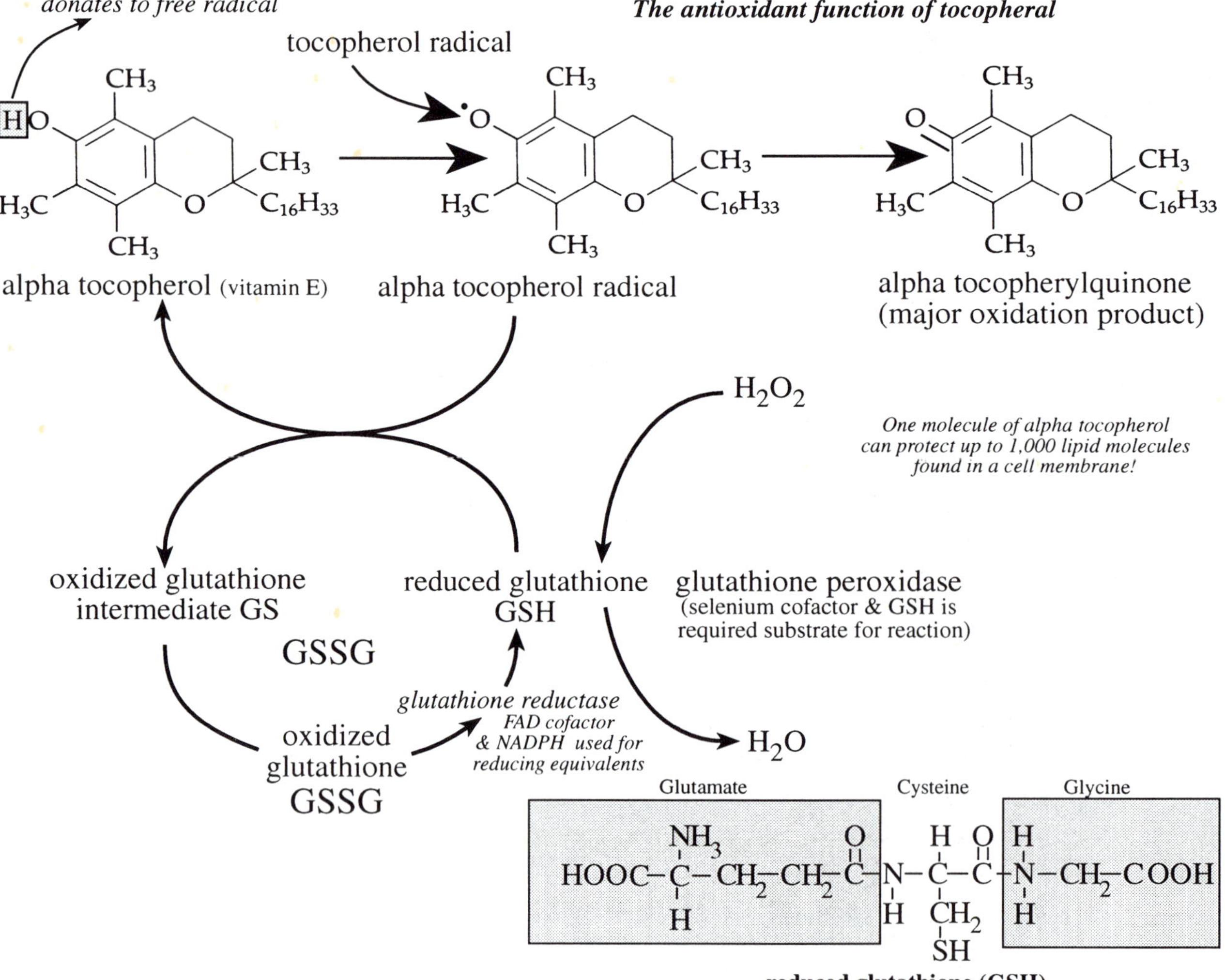

Vitamin E works synergistically with other antioxidant nutrients including selenium, vitamin C, B-carotene and others to quench free radicals, peroxides and other potentially harmful substances. Vitamin E can spare other antioxidants and vice versa.

Red blood cells, because of their high oxygen tension, are particularly susceptible to oxidative damage. Sickle cell anemia has been successfully treated with vitamin E.

**Other antioxidant functions**:

**Nerve and muscle function**–vitamin E is vital for protecting nerve and muscle cell function. In children who had a lack of bile (cholestasis) necessary to absorb fats and vitamin E, it was found that vitamin E was able to protect against damage to Schwann cells, dorsal root ganglia and muscle cells. In adults who are deficient in vitamin E, peripheral nerve degeneration results.

**Premature infants**–develop retrolental fibroplasia or damage to the retina due to their high oxygen exposure. Vitamin E can protect against this damage. In addition, vitamin E can protect the lens of the eye from oxidation, cross linking of the collagen fibers and formation of cataracts.

**Muscular dystrophy–**such diseases have been treated with vitamin E with only anecdotal success.

**Cholesterol peroxidation**–can occur when vitamin E is deficient. In particular LDL cholesterol yields epoxycholesterols which have been implicated in cardiovascular disease (see atherosclerosis p. 243).

**Other functions of vitamin E:**

**Anti-inflammatory effects–**vitamin E inhibits the enzyme lipoxygenase, an enzyme responsible for the formation of leukotrienes which cause inflammation. This can be useful in the treatment of asthma and other inflammatory conditions such as arthritis.

**Anti-platelet aggregation effects**–vitamin E at higher doses has been shown to increase production of prostaglandin I2 which inhibits platelet stickiness.

## IV. Requirements

| | |
|---|---|
| **RDA**–15IU/day | 1mg d-alpha tocopheryl acetate =1.49IU |
| synthetic | 1mg d,l-alpha tocopherol=1 IU |
| | 1mg d-alpha tocopheryl acetate =1 alpha tocopherol equivalent |

**Lab**–Serum tocopherol & RBC hemolysis in hydrogen peroxide

*Optimal daily intake*–600IU, but depends on toxin exposure

Optimal intake level is dependent upon the intake of unsaturated fatty acids. The greater the content of fatty acids in the diet the greater the requirement of vitamin E. Other antioxidant nutrients can, to a certain extent, spare vitamin E. The level of exposure to environmental pollutants such as cigarette smoke, industrial pollution and various other chemicals also determines the ideal requirement for vitamin E. People working in areas where their exposure to toxins is greater, such as a bar, toll booth, print shop, nuclear power plant and many others have an increased requirement for vitamin E as well as other antioxidant nutrients. People receiving chemotherapy and/or radiation have an increased requirement because of the damaging effects of these elements to healthy tissue. Intake should be increased before, during and after therapy with these agents (see surgery preparation in the appendix). Oxyquench is a product that I developed which contains vitamin E as well as other antioxidants including Silymarin (Omnivite Nutrition Inc.). Silymarin has synergistic activity with vitamin E. It is one of the most powerful antioxidants for the liver. It is derived from the plant Silybum marianum.

Storage of vitamin E is limited. The liver briefly stores vitamin E but only in small quantities. Adipose tissue and the adrenal glands do store vitamin E as well. The adipose tissue slowly accumulates vitamin E and then in time slowly releases it as well.

## V. Sources

### Best Food Sources of Vitamin E

| Food | amount | IUs | Food | amount | IUs |
|---|---|---|---|---|---|
| Wheat germ oil | 1 T | 37.2 | Mango | 1 med (200g) | 3.5 |
| Yogurt, Nancy's soy | 1 cup | 33.0 | Avocado | 1 med | 3.5 |
| Sunflower seeds | 1/4 cup | 26.8 | Soy oil | 1 T | 3.5 |
| Mayonnaise, Hellmanns | 1 T | 16.5 | Peanut Oil | 1 T | 3.4 |
| Almonds | 1/4 cup | 12.7 | Brazil nuts | 8 med nuts | 3.2 |
| Sunflower oil | 1 T | 12.7 | Spinach | 2 cups (100g) | 3.0 |
| Pecans | 1/4 cup | 12.0 | Olive oil | 1 T | 2.4 |
| Hazelnuts (filberts) | 1/4 cup (30g) | 12.0 | Lobster | 3 oz | 2.3 |
| Margarine, Mazola | 1 T | 12.0 | Pistachio nuts, dried | 47 nuts (1oz) | 2.3 |
| Wild purslane | 1 cup (50g) | 9.0 | Plums, fresh whole | 3 med | 2.3 |
| Sweet potato | 1 med | 9.0 | Dandelion greens, raw chopped | 1 cup (56gms) | |
| Tempeh | 2 oz | 8.5 | Salmon steak | 3 oz | 2.0 |
| Almond oil | 1 T | 8.0 | Swiss chard, cooked | 1 cup | 2.0 |
| Safflower oil | 1 T | 7.9 | Squash, winter, boiled | 1 cup | 1.9 |
| Flax oil | 1 T | 7.5 | Cherries, fresh | 20 med | 1.8 |
| Wheat germ | 1/2 cup | 6.4 | Cabbage, raw, green | 1 cup | 1.5 |
| Tofu, 2.5 x 2.7 x 1" | 1 med slab | 6.3 | Tomato | 1 med | 1.5 |
| Buckwheat flour | 1/2 cup | 5.8 | Peas, green | 1/2 cup | 1.5 |
| Soybean flour | 1/2 cup | 5.3 | Apricots, dried | 6 halves | 1.5 |
| Peanuts | 1/4 cup | 4.9 | Rice bran | 1 T | 1.4 |
| Corn oil | 1 T | 4.8 | Pear | 1 med | 1.3 |
| Spinach, cooked, chopped | 1 cup | 4.7 | Walnuts, whole | 7 nuts | 1.1 |
| Cod liver oil | 1 T | 3.9 | Brussels sprouts | 1/2 cup (4med) | 1.0 |
| Peanut butter | 2 T | 3.8 | Blackberries | 1 cup | 1.0 |
| Corn oil margarine | 1 T | 3.6 | Currants | 1/2 cup | 0.84 |
| Wheat flour, whole | 1/2 cup | 3.6 | Seaweed, kelp or Kombu raw | 1/2 cup chop | 0.7 |

Different forms of vitamin E and content of selected foods expressed as mg per 100gms food

| Food | α | β | γ | δ | Total |
|---|---|---|---|---|---|
| **Oils** | | | | | |
| Safflower | 34–46 | —[b] | 7–19 | 24 | |
| Sunflower | 49 | — | 5 | 0.8 | |
| Corn | 5–26 | 5 | 44–70 | 1–14 | |
| Soybean | 3–12 | — | 32–63 | 5–25 | 56–109 |
| **Nuts** | | | | | |
| Almonds | 23–32 | 0.3 TM | 0.9 (0.5[a]) | — | |
| Walnuts, pecans | 0.4–1.2 | — | 16–20 | — | |
| Peanuts | 10–11 | — | 7–8 | 1–2 | |
| **Grains** | | | | | |
| Oats, whole | 1.5–2.1 | — | 0.05 | — | |
| Wheat, whole | 1.0–1.4 | 0.7–0.8 (2.5–3.3)[a] | — | — | 0.3–0.5 |
| Rice, brown | 0.3–1.4 | — | 0.3–0.4 | — | |
| **Fruits/vegetables** | | | | | |
| Muskmelon | 10 | — | — | — | |
| Canteloupe | 0.1 | — | — | — | 0.14 |
| Bananas | 0.2–0.5 | — | — | — | 0.4 |
| Orange juice | 0.04 | — | — | — | 0.18 |
| Carrots | 0.5–0.6 | 0.01–0.02 | — | — | |
| Broccoli | 0.5 | — | 0.2 | — | |
| Tomatoes | 0.4 | — | — | — | 0.85 |
| Beans (cooked) | 0.02–0.3 | — | 0.1–7.1 | tr-0.5 | |
| Cauliflower | 0.04 | — | 0.05 | — | |
| **Meats, fish, etc.** | | | | | |
| Butter | 1.7–3.3 | — | 0.14 | — | 1–3.2 |
| Milk | 0.04 | — | — | — | 0.1 |
| Eggs | 0.5 | — | — | — | 1.4 |
| Hamburger | 0.3–0.4 | — | — | — | 0.5–0.6 |
| Haddock | 0.4–0.6 | — | — | — | 1.2 |
| Liver | 0.5–0.6 | — | — | — | 1.6 |
| Margarine | 3.0–33 | — | 29± | 8± | |

From Bauernfeind, JC. Tocopherol levels in common foods. Crit Rev Food Sci Nutr 9:337, 1977.

## VI. Deficiency

Vitamin E deficiency is rare in humans. One study, in which mental patients were supplied with 3 mg of vitamin E, resulted in the hemolysis of their red blood cells. It has also been observed that SIDS babies have blood levels of vitamin E similar to those of premature infants. It is possible that the respiratory stress may be related to lack of antioxidant protection early in life. Premature infants are susceptible to damage of the retina (retrolental fibroplasia) due to the high oxygen tension they are exposed to. Vitamin E can protect against such oxygen-generated damage to the retina and also the lungs as well.

In animal studies central nervous system changes (encephalomalacia) and exudative diathesis occurs. There may also be liver degeneration and reproductive failure affecting both males and females. Muscular dystrophy is another sign of a vitamin E deficiency.

**The signs and symptoms of vitamin E deficiency** are dry skin, easy bruising, decreased clotting time, eczema, elevated indirect bilirubin, psoriasis, elevated heavy metals, PMS, cystic fibrosis, sickle cell anemia, beta thalassemia, cataracts, fibrocystic disease, benign prostatic hypertrophy, poor wound healing, hot flashes, growing pains, and Osgood-Schlatter disease.

## VII. Therapeutics

STUDY–Packer & Lester. *Interaction among antioxidants in health and disease: vitamin E and its redox cycle* Proceedings of the society for experimental biology and medicine. 200:271-276, 1992. Vitamin E inhibits phospholipase A2 activity which prevents release of arachidonic acid (see asthma leukotriene synthesis). Vitamin E also has an inhibitory effect on lipoxygenase and a stimulatory effect on cyclooxygenase. This seems to be the mechanism for its anti-inflammatory effects. In addition, vitamin E and its antioxidant effects seems to protect blood vessels from oxidation and damage, and the lens of the eyes from the damaging effects of ultra-violet light.

### 1) **Nocturnal cramping**–400 IU to 800 IU/day

STUDY–Ayres, Mihan. *Nocturnal leg cramps: A progress report on response to Vitamin E.* South Med. J. 67(11):1308-12,1974. ABSTRACT–103/125 patients with nocturnal leg and foot cramps, over half of whom had suffered for over 5 years, reported complete or nearly complete relief. 20/125 had a moderate to good response and only 2 failed to respond. l/2 responded to 300 IU or less, while half required 400 IU or more. Many had to continue vitamin E to prevent cramps from recurring. Response was usually within 1 week. Similar success was obtained with nocturnal rectal cramps, abdominal muscle cramps, and cramps following heavy exercise.

### 2) **Intermittent claudication**–400 IU-2000 IU/day

STUDY–Haeger. *Longtime treatment of intermittent claudication with vitamin E.* Am J Clin Nut 27:1179, 1974. ABSTRACT–The vitamin E in the muscles of elderly men with peripheral occlusive arterial disease was found to be lower than in normal subjects. During vitamin E therapy the increase in muscle vitamin E content was proportional to the degree of clinical improvement. 47 men were followed for 2-5 years. Each patient received either 300mg of d-alpha tocopherol acetate per day, along with vasodilators, or anticoagulants (dicoumarin). After about 4-6 months of treatment, the increase in walking distance in the vitamin E group was significantly greater than in the non-vitamin E treated groups. 54% of those in the vitamin E group reached the test limit of 1,000 meters of uninterrupted walking, compared to 23% of those treated w/o vitamin E. **Arterial blood flow was significantly better in the vitamin E group, but this difference did not occur until after about 12-18 months.** After 20-25 months, arterial flow to the lower leg had increased by about 34% in the vitamin E group, while no change occurred in those receiving the other therapies.

3) **Restless leg syndrome**–400-800 IU/day–consider using along with Ginkgo biloba and cal/mag and folate.

4) **Muscular dystrophy**–mostly anecdotal stories but outright deficiency leads to M.D.; it makes sense that vitamin E can help heal and protect the muscles because of its antioxidant abilities.

5) **Dysmenorrhea–**75 IU 3x/day; can go up to 400 IU tid.

–Butler & McKnight. *Vitamin E in the primary treatment of primary dysmenorrhea.* Lancet 1:844-47, 1955. ABSTRACT–100 women with spasmodic dysmenorrhea received either alpha tocopherol tabs 50mg 3x/day or placebo for 10 days premenstrually and for the next 4 days. After 2 cycles, 34/50 (68%) in the experimental group improved compared to 9/50 (18%) of the controls.

6) **Fibrocystic breast disease**

7) **Menopause–** can use up to 3,000 IU/day very effective. Some researchers believe the unesterified forms may be more effective.

8) **PMS**

9) **Spontaneous abortions**

10) **Scleroderma & scar tissue–** can use both topically and orally. Apply to surgical wounds once danger of infection has passed. Can use along with Aloe vera, zinc oxide and Herbal Ed Salve (Herb Pharm 1-800-348-4372).

11) **Herpetic lesions and post-herpetic neuralgia**

12) **Raynaud's Syndrome**

13) **Acne**

14) **Seborrheic dermatitis**

15) **Psoriasis**

16) **Osteoarthritis**

STUDY–Machtey, Ouaknine. *Tocopherol in OA: a controlled pilot study.* J. Am Geriat. Soc. 26:328, 1978. ABSTRACT–29 patients, average age 56.5 years, with osteoarthritis received tocopherol 600mg/day and placebo, each for 10 days in a randomized single blind crossover trial. Average duration of symptoms in this group was 9.3 years Patients with inflammatory arthritis were excluded from the study. The effect of tocopherol was assessed by the patients' records, by the physician's examination and interview, and by the amount of analgesics used during the study. A good analgesic effect of tocopherol was noted in 52% of the 29 patients, while only 4% of patients reported such an effect during placebo administration.

17) **Osgood Schlatter's disease–** 400 IU bid use along with selenium 200mcg/day. Can also apply topically along with DMSO and arnica oil. Can also use for "growing pains" (pains in children's legs felt inside or around shins).

18) **Allergy and inflammatory thrombophlebitis**

19) **Anemia, sickle cell anemia & other types of hemolytic anemia**

20) **Cystic fibrosis–**associated with defective absorption of vitamin E because of lack of lipase and formation of chylomicrons. Adding bile salts (Cholecol® from Standard Process) may help.

21) **Retrolental fibroplasia**–in premature infants given $O_2$.

22) **SIDS**–evidence indicates that vitamin E is low in these babies.

23) **Premature infants**–usually are low and have an increased requirement for lungs, etc.

24) **Down Syndrome**–in Down Syndrome there is an increased oxidative problem.

**Cardiovascular Effects**

- Vitamin E 400-2,000 IU/day decreases platelet aggregation.
- Vitamin E causes an increase in HDL.
- Vitamin E decreases vascular fragility.
- Vitamin E may protect the endothelial cells of the arteries from becoming oxidized. In addition it may prevent the oxidation of LDL cholesterol and the formation of epoxycholesterols.

## VIII. Toxicity

1800 IU/day has been shown to cause a prolonged blood clotting time. Vitamin E may interfere with vitamin K.

Hypertension can develop in certain people with sensitivities to Vitamin E. Based upon personal experience, it seems rare. Wilfrid Shute's Vitamin E for Ailing & Healthy Hearts warns that D-alpha-tocopherol if started at too high a dose can increase the contractility of the heart lead to high blood pressure (may also be related to soy allergy). Start out with low doses of vitamin E (100 IU) and gradually work up.

Reports of infant deaths in 1983 due to parenteral administration of vitamin E were found to be related to the solubilizing agent polysorbate instead of vitamin E. This compound was subsequently banned. In premature infants, oral preparation of vitamin E with high osmolality resulted in cases of necrotizing enterocolitis. A few studies have shown larger doses of d,1-alpha tocopherol may ↓ immunity. However, other studies, especially in the elderly, have shown an enhancement of immune function.

Increased triglycerides may be a result of vitamin E toxicity.

Nausea, flatulence, diarrhea may occur from too much vitamin E.

## IX. Interactions

- Iron binds with vitamin E and inactivates it.
- Vitamin E is synergistic with selenium.
- Vitamin A prevents oxidation of vitamin E.
- Large doses of vitamin E may reduce the intestinal absorption of vitamin K and prolong bleeding time. Use with caution in diabetics (retinal bleeding). Balance with vitamin K if using large dose for prolonged period.
- As the amount of polyunsaturated fatty acids goes up in the diet, vitamin E requirements increase proportionally.
- At larger doses, vitamin E may enhance the anticlotting effects of warfarin and coumarin. May need to adjust dose down accordingly.

# VITAMIN K

Vitamin K was first discovered in 1934 by Danish scientist Henrik Dam. The Danish word for coagulation is **K**oagulation. The term vitamin K is used to represent a group of substances belonging to a chemical group known as quinones.

## I. Chemistry

The naturally occurring forms of vitamin K are all fat soluble. They are stored in the liver, though not to any great extent. Stable to heat and reducing agents, they are destroyed by light, acid, alkali, oxidizing agents, and alcohol.

$K_1$–phytonadione or phylloquinone(*Aquamephyton*)–is a natural derivative from fish or plants

$K_2$–menaquinone–fat-soluble form made by intestinal bacteria

$K_3$–menadione–the synthetic water-soluble form tends to have a greater degree of toxicity

O, O, $CH_3$, $CH_2CH{=}C(CH_2CH_2CH_2CH)_3CH_3$ with $CH_3$ branches

*Phylloquinone (vitamin K)*

## II. Metabolism

Vitamin $K_1$ is absorbed in the upper GI tract and requires bile salts for absorption.

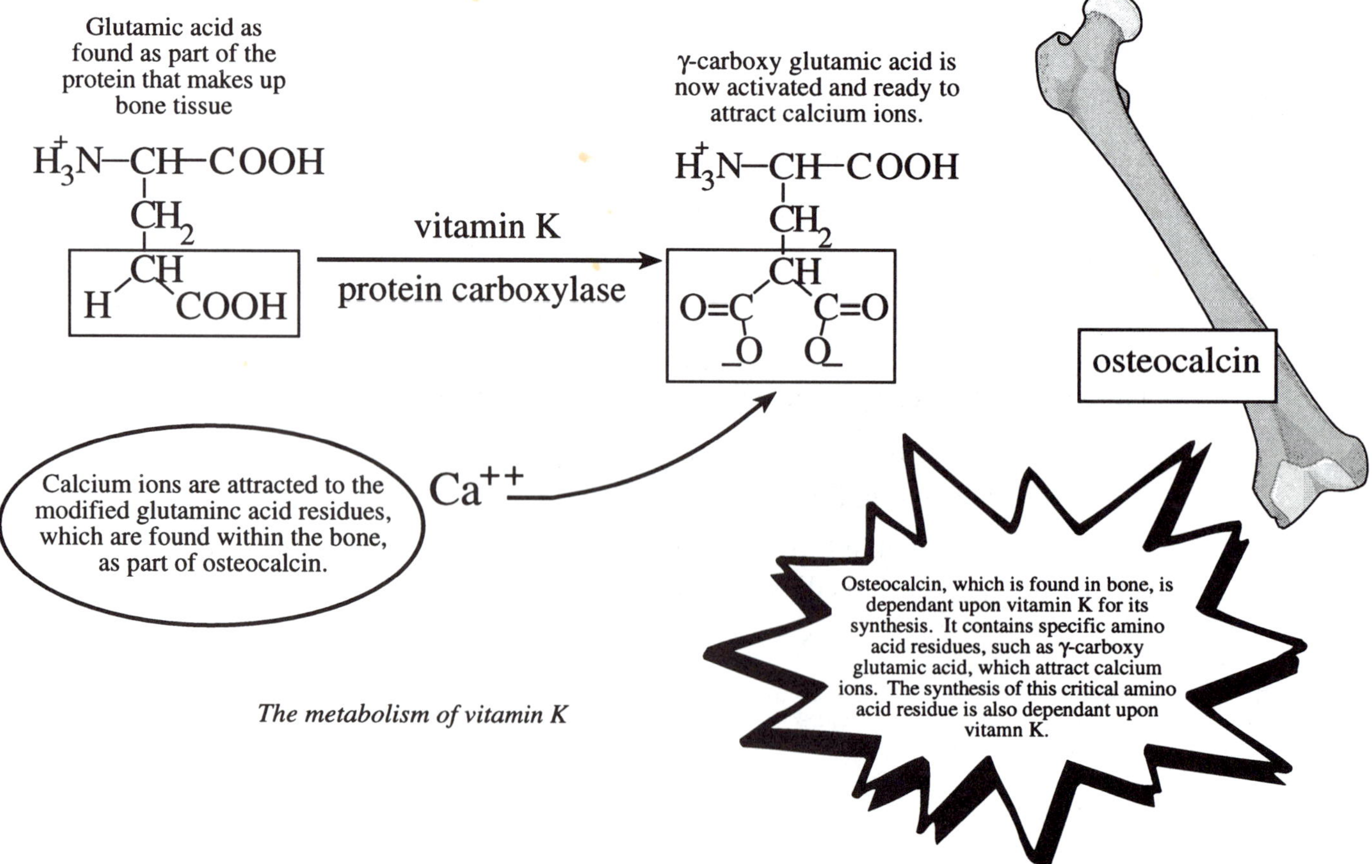


*The metabolism of vitamin K*

## III. Function

1) **Vitamin K acts as a cofactor in the final synthesis of proteins with a modified amino acid residue.**
   This modified glutamic acid residue is:
   a) found in bone proteins and can bind onto calcium ions to cause calcification.
   b) found in the blood and along vessel walls, and along with platelet-derived phospholipid, binds calcium, and is an integral part of the clotting process.
2) **Vitamin K is involved in the synthesis of a protein, osteocalcin,** which is found in high amounts in bone. It allows calcium ions to bind, thus resulting in the calcification of bone.
3) **Vitamin K is involved in the synthesis of a kidney protein** that functions in the **inhibition of Calcium oxalate stone formation** via its ability to bind onto calcium in the kidneys.
4) **Vitamin K is involved in the synthesis of proteins C & S.** These 2 proteins, formed in the liver, promote fibrinolysis and anti-coagulation. Thus, they are involved with reducing inflammation.

## IV. Requirements

No RDA has been established but it is estimated that adults need 70-140mcg/day while infants require 20-100μg. Vitamin K(phytonodione) accumulates in the chlorophyll forming parts of plant leaves and, thus, dark green leafy vegetables are an excellent source. Vitamin $K_2$ (menaquinone) is synthesized by bacteria in the large intestine.

*Optimal daily intake*–750μg

## V. Sources

**Best Sources of Vitamin K**

| Food | Amount | Mcg | Food | Amount | Mcg |
|---|---|---|---|---|---|
| Turnip greens, cooked | 1/2 cup | 471 | Oats, cooked | 150g | 30 |
| Broccoli, cooked | 1 med stalk | 360 | Cheese | 2 oz | 20 |
| Cabbage, cooked | 1/2 cup | 91 | Watercress, chopped | 1/4 cup | 18 |
| Liver, beef | 3 oz | 78 | Peach | 1 med | 15 |
| Green tea | 4t (10g) | 72 | Peas | 1/2 cup | 15 |
| Lettuce, chopped | 1c packed | 71 | Green beans | 1/2 cup | 9 |
| Spinach, chopped, raw | 1c packed | 49 | Milk | 1 cup | 7 |
| Asparagus | 4med spears | 34 | | | |

## VI. Deficiency

1) **Infancy**–*"Hemorrhagic disease of the newborn"* has been related to Vitamin K deficiency. This is due to poor transport across the placenta–especially with premature infants. Also, because of the relatively sterile infant gut, the ability to make vitamin K is impaired.
2) **Easy bleeding in children**–especially spontaneous nose bleeds
3) **Osteoporosis**

STUDY–Hart, Shearer, Klenerman, and Catterall. *Electrochemical detection of depressed circulating levels of vitamin K in osteoporosis.* J Clin Endocrinol Metab vol 60, p.1268-69, 1985. ABSTRACT–16 patients with osteoporosis had mean serum vitamin K levels 35% of age matched controls.

STUDY–Hodges, Pilkington, Shearer, et al. *Age related changes in the circulating levels of congeners of vitamin K2, menaquinone7 & 8.* Clinical Science 78, 63–66, 1990. ABSTRACT–It was found that $K_1$ levels in elderly subjects were not appreciably different from younger ones but when MK8 was looked at the elderly were 2.5 times lower than the younger group.

**NOTE**–There are a number of drugs that interfere with the synthesis of vitamin K in the gut, including anticoagulants (warfarin), anticonvulsants, analgesics, and antibiotics. Consider the elderly at high risk.

## VII. Therapeutics

1) **Blood clotting disorders due to vitamin K deficiency**–as in the case of various malabsorption syndromes, poor diet especially in the elderly who aren't able to chew green vegetables containing vitamin K.

2) **Osteoporosis**–5-10mg/day

STUDY–Tomita. *Post menopausal osteoporosis CA study with vitamin $K_2$.* Clin Endocrinol 19:731-736, 1971. ABSTRACT–**It was found that in osteoporotic women treated with vitamin $K_2$, urinary calcium loss was reduced by 18-50%.**

STUDY–Knapen, Hamulyak, and Vermeer. *The Effect of Vitamin K supplementation on circulating osteocalcin and urinary Ca excretion.* Annals of Internal Med. 111:1001-5, 1989. ABSTRACT–No effect on osteocalcin levels occurred when 1mg of Vitamin K was given to premenopausal women. In postmenopausal women vitamin K induced an increase in serum osteocalcin, a decrease in urinary calcium excretion, and a decrease in urinary hydroxyproline.

3) **Floaters**–may be related to poor clotting in the tiny vessels around the eye and extravasation of RBC's into the vitreous humor. Vitamin K along with bioflavonoids may be helpful.

4) **Nausea and Vomiting of Pregnancy**–May need to be given parenterally 5-10mg along with 100mg of pyridoxine and B-12 or B complex. Usually works immediately and can be repeated a few days consecutively and every 3-4 days afterward. Can also be given orally 5mg vitamin K along with 1gm of vitamin C.

STUDY–Merkel, R. *The use of menadione bisulfite and ascorbate in the treatment of Nausea and Vomiting of pregnancy.* Am. J. Ob & Gyn. Aug 416-418,1952. ABSTRACT–64 out of 70 consecutive cases were helped with complete relief of symptoms in 3 days. 3 cases had the vomiting halted but not the nausea.

5) **Fractures**–Can be given parenterally in people who may have an absorption problem along with vitamin D. Orally 5-10mg/day during the period of healing of the fracture may be helpful when given along with calcium, magnesium and boron.

STUDY–Bouckaert, Said. *Fracture healing by Vitamin K.* Nature 185:849, 1960. ABSTRACT–Vitamin K supplemented to rabbits with fractures produced a significant acceleration of healing even though they were already receiving adequate levels in their diet.

6) **Inflammatory conditions–Rheumatoid Arthritis**

7) **Pruritus-** Generalized idiopathic pruritus may be treated with vitamin K. Can be used IM if fat malabsorption is present.

8) **Prevention of calcium oxalate kidney stones**–Vitamin K helps to synthesize a protein which binds onto calcium

## VIII. Toxicity

Large doses of Menadione, the synthetic derivative, may produce hemolytic anemia and jaundice in the infant. **Most toxicity is associated with IV use** and may be related to allergies to various preservatives or incipients.

## IX. Interactions

- Vitamin E may interfere with the absorption and utilization of vitamin K.
- Lactobacillus acidophilus may inhibit the growth of E. coli, which, in the large intestine, synthesizes vitamin K.
- Dilantin interferes with vitamin K functions and can lead to difficult blood clotting and problems associated with osteoporosis.
- Vitamin K may interfere with the anti-clotting effects of warfarin and coumadin. In people taking either of these medications vitamin K is not necessarily contraindicated but clotting times and prothrombin times should be monitored. In some cases the doses of these medications may need to be slightly raised to compensate for the effects of the vitamin K.

### Notes

---

# THIAMIN, VITAMIN B-1

The disease, beriberi, which literally means, "I can't, I can't," was recognized as early as 2600 B.C. In 1855 a Japanese naval officer, Takaki, was able to cure the 60% of his crew which was suffering from the affliction by feeding them milk and meat. Yet, even as late as 1897, scientists were convinced that beriberi was caused by a bacteria.

To prove this theory of bacterial cause, the Dutch physician, Eijkman, attempted to induce beriberi in chickens by injecting them with "infected blood." He was about to give up when he noticed that all of the chickens in the yard, including the ones he hadn't injected, were swaying as they walked. They exhibited symptoms similar to those of his patients who suffered from beriberi. Upon investigation, he discovered that a lazy cook had fed the chickens polished rice instead of brown rice. Returning brown rice to the poultry feed cured the chickens. From this it was deduced that beriberi was caused by a dietary deficiency.

Later, an accessory food factor was found in the husk of rice. This was named vitamin B. Subsequent investigators showed that there was more than one accessory food factor in rice husks and so the first discovered factor was renamed vitamin B-1. In 1936 R.R.Williams synthesized B-1 and named it thiamine because of the presence of a **thio** sulfur group and an **amine** side chain.

## I. Chemistry

Vitamin B-1 is a crystalline, yellow-white, water-soluble compound that is heat and alkali reactive when placed in solution. In its dry form it is heat and oxygen stable. Acid tends to make it more stable. Black tea, which contains an antithiamine factor (ATF), and chlorinated water tend to destroy B-1. Chlorogenic acid, found both in decaffeinated and caffeinated coffee, also destroys B-1. Thiamine is resistant to freezing.

STUDY–J. Nut. Sci. & Vitamin. Aug, 1979. Rice cooked in chlorinated water had 36% less thiamin than rice cooked in distilled water. Increasing the amount of chlorine decreases the thiamin content even more.

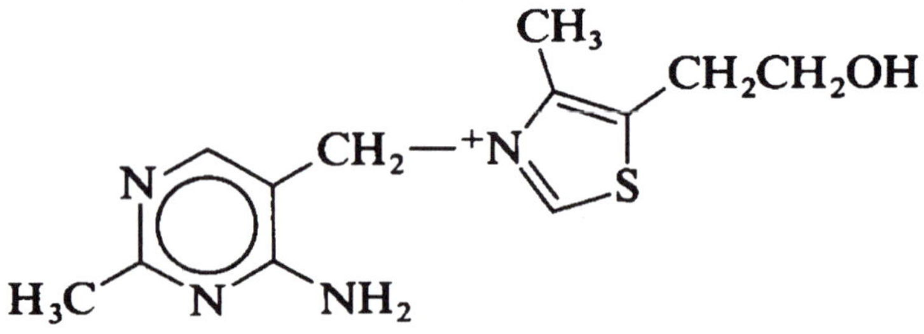

*Thiamin (vitamin B-1)*

## II. Metabolism

Thiamin, which is best absorbed in an acid medium, is passively absorbed in the proximal duodenum. When concentrations are low in the intestine, active transport takes place. In man, thiamin can be synthesized in the large intestine as thiamin pyrophosphate (TPP). TPP is too large a molecule to be absorbed across the intestinal mucosa. It requires the use of an enzyme to cleave the smaller thiamin molecule out of the compound. **Allicin, a substance found in onions and garlic, combines with thiamin and renders it more absorbable.** Small amounts of vitamin B-1 (30-70mg) are stored in the body, primarily in muscle tissue.

## III. Function

The active form, TPP, functions as a co-carboxylase. It is required for the oxidative decarboxylation of pyruvate to form active acetate and acetyl co-enzyme A. It is also required for the oxidative decarboxylation of other alpha-keto acids such as alpha-ketoglutaric acid and the 2 keto-carboxylates derived from the amino acids methionine, threonine, leucine, isoleucine and valine. TPP is also involved as a co-enzyme for the transketolase reaction, which functions for the pentose monophosphate shunt pathway.

TPP has a specific role in neurophysiology separate from its co-enzyme function. It works at the nerve cell membrane to allow displacement so that sodium ions can freely cross the membrane. Thiamin is needed for the metabolism of carbohydrates, fat, and protein. It is especially involved in carbohydrate metabolism in the brain.

## IV. Requirements

**RDA**–1.0-1.4mg

Increase in CHO intake increases the need for thiamin. Alcohol and aging also increase the need for thiamin. Maximum absorption of thiamin occurs at intakes of 5mg/day.

**Lab**–RBC transketolase less than 15% increase is normal.

*Optimal daily intake*–15-30mg

## V. Sources

**Best Food Sources of Thiamin**

| Food | Amount | Mg | Food | Amount | Mg |
|---|---|---|---|---|---|
| Brewer's yeast | 1 T | 1.25 | Rolled oats, cooked | 1 cup | 0.19 |
| Sunflower seeds | 1/4 cup | 0.72 | Brown rice, uncooked | 1/4 cup | 0.17 |
| Soybeans, dried | 1/4 cup | 0.58 | Flour, whole wheat | 1/4 cup | 0.17 |
| Wheat germ, toasted | 1/4 cup | 0.44 | Chick-peas, dried | 1/4 cup | 0.16 |
| Kidney, beef | 3 oz | 0.43 | Salmon steak | 3 oz | 0.15 |
| Navy beans, dried | 1/4 cup | 0.33 | Split peas, cooked | 1/2 cup | 0.15 |
| Flour, soy | 1/4 cup | 0.27 | Flour, dark buckwheat | 1/4 cup | 0.14 |
| Kidney beans | 1/4 cup | 0.24 | Cornmeal | 1/4 cup | 0.12 |
| Liver, beef | 3 oz | 0.22 | Collards, cooked | 1/2 cup | 0.10 |
| Flour, dark rye | 1/4 cup | 0.20 | Asparagus | 4 spears | 0.10 |

USDA Handbook, #8 Series, Washington, DC, ARS, USDA, 1976-1986

## VI. Deficiency

Clinical signs of thiamine deficiency primarily involve the nervous and cardiovascular systems. In adults the symptoms are:

1) Mental confusion, **anorexia,** muscle weakness, calf muscle tenderness, ataxia, indigestion, constipation, tachycardia and palpatations.
2) "Wet Beriberi"–edema starting in the feet progressing upward into the legs, trunk, face, and eventually into the heart where death is caused by heart failure.
3) "Dry Beriberi"–worsened polyneuritis in early stages, difficulty walking, and **muscle wasting**; *Wernicke Korsakoff syndrome* consisting of nystagmus caused by weakness in the 6th cranial nerve, irritability, and disordered thinking.

Commonly, the distinction between wet (cardiovascular) and dry (neuritic) manifestations of beriberi relates to the duration and severity of the deficiency, the degree of physical exertion, and the caloric intake. The wet or edematous condition results from severe physical exertion and high carbohydrate intake. The dry or polyneuritic form stems from relative inactivity with caloric restrictions during the chronic deficiency.

**Infant symptoms appear suddenly and severely, involving cardiac failure and cyanosis.**

The etiology of the deficiency can be traced to an exclusive diet of milled, non-enriched rice or wheat, raw fish consumption (microbial thiaminases), large amounts of tea, alcoholism (impaired absorption and storage), and/or several inborn errors of metabolism.

CLINICAL NOTE–Alcoholics frequently develop a deficiency of thiamin because thiamin is a necessary cofactor in the metabolism of alcohol. Since many alcoholics tend to eat less and drink more and usually their alcoholic drinks are low in thiamin, they frequently develop a thaimin deficiency. In hospitals it is routine for alcoholics when they are admitted to get intramuscular injections of thiamin.

STUDY–J. Am. Geriatrics Society. Oct,1979–In New Jersey a study showed that 25% of 146 elderly people living at an old age home were deficient in B-1.

STUDY–Irish J. Med. vol 149,#3,1980. A study of the elderly showed up to 35% had B-1 deficiency.

STUDY–J. Am. Geriatrics Society. Dividing people into high-intake and low-intake of B-1 found that those with low levels had 2x as many cardiovascular complaints.

STUDY–Majumdar. *Blood vitamin status in patients with alcoholic liver diseases.* Int. J. Vitamin. Res. 52(3):266-71,1982. Out of 41 patients with alcoholic liver disease, all of them were deficient in blood thiamin levels.

## VII. Therapeutics

### 1) Anemia

STUDY–Mangel. *Thiamin dependant beriberi in the "thiamin-responsive anemia syndrome."* NEJM 311:836-38, 1984. ABSTRACT–A 3 month old girl presented chronic symptoms of severe anemia, diabetes, deafness and severe cardiac and neurological disturbances which, despite normal blood transketolase, responded to 100mg of B-1 daily. Symptoms reappeared when treatment was suspended, suggesting that every patient with unexplained anemia deserves a trial high dose B-1.

STUDY–Rogers. *Thiamin responsive megaloblastic anemia.* J. Pediatrics 74(4): 494-504,1969. ABSTRACT–A case of megaloblastic anemia failed to respond to B-12 or folic acid but responded to 20mg thiamin daily. When supplementation was stopped, symptoms returned.

### 2) Depression

STUDY–Brozek. *Psychologic effects of B-1 restriction and deprivation in normal young men.* AJCN. 5(2):109-20,1957. ABSTRACT–5/9 patients placed on a B-1 restricted diet developed marked depression and irritability.

**3) Sensory neuropathy** (diabetic)

STUDY–Mirsky, Stan. Diabetes:Controlling it the Easy Way. Random House, 1981. ABSTRACT–About 80% of patients were found to improve when supplemented with B-1. TPP is involved in the oxidative pathway and may be responsible for the energy required for nerve conduction.

STUDY–Stern. *The intraspinal injection of B-1 for the relief of intractable pain and for inflammatory and degenerative diseases of the CNS.* Am. J. Surg. 34:495, 1938. Intraspinal injections led to dramatic, though transient, improvements.

**4) Sciatica**–50mg given IM with B-12 It is not necessary to give in the area. It has systemic effect.

**5) Trigeminal Neuralgia**

STUDY–Borsook, H., Kremeres, M.Y., Wiggins, C.G. *The relief of symptoms of major trigeminal neuralgia (tic douloureux) following the use of B-1 and concentrated liver extract.* JAMA 1214:1421, 1940.

**6) Glaucoma**

STUDY–Asregadoo, E. R. *Blood levels of thiamin and ascorbic acid in chronic open-angle glaucoma.* Ann Ophthalmol p.1095, 1979.

**7) Insomnia**–A deficiency may decrease the availability of serotonin.

STUDY–AJCN ABSTRACT–20 patients, mostly teenagers, who had a varied array of symptoms classified as anxiety, were studied. These symptoms included irritability, intermittent diarrhea, lack of appetite, fatigue and insomnia . It was found that these patients had a high intake of simple carbohydrates. It was postulated that this increased consumption of carbohydrates resulted in an increased stimulation in the brain. Every one of the subjects studied had a decreased level of serum thiamin. Supplementation of 150-600mg of thiamin completely relieved symptoms in these patients.

**8) Neurosis and anxiety**–100-150mg/day. It has been found that neurotic people have 58% lower levels of B-1. If the patient's diet contains a high carbohydrate content, he/she may require 150-600mg/day of thiamin.

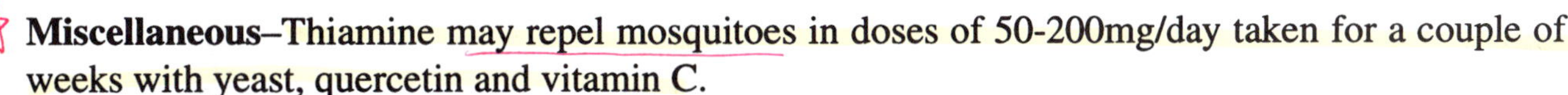

**Miscellaneous**–Thiamine may repel mosquitoes in doses of 50-200mg/day taken for a couple of weeks with yeast, quercetin and vitamin C.

## VIII. Toxicity

There is very little evidence of thiamin toxicity. In monkeys the lethal dose is greater than 350mg/kg body weight.

One anecdotal report tells of a person who took 3gms/day and developed headaches, irritability, weakness, flushing, and itching.

**When thiamin is given by injection either IM or IV, caution must be taken as anaphylactic reactions have been known to occur.**

## Notes

# RIBOFLAVIN, VITAMIN B-2

In the 20s it was known that there was more than one B vitamin since some growth-promoting properties in unmilled rice and wheat were retained after heating had destroyed the anti-beriberi properties. In 1933 Kuhn and coworkers isolated a yellow-green pigment from milk as part of "Warburg's yellow enzyme." In 1935 B-2 was synthesized. It was given the name **Riboflavin** because it was related to a class of compounds called flavins (fluorescent) and this moiety was attached to ribose.

## I. Chemistry

Stable to heat, oxidation, and acid, riboflavin is somewhat soluble in water. Light and alkali destroy it. It should be noted that bottled milk (which has a relatively large amount of B-2) loses a significant amount of B-2 if it is left in the sunlight.

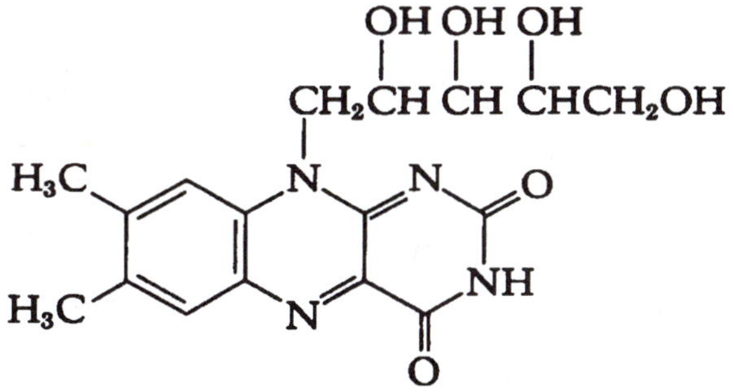

*Riboflavin (vitamin B2)*

## II. Metabolism

Absorption occurs mainly in the upper GI tract. 60% of a 30mg dose is absorbed when taken with meals compared to 15% when taken separately. Synthetic thyroid medication decreases absorption, but thyroid in general increases the absorption. It should be noted that gastric acid is responsible for releasing B-2 from noncovalent bonding in foods so that it may be absorbed.

Tetracyclin and thiazide diuretics increase urinary excretion, as does probenecid, which also decreases absorption. Sulfonamides depress bacterial synthesis. Birth control pills (BCP) have been associated with a reduction in serum levels of vitamin B-2.

Riboflavin is stored to some extent in the liver. However, when supplies are low the liver will only go down to 50% of its maximum storage. Riboflavin is also found in high amounts in the retina of the eye.

## III. Function

1) Riboflavin is involved with production of FMN and FAD, both of which are involved in redox reactions.
2) Riboflavin causes the activation of B-6.
3) Riboflavin is involved in the conversion of tryptophan to niacin.
4) Riboflavin is involved in the conversion of folate to its coenzymes.
5) Riboflavin aids in Beta oxidation in fat metabolism.

6) Riboflavin is involved as a coenzyme component of the dehydrogenases in the first step in glucose metabolism.
7) Riboflavin is needed for the production of corticosteroids; erythropoiesis; gluconeo-genesis; and thyroid enzyme regulation.

## IV. Requirements

**RDA**–1.2–1.6mg/day pregnancy/lactation 1.5-1.7 mg/day

**Lab**–RBC glutathione reductase levels are correlated to adequate status. The Activity Coefficient is determined by addition of FAD to the in vitro mix. 1.0-1.2 is an indication of adequate status, 1.4 is inadequate.

*Optimal daily intake*–5-15mg

## V. Sources

**Best Food Sources of Riboflavin**

| Food | Amount | Mg | Food | Amount | Mg |
|---|---|---|---|---|---|
| Kidney, beef | 3 oz | 4.1 | Brewer's yeast | 1 T | 0.3 |
| Liver, beef | 3 oz | 3.6 | Brie cheese | 2 oz | 0.3 |
| Liver, chicken | 3 oz | 1.5 | Camembert cheese | 2 oz | 0.3 |
| Heart, calf | 3 oz | 1.2 | Roquefort cheese | 2 oz | 0.3 |
| Heart, beef | 3 oz | 1.1 | Rice, wild, raw | 1/4 cup | 0.3 |
| Yogurt | 1 cup | 0.5 | Ricotta cheese, skim | 1/2 cup | 0.2 |
| Broccoli, cooked | 1 stalk | 0.4 | Soybeans, dried | 1/4 cup | 0.2 |
| Almonds | 1/4 cup | 0.3 | Swiss cheese | 2 oz | 0.2 |

USDA Handbook, #8 Series, Washington, DC, ARS, USDA, 1976-1986

## VI. Deficiency

A deficiency of riboflavin usually occurs in concert with other B vitamin deficiencies. However, clinical signs are less dramatic than other deficiencies. Cheilosis and glossitis are classic deficiency symptoms. Dry and scaly skin (seborrheic dermatitis) along with itchy eyes and sensitivity to light are also common. In animals riboflavin deficiencies cause alopecia, anemia, neuropathy, corneal vascularization (precataracts) and congenital malformations.

STUDY–Sauberlich, Judd, Nichoalds, and others: *Application of the erythrocyte glutathione reductase assay in evaluating nutritional status in a high school student population,* AJCN 25:756,1972. ABSTRACT–431 high school students showed 16% of the girls and 6% of the boys had glutathione reductase activity coefficients indicative of inadequate riboflavin intakes. This evidence of deficiency was eliminated by B-2 supplementation at 0.5mg/day for one week.

## VII. Therapeutics

### 1) Acne rosacea

STUDY–Johnson, Eckardt. *Rosacea keratitis and conditions with vascularization of the cornea treated with B-2.* Arch. Ophthamol. 23:899,1940. ABSTRACT–32/36 patients with rosacea keratitis had prompt healing following small doses–1-4.5mg/day orally or by injection of B-2. 9 of these patients also had cutaneous rosacea and 5 of them improved. All of these patients had inadequate dietary B-2 or were hypochlorhydric.

**2) Anemia**–obscure types may be treated with B-2, 30-50 mg/day

**3) Cataracts**–100-150 mg/day in divided doses

**4) Depression**

STUDY–Carney. *B-1, B-2, and B-6 deficiency in psychiatric inpatients.* Br. J. Psychiat. 141:271-72, 1982. ABSTRACT–172 successive psychiatric hospital admissions were determined to have decreased red blood cell aspartate transaminase and glutathione reductase.

## VIII. Toxicity

No toxicity to riboflavin has been found.

### Notes

---

# NIACIN (AMIDE), VITAMIN B-3

It has been known for several centuries that pellagra occurs mainly where people use corn as a staple. It was considered a new disease because it was not recorded in Europe until Columbus brought the first corn plants back from the new world. It was described by Casal of Spain in 1735 and was rampant in Italy (where it received its name meaning "rough skin") at about the same time. Pellagra was first described in the U.S. in the early 1900s. Over 170,000 cases per year were recorded with a fatality rate of 10,000 people per year.

In 1917, the U.S. Bureau of Public Health selected Joe Goldberger to investigate the problem which was rampant in the southern states. Most of the people who died were blacks whose diets were high in cornmeal. Goldberger did a number of studies–one in an orphanage of children who were afflicted with the disease. He supplemented the children's diets with meat, milk, and eggs. They healed miraculously in a short while.

At about the same time another research team announced that one species of fly was spreading the "pellagra microbe" with its sting. The public and most physicians bought this idea of an infectious microbe. Goldberger, who had successfully experimented with prison inmates, was so convinced of his theory that pellagra was a deficiency disease he tried something outrageous. In desperation to prove his theory, he ate the red scales from the legs of diseased people, made a solution of these scales and injected himself and his entire family!! No one became ill. Even with this convincing evidence, it wasn't until 1937, when Elvehjem demonstrated that nicotinic acid cured blacktongue in dogs, that niacin became a dietary essential.

## I. Chemistry

Niacin is extremely stable to heat, light, acid, alkali, and oxidation.

Niacin
(This is the only form that lowers cholesterol and causes vasodilation.)

Niacinamide
(used for arthritis)

Reactive site

**NAD**
(Niacinamide as the active molecule)

## II. Metabolism

Niacin is rapidly absorbed in the proximal small intestine by passive diffusion. Niacin can be synthesized from tryptophan with B-1, B-2, and B-6 as essential cofactors. **60mg of tryptophan yields 1mg of niacin**. (See diagram in pyridoxine and tryptophan chapters).

> **NOTE**–Lime makes the type of niacin found in corn more available. In Mexico it has long been a practice to add lime to corn after it has been ground for tortillas.

**TRYPTOPHAN** ⟶ kynurenine ⟶ 3-hydroxy kynurenine $\xrightarrow{\text{B-6}}$ 3 hydroxy anthranilate ⟶ **NIACIN**
**60mg** **1mg**

## III. Function

1) Niacin is involved in the production of NAD, required for redox reactions in glycolysis and in Kreb's cycle during oxidative phosphorylation. It serves as a coenzyme for a group of enzymes known as dehydrogenases. These dehydrogenase enzymes are responsible for innumerable biochemical reactions in the body including detoxifying alcohol (alcohol dehydrogenase) and utilizing carbohydrates, fats and proteins.
2) Niacin is required in the production of NADPH which is needed for the synthesis of both fatty acids and steroids. It is also involved in the pentose phosphate shunt pathway, which is one way ribose is synthesized. NADPH2 is vital for the regeneration of reduced glutathione from oxidized glutathione (p.137).
3) Niacin is one of the cofactors for A6-6 desaturase in conversion of linoleic acid into GLA.

## IV. Requirements

**RDA–**13mg-18mg/day
**pregnancy and lactation–**15mg and 18mg
LAB–urinary NMN=N-methylnicotinamide
The greater the amount of NMN, the lower the B-3 status.
*Optimal daily intake–*100mg mixed niacin and amide forms.

## V. Sources

### Best Food Sources of Niacin

| Food | Amount | mg Niacin | Trypt/Niacin Equivalent | Total mg |
|---|---|---|---|---|
| Liver, beef | 3 oz | 14.0 | 296 | 21.4 |
| Tuna, canned, water-packed | 3 oz | 11.3 | | |
| Chicken, light meat | 3 oz | 10.6 | 280 | 15.1 |
| Kidney, beef | 3 oz | 9.1 | | |
| Swordfish | 3 oz | 8.7 | | |
| Salmon steak | 3 oz | 8.4 | | |
| Halibut | 3 oz | 7.2 | | |
| Peanuts, chopped | 1/4 cup | 6.2 | 330 | 21.2 |
| Beef, lean | 3 oz | 3.9 | 180 | 6.9 |
| Liver, chicken | 3 oz | 3.8 | | |
| Cod | 3 oz | 2.7 | | |
| Rice, brown | 1/4 cup | 2.4 | | |
| Sunflower seeds | 1/4 cup | 2.0 | 90 | 3.5 |
| Almonds | 1/4 cup | 1.30 | 150 | 3.8 |
| Flour, whole wheat | 1/4 cup | 1.3 | 150 | 3.8 |
| Soybeans, dried | 1/4 cup | 1.2 | | |
| Egg, whole | 1 med | 0.05 | 120 | 2.05 |

USDA Handbook #8 Series Washington, DD, ARS, USDA, 1976-1986

## VI. Deficiency "The 4 Ds!"

1) **Dermatitis** caused by a niacin deficiency is exacerbated by sun exposure. This is known as "mal del sol." This condition is often complicated by other B vitamin deficiencies. The tongue and mouth become inflamed and take on a beefy appearance.
2) **Diarrhea** results from decreased HCL and inflammation of the GI tract.
3) **Dementia** due to a lack of niacin begins with irritability, headaches, and insomnia and is followed by mental confusion, amnesia, hallucinations and severe depression.
4) **Death**–High leucine levels can lead to a niacin deficiency even with normal intake of niacin because leucine blocks NAD synthesis.

Another cause of niacin deficiency is high dietary intake of corn that is not processed with lime. Lime releases tryptophan for bioavailability.

Alcoholism is also a prime cause of B-3 deficiency in this country.

## VII. Therapeutics

**NOTE**–When treating any illnesses with niacin or niacinamide, watch for toxic reactions. The first signs of toxicity are nausea and increased liver enzymes.

1) **Osteoarthritis**–1-3gms/day of niacinamide.

STUDY–Kaufman. *The use of vitamin therapy to reverse certain concomitants of aging*. J. Am. Geriatr. Soc. 3:927,1955. ABSTRACT–663 patients receiving niacinamide were shown to have superior scores on an index of joint range of movement than 842 untreated age-matched patients.

2) **Hypercholesterolemia**–1-6gms/day start out with 100mg t.i.d. with meals. **Use niacin. Niacinamide does not work.**

STUDY–Grundy. *Influence of nicotinic acid on metabolism of cholesterol and triglycerides in man.* J. Lipid research 22:24-36,1981. ABSTRACT–12 hyperlipidemic patients were placed on nicotinic acid for 1 month. During treatment, triglycerides decreased 52%, VLDL decreased 36%, and total cholesterol decreased 22%.

STUDY–Carlson and Oro. *Effect of treatment of nicotinic acid for one month on serum lipids in patients with different types of hyperlipidemia*. Atherosclerosis 18:9,1973. ABSTRACT–188 patients with various types of hyperlipoproteinemia were given 3 gms nicotinic acid daily. Most responsive were patients with Type V. Their cholesterols decreased 70% and triglycerides decreased 90%, followed by Type lll–decreases of 50% and 60% respectively. Both lipids were also reduced in the other types, and even patients with normal lipid levels showed a 10-20% reduction in serum lipids.

STUDY–Canner J. Am. Coll. Cardiol. 5:442,1985; *The coronary drug project research group*. JAMA 213:360,1975. ABSTRACT–Men with 1 or more MI's who took 3 gms/day had a lower incidence of nonfatal MI's and, for several years after the study ended, a lower mortality rate.

3) **Schizophrenia**–500-9,000mg/day. May need to combine with vitamin C. Dr. Abram Hoffer has treated thousands of patients using niacin with considerable success (see *Natural Healing for Schizophrenia*, Eva Edleman). Many contradictory studies

STUDY–Osmond and Hoffer. *Massive niacin treatment in schizophrenia: Review of a nine year study.* Lancet 1:316-20,1962. ABSTRACT–30 patients were randomly divided into 3 groups and received either niacin, nicotinamide, or placebo, usually in addition to Electric Convulsive Therapy, for 33 days. On follow-up, 10 patients in the niacin group 3gms/day were well on an average of 23/26 months and 11 patients in the niacinamide group were well on an average of 26/27 months whereas 9 patients in the placebo group were only well on an average of 11/23 months.

**NOTE**–This study has been criticized on the following grounds:

1) The population was not homogeneous.

2) There were variations in treatments.
3) The control studies were not concurrent.
4) The definition "well" was ambiguous.
5) Readmission to other hospitals was not reported.
6) The niacin flush was not controlled.

STUDY–Hoffer. *Vitamin B-3 dependent child.* Schizophrenia 3:107-113,1971. ABSTRACT–33 children under age 13 with disturbed behavior were placed on nicotinamide with doses increased from 1.5 to 6gms/day along with ascorbic acid 3gms/day and, rarely, very small doses of tranquilizers or anti-depressants. Upon recovery (free of symptoms and signs, performing well in school, getting on well with their families and community), they were switched from B-3 to placebo tablets while the ascorbic acid and other chemotherapy was unchanged. The mother and the author, but not the child, were aware of the switch. Only 1/33 children failed to respond to B-3 therapy. All relapsed within 30 days after the placebo was substituted. They recovered again when B-3 was restarted. The author suggests a trial of niacin for children showing evidence of at least 3 of the following:: 1) hyperactivity, 2) deteriorating school performance 3) perceptual changes and 4) inability to acquire or maintain social relationships.

**4) Anxiety**–500mg b.i.d.

STUDY–Mohler. *Nicotinamide is a brain constituent with benzodiazepine-like actions.* Nature 278:563-65,1979. ABSTRACT–In this animal study nicotinamide resulted in anti-aggressive behavior, anti-conflict, muscle relaxation, and hypnotic actions with effectiveness similar to that of minor tranquilizers. Jonathan Wright, MD, wants to publish an article named, "Valium is an abnormal brain constituent with nicotinamide-like actions." It is postulated that nicotinamide supplementation results in the increased conversion of lactate to pyruvate. Lactate is thought to produce anxiety when it is in high amounts in the body.

**5) Multiple Sclerosis (MS)**

STUDY–Moore. *Treatment of MS with nicotinic acid and Vitamin B-1.* Arch. Int. Med. 65:18,1940. ABSTRACT–Patients showed improvement after IV injections of 100mg B-3 and 60mg of B-1.

**6) Bell's Palsy**–1-3gm/day niacin. Work up to maximum dose, then wean.

STUDY–Kime. *Bell's palsy: A new syndrome associated with treatment by nicotinic acid.* Arch. Otolaryngol. 68:28-32,1958. ABSTRACT–74 consecutive Bell's palsy patients were treated with 100mg to 250mg/day with excellent results noted in all patients within 2-4 weeks.

**7) Trigeminal neuralgia**

**8) Tardive dyskinesia**–100mg-500mg

**9) Diabetes Mellitus type 1**–Niacin or niacinamide may help prevent damage to pancreatic islet cells and preserve endogenous insulin secretion. This may be especially effective in the early onset of type 1 DM. Niacin is precursor for G & F and may in combination with chromium, enhance insulin binding in typical DM.

**10) Insomnia**–100mg/day to treat type A insomnia.

**11) Dysmenorrhea**–niacin, 100mg every 1-2 hours

STUDY–Hudgins. *Vitamin P, C and niacin for dysmenorrhea therapy.* West. J. Surg. and GYN 62:610-11,1954. ABSTRACT–80 patients received 100mg niacin 2x/day and every 2-3hrs during cramps and were followed for up to 3 years. About 90% had at least some relief in their symptoms. The effectiveness of niacin seemed to be enhanced by the addition of rutin 60mg and vitamin C 300mg/day. **Supplementation had to start at least 7-10 days prior to menses to be effective**. Its benefits often remained for several months after discontinuation.

**12) Migraines**–Niacin/100mg must be taken every 15-30 min. at the start of the migraine.

**13) Raynaud's Syndrome**–Use Niacin in conjunction with gingko biloba.

**14) Alcoholism**–consider using along with vitamin B-6 and GLA.

**15) Acne Volgaris**–topical application of 4% niacinamide gel.

**16) Alzheimers**–NAPH, 5mg bid [Cardiovasculer Research (800) 888-4585]

**17) Smoking cessation**–Both lobelia and niacin have been used very successfully in the cessation of smoking.

**Ganglionic Stimulants**

O OH H N H $CH_3$ $CO_2H$ N N N $CH_3$

Lobeline (from lobelia) niacin nicotine

**Figure** *Ganglionic Stimulants*

**Stop smoking–**The above molecules have enough similarity that for people trying to quit smoking they should take lobelia inflata (a botanical that contains lobeline) along with niacin. The lobelia makes cigarettes taste bad while the niacin has a calming effect on the nervous system. Acupuncture is also very helpful.

## VIII. Toxicity

Flushing is the major side effect. Take niacin with meals. The dose can be gradually increased. Time-release formulas can be used but the patient must be monitored because there have been a few reports of fulminant hepatitis with these.

**Use caution with doses of niacin that are greater than 1gm/day.**

Monitor liver enzymes during therapy. Reduce dosage if liver enzymes become elevated. **Nausea is usually the first sign of toxicity with *both* niacin and niacinamide.**

When administering high doses of niacinamide, caution should be taken with diabetic and hypoglycemic patients. Some evidence indicates that it may cause glucose intolerance.

Other possible problems associated with vitamin B-3 are:

- It may increase uric acid, thus increasing the risk of gout in those predisposed.
- Niacin can cause gastrointestinal upset.

## Notes

# PANTOTHENIC ACID, VITAMIN B-5

Vitamin B-5 was first identified as a substance essential for the growth of yeast in 1933. In addition it was found to be essential both in the prevention of dermatitis in chicks and in the graying of hair in rats. Roger Williams and his associates isolated it in 1938 and synthesized it in 1940. It was named Pantothenic Acid (*pantos* means everywhere) because of its widespread occurrence in foods.

## I. Chemistry

Water soluble and stable in moist heat, Pantothenic Acid is unstable in dry heat and acid or basic pH's. Little is lost during normal cooking, however, 50% loss occurs in vegetables when they are frozen and 65% when they are canned. In addition, processed and refined grains lose about 50%, while processed meats lose up to 70% of vitamin B-5.

$$(CH_3)_2\underset{}{\overset{CH_2OH}{\overset{|}{C}}}-\underset{\underset{OH}{|}}{CH}\overset{O}{\overset{\|}{C}}-NHCH_2CH_2\overset{O}{\overset{\|}{C}}OH$$

*Pantothenic Acid (vitamin B-5)*

$$(CH_3)_2\overset{CH_2OH}{\overset{|}{C}}-\underset{\underset{OH}{|}}{CH}-\overset{O}{\overset{\|}{C}}-NHCH_2CH_2\overset{O}{\overset{\|}{C}}NHCH_2CH_2SH$$

*Pantotheine*

## II. Metabolism

Pantothenic acid is readily absorbed from the gastrointestinal tract. About 70% of absorbed pantothenic acid is excreted in the urine. Before pantothenic acid gets utilized it must first be converted to the sulfur containing **pantotheine.** It is stored in high amounts in the adrenal glands.

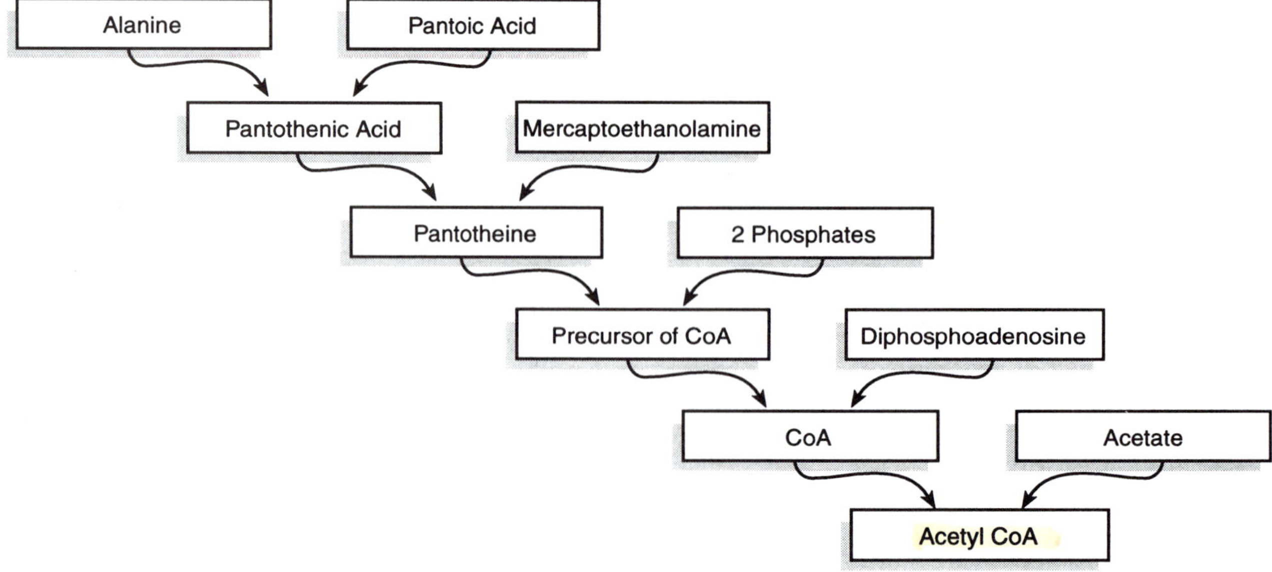

## III. Function

1) The active form of B-5, coenzyme A, is involved in the Kreb cycle in the production of ATP. It is required for proper functioning of adrenal glands.
2) Pantothenic acid, upon being converted to 4'-phosphopantetheine, binds to a protein to form acyl carrier protein (ACP). This ACP is involved in the synthesis of fats including cholesterol.
3) Pantothenic acid provides acetyl groups for the formation of acetylcholine, which is needed in the transmission of nerve impulses and for the detoxification of certain drugs.
4) It is essential for the formation of porphyrin (hemoglobin synthesis).
5) **Pantothenic acid is required for the synthesis of certain steroids produced in the adrenal glands via the action of Coenzyme A.**

## IV. Requirements

No RDA for Vitamin B-5 has been established but the estimated requirement is approximately 4-7mg/day. The average American intake is 5-20mg/day.

**LAB**–normally whole blood=100-180mg%
Average intake of teenagers is about 4.7mg/day
*Optimal daily intake*–100mg

## V. Sources

**Best Food Sources of Pantothenic Acid**

| Food | Amount | Mg | Food | Amount | Mg |
|---|---|---|---|---|---|
| Liver, beef | 3 oz | 4.8 | Rice, brown, cooked | 1 cup | 0.8 |
| Liver, chicken | 3 oz | 4.6 | Sweet corn | 1 med ear | 0.8 |
| Kidney, beef | 3 oz | 2.6 | Beef, lean | 3 oz | 0.7 |
| Turkey, dark meat | 3 oz | 1.1 | Sweet potato | 1 med | 0.7 |
| Brewer's yeast | 1 T | 1.0 | Cashews | 1/4 cup | 0.6 |
| Peanuts or Peas, dried | 1/4 cup | 1.0 | Soy flour | 1/4 cup | 0.6 |
| Chicken, dark meat | 3 oz | 0.9 | Buckwheat flour | 1/4 cup | 0.4 |
| Egg, hard cooked | 1 large | 0.9 | Rye flour | 1/4 cup | 0.4 |

USDA Handbook #8 Series, Washington, DC, ARS,USDA, 1976-1986

## VI. Deficiency

A deficiency of pantothenic acid is uncommon because of its wide distribution in foods. Experimentally induced human Vitamin B-5 deficiency has caused insomnia, leg cramps, paresthesias of the hands and feet, mental depression, decreased antibody formation, easy fatigue, postural hypotension, GI disturbance, and upper respiratory infections. In sever deficiency may get "burning foot syndrome."

Dr. Roger Williams conducted a study with 2 groups of mice. They were fed identical diets, but one group received pantothenic acid in their drinking water. The supplemental group lived on the average 19% longer. This translates into about 14 years more for a human living 75 years.

# VII. Therapeutics

### 1) Osteoarthritis

STUDY–*Calcium pantothenate in arthritic conditions.* A report from the general Practitioner Research Group. Practitioner 224:208-11,1980. ABSTRACT–47/94 patients with arthritic conditions (63% with OA) who were previously untreated or who had not responded to previous drug treatment were randomly chosen to receive 2gms daily of Calcium pantothenate while the rest received placebo. Patients were permitted to take paracetamol to relieve pain but no other medications. After 2 months, daily records kept by patients failed to show significant reductions in the duration of morning stiffness or degree of disability in either the experimental or control groups. Both groups reported significant pain relief but neither resulted in any significant reduction in requirements for pain medication. There was no significant difference between groups and overall assessment by the doctors at the end of the trial gave similar results for active and placebo medications. There was, however, evidence that the subgroup of patients with rheumatoid arthritis may have benefited.

STUDY–Annand. J. Coll Gen Practrs. *Pantothenic acid and OA*. Lancet 2:1168,1963. ABSTRACT–Patients treated with 12.5 mg 2x/day of pantothenate demonstrated a limited, variable improvement starting in 1-2weeks and ending upon discontinuation of the supplementation.

### 2) Rheumatoid Arthritis

STUDY–Note above study in Practitioner 1980 showed that of 18 patients with rheumatoid arthritis, there was a significant subjective reduction in the duration of morning stiffness, degree of disability, and severity of pain compared to baseline. Controls failed to report significant improvements.

STUDY–Barton-Wright, Elliott. *The pantothenic acid metabolism of rheumatoid arthritis.* Lancet 2:862-63,1963. ABSTRACT–The mean level of whole blood pantothenic acid for 66 patients was significantly lower (45% lower) than that for 29 normals. Moreover, the lower the level of pantothenic acid, the greater the symptom severity (when pantothenate was 400% less than the mean level, patients showed the most severe symptoms; 2 were bedridden). Vegetarian normals had a much higher pantothenate level than did normals consuming a usual "balanced diet". **It should be noted that attempts to supplement pantothenic acid resulted in a short term improvement after 7 days but then stopped.** 20 patients received 50mg Calcium-D-pantothenate IM daily which lead to a temporary alleviation of symptoms after 7 days along with an increase in whole blood pantothenate. Another 21 days of injections failed to result in further improvement. After discontinuation, blood levels fell to their initial values by the end of one month with concomitant reappearance of symptoms, suggesting that abnormal pantothenate metabolism is due to some other factor. Since royal jelly is rich in pantothenic acid in its free state as well as in other 10 carbon chain fatty acids, 20 patients received a mixture of royal jelly and pantothenic acid–50mg of each IM daily. By 28 days, 14 patients noted an improvement in general condition and joint mobility along with a fall in ESR coincident with rising blood levels. This lasted until blood levels returned to previous values 2 months following discontinuation of the injections. 10 vegetarians with rheumatoid arthritis all improved on the same regime by 14 days with greater rise in whole blood pantothenate levels than in the nonvegetarian arthritics. Preliminary results with oral supplementation have been encouraging.

**3) Contact dermatitis**–2% panthenol ointment (Scientific Botanical Inc.) improved symptoms of Lichen planus (vaginitis). Wade Boyle, N.D. swears by it.

**4) Eczema**–Especially related to allergic atopic eczema.

### 5) Anemia

STUDY–McCurdy. *Is there an anemia responsive to pantothenic acid?* J AM Geriatr Soc 21(2):88-91, 1973 ABSTRACT–A 53 year old black female was admitted with anorexia, weight loss, lethargy, incontinence and hypochromic anemia with increased iron storage in the bone marrow. After an unsuccessful trial of B6, all symptoms and signs improved dramatically following administration of pantothenic acid 50-200mg IM daily. Several years later a similar clinical picture developed. There was a clinical, but probably not hema-tologic, response to a multivitamin preparation containing large amounts of B5 suggesting that lethargic patients with iron-loaded hypochromic anemia unresponsive to B6 might benefit from a trial of B5.

**6) Systemic Lupus Erythematous**–2 studies, 1 yes the other no.

**7) Allergies**–Szorady conducted allergy skin tests on 24 children injecting them with histamine. Pantothenic acid reduced the intensity of skin reaction by 20-50% in all children.

**8) Stress**–A study in the 30's revealed that rats fed deficient, adequate and high pantothenate levels could swim 16, 29 and 62 minutes respectively.

STUDY-Szegszardy T, Gazdagh I, and Szorady I–*Beobachtungen uber die gemeinsame Strahlenschutzwirkung on Pantothensaure und Aminoathylisothiuronium.* Radiobiol-Radiother 3/72.. ABSTRACT–Mice were broken up into 3 groups. There was one control, a group that received pantothenic acid alone and a third group that received a combination of aminoethylisothiuronium and pantothenate. Mice were exposed to full body irradiation and it was found that the mice that were supplemented with the pantothenate and aminoethylisothiuronium had a much longer survival time. In addition, their body w.

STUDY–Ralli, Dumm. NYU Bellevue Med Center 1952. ABSTRACT–Men were immersed in 48 degree water for 8 minutes. White blood cells and vitamin C levels were measured and then the men received 10gms of B5 every day for 6 weeks. They were then subjected to the same dunking. The supplemented period resulted in a less pronounced drop in their white blood cells and vitamin C levels. Cholesterol levels were also lower in the pantothenic acid group.

STUDY–Am J of Surg 50 patients undergoing abdominal surgery were given 500mg of B5 the day of surgery and for 5 days afterwards. Another 50 patients were not given B5. The B5 group had a more "benign postoperative course."

STUDY–Szorady I. University Med. School Szeged, Hungry Acta Paediatrica Hungarice ABSTRACT–200 mice divided into 4 groups with one group receiving pantothenate for a week before total body irradiation. 1/2 were still alive after 21 days but of the non supplemented groups 1/2 were dead within 8 days.

**9) Atherosclerosis**–300mg t.i.d. Several studies show an increase in HDL and an inhibition of platelet aggregation.

STUDY–*Pantetheine treatment of hyperlipidemia.* Clin Ther 8:5637,1986. ABSTRACT–24 patients (average age 51 years) with types llA, llB or IV hyperlipidemia received pantetheine 300mg 3x/day. After one year there was a highly significant reduction of about 17% in mean serum cholesterol levels which had become evident within one month and persisted thereafter. Mean HDL cholesterol levels increased by about 15% and mean triglyceride levels fell by 48%. No significant side effects.

STUDY–Cattin. *Treatment of hypercholesterolemia with pantetheine and fenofibrate: An open randomized study on 43 patients.* Current Ther Res. 38(3):386-95,1985. ABSTRACT–In an open randomized study of hypercholesterolemic patients pantetheine was as effective as fenofibrate in lowering total and LDL cholesterol levels but without the side effects of the drug.

STUDY–Galeone. *The lipid lowering effect of pantetheine in hyperlipidemic patients: A clinical investigation.* Current Ther Res 34:383-90,1983. ABSTRACT–Following supplementation normal values were obtained in 83% of hypercholesterolemic patients and 35.7% of hypertriglyceride patients.

STUDY–Da Col, P.G. *Pantetheine in the treatment of hypercholesterolemia: A clinical investigation.* ABSTRACT–Supplementation was ineffective for patients who had previously failed to respond to a combined drug/diet

## Notes

# PYRIDOXINE (B-6)

In 1934 pyridoxine was first identified as adermin, a substance that was capable of curing a characteristic dermatitis in rats who did not respond to any of the 3 factors then known in the B complex. It was isolated in 1938 and named by Szent-Gyorgy.

## I. Chemistry

Pyridoxine is water-soluble and stable to heat in acid mediums. It is unstable in alkaline solutions and very unstable to light. Freezing of vegetables decreases B-6 by 20%, canning by 54%, and processing of grains by 40-90%

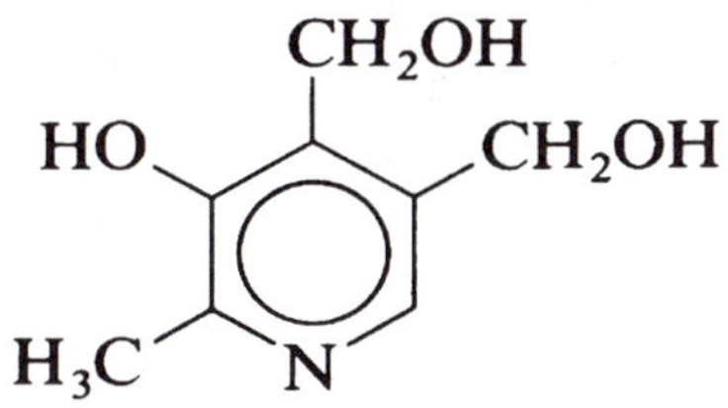

$CH_2OH$ HO $CH_2OH$ $H_3C$ N

*Pyridoxine (vitamin B-6)*

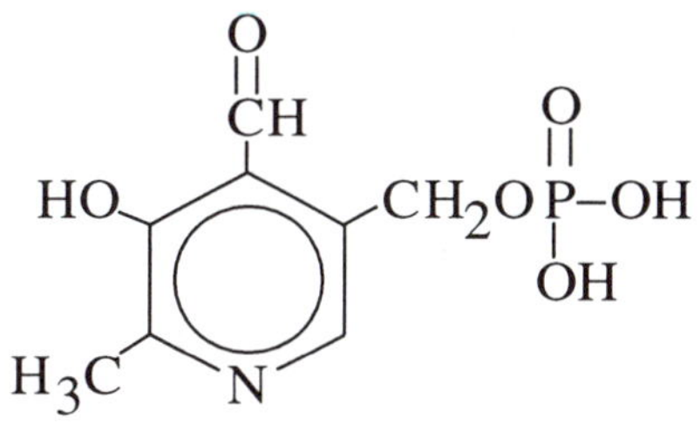

O CH O HO $CH_2O$ P–OH OH $H_3C$ N

*Pyridoxal 5' Phosphate (active form)*

## II. Metabolism

Pyridoxine is absorbed in the upper small intestine by simple diffusion.
**The more acidic the milieu, the greater the absorption.**

## III. Function

Its active form is pyridoxine 5 phosphate (P5P or PLP). It is involved in:

1) Transamination–the transfer of $NH_2$ to other amino acids.
2) Deamination–removal of amino groups from certain amino acids to be used for an energy source.
3) Desulfuration–transfer of the sulfhydryl group (HS) from one amino acid, methionine, to another, serine, to form cysteine.
4) Decarboxylation–the removal of COOH groups from certain amino acids to form another compound. Required in the synthesis of the neurotransmitters serotonin, norepinephrine, and histamine from tryptophan, tyrosine, and histamine, P5P can be highly concentrated in the brain even when low levels exist in the blood. It is thought that dementia is associated with reduced transport.
5) Required for the formation of alpha aminolevulinic acid, a precursor of heme in hemoglobin.
6) **Tryptophan** ⟶*Pyridoxine 5 Phosphate* ⟶**Niacin**
   **Tryptophan load test**–In a deficiency of Pyridoxine, excess xanthurenic acid will be produced from kynurenine (see next page diagram).
7) Promotes release of glycogen from liver and muscle as glucose-1-phosphate.

8) Linoleic acid $\xrightarrow{B\text{-}6}$ GLA ⟶ DHGLA ⟶ PGE1 & small amounts of arachidonic acid.

9) Vital for the formation of sphygolipids involved in the development of the myelin sheath surrounding nerve cells.

10) Involved with the synthesis of the intrinsic factor.

## IV. Requirements

**RDA**– 2.0mg **Pregnancy/Lactation**– 2.2mg/2.1mg

*Optimal daily intake*–35mg for males and 50mg for females

In view of the fact that there are so many antagonists, it seems likely that our requirements must be greater.

**Lab evaluation of vitamin B-6 status**

**a) Tryptophan Load Test**–This test involves giving a 2gm dose of tryptophan and then measuring the amount of xanthurenic acid in the urine. Since converting 3-Hydroxykynurenine into xanthurenic acid is an easy step which doesn't require much vitamin B-6, a B-6 deficiency will produce an excess amount of xanthurenic acid appearing in the urine.

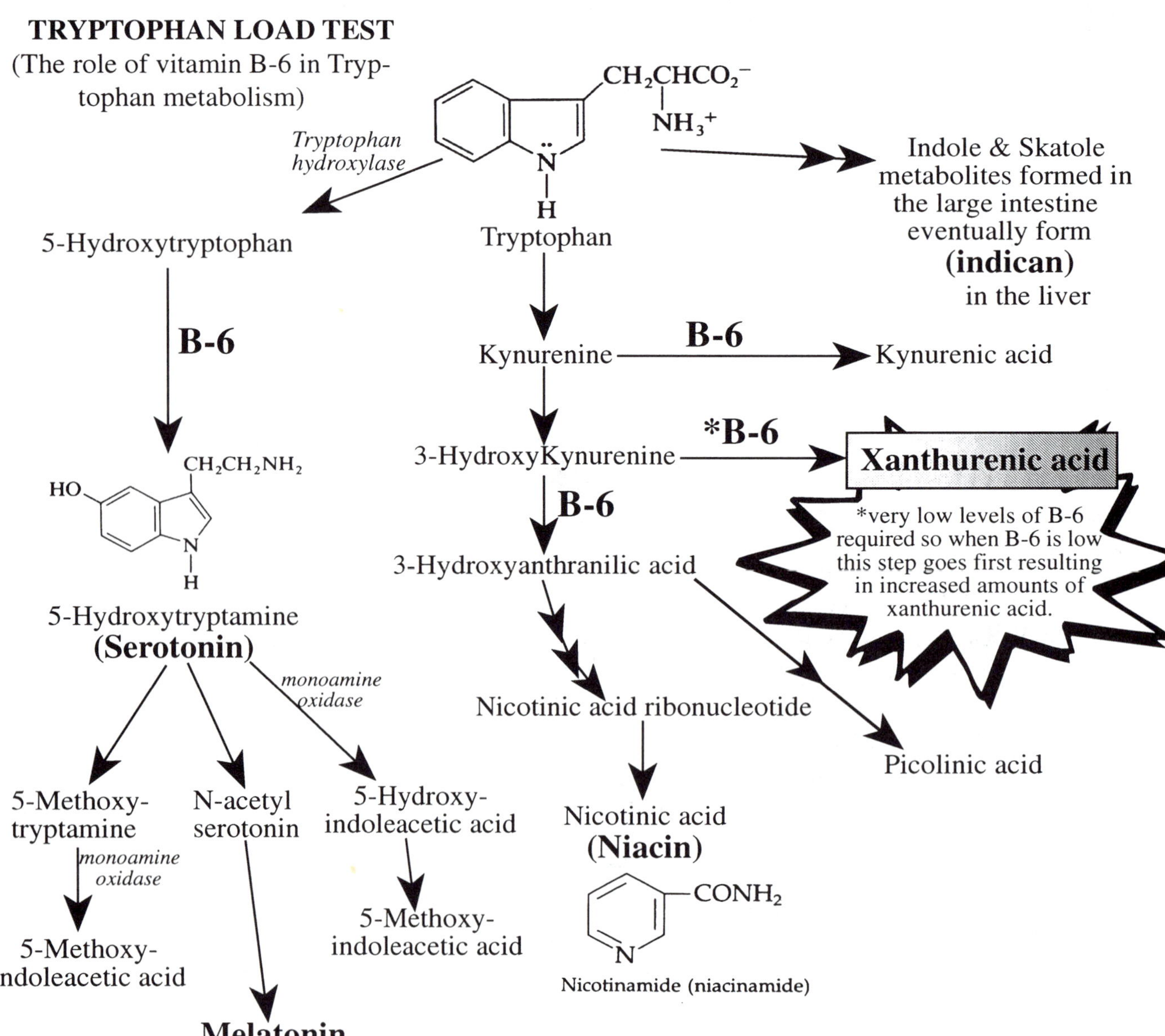

**b) Erythrocyte Glutamate Oxaloacetic Transaminase Test (EGOT test)**–A functional test for measuring vitamin B-6 status, it measures the activity of the EGOT enzyme as the daily intake of vitamin B-6 is increased. As the dosage of vitamin B-6 rises, the activity of EGOT goes up. When the daily dose of vitamin B-6 no longer increases the activity of the enzyme, the maximal functional dose has been reached (Meridian Labs).

## V. Sources

**Best Food Sources of Pyridoxine (vitamin B-6)**

| Food | Amount | Mg | Food | Amount | Mg |
|---|---|---|---|---|---|
| 100% bran cereal | 1 cup | 12.1 | Potato, raw | 1 med | .38 |
| 40% bran cereal | 1 cup | .80 | Tuna, canned | 3 oz | .36 |
| Pork loin chop, broiled | 3 oz | .78 | Herring, Atlantic, raw | 3 oz | .34 |
| Watermelon | 1 slice | .69 | Turkey, dark w/o skin | 3 oz | .32 |
| Banana | 1 med | .66 | Chicken, dark w/o skin | | |
| Salmon, raw | 1 med | .66 | Broccoli, raw | 1 med stalk | .29 |
| Avocado | 1 med | .56 | Brown rice, uncooked | 1/4 cup | .28 |
| Chicken, light w/o skin | 3 oz | .51 | Sirloin, beef | 3 oz | .26 |
| Turkey, light w/o skin | 3 oz | .48 | Chick-peas, dried | 1/2 cup | .27 |
| Liver, beef | 3 oz | .47 | Crab | 3 oz | .26 |
| Tomato juice | 1 cup | .47 | Clam chowder | 1 cup | .26 |
| Rainbow trout, raw | 3 oz | .45 | Kidney, beef | 3 oz | .24 |
| Steelhead, raw | 3 oz | .45 | Pineapple juice | 1 cup | .24 |
| Mackerel, Atlantic, raw | 3 oz | .45 | Walnuts, English | 1/4 cup | .22 |
| Sunflower seeds | 1/2 cup | .45 | Veal | 3 oz | .22 |
| Granola cereal | 1 cup | .43 | Ocean perch | 3 oz | .21 |
| Soybeans, dry | 4 cups | .43 | Brewer's yeast | 1 T | .20 |
| Pork, cured, cooked | 3 oz | .40 | Cod, raw | 3 oz | .20 |
| Halibut, raw | 3 oz | .39 | Brussels sprouts, raw | 4 | .19 |
| Sweet potato, raw | 1 med | .39 | Filberts, shelled | 1/4 cup | .18 |

USDA Handbook #8 Series Washington, DD, ARS, USDA, 1976-1986

## VI. Deficiency

Adults given deoxypyridoxine (antagonist) developed depression, nausea, vomiting, mucous membrane lesions, seborrheic dermatitis and peripheral neuritis. Also ataxia, hyperacusis, hyperirritability, altered mobility and alertness, abnormal head movements and convulsions.

Analysis of our food supply indicates that many of us are consuming less than the RDA amount. This is due to practices of milling that remove up to 90% of B-6. As yet, there are no laws requiring the enrichment of milled grains with pyridoxine.

Probably the biggest cause of deficiency (or an increased requirement) is the addition of antagonists in the environment over the last 50 yrs. Among the antagonists are:

**HYDRAZINE COMPOUNDS**:

1) Hydrazine compounds used in medicine INH (isonicotinic acid hydrazine), and hydralazine, which is high in store-bought mushrooms. *Hydralazine* is a medication that is used to treat hypertension and has been linked to a few cases of peripheral neuritis which is associated with pyridoxine deficiency. *Phenelzine* is a drug used to treat depression and some people taking it have been found to experience pronounced edema especially in the legs.

*Succinic acid 2,2-Dimethylhydrazide* is another chemical used in the U.S. and Canada to speed the ripening of fruits. It is sprayed on such fruits as peaches, nectarines, tomatoes, brussels sprouts, cherries, grapes and apples and residues remain on these fruits after harvesting.

*Maleic hydrazide* is another derivative of hydrazine used in agriculture as a plant growth inhibitor and herbicide (potato chips have particularly high levels maleic hydrazide with as high as 25mg per 6 oz bag of chips).

2) Antioxidants in the petroleum industry and plating materials and anti-tarnish agents used in metal manufacturing.

3) Tartrazine (yellow dye #5)– From 1949-1970 nearly 1 million pounds/year were used in foods and medications.

4) Peroxides and free radicals found in abundance in our food supply as oxidized fats. Foods such as barbequed foods, fried foods, potato and corn chips, all foods processed with fats or oils which includes most restaurant prepared foods.

5) Birth Control Pills (BCP)– are well known B-6 antagonists. 15-20% of women on oral contraceptives show deficient levels of pyridoxine on tryptophan load tests and many suffer deficiency symptoms. It should be noted that 10-30mg/day of B-6 corrected both the load test and relieved the symptoms in most of these women.

6) PCB's–polychlorinated biphenols–Although they have been banned, there are still incredible amounts in the environment. They have been found in 99% of all Americans tested and 100% of all Canadians. Fish taken from contaminated waters are the primary source of PCB's. In 1975 69% of all breast milk tested positive and in Michigan, of more than 1000 women tested, 100%were positive.

7) Environmental toxins– rocket or jet fuel produces hydrazines which can persist for weeks after its production. Tobacco smoke contains significant amounts as well as the tobacco itself thus chewing tobacco will increase the need for more B-6.One study on the birth weight of newborns showed that the normal growth inhibition that occurs with exposure in utero to tobacco smoke could be inhibited with the addition of 15mg of B-6/day.

8) L-canavanine–compound found in alfalfa sprouts.

9) Other non-hydrazine medications that act as pyridoxine antagonists include penicillamine and cycloserine.

10) Alcohol– has been shown to deplete B-6 stores.

11) Caramel coloring– acts as an antagonist to B-6 and has been found to prevent B-6 from entering into the brain. Caramel coloring is produced from the heating up of certain sugars. Other foods that contain lysine (an essential amino acid found in many foods) that have been processed with heat have been found to antagonize B-6.

> Note– many other compounds that have been recently introduced into our environment can act as vitamin B-6 antagonists. It seems likely that our requirements have greatly exceeded the RDAs.

Other causes of deficiency are:

**Pregnancy**–Up to 50% of pregnant women may suffer vitamin B-6 deficiencies on normal diets according to tryptophan load test studies. It is known that B-6 is actively transported to the fetus and concentrated up to 4 times the normal level.

**Malabsorption**–Celiac disease, Crohn's disease, etc.

**Age-related**–several studies of Danes and Americans showed low B-6 status corresponding to age.

# VII. Therapeutics

## Women's Health Problems

**1) PMS**–Pyridoxine relieves edema associated with menstrual cycle, irritability, depression, headaches, swollen breasts, abdominal bloating, nausea, constipation, acne, and lack of coordination. 70-90% of menstruating women have PMS and an estimated 20-40% have it severely. Recently 2 court cases reduced charges because of PMS. It has been found that B-6 can increase levels of progesterone, dopamine, and serotonin all of which are believed to be low in women with PMS.

STUDY–Biskind, Morton, Gerson, Gerson, Leonard. *B-6 deficiency in the Etiology of Menorrhagia, Metrorrhagia, Cystic Mastitis, and Premenstrual Tension.* Surgery, Gynecology and Ob, Jan. 1944, pp49-57. ABSTRACT–Biskind discovered that when he fed rats a diet deficient in B vitamins they lost the ability to metabolize estrogen at normal rates. Suspecting that women who had a deficiency in B vitamins might have symptoms associated with excess estrogen–such as heavy menstrual flow, irregular bleeding, cystic breasts, and premenstrual tension–he surveyed B vitamin deficient women. Of 39 women questioned, 37 had gynecological problems. In treating their B vitamin deficiency, he found that they also experienced dramatic relief of their gynecological symptoms. In another 52 patients without obvious B vitamin deficiency he gave B vitamins for one or more gynecologic complaints and these women also experienced great relief.

STUDY–Abraham and Hargrove. *Effect of Vitamin B-6 on premenstrual symptoms in women with PMS. A double blind crossover study.* Infertility, Vol 3(**2**),1980,pp.155-65. ABSTRACT–25 women with moderate to severe PMS were studied for 6 menstrual cycles. During 3 of these cycles they received a single sustained-release tablet containing 500mg of B-6 each day. During the other 3 cycles they were given an inert placebo that appeared identical to the B-6 tablets. Throughout the entire 6 month period women kept a symptom diary. A total of 19 symptoms were rated using a 4 point scale. The daily symptom score was totalled for each day and for each 3 month cycle. **At the end of the** study, **21 of 25 subjects had lower PMS scores while taking the vitamin B-6 compared to the placebo. In each case the difference was statistically significant.**

**2) Nausea of Pregnancy**–IV B-6 with B-12 and Vitamin K

STUDY–Willis Dept of OB, Baylor College of Medicine. ABSTRACT-Administration of 25-50mg B-6 IV or IM to 37 women resulted in complete or partial relief of symptoms. The following year other physicians confirmed these results. Complete relief was experienced by 38/40 women treated with IV B-6. Oral doses of 30-80mg were of no use. Improvement generally occurred within 6 to 24 hours after the first injection. 22 patients experienced complete and permanent relief after the first injection. Also, 6 patients with seborrheic dermatitis noted great improvement in their skin.

STUDY–Weinstein *Oral Administration of B-6 in the treatment of nausea and vomiting of pregnancy.* Am. J. Obs. Gyn. 47:389-94,1944. ABSTRACT–78 women were treated first with 100mg IM then by mouth. Nearly all women responded in 1-3 days. Of the 10 patients with the most severe nausea and vomiting, 8 lost their symptoms entirely after this treatment.

STUDY–Gant, Von. *Vitamin B-6 depletion in women with Hyperemesis Gravidarum.* Wiener Klinische Wochenschrift, Sept 5, 1975 p. 510. ABSTRACT–20 women with nausea and vomiting were treated with 200mg/day B-6 and their symptoms cleared promptly. The serum levels of B-6 were quite low, possibly due to vomiting.

**NOTE**–Benedictin–This drug was used for many years in the treatment of nausea of pregnancy but was taken off the market for allegedly causing birth defects. It consisted of 15mg of pyridoxine and another drug. The B-6 seemed to be the active ingredient in the drug. The correlation with birth defects seemed weak at best.

**3) Toxemia of Pregnancy**– May need to give IV along with magnesium in more severe cases of toxemia. Can have a pronounced effect on removing excess fluid and decreasing blood pressure.

STUDY–Wachstein, Graffeo. *Influence of B-6 on the incidence of preeclampsia.* Gyn.8: 177, 1956. ABSTRACT–820 middle income women were divided in half. 410 received a multivitamin without B-6 and 410 received the multivitamin with 20mg B-6. The B-6 half developed toxemia at a rate of 1.7% while the group without B-6 had an incidence of 4.4%.

STUDY–Ellis. 225 pregnant women were treated for edema with between 50-450mg B-6/day. In a few cases IM injections were used. Only 6 out of the 225 failed to respond. Some of the women lost between 10-15 lbs in 2 weeks. It was recommended that the B-6 be given with magnesium. Ellis believes pregnant women should get 50mg B-6 per day throughout pregnancy.

**Neurological Problems**

4) **Carpal tunnel syndrome (CTS)**–In 1950 George Phalen, M.D., who was a pioneer in the surgical treatment of CTS, presented his first 11 cases of CTS at the 99th annual meeting of the Am. Med. Assoc. Until then few physicians were familiar with the condition. Years later in the 60s Dr. John Ellis successfully pioneered the treatment of CTS with vitamin B-6 treatment. 85% of patients respond in a few weeks, but some may take 8-12 weeks. Try P5P if pyridoxine doesn't work. Magnesium may also be effective. Consider using the EGOT to evaluate higher doses of therapeutic pyridoxine.

STUDY–Ellis. *Response of Vitamin B-6 deficiency and the CTS to pyridoxine.* Proceedings of the National Academy of Sciences, Dec 1982 pp.7494-7498. ABSTRACT–7 patients suffering from CTS were treated with B-6 or placebo, each for 12 weeks. Prior to the study, all 7 patients showed biochemical evidence of B-6 deficiency. When the patients received B-6 their symptoms improved significantly. While on the placebo no improvement was noted. Symptoms were relieved with B-6 even in patients who had symptoms for as long as 8 years.

5) **Infant seizures**–several studies showed benefits. 20-50mg/kg/d in divided doses with results in 3-6 days.

6) **Rheumatism**–50mg t.i.d. **consider panniculofibrositis**–numbness, swelling, tingling, reduced sense of touch in the fingers and hands, and pain in the finger joints resulting in impaired hand movements and weakened grip. Sometimes the symptoms include stiffness in the shoulders, chest, elbows, knees, and feet, also muscle spasm of legs. Most effective in middle aged women with Heberden's nodes.

7) **Tardive Dyskinesia**–from long term overdosing of L-dopa, B-6 supplementation decreased involuntary movements.

8) **Diabetic neuropathy**–50-100mg/day has been shown to decrease glycosylation of hemoglobin. It is thought that glycosylated hemoglobin is what may be responsible for the end organ damage that results from diabetes.

**Mental Problems**

9) **Depression**–100-500mg/day– B-6 is a cofactor for the conversion of tryptophan to serotonin. B-6 is a cofactor for the synthesis of norepinephrine. B-6 has been found to be quite low in patients admitted to the hospital for depression. Wright claims that whenever women have depression and insomnia, B-6 and tryptophan work almost all the time.

STUDY–Baublatt and Winston. *B-6 and the pill.* Lancet April 18,1970, pp.832-33. ABSTRACT–58 women depressed and taking BCP were treated with vitamin B-6 in doses of 25mg 2x/day at the first sign of any premenstrual depression. After 3 months of therapy, more than 75% of the women reported either complete relief or considerable improvement in their symptoms. The 44 women who appeared to respond to the B-6 were then asked to discontinue it for a while to see if symptoms would return. All of the women refused.

**10) Dementia**–B-6 is often found to be deficient in elderly Alzheimer patients as compared to controls. It has been found that there is an age-related fall in dopamine receptors which parallels a decline in plasma B-6 levels.

**11) Hyperkinetic behavior**– Studies indicate that if there is a decrease level of serotonin in the blood, then B-6 may be helpful at a dosage of 20-30mg/kg/d.

**12) Schizophrenia**–mixed reviews. Most control studies don't show benefits.

**Dermatological Problems**

**13) Seborrheic dermatitis**

**14) Acne**

STUDY–Snider, Dieteman. *B-6 therapy for premenstrual acne flare.* Letter to Ed. Arch. Dermatol. 110:130-131,1974). ABSTRACT–106 young female patients received vitamin B-6 50mg/day for 1 week prior to and during menses. 72% improved.

Jonathan Wright, M.D. recommends topical B-6 cream.(Scientific Botanicals)

**Anemia**

**Sideroblastic anemia is the major type of anemia that responds to B-6 therapy. Inherited sideroblastic anemia responds much more readily than the acquired type. Doses >200mg/day are required.**

B-6 is the coenzyme for the enzyme delta-aminolevolinic acid synthetase, which catalyzes an important step in hemoglobin synthesis.

**15) Iron-resistant**–Parenteral PLP 25-50mg 4x daily for 8-10 days

STUDY–Hines, Love. *Vitamin B-6 metabolism in sideroblastic anemia: Effect of pyridoxal phosphate therapy.* Clin Res. 23:403A, 1975. ABSTRACT–18/34 patients with sideroblastic anemia unresponsive to vitamin B-6 and folate had subnormal concentrations of serum and red blood cell PLP and in vitro evidence of defective phosphorylation of pyridoxine and pyridoxal to P5P. Treatment of these patients with parenteral PLP 25-50mg 4x daily for 8-10 days produced significant elevation of hemoglobin in 11 cases.

**16) Sickle cell anemia (SCA)**–50mg B-6 2x/day for 2 months

STUDY–Natta, Reynolds. *Apparent Vitamin B-6 deficiency in SCA.* Am J Clin Nutr 40:235-9,1984. ABSTRACT–16 patients with SCA had significantly lower plasma pyridoxal phosphate than controls while their red blood cell PLP was significantly elevated, possibly reflecting a greater affinity of PLP to sickle hemoglobin chain than to the normal beta chain. Oral supplementation of 5 patients with 50 mg 2x/day for 2 months resulted in increased plasma and red blood cell PLP levels and a slight, insignificant increase in red blood cell number, Hemoglobin concentration, and hematocrit. One subject also experienced reduction in the frequency and duration of painful crises.

**17) Asthma**–300mg/day in divided doses

STUDY–Reynolds, Natta. *Depressed plasma B-6 concentrations in adult asthmatics.* Am J. Clin. Nutr 41:684-8,1985. ABSTRACT–15 patients had significantly lower levels of plasma and red blood cell P5P than non-asthmatics. 7 patients and 6 controls received 50mg B-6 2x/day. Both plasma and red blood cell pyridoxal phosphate levels only increased significantly in the controls. However, all asthmatics reported a dramatic decrease in the frequency, duration and severity of asthmatic attacks and wheezing ceased in about one week.

STUDY–Collip. *B-6 treatment of childhood bronchial asthma.* Ann. Allergy 35:93-97, 1975. ABSTRACT–76 asthmatic children who received B-6 200mg daily demonstrated significant symptom improvement and a reduction in dosage of bronchodilators and cortisone required to relieve symptoms.

**Miscellaneous**

**18) MSG sensitivity**–50mg/day will decrease sensitivity

**19) Kidney stones**–25-50mg/day with magnesium prevents the formation of calcium oxalate stones.

**20) Diabetes**

## VIII. Toxicity

See journal articles. In one case it was determined that 200mg/day resulted in peripheral neuropathy. This was an anecdotal study done by Katrina Dalton. Normally 2-5gms per day over a few months is the dose required to get toxic symptoms consisting of numbness and tingling in the extremities. These symptoms usually disappear once the vitamin B-6 is discontinued, but may linger for a few months if severe.

**CAUTION**

If the patient is on L-Dopa for Parkinson's disease and you give B-6, it will convert the L-dopa into dopamine outside the blood brain barrier. This will render the L-dopa ineffective because dopamine can not pass the blood brain barrier.

If the patient is on Sinemet (combo of L-dopa and Carbidopa), B-6 may actually have a synergistic effect. Carbidopa stops conversion of L-dopa outside the blood brain barrier. The vitamin B-6 would then cross the BBB along with the unchanged L-dopa. Once inside the BBB vitamin B-6 would then convert the L-dopa into dopamine where it could then effectively be used by the brain.

**Synopsis of an editorial that Dr. Alan Gaby wrote in the Townsend Newsletter, May 1988.**

In 1983 Schaumburg reported the first cases of pyridoxine toxicity. He reported 7 cases of sensory neuropathy with a stocking glove distribution. In a few cases a biopsy had revealed axonal degeneration of the sensory nerves. When the people stopped taking their B-6 their symptoms went away gradually except for a few cases where mild symptoms remained after 2 years. These symptoms were attributed to B-6 because: 1) animal experiments showed that large doses could cause neuropathy, 2) no other cause was found and 3) symptoms went away when B-6 was discontinued. Patients had taken usually 2-5gms on a long term basis.

In 1987 Dr. Katherina Dalton, a physician well known for treatment of PMS with progesterone for over 30 years, reported a number of cases of B-6 induced neuropathy at doses much lower than Schaumburg. In a study published in the Acta Neurol Scand 78:3, 1987, *Characteristics of pyridoxine overdose neuropathy,* Dr. Dalton measured B-6 levels in all women attending her PMS clinic. In 172 patients, above normal B-6 levels were found (although "normal" levels had been spuriously established), and in these patients, 103 (60%) complained of neurological symptoms. The average daily B-6 intake was 117mg per day for an average duration of about 3 years. 20% of these women were taking less than 50mg per day and one only 20mg. Symptoms included paraesthesia, hyperaesthesia, bone pain, muscle weakness, numbness, and fasciculations. All women were advised to discontinue B-6. 3 months later 55% of these 103 women reported partial or complete relief of symptoms and, after 6 months, all of the women were asymptomatic. 7 patients who did not discontinue their B-6 still had symptoms. This study caused a great deal of alarm and was widely publicized both in public media and academia. This was unfortunate as Dr. Dalton's scientific methodology seemed quite poor. There were absolutely no reasonable conclusions that could be made from her study.

All the symptoms these women were experiencing are not uncommon, particularly in those who have PMS. These symptoms may be related to a number of other causes such as allergies, excess consumption of alcohol or caffeine, etc. Dr. Gaby points out that these symptoms are quite common in women not taking B-6 and who don't have PMS. Just because they happened to be taking B-6 and they have these symptoms does not mean anything. Dr. Dalton could probably have found a number of things that were just as commonly being taken, such as vitamin C. It also is not surprising to see serum B-6 higher than normal in women who were taking B-6 supplements. The normal ranges were generated from people who were not taking vitamins. No evidence was produced in her study that the "higher" levels were harmful. Dalton did not compare symptoms between B-6 users and nonusers, so she never really established that there was an increased incidence of symptoms. The fact that women improved after stopping the B-6 was also not surprising. Here was a physician treating PMS for over 30 years. When they were taken off the B-6, they were also undergoing therapy to treat their PMS symptoms. Why wouldn't one expect their symptoms to go away? The fact that they had also stopped taking B-6 was merely a coincidence. The women who still had symptoms and continued to take B-6 after they were asked to stop may also have been in non compliance with other parts of the treatment program.

In summary, Dalton failed to show that moderate B-6 intake causes neurological symptoms. The fact that this study was awarded a prize for research excellence is perplexing and just shows that the "powers that be" have something to gain by attacking a particularly popular vitamin therapy. Certainly Schaumburg has brought to light some caution in the use of B-6 supplements but there certainly should not be a hysterical reaction against a treatment that has been studied extensively and has shown significant therapeutic effectiveness. From my 13 years of practice and from the experience of many of my colleagues who have routinely prescribed 100-300mg per day for extended periods of time without side effects, except for occasional vivid dreams and additional energy, it seems far fetched that such a dramatic rash of symptoms could possibly be attributed to pyridoxine.

## Notes

---

# COBALAMIN, Vitamin B-12

Pernicious anemia, a fatal disease of unknown origin, characterized by neurological damage and a megaloblastic anemia, took a toll of 10,000 deaths per year until 1926 when Minot and Murphy established that the condition could be cured if the patient was fed large amounts of raw liver (2/3 lb per day!). In 1934 they were awarded, along with Whipple, the Nobel Prize in medicine for this treatment. In the same year ,1926, Castle noted that pernicious anemia patients had a low HCL secretion and certain cases seemed to not respond to purified liver extracts. He postulated that the antipernicious anemia substance was formed from an "intrinsic factor" present in gastric secretions and an "extrinsic factor" present in food, especially liver. It was later found that these unresponsive cases were actually related to a folate deficiency and the purified extracts that were being used had the folic acid removed. It wasn't until 1948 that B-12 was actually isolated. This discovery of vitamin B-12, the antipernicious anemia substance, was eventually recognized as "Castle's extrinsic factor." The intrinsic factor was found to only be necessary for absorbing the vitamin B-12.

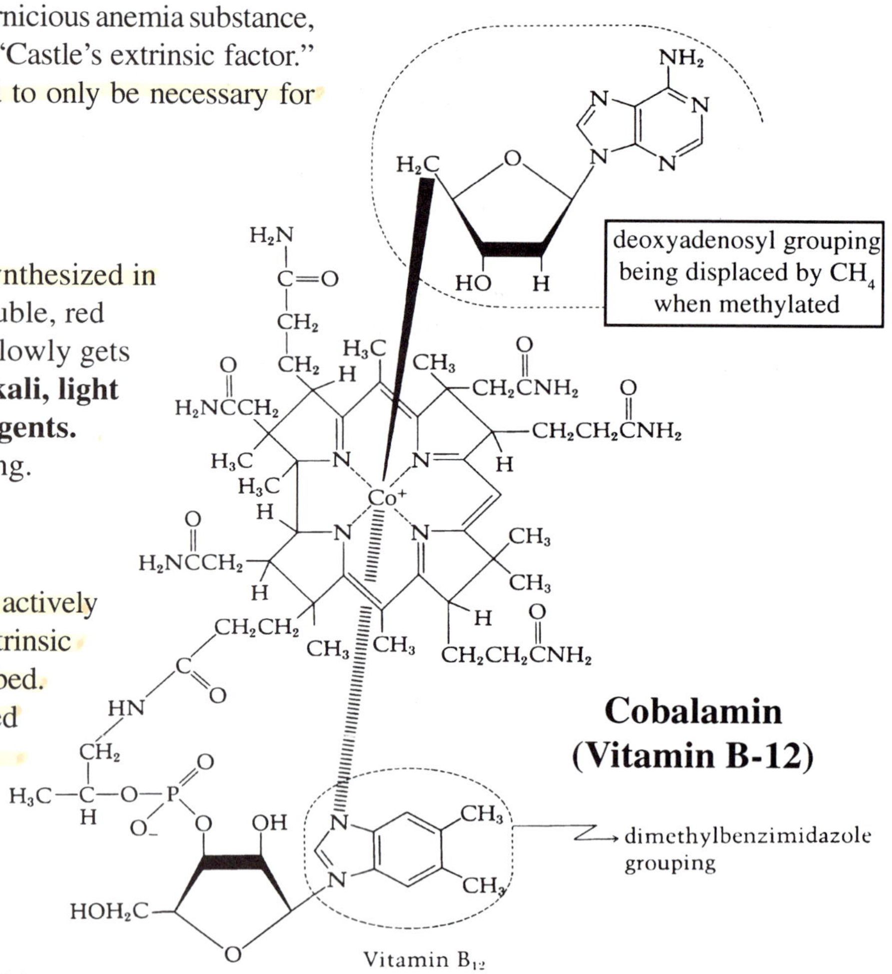

deoxyadenosyl grouping being displaced by $CH_4$ when methylated

## I. Chemistry

Cobalamin was not synthesized in the lab until 1973. Water soluble, red from the cobalt molecule, it slowly gets **destroyed by dilute acid, alkali, light and oxidizing or reducing agents.** 30% gets destroyed by cooking.

## II. Metabolism

Cobalamin is normally actively transported but, without the intrinsic factor, it is very poorly absorbed. The intrinsic factor is produced by the parietal cells. B-12 from foods gets released from the protein complex that it comes from via the action of hydrochloric acid and proteases. The secreted intrinsic factor then binds itself to the B-12. This complex travels down to the ileum where it attaches to the terminal aspect. At this point it is actively transported into the blood. B-12 is stored in the liver after it is absorbed. Stored for as long as 3 years, the excess is excreted in the urine.

**Cobalamin (Vitamin B-12)**

dimethylbenzimidazole grouping

Vitamin $B_{12}$

## III. Function

Cobalamin is involved as a cofactor in the transfer of methyl groups. It is needed to remove the methyl group from methyl tetrahydrofolate so that THF can be used for the synthesis of DNA.

The methyl-B-12 is used to transfer the methyl group onto homocysteine to form methionine. Methionine is important in methyl transfers and is necessary for the synthesis of myelin sheaths. In the absence of B-12, DNA is not produced and the cells grow without dividing, becoming megaloblasts.

B-12 is also involved in carbohydrate metabolism. It has been noted that lactic acid and pyruvate increased from 50% to 100% during B-12 deficiency. Neurological problems often occur when there is a B-12 deficiency because the nervous system relies on carbohydrates as its main source of fuel.

## IV. Requirements

**RDA**–3mcg

*Optimal daily intake*– 100–500mcg

**LAB**–serum B-12 (microbial assay) normal >100pg/ml, appears to be the most widely used and considered the most accurate. (Dr. Herman Baker of New York, one of the world experts in vitamin measurements, claims most all assays tend to analyze inactive metabolites.) Pregnancy, large doses of vitamin C, and folate deficiency may result in a falsely reduced B-12 assay.

Serum B-12 (RIA) is not as accurate, since it picks up all forms of cobalamin including those that are inactive.

24 hour urine MMA–Methylmalonic acid requires B-12 for conversion to succinic acid and, without B-12, it increases in the urine. This test is very sensitive and also very expensive.

**SCHILLING TEST**–This test can be used to assess the etiology of deficiency.

1) Ingest 1µg radioactive B-12 without intrinsic factor (IF). Next give a large "flushing" dose of non-labeled B-12 via IM and collect 24-48 hour urine.
   If > 7% *B-12 in urine = OKAY.
   If < 7% *B-12 in urine = Deficient B-12 due to **malabsorption** or **lack of IF**.
2) Ingest radioactive B-12 with IF and find *B-12 in urine = **pernicious anemia**.
3) Ingest radioactive B-12 with IF and find no *B-12 in urine= **malabsorption**.

**NOTE**–50-75% of patients with pernicious anemia have antibodies to IF–Heidelberg.
Hypersegmented neutrophils–**takes 1-2yrs for MCV to become elevated.**

* Indicates radioactive label.

## V. Sources

**Best Sources of Vitamin B-12 (animal sources)**

| Food | Amount | µg | Food | Amount | µg |
|---|---|---|---|---|---|
| Liver, beef | 3 oz | 93.5 | Tuna, canned, drained | 3 oz | 1.8 |
| Clams | 3 oz | ~60.0 | Cheese | 3 oz | 1-2 |
| Salmon steak | 3 oz | 3.0 | Milk (whole or skim) | 8 oz | 0.9 |
| Lamb | 3 oz | 2.6 | Halibut | 3 oz | 0.8 |
| Lobster | 3 oz | 2.6 | Egg | 1 large | 0.6 |
| Beef | 3 oz | 2.0 | Chicken | 3 oz | 0.3 |

**Sources of Vitamin B-12 (non-animal sources)**

| | Food | Amount | µg |
|---|---|---|---|
| | Brewer's yeast | 2 T | 2.0 |
| *Sea Vegatables* | Nori | 2 sheets | 2.0 |
| | Wakame | 3 wet oz | 1.9-5.3 |
| | Kombu | 3 wet oz | 1.5-4.1 |
| | Arame | 3 wet oz | 0.09-0.15 |
| *Micro-algaes* | "Super Blue Green" | 3g | 23.1 |
| | Chlorella | 3g | 4.0 |
| | Spirulina | 3g | 1.2 |

*"Super Blue Green" algae source of B-12 confirmed by Dr. Herman Baker, Brooklyn, New York.*

USDA Handbook #8 Series Washington, DC, ARS, USDA, 1976-1986

**NOTE**–There is debate over the reliability of non-animal sources of Vitamin B-12. An excellent review of this controversy, "The Myth of the Vegetarian B-12" by Gene Bruce, is presented in the *East West Journal,* May, 1988 issue. In summary, it was found that people on macrobiotic diets had lower levels of serum B-12 levels than the general population. In particular, infants breast fed or fed a macrobiotic diet directly are at a great risk of developing B-12 deficiency.

Non-animal sources which claim to have significant amounts of B-12–such as tempeh, micro-algaes (spirulina, chlorella), miso, tamari, and sea vegetables (nori, arame, kombu, wakame)–have been found to have negligible amounts or B-12 analogues that show up on lab tests, but don't have the activity of real B-12.

It should be noted that there are different techniques for measuring the B-12 content of foods. The radio immune assay measures only the active B-12 molecule. The microbiological test measures both the active B-12 and the inactive analogues. This latter test involves feeding a sample of the food being tested to certain bacteria which grow only when fed B-12. The bacteria growth rate determines the quantity of B-12. One problem with this test is that the bacteria will grow when fed a number of substances similar to B-12. Not only can these B-12 analogues falsely elevate the reported content of B-12 in foods, but they can have an antagonistic effect on the B-12 that may be present, thus making a deficiency more pronounced!

Also, the B-12 content in fermented foods, such as tempeh, may be different due to the production techniques. In Indonesia traditionally produced tempeh is loaded with B-12 producing bacteria which grows on the molds commonly growing on the food. In the U.S., however, large scale production and improved sanitation decreases the mold and bacteria and the subsequent B-12 content of the food. The most reliable non-animal source of B-12 seems to be brewer's yeast. However, the yeast must be grown on a medium containing the vitamin or else added during the final processing in order to get significant amounts.

## VI. Deficiency

The etiologies vitamin B-12 deficiency are:

1) Deficiency of intrinsic factor
2) Gastrectomy, especially of the cardiac or fundus
3) Pregnancy
4) Malabsorption (celiac disease, colitis, etc.)
5) Achlorhydria
6) Elderly
7) Vegans
8) Tapeworms
9) Excessive antibiotics or anti-convulsants
10) Megadoses of vitamin C and/or copper
11) Liver disease or cancer

## VII. Signs and Symptoms

Signs and symptoms of B-12 deficiency include: classic pernicious anemia due to lack of intrinsic factor; progressive peripheral neuropathy with pronounced anemia; fatigue, depression, confusion, memory loss, psychosis, glossitis, achlorhydria, impaired lymphocyte response, decreased phagocyte and PMN response, spinal degeneration and macrocytic cells.

## VIII. Therapeutics

**1) Pernicious Anemia**–B-12 IM

**2) Anemia of Pregnancy**–best to give B-12 with iron and folate as a larger increase of hemoglobin was noted with combined treatment.

**3) Anemia**

**Immune Problems**

**4) Allergies**

**a) asthma–**1-3mg/day of hydroxycobalamin IM. Repeat daily for 3 days then every other day and eventually every other week (Jonathan Wright). Since learning about this treatment from Dr. Wright, I have found it is almost always helpful in children. In adults it tends to be much less effective unless sulfate sensitive.

**b) contact dermatitis**

**c) atopic dermatitis**

**5) Canker sores**

**6) Viral hepatitis**

STUDY–Jain, Mukerji. *Observations on the therapeutic value of intravenous B-12 in infective hepatitis*. J Indian Med Assoc. 35:502-5,1960. ABSTRACT–13/26 patients with viral hepatitis selected alternately received B-12 100mcg IV daily in addition to standard treatment. While liver function tests were unmodified, the experimental group had less anorexia and jaundice and the mean duration of illness was 34.5 days compared to 45.8 days in the controls.

STUDY–Campbell, Pruitt. *Vitamin B-12 in the treatment of viral hepatitis*. Am J.Med Sci. 224:252,1952. ABSTRACT–IV B-12 brought about rapid return of appetite and liver size to normal in patients with viral hepatitis. In addition, the serum bilirubin returned to normal earlier (in 10 weeks compared to 18), and the mean duration of illness was reduced from 54 to 48 days.

**7) Herpes zoster**–1-3mg/day IM. According to Jonathan Wright, B-12 given IM (2-3mg) along with thiamin (50mg) and adenosine monophosphate (50-75mg) works 80% of time to relieve pain symptoms. The treatment may need repeating daily and then again 3-4 days later. B-12 may also be used topically with vitamin B-1, AMP, and DMSO for relief of pain.

**Dermatology**

**8) Psoriasis**

STUDY–Carslaw, Neill. *Vitamin B-12 in psoriasis*. Letter to the editor. Brit. Med J. 1:611,1963. ABSTRACT–Vitamin B-12, saline or triamcinolone were infused into psoriatic lesions (epidermis and mid-dermis) with a hypodermic needle. Triamcinolon caused rapid regression of lesions, while normal saline had no effect. Of the 8 patients who received the B-12, 6 showed regression of the lesion.

**9) Seborrheic dermatitis**

**10) Acne**

**Neurological Problems**

**11) Diabetic neuropathies**

**12) Neuralgias**

**General**–can be used for poor energy and inability to concentrate.

**13) Senile dementia & Alzheimer's disease-**Patients with dementia or Alzheimer's disease frequently have low levels of vitamin B-12. Certainly a trial of vitamin B-12 given IM may dramatically improve mental functioning in these patients. It is best to treat early on in their condition.

STUDY–Lindenbaum J, et al. *Neuropsychiatric disorders caused by cobalamin deficiency in the absence of anemia or macrocytosis.* NEJM 318:1720-28, 1988. ABSTRACT–141 consecutive patients with neuropsychiatric abnormalities, that were attributed to vitamin B-12 deficiency, were evaluated via hematocrit or MCV. It was found that 40 of them had normal values of hematocrit, MCV or both. They all had serum cobalamin levels of below 200pg/ml and serum MMA and homocysteine were markedly elevated. These 40 patients treated with B-12 all responded favorably to treatment with B-12 and all showed a dramatic drop in MMA and homocysteine levels (one patient did die during the first week of treatment not attributed to the B-12 therapy).

**14) Fatigue**– 1-3mg given once every few days or few months depending upon response.

STUDY–Ellis, Nasser, *A pilot study of B-12 in the treatment of tiredness.* Brit J Nutr. 30:277-83,1973. ABSTRACT–28 men and women who complained of tiredness but had normal serum B-12, hemoglobin, and folate levels were divided into 2 groups One group was given injections of hydroxycobalamin 5mg 2x day for 2 weeks followed by a 2 week rest period and then a similar course of placebo injections and the other group was treated with the placebo first.. Those who received placebo first felt significantly better in regard to "general well being" when they started the second period of receiving the B-12. Their improvement in symptoms of fatigue was borderline. The other group felt better immediately but recorded no less improvement during the second series of placebo shots (they felt no difference). This was probably due to the fact that they were storing significant amounts of B-12 and their levels had not dropped off yet.

**15) Bursitis**–Can use with ultrasound or give IM daily for up to 2 weeks. Dr. Jonathan Wright swears by it.

STUDY–Klemes. *Vitamin B-12 in acute subdeltoid bursitis.* Indust. Med. Land Surg. 26:290-2,1957. ABSTRACT–40 acute patients received vitamin B-12 1000mcg daily for 7-10days; then 3x weekly for 2-3wks; and finally 1-2x weekly for 2-3wks (depending upon their rate of progress). All but 2 or 3 improved with rapid relief of pain and subjective symptoms, sometimes within a few hours. Complete relief was often noted in several days. Follow-up radiographs of cases of calcific bursitis showed considerable resorption of calcium deposits.

**16) Sciatica**–1-3 mg with 50mg thiamin IM daily for 4-7 days or until pain much better. Can then spread IM injections out to 1x every 4-7 days (Jonathan Wright).

**17) Insomnia–**as needed IM 1-3mg

**18) Depression**

**19) Bone spurs in feet–** 1-3mg daily until pain gone (Jonathan Wright).

**20) Stop smoking**–can inject along with homeopathic nicotine and lidocaine into acupuncture ear points. Can also do IM and orally along with B complex to calm nerves.

**21) Heart disease or osteoporosis related to elevated levels of homocysteine-**It has been found that vitamin B-12 can significantly reduce the levels of homocysteine if elevated.

**NOTE**–on IM injections, hydroxo or hydroxy cobalamin may be the most helpful form as it tends to elevate tissue levels more than cyanocobalamin.

## IX. Interactions

In food, B-12 is destroyed by large amounts of vitamin C. This is contested by Russell Jaffe, M.D. from the *Brain Bio Center* in New Jersey. Dr. Jaffe says that the change in color which happens to vitamin B-12 when put into solution with vitamin C isn't a destruction of B-12, but rather a change of the ion structure surrounding the B-12. There is no breakage of the ring and the activity of the B-12 is still present.

If very large doses of vitamin C (100gms) are stored in solution with vitamin B-12, there may be some destruction over 3 weeks time. Also the combination of copper, vitamin C, and thiamin may destroy vitamin B-12 as well.

If macrocytic anemia is present due to either vitamin B-12 or folate deficiency, it is wise to give **both** folate and B-12 by injection.

## X. Toxicity

Use hydroxycobalamin as an injectable. Some evidence indicates that the cyano part of cobalamin is toxic to cells (related to cyanide). This is probably a more theoretical consideration and has not been actually substantiated.

## Notes

---

# FOLIC ACID (FOLATE)

Folic acid was discovered during the search for the factor which makes liver effective in curing pernicious anemia. Folacin was first isolated from green leafy vegetables (spinach) in 1941. It has been established as an essential nutrient for humans, many animals, and microorganisms including Lactobacillus casei.

## I. Chemistry

Folic acid is water-soluble with some forms stable to heat and others quite sensitive. Some forms are stable to acid and others destroyed. **Vegetables stored at room temperature suffer considerable loss of folic acid**. Dried milk has virtually all of the folate destroyed.

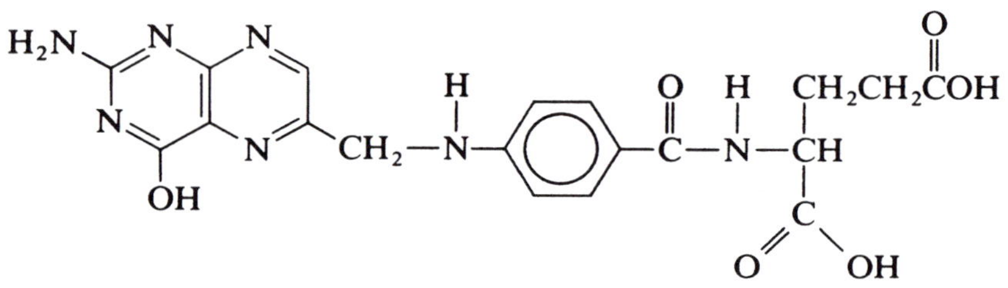

$H_2N$ N N H O H $CH_2CH_2\overset{O}{\overset{\|}{C}}OH$

N N $CH_2$—N—⟨benzene⟩—C—N—CH

OH C

O OH

*Folacin (folic acid)*

## II. Metabolism

Folacin, usually present in the polyglutamate form in food, is broken down to the monoglutamate form by folyl conjugase from the pancreas and mucosal conjugase from the intestinal wall. It is absorbed by both active transport and diffusion in the proximal small intestine. There is decreased absorption in an alkali medium and with added zinc.

**polyglutamate** $\xrightarrow[\text{(pancreas \& Small Intestine)}]{\textit{folyl conjugase}}$ monoglutamate ⟶ methyltetrahydrofolate

*stored up to 4 month*

*supply–10mg*

## III. Function

1) Folic acid facilitates the synthesis of purines: guanine & adenine and pyrimidine thymine.
2) It is essential for the formation and maturation of red and white blood cells.
3) Folacin is the single carbon carrier in the formation of heme.
4) histidine ⟶ urocanate ⟶ **Formiminoglutamate** ⟶ glutamic acid
5) phenylalanine ⟶ tyrosine

## IV. Requirements

**RDA**–200mcg (this has recently changed taking into account increased folate activity)
Pregnancy–400mcg., lactation–300mcg
*Optimal daily intake*–2mg
**LAB**
**1) Serum folate (RIA)**
2) **Hypersegmented neutrophils**–With levels at 25% and above, the likelihood of a folate deficiency should be considered. However, this could be caused by hypochlorhydria. Pernicious anemia should also be considered.
**3) FIGLU**–Formimino glutamic acid. Since folate is essential in the conversion of histidine to glutamic acid, FIGLU, an intermediary product, is built when folate is deficient. It is then excreted in the urine.
**4) Macrocytic red blood cells**

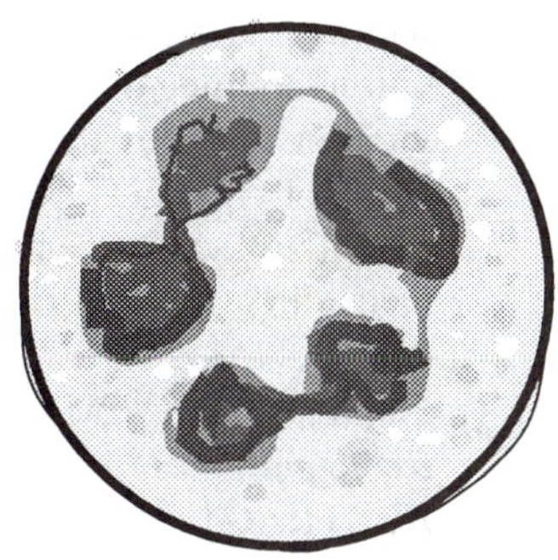

*Hypersegmentation of neutrophil*

## V. Sources

**Best Food Sources of Folate**

| Food | Amount | mcg | Food | Amount | mcg |
|---|---|---|---|---|---|
| Liver, chicken | 3 oz | 654 | Dandelion greens, cooked | 1 cup | 82 |
| Brewer's yeast | 1 T | 313 | Leeks, fresh chopped | 1 cup | 67 |
| Blackeyed peas | 1/2 cup | 280 | Broccoli, fresh chopped | 1 cup | 62 |
| Lentil beans, cooked | 1/2 cup | 180 | Bok choy fresh shredded | 1 cup | 57 |
| Turnip greens fresh | 1 cup | 171 | Swiss chard, cooked | 1 cup | 57 |
| Lima beans | 1 cup | 137 | Parsley fresh chopped | 1/2 cup | 55 |
| Orange juice | 1 cup | 136 | Squash, Acorn | 1 cup | 46 |
| Liver, beef | 3 oz | 123 | Rice, wild | 1 cup | 43 |
| Kidney beans | 1/2 cup | 115 | Tomato sauce | 1 cup | 39 |
| Peanuts | 1/2 cup | 106 | Tofu, firm | 1/2 cup | 37 |
| Lettuce Romaine | 1 cup | 100 | Brussels Sprouts | 4 medium | 28 |
| Peas, sprouted | 1/2 cup | 87 | Oat bran | 1/2 cup | 25 |

USDA Handbook #8 Series Washington, DC, ARS, USDA, 1976-1986

## VI. Deficiency

Folate deficiencies result in poor growth, megaloblastic anemia and other blood disorders, glossitis, and GI tract disturbances. Since the main metabolic consequences of folic acid deficiency are changes in cellular nuclear morphology, rapidly multiplying cells, such as the epithelial cells of the stomach, intestines, vagina, and cervix, are most affected. In pernicious anemia, folic acid administration will produce marked alleviation of the anemia but the GI signs and symptoms and the neurologic lesions continue to progress.

The drugs Aminopterin–used to treat leukemia–and sulphasalazine–used for ulcerative colitis–can create folate deficiency. Anticonvulsant drugs may also cause folate deficiency.

**NOTE–Estimates of folate deficiency are as high as 60% in pregnancy!**

STUDY–Herbert Victor. Veterans Hospital Bronx, N.Y. Am J of Ob & Gyn. ABSTRACT–A study of 110 pregnant women from low income families in NYC found that 16% had definite folate deficiency and another 14% had marginal folate levels.

# VII. Therapeutics

### 1) Megaloblastic anemia–RBCs become large and ineffective.

### 2) Neural Tube Defects–360mcg of folate/day

**NOTE**–It requires $250,000/yr to care for a spina bifida patient.

STUDY–Smithells, Sheppard, and Schorah. *Vitamin deficiency and neural tube defects.* Archives of Disease in Childhood, Dec.1976, pp944-50. ABSTRACT–438 women who had previously given birth to babies with neural tube defects were studied. One group of 178 mothers took a multivitamin formulation providing **360mcg of folate/day**. Another group of 260 took no vitamins or started them later on. The daily vitamin also provided 4000 IU of vitamin A, 400 IU vitamin D, 1.5mg of B-1, 1.5mg B-2, 15mg of B-3, 40mg of vitamin C, 75mg Fe, and 480mg of calcium (note that neural tube closure occurs at four weeks). Out of 260 women who did not take vitamins, 5% of the babies were born with neural tube defects. Out of the 178 women who took the vitamins, only one baby or .6% of the group developed neural tube defects.

STUDY–Laurence, James, Miller, Tennant, Campbell. *Double-blind randomized controlled study: A trial of Folate treatment before conception to prevent recurrence of neural tube defects.* Br. Med J. 282:1509,1981. ABSTRACT–Women from South Wales who previously had babies with neural tube defects were broken into 2 groups. 60 women were asked to take 4mg of folate/day before conception and during early pregnancy. 44 of these women actually complied. 51 women were in the placebo group. One woman in the folate-supplemented group, one in the non-compliers, and four in the placebo group had babies who developed a neural tube defects. At first there was no statistical significance. Then the woman in the folate-supplemented group whose baby was born with a neural tube defect admitted that she had not been taking her folate.

### 3) Cleft Palate

STUDY–Tolarova. *Periconceptional suppl. with vitamin and folic acid to prevent recurrence of cleft lip.* Lancet; 2:217,1982. ABSTRACT–297 women were studied who had one child with unilateral harelip with or without cleft palate and other family symptoms of orofacial clefts. They were invited to participate in a trial of periconceptional vitamin supplementation. The daily supplement consisted of 10mg folate, 6000 IU vitamin A, 3mg of B-3, and 3mg of pantothenate. The women were asked to take these vitamins from 3 months prior to conception until the end of the first trimester of pregnancy. In the 85 women who took the vitamins, there was one recurrence (1.2%) and in the 212 unsupplemented pregnancies there were 15 recurrences (7.4%).

### 4) Restless Leg Syndrome–35-60mg/day There are two types:

1) The familiar mixed sensorimotor form is characterized by pain, numbness, and lightning stabs of pain in the lower or upper limbs. This pain is relieved by movement of the legs. Patients move their legs irresistibly in the night. About one-third of these patients respond to folate therapy. Pregnant women frequently develop this condition near the end of pregnancy as stores get used up.

2) The pure motor or myoclonic form, which does not have a sensory component, is characterized by leg jerks lasting less than ten seconds. The patient is unaware of the problem but complains of frequent nocturnal awakenings or excess daytime sleepiness.

STUDY–Botez, Cadotte, Beaulieu and Pichette. *Neurologic Disorders Responsive to Folate Therapy* Can Med AssocJ. 115:217-23,1976. ABSTRACT–3 women with acquired folate deficiency had mild signs and symptoms of restless legs, depression, muscular and mental fatigue, depressed ankle jerks, diminution of vibratory sensation in the legs, a stocking-type hypoesthesia, and chronic constipation. All 3 recovered with folate treatment.

STUDY–Botez. Nut Reports International. ABSTRACT–21 pregnant women were randomly examined. It was found that 8/10 women not receiving supplemental folate had restless legs syndrome. Only one of eleven taking folate had the problem. 3 of these women with the most severe restless legs were given 10 mg folate daily. Their signs and symptoms disappeared after 8 days.

**5) Cervical dysplasia**–10mg/day, can use orally and topically.

**BCP's interfere with folate**

STUDY–Butterworth, Hatch, Gore, Mueller, Krudmieck. *Improvement in cervical dysplasia associated with folic acid therapy in users of oral contraceptives.* Am J. Clin Nut. 35:73, 1982. ABSTRACT–47 women with mild or moderate cervical dysplasia took folate 10mg/day or placebo for 3 months. All had taken combination oral contraceptives for at least 6 months and continued them during the study. After treatment, biopsy and PAP smear scores were significantly better in supplemented women, but unchanged in the placebo group.

STUDY–Whitehead, Reyner, and Lindenbaum. *Megaloblastic changes in cervical epithelium associated with oral contraceptive therapy and reversal with folate.* JAMA 226;1421,1973. ABSTRACT–22 of 115 women taking oral contraceptives had megaloblastic changes in cervical cells, compared to none of 51 controls. Eight women with the abnormal cervical cytology took 10mg/day folate for 3 months and all had complete remission or marked improvement.

**6) Depression**

**NOTE**–Epileptics who are on anticonvulsant drugs must be cautious about higher doses of folate which may interfere with the effectiveness of the anticonvulsant drugs.

STUDY–Ghadirian. *Folate deficiency and depression.* Psychosomatics 21(11):926-9,1980. ABSTRACT–A study of 48 psychiatric in-patients showed that serum folate levels in depressed patients were significantly lower than in non-depressed patients who were either medically or emotionally ill. These levels negatively correlated with the degree of depression.

STUDY–Coppen. *Folic acid enhances lithium prophylaxis.* J Affective Disorders 10:9-13, 1986. ABSTRACT–42 patients undergoing lithium therapy for affective disorders received either folate 200mcg/day or placebo. After one year, there was a small but insignificant change in the affective morbidity index (AMI) in both groups. However, depression scores were significantly lower in the folate-supplemented group. When the supplemented group was broken down according to mean folate levels at the end of the study, it was found that the half with the highest mean folate levels had the best scores for both AMI and depression.

**7) Malabsorption and GI inflammation**–3-10mg/day. Since some of the fastest turnover of cells occurs in the GI tract, folate is a critical nutrient for the regeneration of new cells. Diarrhea can seriously impair the absorption of folate.

**8) Increased fracture of chromosomes**–It was found that the "fragile X chromosome" fractures more often when there is a folate deficiency. When supplemented, the number of fractures goes down. Also, coffee, even in moderate amounts, increases the fracture rate of these X chromosomes.

**9) Gingivitis or periodontal disease**–A few drops Folirinse (Scientific Botanicals), along with other nutrients (zinc, quercetin & co-enzyme Q), and botanicals (IPSAB, sanguinaria & hawthorne)

**10) Gout**– 25-75mg/day–along with vitamin C may inhibit xanthine oxidase and thus lower serum uric acid levels.

## VII. Toxicity

Be aware that a B-12 deficiency may mask neurological signs and symptoms even though it corrects the anemia in pernicious anemia.

Folate may interfere with anticonvulsant drugs in large doses greater than 10-15mg/day.

There is no other known toxicity.

Some experts are divided on supplementation of folate during chemotherapeutic use of methotrexate, a drug which antagonized folate. I believe a small amount, 1 mg or so, does not interfere with the positive effects of methotrexate.

## Notes

# BIOTIN

Biotin was recognized as a growth factor for microorganisms in 1924. It was originally named Bios II, one of 3 growth factors. The other factors were named vitamin H & coenzyme R. Later, it was found the 3 factors were all the same. Biotin was synthesized in 1943 and recognized as a compound which protected rats against "egg white injury." Rats fed raw egg whites developed eczema and alopecia around the eyes. A substance in egg white, "avidin," was found to cause the illness.

## I. Chemistry

Stable to heat and water soluble, biotin is sensitive to alkalai and oxidation.

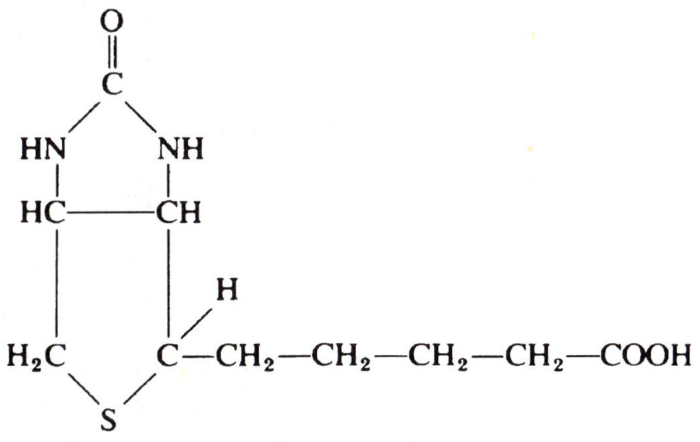

```
          O
          ‖
          C
        /   \
     HN       NH
      |        |
     HC ------ CH
      |        |
      |        |    H
      |        |  /
    H₂C        C—CH₂—CH₂—CH₂—CH₂—COOH
       \      /
          S
```

*Biotin*

## II. Metabolism

Biotin is rapidly absorbed, chiefly intact, throughout the small intestine.

## III. Requirements

**RDA**–100-200mcg
**Lab**–microbial assay–blood and urine–has a wide variation.
*Optimal daily intake*–300mcg

## IV. Function

1) Biotin is a cofactor required in the synthesis and oxidation of fatty acids.
2) It is involved in the deamination of amino acids such as serine, aspartic acid, and threonine.
3) Biotin is essential for carboxylation–the addition and removal of C02 from certain active compounds.
4) It is required for the synthesis of pancreatic amylase and niacin.
5) Biotin may be involved in the synthesis and release of insulin.

## V. Sources

**Best Food Sources for Biotin**

| Food | Amount | μg |
|---|---|---|
| Liver, chicken | 3 oz | 146 |
| Liver, calf | 3 oz | 45 |
| Kidney, lamb | 3 oz | 36 |
| Rolled oats, uncooked | 1/2 cup | 16 |
| Egg, hard cooked | 1 large | 10 |
| Haddock | 3 oz | 5 |
| Milk | 1 cup | 5 |
| Halibut | 3 oz | 4 |
| Camembert cheese | 2 oz | 3 |
| Chicken, dark meat | 3 oz | 3 |
| Cod | 3 oz | 3 |
| Salmon | 3 oz | 3 |
| Tuna, canned | 3 oz | 3 |
| Orange | 1 med | 2 |
| Tomato | 1 med | 2 |
| Whole wheat bread | 1 slice | 2 |

USDA Handbook #8 Series Washington, DD, ARS, USDA, 1976-1986

## VI. Deficiency

Biotin deficiency causes early changes to occur in the skin. Signs and symptoms are similar to B1 deficiency. Dermatitis, characterized by scaliness or hardening, which frequently starts in the region of the eye, is often the first symptom. Other signs and symptoms are anorexia, lassitude, and nausea. Loss of hair and muscular atrophy follow. There is evidence that deficiency also results in the elevation of both glucose and cholesterol levels.

## VII. Therapeutics

1) **Case Study**–NEJM, April 2, 1981. A baby at age 3 months began to have seizures (around 10/day). Many things were tried. By 14 months, all of her hair had fallen out, even her eyebrows and eyelashes. A red, scaly rash covered her body and her eyes were edematous and inflamed. She became irritable and sleepy as her muscles grew weak and her gait unsteady. Lactic acid levels rose to 2x normal. 12 hours after administering 10mg biotin orally, blood levels of lactic acid dropped to normal. Within 48 hours all blood chemistries returned to normal and, over the next 4 months, her entire development returned to normal.

2) **SIDS**–The livers of SIDS infants contained considerably lower levels of biotin than normal. Researchers in Australia and Great Britain have found that SIDS closely resembles a disorder in which marginally biotin deficient chickens die when subjected to mild stress. The chickens did not display any typical biotin deficient signs and symptoms but had low levels of biotin in their livers.

**3) Diabetes mellitus**

STUDY–Coggeshall. *Biotin Satus and Plasma Glucose in Diabetics.* Annal N.Y. Acad Sci 447:389-92,1985. ABSTRACT–Patients with insulin-dependant diabetes mellitus were removed from insulin therapy and treatment with biotin 16mg daily or placebo for one week. Fasting blood sugar levels fell significantly in patients on biotin, while they rose as expected in patients on placebo. Since biotin levels typically are elevated in diabetics, the authors speculate that it may be abnormally bound and/or biologically unavailable.

**4) Seborrheic dermatitis**–5-10mg in infants (can be used for "craddle cap" topically and orally in infants)

STUDY–Nisenson. *Treatment of Seborrheic Dermatitis with Biotin and Vitamin B Complex.* Letter to Ed. J. Pediat. 81:630-31,1972. ABSTRACT–Infants with extensive seborrheic dermatitis unresponsive to local treatment were fed liver and egg yolk (both of which have very high biotin levels in them; biotin was unavailable at the time). They were fed early in the first month or two of life, with good clinical improvement. Those infants with more widespread involvement improved more rapidly when B complex was added to the regime (1cc 1x or repeated every week).

**5) Cardiovascular disease**–Biotin has the effect of lowering cholesterol.

**6) May strengthen nails and stimulate hair growth.**

## VIII. Toxicity

None known to date

## Notes

# VITAMIN C (ASCORBIC ACID)

In ancient Rome, Egypt, and Greece military crews usually developed scurvy during long voyages at sea. During the middle ages, "The Black Death" was a fulminating, virulent epidemic of a bacterial disease, bubonic plague, concurrent with pulmonary infection superimposed on scurvy which claimed one fourth of the population of Europe (some 25 million deaths!).

**1497**–Vasco De Gama lost 100 of 150 crew members to scurvy.

**1536**–French Explorer Jacques Cartier survived with advice from the Newfoundland Indians who told him about tea from Spruce Tree Needles.

**1556-1857**–114 scurvy epidemics were reported especially in winter and spring. In 1593 Admiral Sir Richard Hawkins protected sailors, aboard the British ship "*The Dainty*", with oranges and lemons against the dreaded scurvy plague.

**1720**–Kramer prescribed fresh herbs or lemons to Austrian soldiers fighting the Turks.

**1747–James Lind performed a famous experiment on 12 men who were severely ill with scurvy. Six groups of "2" received the following foods:**

1) Cider 1 qt tid 2) 2 teaspoons of vinegar tid
3) Oil of vitriol dilute tid 4) 1/2 pint seawater tid
5)1 lemon and 2 oranges 6) Garlic, mustard seed, horseradish, gum myrrh & balsam of Peru

Sailors receiving the lemons & oranges were cured and James Lind recommended that all sailors receive lemons & oranges.

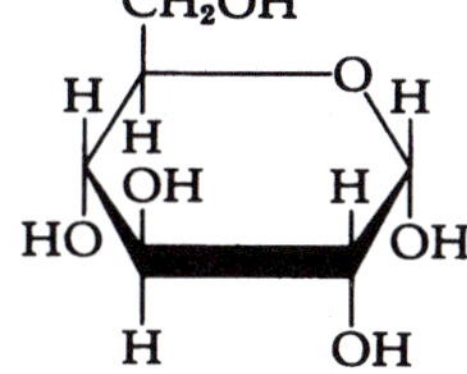

*Hayworth view of ascorbic acid*

**1795**–The British Admiralty finally adopted Lind's recommendation. 100,000 lives had been lost to scurvy since his discovery.

**1865**–The British Board of Trade adopted precautions, citing the records of merchants delivering lemons who died while transporting them.

**1865**–American Civil War had 30,000 cases of scurvy. The U.S. didn't adopt precautions until 1895.

**1913**–**Casimir Funk** developed the experimental hypothesis that pellagra, rickets, beriberi, and scurvy are all deficiency diseases.

**1928–Albert Szent-Gyorgyi** first isolated Vitamin C from ox adrenal glands.

**1932–Albert Szent-Gyorgyi** proved the isolate to be vitamin C.

## I. Chemistry

**Vitamin C** is water soluble and easily oxidized in solution and with heat. **Iron, copper, and alkaline pH increase oxidation.**

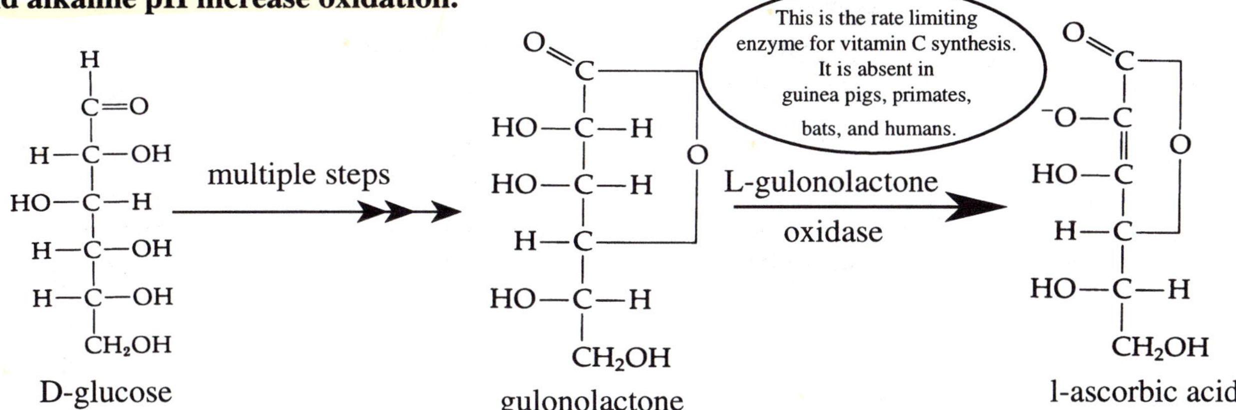

*Conversion of glucose into ascorbic acid.*

## II. Function

1) **Collagen synthesis**–hydroxylation of proline–Prolylhydroxylase & lysyl hydroxylase–Both of these enzymes hydroxylate lysine and are essential for the hydroxylysine cross-links in collagen. Ascorbic acid acts as a reducing agent and keeps both of the above enzymes active. These connective tissues include cartilage, dentin, skin, and bones.

In the diagram at the right vitamin C is used by fibroblasts to generate collagen components.

From Pot, G, & Gerlack. Enzyme 25:394, 1980.

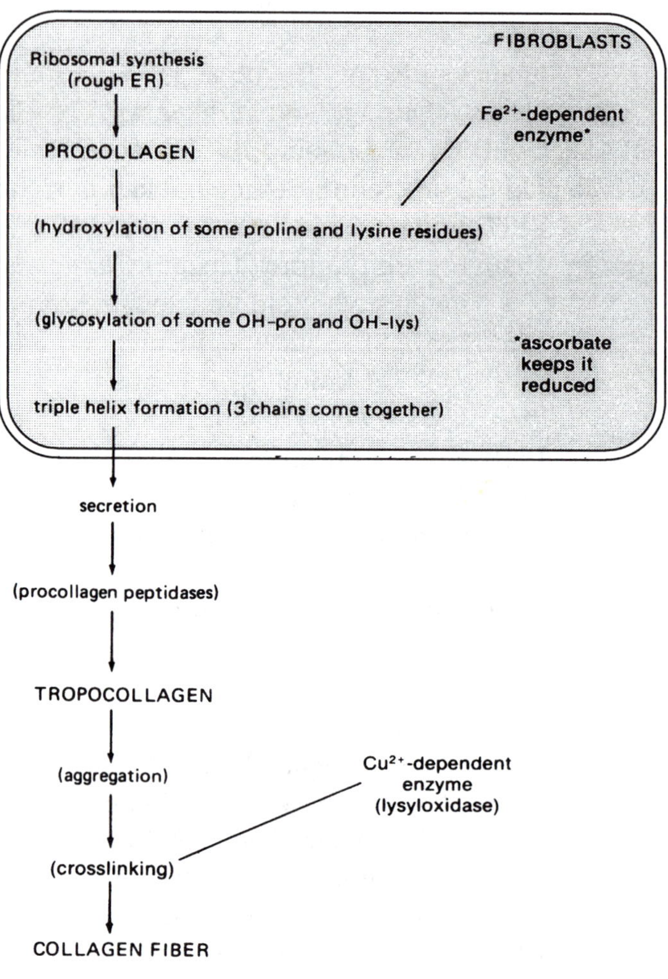


STUDY–British J Nut, 1972 ABSTRACT–double blind controlled trial–20 surgical patients suffering from pressure sores were treated with either placebo or one gm vitamin C. 43% of placebo patients had improvement compared to 84% of vitamin C group.

STUDY–British J Derm, 1975 ABSTRACT–In a double blind, placebo-controlled experiment ß-thalassemia patients were treated with 3gms vitamin C or placebo for leg sores. It was found that there was a markedly significant increase in partial or complete healing of sores.

2) **Norepinephrine synthesis**

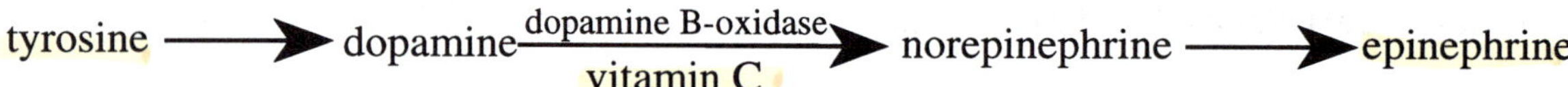


STUDY–Injections of vitamin C into brains increases the conversion of dopamine to epinephrine. It may be valuable in the treatment of schizophrenia, chorea, dyskinesia.

STUDY–Brit J Psych– Schizophrenics responded well to vitamin C one gm /day.

**NOTE**–Schizophrenics metabolize vitamin C 10x faster than normals (Vanderkamp '66).

3) **Aid the absorption of iron**–vitamin C works by reducing ferric iron to ferrous iron. It works best when taken with foods containing iron or iron supplements. In addition it blocks the degradation of ferritin to hemosiderin, a form of iron storage that is a considerably less bioavailable form. It thus provides a more easily available source of iron.

4) **Steroid hormone synthesis**-ACTH stimulation causes marked loss of ascorbic acid from the adrenal cortex. ACTH is primarily involved with glucocorticoids-cortisol.

5) **Antioxidant**–Vitamin C is a powerful reducing agent and seems to work synergistically with other antioxidants such as glutathione and vitamin E. At the branched sites of arteries where atherosclerotic plagues are the most abundant vitamin C levels are the lowest.

6) **Drug metabolism & detox**

7) **Carnitine synthesis**

8) **Degradation of cholesterol**

9) **Regulates cellular humoral immune function & increase macrophage activity**

10) **Cancer prevention**

11) **Activates certain vitamins into their active forms**–conversion of folacin to tetrahydrofolic acid, tryptophan to 5-hydroxytryptophan and eventually serotonin.

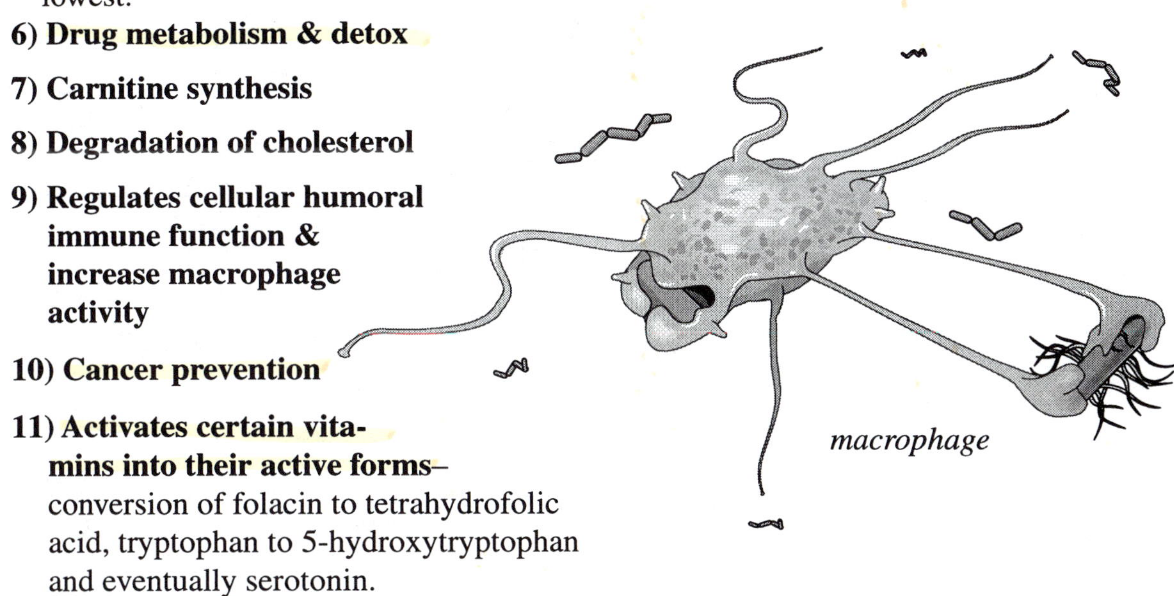
*macrophage*

12) **Antihistamine effects**–at doses over 6-8gms per day.

## III. Requirements

**5mg/day prevents scurvy**

**RDA**–60mg/day (RDA increased from 45 mg in 1974) saturates RBC's but not serum (only 75mg/dl)
400mg/day results in maximum serum level–>1.4mg/dl
Beyond 400mg/day results in increased tissue levels of vitamin C. The concentration of vitamin C in the adrenals is 50x that of the serum.
*Optimal daily intake*–1-9gms depending upon individual
**Irwin Stone**–Committee on Animal Nutrition from *The Healing Factor; Vitamin C Against Disease, 1972.*

1) Nutrient requirements of lab animals:
   a) Monkeys–4 gms vitamin C on an equivalent body weight basis of 150lbs.
   b) Guinea pigs–3-12 gms equivalent body weight.
2) Adult Gorillas in wild eat 4.5 gms/day.
3) Rats synthesize 2-4 gms equivalent if under little or no stress.
   Rats synthesize 15 gms/day equivalent if under moderate stress.
   Goats synthesize 13 gms/day equivalent if under moderate stress.
   Mice, cats, dogs, and cattle all synthesize 10gms/day equivalent body weight.
4) Pauling calculated from raw plant foods that 2-9gms/day could be eaten.

The only animals that can not synthesize ascorbic acid are guinea pigs, a rare species of bats and primates–gorillas, chimps, monkeys and humans.

## IV. Sources

**Best Food Sources for Vitamin C**

| Food | Amount | Mg | Food | Amount | Mg |
|---|---|---|---|---|---|
| Acerola berries | 10 med | 900 | Orange | 1 med | 50 |
| Orange juice | 1 cup | 124 | Cauliflower | 1/2 cup | 45 |
| Guava | 1 med | 110 | Turnip greens, cooked | 1/2 cup | 45 |
| Pepper, red chili | 1 med | 109 | Strawberries | 1/2 cup | 44 |
| Green peppers | 1/2 cup | 96 | Tomato juice | 1 cup | 39 |
| Pepper, sweet | 1 med | 95 | Baked potato, with skin | 1 med | 31 |
| Grapefruit juice | 1 cup | 93 | Tomato | 1 med | 28 |
| Watermelon | 2 med slice | 92 | Sweet potato | 1 med | 28 |
| Cantaloupe | 1/2 med | 90 | Kale | 1/2 cup | 27 |
| Honeydew melon | 1/4 med | 90 | Potato baked, then peeled | 1 med | 26 |
| Papaya | 1/2 med | 85 | Cabbage, raw | 1/2 cup | 21 |
| Grapefruit | 1 med | 82 | Mustard greens, cooked | 1/2 cup | 18 |
| Grapefruit | 1 med | 74 | Blackberries | 1/2 cup | 15 |
| Kiwi | 1 med | 74 | Spinach, raw | 1/2 cup | 14 |
| Brussels sprouts | 4 med | 73 | Blueberries | 1/2 cup | 10 |
| Cauliflower, cooked | 1 cup | 70 | Potato, peeled then boiled | 1 medium | 10 |
| Broccoli, chopped, raw | 1/2 cup | 66 | Cherries | 1/2 cup | 8 |
| Mango | 1 med | 57 | Mung bean sprouts | 1/4 cup | 5 |

## V. Deficiency

Symptoms of severe vitamin C deficiency, or scurvy, include listlessness, fatigue, weakness, shortness of breath, muscle cramps, aching bones, joints and muscles, and anorexia. Other symptoms are dry skin, fever, hemorrhage, easy bruising and secondary infections.

Experimentally induced vitamin C deficiency causes hypertrophy of the cornea, congestion of follicles or ducts, swollen joints, bleeding gums, muscle aches and fatigue.

**Lab**–decreased glucose tolerance and elevated cholesterol levels combined with impaired physical performance. There is also a salivary test that measures tissue levels of vitamin C but appear to be a rather crude assessment of vitamin C status.

## VI. Therapeutics

Vitamin C is considered a nutrient that is involved with stress. As stress, both physical and mental, goes up the amount of vitamin C that is produced goes up correspondingly in all animals that produce it.

The experiment represented on the right was performed on rats exposed to cold illness. Their normal response is to greatly increase synthesis, in the liver, of vitamin C. This is pretty typical of most animals who make their own ascorbic acid.

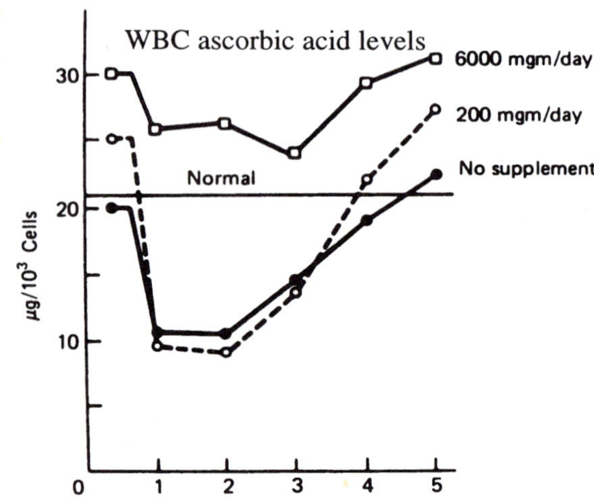


From Anderson, TW. *Nutrition Today Magazine*, Jan/Feb 1, 1977

1) **Viral or Bacterial infections**–use to bowel tolerance then cut back on dose. Take 1-2 gms every hour or every other hour. Often, if treating someone who has infection, patient can tolerate higher doses before they get diarrhea. It has been reported that some people can tolerate up to 200gms orally of vitamin C before they get diarrhea! Buffered vitamin C is tolerated better and smaller doses given more frequently is alsobetter tolerated.

    Can also use intravenously up to 100 gms (see Robert Cathcart protocol appendix B & C in *Antioxidant Adaptation: Its role in Free Radical Pathology* Levine & Kidd). Can use for any type of infection such as Candida, colds, hepatitis, influenza, mononucleosis, viral pneumonia, herpes simplex and zoster to name a few.

2) **Decrease triglycerides and platelet adhesiveness**

3) **Allergies**–greater than 6gms per day
    - increases epinephrine
    - decreases histamine levels
    - stabilizes mast cell membranes

4) **Cancer**–can use prophylactically or in treatment. For treatment must use high doses, greater than 8gms.

STUDY–Pauling and Cammeron–100 terminal cancer patients increased survival by 4-fold at 10gms/day. More than 5gms vitamin C increased survival 105 days. Less than 4gms C increased survival 35 days.

5) **Wound healing**–1-6gms per day. (See protocol for surgery in appendix). Dose up before during and after for maximum effect. Can use for both internal wounds such as ulcers of the intestines and also of the skin. Can use for any condition in which epithelial cells are involved such as periodontal disease, macular degeneration, gingivitis, canker sores, easy bruising, ulcerative colitis, and cervical dysplasia.

6) **Low back pain**–especially if have disc degeneration, 1-3gms per day long term.

7) **Improve soreness after physical activity**–1-3 gms when taken before and after has been shown to decrease soreness and lessen the time of recovery compared to placebo.

8) **Diabetes mellitus**–Localized tissues in diabetics are often very low in vitamin C. It has also been shown that vitamin C decreases glycosylation of albumin, which can significantly reduce the risk of development of atherosclerosis and generally protect other tissues susceptible to damage.

9) **Heavy metal detox**–large doses of vitamin C have been shown to increase excretion of heavy metals and other toxins such as nicotine.

10) **Gout**–start with 1 gm and then increase dose to 1gm tid can reduce urine acid levels. Vitamin C promotes urinary excretion of uric acid. It is best to start off at lower doses as to not mobilize uric acid too quickly and precipitate kidney damage or gout attack.

11) **Infertility**–especially if there is a lot of agglutination of sperm

12) **Schizophrenia**–and other mental disorders. Abram Hoffer has done extensive work in this area (Refer to A Physician's Handbook on Orthomolecular Medicine, Roger Williams & Dwight Kalita).

**13) Cataracts**–Vitamin C has been shown to lower sorbitol levels in RBCs within 30 days. In addition vitamin C is a powerful antioxidant which can directly protect the lens of the eye against oxidative damage.

**14) Premature rupture of placenta**–1-3 gms when taken before and after has been shown to decrease soreness and lessen the time of recovery compared to placebo.

**15) Antiinflammatory**–Use both topically, as Derm C (from Interplexus a topical form of vitamin C which can actually get transported directly across the skin into the tissues directly) and orally 1-4 grams per day. Vitamin C has mild antiinflammatory and membrane stabilizing properties which can decrease swelling and enhance the body's natural healing process involved with making collagen and connective tissue for repair.

## VIII. Toxicity

- Vitamin C in large doses, 6-10gms or greater, usually results in diarrhea.
- Vitamin C has been shown to increase uric acid excretion and has been implicated in possibly precipitating gout. This increased excretion of uric acid however may actually be beneficial. For example, Probenecid, a drug used to treat gout, actually increases excretion of uric acid. It is best to increase the dose slowly after starting with lower doses such as 500mg. There are individuals who have a defect in oxalate metabolism and may be susceptible to stones.
- Another claim that is often made about vitamin C's toxicity is that it can raise oxalic acid levels in the urine and possibly cause kidney stones. It should be noted, however, that when you put vitamin C in water or urine and let it sit, it will normally turn to oxalic acid. You can prevent this reaction by acidifying the urine during collection. Labs normally don't take the precaution of acidifying the urine so any present vitamin C will turn into oxalic acid and falsely elevate the value. To date the connection between large doses of vitamin C and oxalic acid kidney stones is only conjecture. It has never been proven in any controlled studies. There is an exception, 1 of every 400 people have a genetic defect in which large doses of vitamin C (4-10gms orally) will cause their oxalic acid to rise dramatically. This may or may not be a problem, however, as vitamin C tends to bind onto calcium, which causes it to be excreted in urine. This renders it unavailable for making calcium oxalate stones. A study done by Jonathan Wright has shown that one form of vitamin C, "Ester C," does not cause this rise in oxalate. Considering the number of people taking large doses of vitamin C and the lack of reports of kidney stones, it seems unlikely that there is much validity to this accusation.
- Increased absorption of iron results with vitamin C increases and could result in iron overload.
- Lastly, it is often reported in textbooks that rebound scurvy can occur in infants if the mother takes "megadoses" of vitamin C during gestation. This is largely based on one poorly controlled study done in 1965 on 2 babies. The study involved two women who had each taken 400mg of supplemental vitamin C during pregnancy. The vitamin C was discontinued after the births. Their babies were on formula and it was "presumed" that the formula had adequate levels of vitamin C. However, there was absolutely no analysis of the vitamin C content in the formula. Neither was any attention given to the storage, preparation or administration of the

similar cases documented, I believe the risk is extremely low–if existent at all. Below is the study that this rebound scurvy is based upon.

STUDY–Cochrane, W.A. *Overnutrition in prenatal and neonatal life: a problem?* Can Med Assoc J 93:893, 1965.

- Large doses may interfere with lab tests such as occult blood in stools and uncommonly urine glucose tests.

**Note**–Much has been talked about the allergenicity of vitamin C because it can come from corn. Many times the actual amount of corn that is in the product is extremely small and chances are very unlikely that even someone with a corn allergy will have a reaction. There are forms of vitamin C that have significant amounts of corn in them as fillers or incipients and they usually will specify on the label. The use of Sago palm as a source of vitamin C because it does not have any corn in it is mostly hype. Usually there is no guarantee that you are getting 100% sago palm as your source of vitamin C.

## Notes

---

# NUTRITIONAL TREATMENTS FOR SPECIFIC CONDITIONS

In this section conditions are discussed with regards to the nutritional etiology, diagnosis, signs & symptoms and treatment. Each condition has a brief overview in which the incidence, epidemiology and unique aspects are discussed. This is followed by etiology, signs & symptoms, diagnosis, and therapeutics. Each of this sections focuses in on the nutritional aspects unique to the condition. When lab tests are discussed there is usually a mention of specific nutritional tests that may be employed to add in the understanding of nutritional treatments of the condition. Often times in convention medicine nutritional diagnosis is mostly left out or mentioned as ineffective afterthought. Here in this text it is not relegated to such an inferior role of the treatment but rather it is elevated as the most important aspect. Conventional treatments are discussed briefly, but the focus of the treatment plan is almost entirely nutritional. The nutritional treatment involves the use of foods, dietary changes, vitamins, minerals, amino acids, glandulars, accessary nutritional factors, and botanicals. Botanicals are included because they are so closely related to foods and indeed they are often foods which can be used to treat a particular condition. Botanical medicine is such a large field in itself, and I regret that only a very superficial discussion of their use is talked about in the therapeutics section. Mostly the more popular botanicals are included as treatments.

Under the section on therapeutics, treatment usually lists dietary treatments first, followed by food related substances, vitamins, minerals and then other materials. The treatment plan is usually numbered in order of importance, with the lesser items appearing at the end of the treatment plan. The treatment plan is designed to give the health care practitioner an over view of all the treatments possible and is usually not meant to be employed all at once. In other words each individual case must be evaluated and the treatments should be specific to the individual person. Some people may require more and others less depending upon motivation to do other things or else the severity of the condition. At times the treatment for a particular condition may be better discussed in another source and usually that source will be listed where appropriate. Although homeopathics are not usually listed as part of the treatment plan, they are often quite helpful to use in conjunction with nutritional treatments and often enhance the action of the nutritional therapies. Of course the nutritional therapies may also enhance the effectiveness of the homeopathics as well. Other miscellaneous therapies are also included such as light therapy, acupuncture, chiropractic techniques, exercise and hydrotherapy as well. For a list of all the conditions, please refer to the table of contents which has a complete listing of all the diseases here in the condition section.

# CARDIOVASCULAR DISEASE–ATHEROSCLEROSIS

- Cardiovascular diseases–including atherosclerosis, myocardial infarction, and degenerative and arteriosclerotic heart diseases–are the number one killers in the United States. 20% of all deaths are caused by myocardial infarction. Degenerative and arteriosclerotic heart diseases account for another 33% of the national death rate.
- While dietary and lifestyle changes appear to be the only effective cures for atherosclerosis–a degenerative arterial condition in which intimal thickening occurs due to the localized accumulation of lipids–more than 56 billion dollars per year are spent on health care for atherosclerosis alone.
- Rampant in the United States and throughout the industrialized nations, it is commonly accepted that the Western diet and lifestyle brings about the risk factors that lead to cardiovascular disease.
- A 1984 study by the Kellogg Foundation revealed that 98% of 7-12 year olds showed at least one major risk factor for heart disease. 54% had 3 or more risk factors! Abnormally high cholesterol levels were recorded in 42% of the children.

## I. Etiology

The causes of cardiovascular disease are:

**1) Injury to the endothelial cells via physical, mechanical, hemodynamic, viral, chemical, and drug factors(see diagrams on pgs 45 & 46).**

a) Disruption of the endothelial cells result in an increased permeability to plasma constituents, especially lipoproteins (LDL cholesterol and epoxycholesterol). Oxidized LDL attracts monocytes and macrophages which attempt to engulf the detritus. The engorged macrophages may result in fatty streaks along with foam cells. As this process continues, the macrophages themselves may be poisoned and may release the oxidized LDL which can further damage the inner aspect of the endothelial cells.

b) The damaged endothelial cells decrease PGI2 (prostacyclin) which normally inhibits platelet aggregation. Activation of platelets causes the release of TXA2 (thromboxane A2) which stimulates further aggregation and PDGF (platelet-derived growth factor). This causes smooth muscle cells to migrate from the media into the intima of the vessel wall where they tend to proliferate. Monocytes then enter the area and can contribute to the local synthesis of cholesterol. Much of the accumulated cholesterol comes in the form of LDL.

c) At some point the endothelial cells become damaged to the extent that gaps develop between them. This stimulates adherence of blood platelets to the scarred surface. LDL cholesterol carries more fats and cholesterol into the area and scar tissue is laid down in the intima. This traps extracellular lipid and cells further from the lumen. Collagen and elastin are secreted by the smooth muscle cells which have proliferated. Part of the trapped lipid is oxidized cholesterol. Trapped cells eventually die and necrotic cellular debris accumulates within the plaques. A fibrous cap, composed of collagen, elastin, necrotic debris, oxidized cholesterol products and glycosaminoglycans forms.

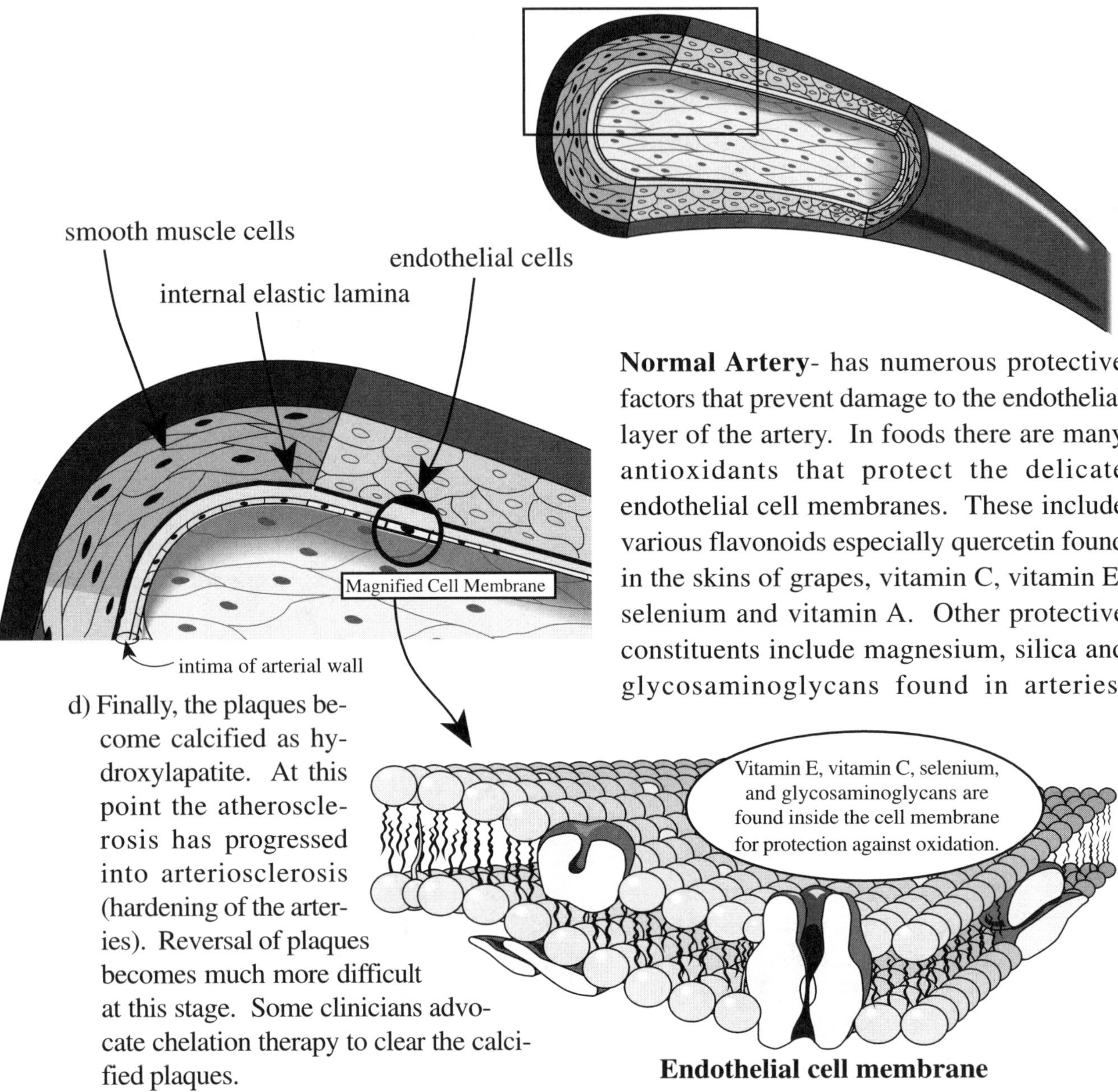


**Normal Artery**- has numerous protective factors that prevent damage to the endothelial layer of the artery. In foods there are many antioxidants that protect the delicate endothelial cell membranes. These include various flavonoids especially quercetin found in the skins of grapes, vitamin C, vitamin E, selenium and vitamin A. Other protective constituents include magnesium, silica and glycosaminoglycans found in arteries.

d) Finally, the plaques become calcified as hydroxylapatite. At this point the atherosclerosis has progressed into arteriosclerosis (hardening of the arteries). Reversal of plaques becomes much more difficult at this stage. Some clinicians advocate chelation therapy to clear the calcified plaques.

**Endothelial cell membrane**

2) **The monoclonal hypothesis**–This states that mutation causes benign monoclonal neoplastic growth which subsequently creates intimal plaque. The mutagens may be exogenous (chemicals), endogenous (cholesterol oxidation products), or viruses.

3) **Excess fats, especially from animal sources**

4) **Excess simple carbohydrates, especially sucrose (Yutkin)**

*Other causes of endothelial toxicity:*

5) **Xanthine oxidase**–Kurt Oster from Bridgeport, CT has shown that homogenized milk contains the enzyme xanthine oxidase. This enzyme has been found in the atherosclerotic plaques of humans. Shown to be very damaging to the epithelial cells, it is thought that the homogenization process protects the enzyme from being destroyed by stomach acid. Skim milk and cheeses do not contain significant amounts of this enzyme

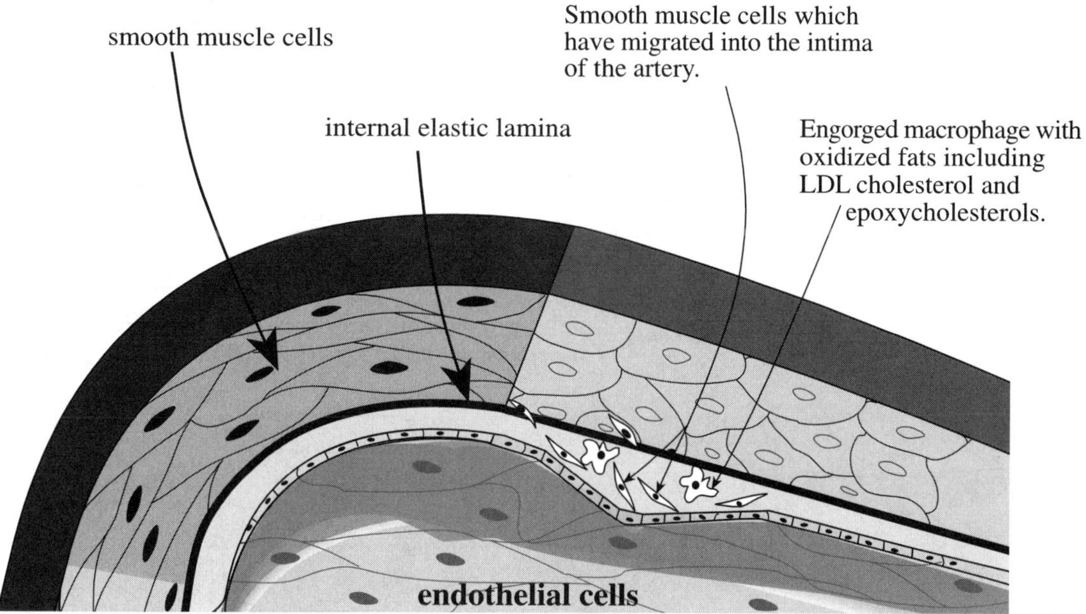


6) **Homocysteine**–Formed from methionine, homocysteine is toxic to arterial walls. Western diets tend to be high in methionine due to the generally high intake of protein and more specifically animal protein which generally has high levels of methionine. 2% of healthy individuals are heterozygous for homocystinuria, a mild deficiency of cystathionine synthase which causes increased levels of homocysteine. There is an increased incidence of homocystinuria in women after menopause. In males with advanced atherosclerosis 25-30% have been found to have higher than normal levels of homocysteine (see amino acids, methionine metabolism, p. 89).

7) **Environmental toxins (especially lead)**–In humans, increased amounts of environmental toxins lead to the increased incidence of hypertension, strokes and myocardial infarctions. In animals, even low levels have been shown to produce these effects. Also, any substances that may induce free radical formation in the body–environmental toxins including cigarette smoke, car exhaust, factory pollution, water pollution, iron, cadmium, etc.–may damage blood vessels by initiating free radical formation. Certain substances may act as a direct toxin to the endothelial cells such as alcohol, chlorine and xanthine oxidase.

8) **Oxidized cholesterol**–This may occur both inside and outside the body as epoxycholesterols and oxidized fats found in various foods. Sources of these exogenous oxidized fats are found in smoked meats, barbecued foods, deep fat and regular fried foods, improperly stored oils or foods containing oils.

Note–Vietnam era soldiers (even very young ones) were found to have a high incidence of atherosclerosis. This may have been due to the very high levels of chlorine in their drinking water. In epidemiological studies, it has been found that in areas of the world where there is little or no chlorine in the drinking water, the incidence of atherosclerosis is usually low. Conversely, in areas of the world where the water is routinely chlorinated, the rates of heart disease are always relatively high.

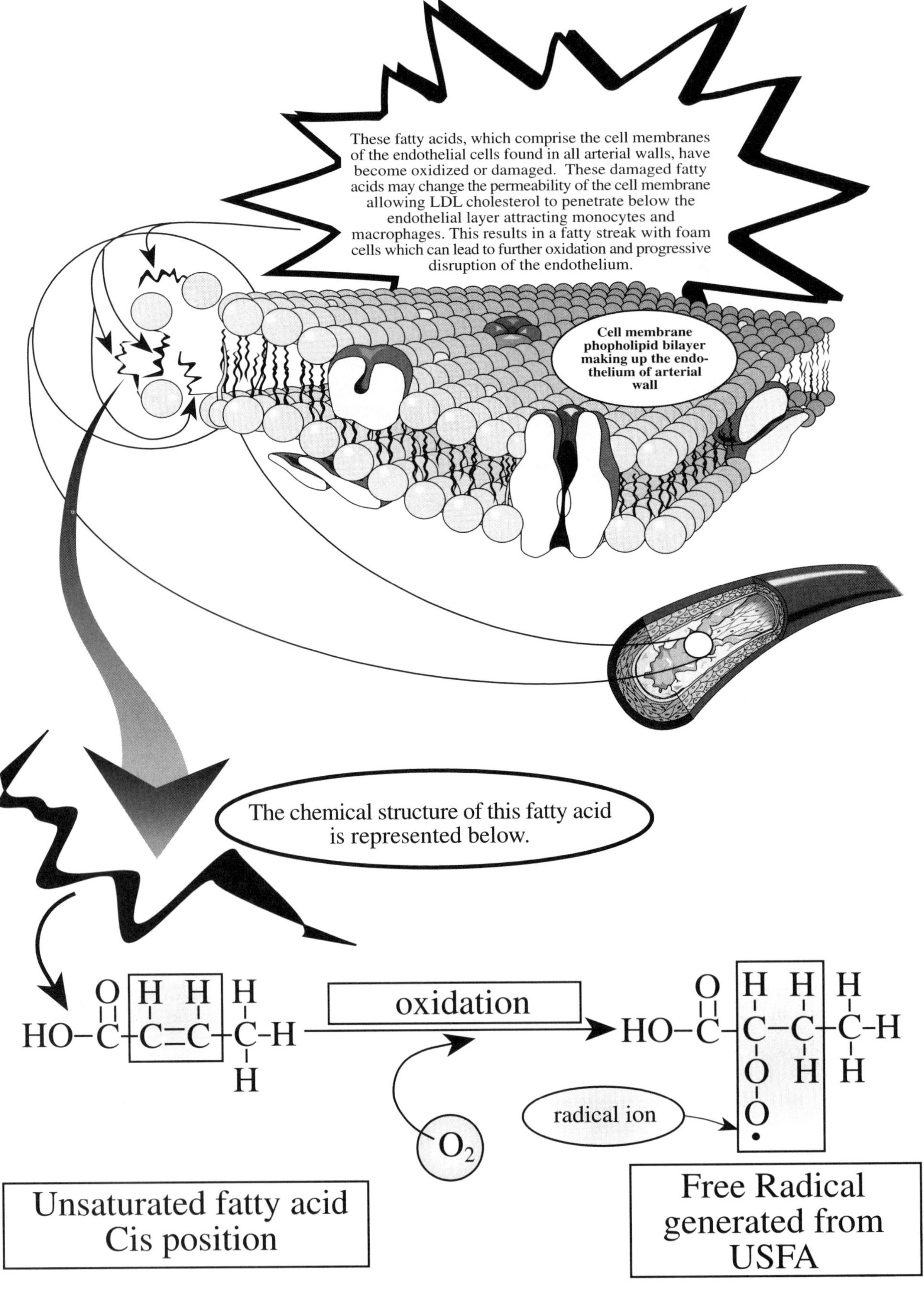
These fatty acids, which comprise the cell membranes of the endothelial cells found in all arterial walls, have become oxidized or damaged. These damaged fatty acids may change the permeability of the cell membrane allowing LDL cholesterol to penetrate below the endothelial layer attracting monocytes and macrophages. This results in a fatty streak with foam cells which can lead to further oxidation and progressive disruption of the endothelium.
Cell membrane phopholipid bilayer making up the endothelium of arterial wall
The chemical structure of this fatty acid is represented below.
oxidation
$O_2$
radical ion
Unsaturated fatty acid Cis position
Free Radical generated from USFA

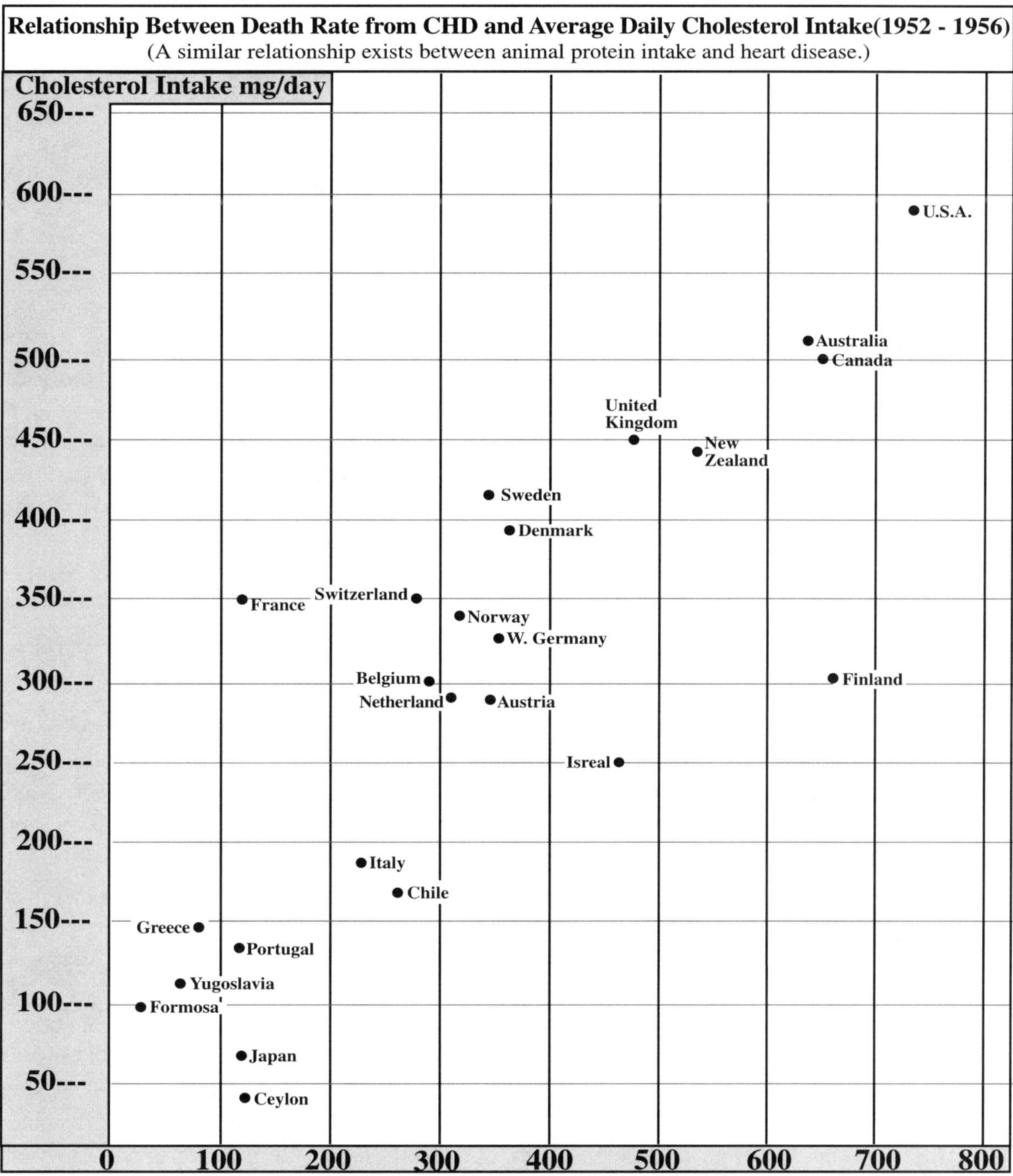

From Conner WE (1980): *In Garry PJ*, ed: Human nutrition, clinical and biochemical aspects. Washington, DC: American Association for Clinical Chemistry, p44.

**9) Hemochromatosis**-The abnormal gene that causes hemochromatosis has a heterozygous frequency of one in ten. Elevated iron is associated with an increased risk of CAD.

**10)** Some individuals who have died of myocardial infarction have been found to have clean vessels. This indicates that there are factors other than simple occlusion that are involved with cardiovascular disease. Magnesium deficiency may be related to MIs without plaques.

## II. Signs and Symptoms

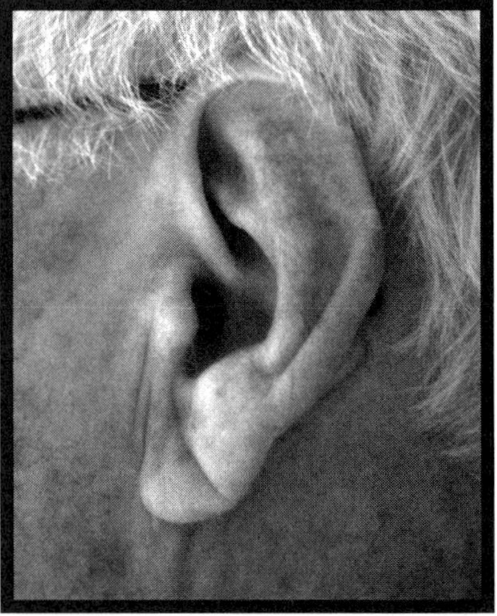

Generally, atherosclerosis is an insidious disease. Atheromatous plaques may develop over many years without signs and symptoms.

The following are nutritional signs that I look for:

**1)** "Silver wire" changes in the retinal arteries (advanced)

**2)** Atrophic changes in the skin and loss of hair on the legs and dorsum of the feet and toes. Also, look for violaceous mottling of the skin of the lower legs.

**3) Diagonal ear lobe creases, especially in males**. In one study of 205 random patients the ear lobe crease showed an 82% accuracy with a false positive rate of

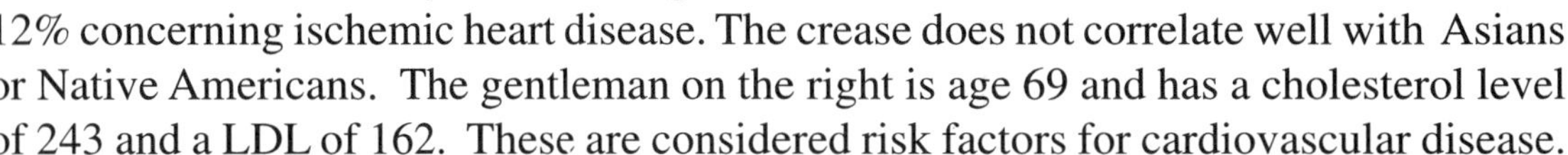

12% concerning ischemic heart disease. The crease does not correlate well with Asians or Native Americans. The gentleman on the right is age 69 and has a cholesterol level of 243 and a LDL of 162. These are considered risk factors for cardiovascular disease.

**4)** Ringing in ears (sign of decreased blood flow).

**5)** Dry skin and ear canals indicating an EFA deficiency. Excessive dark earwax also indicates EFA deficiency.

**6)** Poor circulation, especially in the extremities

**7)** Waist hip ratio (WHR)–a negative correlation (highly significant) exists for heart disease and apolipoprotein A: In addition, there is a significant **"positive"** correlation with glucose intolerance if the waist-to-hip ratio is greater than 1.2, which indicates upper-body heaviness. In females this means small hips and a larger abdomen; for males, a small waist and a protuberant stomach/abdomen area. There is a seven times increased risk of developing diabetes in mid to late life when the WHR is greater than 1.2.

## III. Diagnosis

**1) Signs and symptoms** (above)

**2) Chem screen**–lipid score including cholesterol, HDL, LDL, apolipoproteins A & B, lipoprotein A (LpA, not the same as apolipoprotein A), and triglycerides (Metpath does a lipid score, age related risk %). Higher LpA levels have been correlated to increased risk of CHD where as apolipoprotein A is protective. Make sure ferritin is included to determine iron storage problems (heterozygous frequency in the U.S. is 10% of the population!). If there is a very strong family history, consider homocysteine levels (see "Cardiovascular Assessment for patient" appendix).

STUDY–Framingham Heart Study reported any cholesterol values above 150 increased the risk of cardiovascular disease.
Cholesterol levels of over 300mg/dl–90% will develop coronary heart disease (CHD) in the next 25yrs.
Cholesterol levels of 225mg/dl–40% will develop CHD.
Cholesterol levels of between 150-200mg/dl–20% will develop CHD.

**HDL cholesterol differentiation:**

**Cholesterol levels under 200 but with HDL levels of under 40mg/dl had the same relative risk as people with cholesterol levels of 260mg/dl, (almost 50% will develop CVD in 5 years).**
**Cholesterol levels of 260mg/dl and HDL levels of between 50-59mg/dl still run a significantly increased risk of CVD.**

**NOTE**–Cholesterol is not affected by whether subject is fasting or not, but the time of collecting blood issignificant.

STUDY–Castilli, W.P. *The folly of questioning the benefits of cholesterol reduction.* Am Fam Phys 41:3, 567-74, 1994. Dr. Castelli, director of the Framingham study, one of the largest and most comprehensive studies on cholesterol levels and cardiovascular disease, "Patients with ratios over 4.5 are at high risk of coronary heart disease and require aggressive therapy. A well-monitored low-fat diet and an exercise program are recommended for patients with ratios between 3.5-4.5."

3) **Stress EKG**–A treadmill stress test is much more sensitive compared to a stationary EKG. Thallium stress test or angiography studies are probably the most sensitive but they are considerably more invasive than a conventional treadmill stress test.

4) **Ionic magnesium or sublingual smear** –Drs. Burton and Bella Altura at the Down-State University of New York at Brooklyn [(718) 270-2194] have found ionic magnesium to be the most accurate way to measure intracellular levels of magnesium. Another technique developed by Dr. Burton Silver uses X-ray analysis of a sublingual cell smear [Intracellular Diagnostics Inc. (800)874-4804]. It appears for measuring intracellular magnesium that both these methods are considerably more accurate than measuring WBC or RBC magnesium levels.

5) **Homocysteine levels** (1.5-2% of the general population in the U.S. is heterozygous for homocysteinuria/homocysteinemia; see evaluation of cardiovascular disease risk append.) This certainly should be measured if there is a strong history of early age heart disease in the family.

STUDY–Glueck, C.J. *Evidence that homocysteine is an independent risk factor for atherosclerosis in hyperlipidemic pts.* Am J Cardiol 75:132-36, 1995. ABSTRACT–482 hyperlipidemic patients were studied and 3.7% had high homocysteine levels. Of these 18 patients, 72% had atherosclerotic vascular diseases compared to 44% of those with normal homocysteine levels (p=0.02). Homocysteine was found to be an independent risk factor for atherosclerosis.

STUDY–Perry, I.J., et al. *Prospective study of serum total homocysteine concentration and risk of stroke in middle aged British men.* Lancet 346:1395-1398, 1995. ABSTRACT–In a case-controlled study of 5,661 randomly selected British men aged 40-59 yrs, serum total homocysteine concentrations were significantly higher in men who subsequently developed a stroke compared to those who did not. As higher homocysteine levels were found, the risk of stroke went up proportionally. The study concluded that homocysteine was a strong independent risk factor.

6) **Lipid hydroperoxides and endoperoxides, circulating sulfhydryls, including glutathione.** [DiagnosTechs Labs,(800)878-3787; Antibody Assay Labs (800)522-2611, Metametrix (800)221-4640].

7) **Hair analysis**–for heavy metal toxicity, especially lead and cadmium

8) **Platelet aggregation** (Meridian Labs)-This test is different than clotting time and is a technique for evaluating how sticky the platelets are. Hospitals may be able to run this test as well.

## IV. Therapeutic Considerations

**Miscellaneous**–In the Am. J. Epidem, it was noted that from 1976-80 there was a marked drop in MIs and strokes. 1976 was the year that unleaded gas becamen readily available.

STUDY–Speich, M. *Low lead doses and atherogenic diet in rabbits: biochemical results in blood.* Atherosclerosis 27:521, 1983. ABSTRACT–It was found that the introduction of small amounts of lead in the diets of rabbits could produce significant atheromatous lesions in the arteries.

One study with animals showed that a high fat diet may cause nutrient deficiencies, especially of magnesium. Normally high fat diets induced atheromas. However, if magnesium was increased by 4x normal intake, then no atheromas developed.

**NOTE**–JAMA, 1984 (Biggest study)–The National Institute of Health issued a consensus opinion on the effectiveness of cholesterol-lowering drugs such as Gemfibrizol(Lopid®) & Levostatin(Mevacor®), "They decrease the incidence of death by MI by 19%, and for every 1% decrease in cholesterol, cardiac mortality goes down 2%." The other side of the story is that there were 3x as many deaths due to homicide, suicide and accidents in the people that took these drugs. The net result is that there is no change at all in overall mortality. This so-called "artifact" occurred in another large study as well. Both times it was dismissed as coincidence even though the P value for this happening by chance came out to .0001. It should be noted that both Lopid®, Clofibrate, and Mevacor® have been shown to be carcinogenic in animals. Mevacor® is a HMG reductase inhibitor and has also been found to decrease coenzyme Q 10 in the blood. Cholestyramine works differently to lower cholesterol and may actually have side benefits by binding endotoxins.

**NOTE**–One Italian pathologist has studied asymptomatic people whose coronary blood vessels were almost entirely occluded. He found, on autopsy, that these people had extensive micro-collateral circulation that had not been picked up by angiographic studies (the vessels were found to be less than 2 microns in diameter). Why were these people asymptomatic?

**NOTE**–Masei warriors have been shown to have a very high fat diet and significant atherosclerosis. However, they also been shown to have extensive collateral circulation and, as a result, very few cardiovascular problems. This may be due to in part to their very active lifestyle.

## V. Treatment

### 1) Consumption of water-soluble fibers such as pectin, guar gum, oat bran, rice bran etc.

STUDY–Bell, L.P., Hectorne, K., Reynolds, H., Balm, Hunninghake. *Cholesterol-lowering effects of psyllium hydrophilic mucilloid: adjunct therapy to a prudent diet for patients with mild to moderate hypercholesterolemia.* JAMA 261; 3419-23, 1989. ABSTRACT–75 hypercholesterolemic patients followed a diet and received either 3.4gms of psyllium (equivalent to one teaspoon of Metamucil) 3x a day or a placebo for 8 weeks. Compared to placebo, psyllium achieved an additional 4.8% reduction in total cholesterol, an 8.5 reduction in LDL-cholesterol, and an 8.8% reduction in apolipoprotein B level (all significant differences).

**NOTE**–There have been reports of patients who significantly lowered their cholesterol levels by switching from olive oil or safflower oil to **rice bran oil**.

STUDY–Cerda, J.C. et al. *The effect of grapefruit pectin on patients at risk for coronary heart diseases without altering diet or lifestyle.* Clin Cardiol 11(9):589-94, 1988. ABSTRACT-27 patients aged 32-65 with a mean cholesterol level of 275 mg/dl took a 5 gm cap of grapefruit pectin or placebo 3x per day. After 8 weeks, while patients on placebo failed to demonstrate changes in lab values, serum cholesterol levels in experimental pts. had dropped a mean of 7.6%, LDL cholesterol by 10.8%, and the LDL/HDL ratio by 9.8%. About 42% of patients demonstrated improvements greater than 10% and up to a 20%↑ in these parameters.

STUDY–Leven, E.G. et al. *Comparison of psyllium hydrophilic-mucilloid and cellulose as adjuncts to a prudent diet in the treatment of mild to moderate hypercholesterolemia.* Arch Intern Med 150:1822-7, 1990. ABSTRACT–96 patients with hypercholesterolemia were fed either 5.1 gms psyllium powder daily or placebo in conjunction with a "prudent diet." After 16 weeks psyllium supplementation was associated with a 5.6% reduction in total cholesterol and a 8.6% reduction in LDL cholesterol. HDL cholesterol levels, which initially decreased, had returned to their original levels and triglyceride levels were unchanged.

### 2) Consumption of soy and other vegetable protein

STUDY–Check, W. *Switch to soy protein for boring but healthful diet.* JAMA 247:3045-6, 1982. ABSTRACT–Subjects with elevated lipid levels showed reduction in cholesterol and triglycerides when 500ml of 2% fat soy drink product was substituted for 2% fat cow's milk.

STUDY–Terpstra, A. *A longitudinal cross-over study of serum cholesterol and lipoproteins in rabbits fed on semi-purified diets containing either casein or soya bean protein.* Br. J. Nutr. 47(2):213-21,1982. ABSTRACT–Rabbits in one group were placed on a diet containing 400mg of casein protein for 20 days. Their cholesterol was measured at 3068mg/L. Another group of rabbits was fed a diet containing 400mg of soy protein. Their cholesterol was measured at 800mg/L. The 2 groups were crossed over and by day 10 the cholesterol levels of the 2 groups had also crossed over.

### 3) Increase complex carbohydrates and decrease fats down to 12% of total calories

The level of the cholesterol in the blood should determine the appropriate percentage of fat in the diet.

> **NOTE**–There have been several studies done on people with chronic heart disease where they were placed on a 30% fat diet. The result was a progression of the disease. This indicates that the recommendations by the American Heart Association may not be strict enough. It seems likely that there are other factors, such as the type of fat eaten, but 30% is undoubtedly too high for many people and the AHA should probably reevaluate their recommendations.

STUDY–Edigton, J. et al. *Serum lipid response to dietary cholesterol in subjects fed a low fat, high fiber diet.* AJCN 50:58-62, 1989. ABSTRACT–Reducing fat calories to 30% of total and **varying cholesterol intake between 90 and 4300mg/day** in 58 patients led to small and **statistically insignificant** changes in serum cholesterol levels.

STUDY–Rosenthal, M. *Effects of a high complex carbohydrate, low fat, low cholesterol diet on serum lipids and estradiol.* Am. J. Med. ABSTRACT–21 patients followed a high complex carbohydrate, low fat (12%), low cholesterol diet for 26 days and both their mean serum estradiol and triglycerides fell by 50%. Serum cholesterol fell by 21%.

STUDY–Kush, L. *Diet and 20 year mortality from CHD. The Ireland-Boston Diet-Heart study.* NEJM. 312(13):811-18,1985. ABSTRACT–3 groups of men were studied starting in 1959: 1) men born and living in Ireland, 2) men born in Ireland who migrated to Boston, and 3) men born in Boston to Irish immigrants. Subsequent mortality in 1982 was studied and it was found that those who died of coronary heart disease ate significantly less total carbohydrate, fiber, starch, and vegetable protein. Overall it was determined that the nutritional change that was most closely linked to the increased mortality rate from coronary heart disease was a decrease in complex carbohydrate rather than the changes in the consumption of dietary lipids.

STUDY–Ornish, D., et al. *Can lifestyle changes reverse CHD?* Lancet 336:129-33. 1990. ABSTRACT–28 people with documented coronary artery disease were put on an extremely low fat diet (6.8% calories from fat) plus stress management training, exercise, and no smoking for a year. A paired control group of 20 people was also watched during the same period. In the experimental group, there was a 22 lb average weight loss, a 40% drop in LDL levels, a reduction in symptoms of angina and a **statistically significant reperfusion of coronary vessels measured by angiography**. The control group became more atherosclerotic during the same period. Patients with the most severe stenosis went from 61.1% to 55.8%, while the equivalent subset of the control group saw an increase of their stenosis from 61.7% to 64.4%

> **NOTE**–There is evidence that a very low fat diet not only decreases total cholesterol but also decreases HDL cholesterol. A higher fat diet with specific beneficial fats may be indicated in certain circumstances.

STUDY–Sacks, F.M., et al. *More on chewing the fat: the good fat and the good cholesterol.* Editorial N Engl J Med 325(24):1740-2, 1991. ABSTRACT– The traditional "Mediterranean diet" is made up of 30-40% of calories from fat but mostly monounsaturated fat from olive oil. These MUSFA do not lower HDL levels and people that follow such diets have been found to have the lowest rates of CHD relatively speaking(see chart on CHD p.247).

STUDY–De Lorgeril, M., et al. *Mediterranean alpha linolenic acid rich diet in secondary prevention of CHD.* Lancet 343:1454-59, 1994. ABSTRACT–About 600 patients who had suffered an MI were randomly divided into 2 groups, a control and an experimental group. The experimental group was given a diet of more bread, root and green vegetables, fruit, and fish with less meat. Butter and cream were replaced by margarine that was high in oleic acid (48%) and alpha linolenic acid (4.8%). Serum lipids, blood pressure and body mass index remained the same in the 2 groups. After a mean period of 27 months, there were 73% fewer fatal and nonfatal MIs and a 70% reduction in overall mortality in the experimental group compared to the control.

4) **Avoid sucrose and other simple sugars**–It has been shown that sucrose can induce hyperinsulinism, abnormalities in platelet electrophoretic motility, a decrease in HDLs, and an increase in serum triglycerides, as well as an increase in excretion of chromium (see Yudkin).

5) **Avoid hydrogenated oils and trans-fatty acids**–From 1900-1930 the rate of multiplied. Significantly, margarine was introduced as a butter replacement in 1925(see Kummerow).

STUDY–Jackson, R. *Influence of dietary trans-fatty acids on swine lipoprotein composition and structure.* J. Lipid Res.18:182,1977. ABSTRACT–Swine fed a hydrogenated fat which contained 50% trans fatty acids had serum cholesterol levels 14mg/dl higher than those fed animal fat containing 25% or more saturated fatty acids.

STUDY–Hill, E. *Intensification of EFA deficiency in the rat by dietary trans-fatty acids.* J. Nutr. 109:1759-67, 1979. ABSTRACT–It was found that hydrogenating vegetable oils elevates serum cholesterol levels while oils in the natural cis state lowers them.

STUDY–Mensink, R.P., & Katan, M.B. *Effect of dietary trans-fatty acids on HDL & LDL cholesterol levels in healthy subjects.* NEJM 323:439-45, 1990. ABSTRACT–54 young adults were placed on identical 3 week diets except that 10% of the calories were either monounsaturated, a common trans fatty acid, or a saturated fatty acid The trans fatty acids did more damage to the serum LDL/HDL ratio than did the saturated fat. Not only did LDL increase 14 mg, but HDL dropped 7 mg.

6) **Avoid oxidized fats**–Fast foods, deep fried fat, ghee (clarified butter), beef jerky, egg beaters, sprayed eggs, etc. are full of oxidized fats.

STUDY–Jacobson, M. *Cholesterol oxides in Indian Ghee: possible cause of unexplained high risk of atherosclerosis in Indian immigrant populations.* Lancet 2:656, 1987.

STUDY–Imai, H. *Angiotoxicity and arteriosclerosis due to contaminants of USP-grade cholesterol.* Arch. Pathol. Lab. ABSTRACT–Heating of fats containing cholesterol oxidizes it to 25-hydroxy cholesterol which has been shown to accelerate the degeneration of smooth muscle cells in arterial tissue.

7) **Eat cold water fish**–Cold water fish contain omega-3 EPA type fatty acids which have been shown to decrease platelet aggregation, increase HDL, and lower triglycerides. Certain fish may provide a higher ratio of DHA to EPA. There is some evidence that fish which have a higher ratio of DHA to EPA may have a greater effect at raising HDLs and lowering LDLs.

STUDY–Singer, P. *Influence on serum lipids, lipoproteins and blood pressure of mackerel and herring diet in patients with type 4 and 5 hyperlipoproteinemia.* Athero 56(1):111-118,1985. ABSTRACT–8 patients with type 4&5 hyperlipoproteinemia were put on mackerel and herring diets for 2 weeks each. After mackerel, triglycerides and total cholesterol were significantly lower, returning to basal levels 3 months later, while HDL was slightly increased. After herring, which has half the EPA content of mackerel, the differences were minor.

8) **Fish oil capsules containing (EPA/DHA)**–1.5-4gms/day EPA/DHA–Most capsules are 300mg EPA/DHA, although 500mg capsules can be found. May increase HDL levels but its most reliable effect is in lowering high serum triglycerides.

STUDY–Saynor, R. *Effects of omega-3 fatty acids on serum lipids.* Lancet 2:696-7,1984 ABSTRACT–16 male patients consumed 5gms of MaxEPA (1.5gms of EPA/DHA) daily for 2 months then switched to 5gms omega-6 rich vegetable oil/day. After the EPA, total cholesterol and triglycerides significantly went down while HDL significantly went up. There were only minor improvements in the vegetable oil trials.

STUDY–Childs, M., et al *Divergent lipoprotein responses to fish oils with various ratios of EPA and DHA.* AJCN 52: 632-9, 1990. ABSTRACT–A high ratio of EPA to DHA raised LDLs and oils with higher DHA levels, reduced LDLs and Apolipoprotein B ( See handout on EFA ratios p.259).

9) **Flavonoids from diet**–Flavonoids have been found to be potent antioxidants to protect arterial endothelial cells from damage against LDL and other toxins. The flavonoids: quercetin, Proanthocyanidins (procyanidolic oligomers or PCO), and catechin are primary ones.

STUDY–Hertog M. et al *Dietary antioxidant flavonoids and risk of coronary heart disease: the Zutphen elderly study.* Lancet 342: 1007-11, 1993. ABSTRACT–805 elderly men were studied and it was found that there was an inverse relationship with the level of flavonoid intake (in the form of tea, onions and apples) and the rate of CHD.

STUDY–Knecki, P., et al. *Flavonoid intake and coronary mortality in Finland: a cohort study.* Brit Med J 312: 478-81, 1992. ABSTRACT–A positive correlation was found between low flavonoid intake and increased CVD.

**10) Legumes** decrease cholesterol (especially soybeans) and have a low glycemic index. Soaking beans and sprouting them will break down some of the gas-forming sulfur-containing proteins. Tofu, a fermented soybean product, can be very useful to add to many foods and even desserts. As a legume, it tends to be well-tolerated by the digestive tract.

STUDY–Nervi, F. et al. *Influence of legume intake on biliary lipids and cholesterol saturation in young Chilian men.* Gastroenterology 96:825-30, 1989. ABSTRACT–1/4 lb or 120gms of beans for one month led to a 110%-160% increase in bile saturation in 20 young men in a controlled (but obviously not blinded) study.

**11) Yogurt**–There may be some unidentified substances in fermented milk which decrease cholesterol. Even yogurt with higher fat content has been shown to reduce cholesterol.

STUDY–Hepner, B. *Hypocholesterolemic effect of yogurt and milk.* Am. J. Clin. Nutr. 32:19-24,1979. ABSTRACT–5 men and 6 women ate 3 cups of yogurt daily. After the first week, the average cholesterol level decreased from 252 to 230. It stayed at 230 for the final 11 weeks of the study.

**12) Garlic and onions** inhibit platelet aggregation by blocking thromboxane synthesis for several hours.

STUDY–Doullin, D. *Garlic as a platelet inhibitor.* Lancet 1:776-7,1981. ABSTRACT–100-150mg/kg of fresh garlic completely inhibited platelet aggregation for up to 2.5 hours after ingestion.

**13) Alfalfa**–5 cups or more increase HDL by significant amounts. Use caution as alfalfa can act as an antagonist to B-6.

**14) Decrease coffee intake**–Some studies show that more than 11/2 cups/day increases cholesterol. One study has shown that greater than 5 cups/day increases the risk of heart disease by 50%. Studies have shown that the method of brewing is important. Paper filtering is much better than boiling, percolating or other types of filtering which seem to increase the risk of coronary heart disease.

STUDY–Grobbee, D.E., et al. *Coffee, caffeine, and cardiovascular disease in men.* NEJM 323:1026-32, 1990. ABSTRACT–45,000 American men 40-75years old were studied for 2 years to see if there was a correlation between coffee intake and MI, strokes, etc. Greater than 4c/day of caffeinated coffee intake was not paired with cardiovascular disease. High intake of decaffeinated coffee, however, was associated with a relative risk of 1.63. Allowing for diet and smoking did not effect these findings.

STUDY–La Vecchia, C., Gentile, A., Negri, E., Parazzini, F., Francheschi, S. *Coffee consumption and MI in women.* AM J. Epidemiol 130:481-85, 1989. ABSTRACT–In a case control study of women, there was a positive association between heavy coffee drinking and risk of MI. Relative risk was 2.7x when 4 or more cups were consumed. After allowing for smoking and other relevant variables, relative risk was not elevated for consumption of 1-3c/day, but was 1.7x for 4 or more c/day (p=0.022).

**15) Small amounts of alcohol**–There is conflicting evidence. However, alcohol is a known angiotoxin. Studies that show small amounts of alcohol to be protective against atherosclerosis are misleading. Groups of people who were asked whether they drank or not were divided up. In the group that *did not drink at all*, part of the group consisted of people who drank large amounts of alcohol for years, but then stayed strictly off it. As a result, the non-alcohol group may have had a greater incidence of atherosclerosis due to this inclusion of ex-heavy drinkers (see next page for note on "The French Paradox").

STUDY–Eichner, E. *Alcohol versus exercise for coronary protection.* Am. J. Med. 79(2): 231-40, 1985 ABSTRACT–Moderate alcohol ingestion raises HDL3 levels but not HDL2. HDL3 levels have no beneficial effects. In addition, alcohol has a detrimental effect on blood pressure, body weight, and glucose tolerance.

**NOTE**–The so-called "French Paradox" in which the French people eat a high fat diet, exercise very little and tend to smoke a lot, yet have a relatively low incidence of CVD was once thought to be due to alcohol consumption because they drink 10x more wine per capita than U.S. counterparts It is probably due more to the increased flavonoid intake coming from the wine, fruits and vegetables they consume (red wine is fairly high in quercetin, see flavonoids #9). In addition, they tend to eat less calories in general.

**16) Niacin**–1-3gms–Use caution as some time-release niacin has precipitated fulminant hepatitis. It is better to use niacin hexicinate because it doesn't flush and is much less toxic. However, its effect is not as strong as straight niacin.

STUDY–Carlson, L. & Oro, L. *Effect of treatment of niacin for one month on serum lipids in patients with different types of hyperlipidemia.* Atherosclerosis 18:1-9,1973. ABSTRACT–188 patients with various types of hyperlipoproteinemia were given 3 gms niacin/day. Most responsive were patients with type 5 whose cholesterols decreased 70% and triglycerides decreased 90%, followed by type 3 whose cholesterol dropped 50% & 70% respectively. Both lipids were reduced in the other types, and even patients with normal lipid levels showed a 10-20% reduction in serum lipids.

STUDY–Luria, M. *Effect of low dose niacin on HDL and total cholesterol/HDL ratio.* Arch Intern Med 148:2493-5, 1989. ABSTRACT–55 cardiovascular patients were given only one gm of "long-acting" niacin/day for an avg of 6.7 months in a controlled but not blinded trial. Total cholesterol to HDL ratio was reduced by 27% due to HDL increase (with no change in the control group). 40% dropped out due to the side effects and one became diabetic.

*STUDY–Urberg, M. et al. *Hypocholesterolemic effects of nicotinic acid and chromium suppl.* J Fam Practice 27(6):603-6, 1988. ABSTRACT–2 women whose cholesterols were 399 and 337mg/dl to start had a **drop in cholesterol by 25-30% with very low doses (100mg/d) of niacin when combined with 200mcg of chromium.** This drop took 4 weeks initially and improved even further at 4 months. One of the women stopped the supplements for a period of 3-4 weeks and her cholesterol rose by 25mg/dl. Once she resumed, her cholesterol dropped again. Patients were followed for one year.

**17) Pyridoxine**–40mg–**folate**–5-10mg & **vitamin B-12**–It appears as though folate has the most potent effect at lowering homocysteine levels. It works with vitamin B-12 to methylate homocysteine back to methionine (see amino acids and methionine). Pyridoxine, on the other hand, promotes the conversion of homocysteine to cystathionine. Homocysteine is thought to be toxic to arterial walls and is an independent risk factor in cardiovascular disease. It is estimated that the incidence of *heterozygous homocystinuria due to cystathionine synthase deficiency occurs in about 1.4% of the overall population.* **People who have cardiovascular disease at an early age (or with parents who had MIs early in life) have been found to have this defect 30% of the time!** Methionine is an amino acid that is converted to homocysteine and found in relatively high amounts in western diets (meat eaters have higher intakes). Betaine may also be of value in lowering homocysteine.

STUDY–Ubbink, J.B., et al. *Hyperhomocysteinemia and the response to vitamin supplementation.* Clin Invest 71: 993-98, 1993. ABSTRACT–22 males with moderately high homocystinuria reduced plasma homocysteine levels by 55% with supplementation of folate 1mg, B-6 10mg, and B-12 50mcg after 6 weeks. About 4 months after discontinuing therapy only 7 of the 22 had homocysteine levels below the original cutoff point. It took another 6 weeks to normalize the homocysteine levels after supplementation was started again. This study concluded that supplementation was necessary to reduce homocysteine levels and that general dietary recommendations were not sufficient.

STUDY–Brattstrom, L.E., et al. *Folic acid, an innocuous means to reduce plasma homocysteine.* Scand J Clin Lab Invest 48: 215-221, 1988. ABSTRACT–42 healthy volunteer men age 51 yrs old consumed 1mg B-12, 5mg folate, and 40mg of B-6 separately. Folate reduced homocysteine levels by 52%, while the B-12 and B-6 had no effect.

**18) Vitamin C**–3gms/day–Vitamin C can significantly reduce cholesterol in 3 weeks as well as improve platelet aggregation. It has been found that the branching regions of arteries, where the greatest stress and the greatest chance for damage exists, have decreased levels of vitamin C locally. These are the most common areas where atheromas are found.

**19) Vitamin E**–800-1800IU/day

STUDY–Anastasi, J., et al. *Effect of vitamin E:an inhibitor of the platelet release reaction.* Am J Clin Nut 29:467, 1976. ABSTRACT–Alpha-tocopherol acetate dose dependently reduced the maximal aggregation response of human platelets to collagen or ADP. At a dose of 1800IU/day, collagen-induced aggregation was reduced by 50%. No further reduction in platelet aggregation was produced by doses higher than 1800IU per day.

STUDY–Rimm, E.B., et al. *Vitamin E consumption and the risk of coronary heart disease in men.* N Engl J Med 328:1450-56, 1993. ABSTRACT– In 1986, 39,910 male health professionals who were free of coronary heart disease, diabetes mellitus, and hypercholesterolemia were studied by questionnaire. After controlling for age and other CHD risk factors, it was found that the higher the intake of vitamin E the lower the risk of CHD. For men consuming > 60IU/day of vitamin E the risk of CHD was almost half as much as those who were consuming < 7.5IU/day.

STUDY–Hodis, H.N., et al. *Serial coronary angiographic evidence that antioxidant vitamin intake reduces progression of coronary artery atherosclerosis.* JAMA 273:1849-54, 1995. ABSTRACT– It was found that vitamin E > 100IU/day significantly reduced the risk of CHD in men after 2 years. This effect was enhanced by the meds colestipol and niacin.

**20) Magnesium aspartate**–500-800mg/day–Magnesium is found concentrated in the heart 18x higher than in the blood. It promotes efficient metabolic functioning of the heart muscle by its involvement with ATP production. People with cardiomyopathy have 1/3 the levels of magnesium compared to normals. Some animal studies have shown that magnesium has a prophylactic effect against a high fat diet. Magnesium decreases platelet aggregation, prevents spasm of smooth muscle, and is a good calcium channel blocker (comparable to Verapromil). It also has been shown to increase HDL and has fibrinolytic activity (similar to the drug Streptokinase). IV magnesium at the onset of an MI or stroke is often very effective at limiting the amount of damage. It should be noted that magnesium tends to not be absorbed very well. In more advanced disease states it is necessary to give IV or IM. Magnesium in the form of aspartate appears to be the better absorbed. The practitioner must be aware that supplemental calcium interferes with absorption if used in large amounts.

STUDY–Rasmussen, H.S., et al. *Intravenous magnesium in acute myocardial infarction.* Lancet 1:234, 1986. ABSTRACT–In a double-blind placebo-controlled study, 273 patients with suspected acute MIs were randomized to receive either magnesium (Mg) intravenously or placebo, immediately on admission to the hospital. The Mg group was given 50 mmol of elemental Mg (as Mg chloride) during the first 24 hours and an additional 12 mmol during the second 24 hours. Of the 130 patients with proven MI, 56 received Mg and 74 received placebo. During the first 4 weeks after treatment, mortality was 7% in the Mg group and 19% in the placebo group. In the Mg group, 21% of the patients had arrhythmias that required treatment, compared to 47% in the placebo group. There were no side effects attributable to Mg therapy.

**21) Selenium**–200-300µg/day There has been found to higher rates of CVD in areas in the country where soil selenium levels are the lowest. As a potent antioxidant selenium may help protect the delicate endothelial cell wall.

**22) Bromelain** can be useful to decrease platelet aggregation and to break down arteriosclerotic plaques.

**23) Molybdenum**

**24) Chromium**–200-1500µg/day (can use brewers yeast)–Most studies use chromic chloride which doesn't get absorbed very well. Alan Gaby recommends chromium aspartate.

STUDY–Railes, R., Albrink. *Effect of chromium supplementation on Glucose tolerance and serum lipids including HDL.* Am. J. Clin. Nut 34:2670-8,1981. ABSTRACT–13/23 healthy young men received 200mcg/day of chromium while the rest received placebos. After 12 weeks, the chromium-supplemented men demonstrated decreased serum triglycerides and total cholesterol, along with an increase in HDL and improved glucose tolerance.

STUDY–Abraham, A. *The effect of chromium on established atherosclerotic plaques in rabbits.* Am. J. Clin. Nutr. 33:2294-98, 1980. ABSTRACT–Rabbits with established atherosclerotic plaques had significant plaque regression when supplemented with chromium.

**25) Zinc**–Studies on rats have shown that zinc supplements can lower serum cholesterol, however in humans excessive zinc supplementation can raisetotal cholesterol and lower HDL cholesterol. It is thought that excess zinc causes adverse effects on cholesterol metabolism due to a lowering of copper which is critical for cholesterol metabolism.

STUDY–Hooper, P. *Zinc lowers HDL levels.* JAMA 244:1960, 1980. ABSTRACT–12 healthy young men received 160mg elemental zinc/day. 12 matched controls received placebos. By the 7th week the zinc-supplemented men experienced a marked decrease in HDL. Cholesterol, triglycerides, and LDL remained the same.

STUDY–Goodwin, J. *Relationship between zinc intake, physical activity and blood levels of HDL in healthy elderly population.* Metabolism 34(6): 519-23,1985. ABSTRACT–Healthy elderly volunteers failed to experience an increase in HDL from exercise so long as they supplemented their diets with over 15mg zinc/day. Cessation of zinc supplementation for 8 weeks resulted in an exercise-related increase in HDL.

**26) Copper**–2mg/day–Decreased copper levels in the body can cause marked elevations in serum cholesterol. In addition, it has been found that people dying from aneurysms have 1/4 as much copper in their tissues compared to normals.

STUDY–Klevay, L. & Fischer, P. *Interactions of copper and zinc in CVD.* Ann N.Y. Acad. Sci. 355:140-151, 1980; *The effect of dietary copper and zinc on cholesterol metabolism.* Am. J. Clin. Nutr.33:1019-25, 1980. ABSTRACT–The contradictory findings of zinc supplementation and the lowering of HDL levels may be a result of copper deficiency, especially considering that **there is marginal copper intake in the U.S.**

**27) Pantethine**–600-1200mg/day–A metabolic intermediary of pantothenic acid, pantethine (also pantetheine) is precursor of Coenzyme A. It raises HDL 10-30%, decreases cholesterol 10-20%, and decreases triglycerides 30-60%.

STUDY–Maioli, M., et al. *Effect of pantethine on the subfractions of HDL in dyslipemic patients.* Curr Ther Res 35:307, 1984.

**28) L-carnitine**–3gms/day–increased exercise tolerance, and may increase HDL in patients with normal cholesterol and low HDL.

STUDY–Cherchi, A., et. al.. *Effects of L-carnitine on exercise tolerance in chronic stable angina: a multicenter, double-blind randomized, placebo-controlled crossover study.* Int J Clin Pharm Ther Toxicol 23;569-72, 1985. ABSTRACT–44 men with chronic stable exercise-induced angina received 1gm bid L-carnitine or placebo each for 4 weeks in a double-blind crossover trial. Compared to placebo, carnitine significantly increased the level of work required to induce angina symptoms. Carnitine was significantly more effective than placebo at preventing angina symptoms and ST segment depression at a given work load.

STUDY–Orlando, G., Rusconi, C. *L-carnitine in the treatment of chronic cardiac ischemia in elderly patients.* Clin Trials J 23:338-44, 1986. ABSTRACT–30 patients experiencing symptoms such as palpitations, asthenia, and precordial pain were treated with 2gms carnitine tid for 2 months. Via the NYHA functional class evaluation, 4 of these patients improved significantly. In 30% of the patients, EKG and echocardiographic evidence showed improvement. Most of the patients showed significant improvement in their symptoms.

STUDY–Pola, P., et al. *Statistical evaluation of long term L-carnitine therapy in hyperlipoproteinemias.* Drugs Exptl Clin Res 9:925-34, 1983. ABSTRACT–39 patients aged 50-60yrs of age with Fredrickson's type II, IV, or V hyperlipoproteinemia were studied. 1/3 of these patients were unresponsive to previous therapy with cholesterol lowering drugs. Patients were treated with 1gm per day and after 4 months serum cholesterol fell from 295 to 234 and HDL increased by 15%. TGs fell from 345 to 208 (40% reduction) in type IV patients and from 170 to 124 in type II patients. In 3 type V patients TG levels of 950 avg. fell rapidly to below 400. The L-carnitine eventually brought cholesterol levels down below 240 in 90% of the patients, 66% of them in 4 months.

STUDY–Davini, P., et al. *Controlled study on L-carnitine therapeutic efficacy in most MI patients.* Drugs Exptl Clin Res 18:355-65, 1992. ABSTRACT–160 patients following MIs were randomly assigned to receive either 4g/day of carnitine in addition to standard treatment or standard treatment alone. During the follow-up period the next year, the carnitine group had significant reductions in blood pressure, fewer anginal attacks and a significant reduction in cholesterol levels. The mortality rate in the carnitine group was 1.2% compared to 12.5% in the control group (p=0.005).

**29) Phosphatidyl ethanolamine**–2 T or 12-20 caps/day–It appears that phosphatidyl ethanolamine mostly increases HDL and doesn't effect cholesterol.

STUDY–Knuiman, J., et. al. *Lecithin intake and serum cholesterol.* Am J Clin Nutr 49:266-8, 1989 (review). A review of 24 studies showed that the main effect of most lecithin supplementation, in terms of lowering cholesterol, comes from linoleic acid.

**30) Treat hypothyroidism–(See hypothyroidism)**

**31) Vanadium–**.5-1mg/day–lowers cholesterol

**32) Saturated solution of potassium iodine (SSKI)**–A book about the many uses of iodine by Dr. Richard Kunin should be available in early 1999 (call Jonathon Wright via Meridian labs).

**NOTE**–More than 300mg/day of iodine inhibits thyroid.

STUDY–Abrahamson, I.A., et al. *Ophthalmoscopic warning of system diseases: treatment of retinal arteriosclerosis and hemorrhages.* EENT Digest 30:48, July, 1968. ABSTRACT–135mg/day of sodium iodide reversed atherosclerotic changes in eyes. It seems that niacin protects against the baleful effects of iodide.

**33) Remove chlorine from drinking water-**According to epidemiological studies, areas in the world where they do not chlorinate their water, the indigenous people have the lowest heart disease rate compared to their chlorinated counterparts. In fact chlorinated water correlates closely to the incidence of heart disease and almost no areas that chlorinate their water do they have a low rate of heart disease.

STUDY–Zeighami, E.A., Watson, A.P., and Craun, G.F., *Chlorination, water hardness and serum cholesterol in 46 Wisconsin communities,* Int. J. Epid. 19(1):49-58, March 1990. ABSTRACT–46 small Wisconsin communities, 24 with chlorinated water and 22 without were studied. A total of 654 male and 866 female volunteers participated. Residents between the ages of 40 and 70 who had lived in the area for at least 10 years were invited for interviews. Accounting for other factors such as smoking, lifestyle, diet, etc., it was found in the men who drank the chlorinated water their cholesterol went up 4mg/dl and the women 11mg/dl.

**34) Hard water (silicon and magnesium)**–It has been demonstrated in a number of epidemiological studies that areas with harder water have a lower incidence of CVD in the population. It is postulated that hard water has significant amounts of magnesium as well as silicon which have been found to be protective against CVD.

STUDY–Karppanen, H. *Epidemiological study on hardness of drinking water and CVD.* Artery 9:190, 1981.

**35) Ginger**–may cause a decrease in platelet aggregation and also lower cholesterol levels.

**36) Estrogen**–"Triple estrogen formula" is probably the best for avoiding deleterious effects. Estrogen may increase HDL and lower cholesterol and prevent the oxidation of LDL. Dr. J. Wright has recently formulated an optimal ratio of estrone, estradiol and estriol(over 90%). Progesterone may also be of benefit.

**37) DHEA**–Especially consider in the elderly.

**38) Chondroitin polysulfate**

STUDY–Nakazawa, K., Murata, K. *The therapeutic effect of chondroitin polysulfate in elderly atherosclerotic patients.* J Int Med Res 6(3): 217-25, 1978. ABSTRACT–50% of 46 elderly patients received 3 gms chondroitin polysulfate daily while the other half received placebo. After .5-5 yrs serum cholesterol in the treated group fell to 10-20% lower and serum TG's fell to 27% lower than controls. After 3 months clotting time was prolonged by 50%.

**SPECIAL NOTE**–Many nutritional or alternative therapies for heart disease are are considered "quack therapies." The use of snake oil in the treatment of various ailments is the classic depiction of quackery: "*The Snake oil Salesman.*" Interestingly enough, the use of both snake oil and snake venom have recently been found to have some powerful therapeutic value in the treatment of various cardiovascular conditions. Snake oil also has a powerful platelet anti-aggregating effect because of its high content of EPA. A drug, Ancrod (Arvin® is tradename), has been used in Europe and Canada for over 20 years for the prevention of strokes. It is basically a purified extract of the venom from the Malaysian pit viper and it functions to inhibit blood clotting.

## Notes

## FATTY ACID COMPOSITION OF FOODS

(concentration of fatty acids expressed in % by weight of total fatty acid content)

| Source | Oleic acid | Linoleic acid | **Arach–idonic acid** | Alpha linolenic acid | Eicosa -penta-enoic a. | Docosa-hexa-enoic a. | Saturated fats | **Cholesterol (in mgs per 3 oz** |
|---|---|---|---|---|---|---|---|---|
| | 18:1 omega 9 | 18:2 omega 6 | 20:4 omega 6 | 18:3 omega 3 | 20:5 omega 3 | 22:6 omega 3 | | |
| Atlantic cod | 4.0 | 1.2 | | 0.8 | 12.4 | 21.9 | 36 | 47 |
| Pacific Halibut | 25.7 | 0.9 | | 0.3 | 1.0 | 7.9 | 19 | 35 |
| Lake Herring(Fresh) | 18.1 | 4.3 | | 3.4 | 5.9 | 13.3 | 25 | 54 |
| Pacific Herring | 16.9 | 1.6 | | 0.6 | 8.6 | 7.6 | 26 | 81 |
| Mackerel | 19.3 | 1.1 | | 1.3 | 7.1 | 10.8 | 34 | 62 |
| Ocean perch | 22.0 | 9.5 | | 0.6 | 9.3 | 12.0 | 18 | 53 |
| Chinook Salmon | 29.1 | 4.3 | | 3.4 | 8.2 | 5.9 | 21 | 54 |
| Chum Salmon | 21.4 | 2.0 | | 1.0 | 6.7 | 16.1 | 20 | 54 |
| Coho Salmon | 18.6 | 1.2 | | 0.6 | 12.0 | 13.8 | 15 | 42 |
| Pink Salmon | 17.6 | 1.6 | | 1.1 | 13.5 | 18.9 | 15 | 44 |
| Tuna, can in water | 17 | 2 | | 2.0 | 8 | 21 | 27 | 35 |
| Rainbow Trout(fresh) | 19.8 | 4.6 | | 5.2 | 5.0 | 19.0 | 15 | 45 |
| **SHELLFISH** | | | | | | | | |
| Blue Crab | 17.6 | 1.9 | | 1.2 | 13.4 | 11.0 | 19 | 78 |
| Littleneck Clam | 10.8 | 1.4 | | 1.6 | 10.0 | 14.5 | 28 | 57 |
| Shrimp | 10 | 2 | | 1.0 | 16 | 13 | | 166 |
| Pacific Oysters | 8.5 | 1.2 | | 1.6 | 21.5 | 20.2 | 25 | 93 |
| Sea Scallops | 5.2 | 0.6 | | 0.3 | 21.3 | 26.2 | 26 | 28 |
| Shark | 16 | 0.3 | 5.0 | 0.0 | 10* | 10* | | |
| **OILS** | **Oleic** | **Linoleic** | **Arach.** | **Linolenic** | **EPA** | **DHA** | **Saturated** | **Cholesterol** |
| Butter | 25 | 2.0 | | 1.0 | 0 | 0 | 70* | |
| Flax seed | 17 | 15 | | 55.0 | - | - | **13** | - |
| Cod liver | 23 | 2.0 | 0.7 | 1.0 | 9.5 | 9.5 | 19 | - |
| Safflower | 12.5 | 79 | | 0.5 | - | - | 8 | - |
| Corn | 29 | 54 | | 1.0 | - | - | 17 | - |
| Cottonseed | 24 | 50 | | 0.4 | - | - | 26 | - |
| Sesame | 46 | 41 | | | - | - | 13 | - |
| Sunflower | 26 | 66 | | 0.3 | - | - | 8 | - |
| Olive oil | 82 | 10 | | 0.7 | – | - | 8 | - |
| Soybean | 28 | 58 | | 7.0 | - | - | 14 | - |
| Peanut | 51 | 29 | 2.2 | 1.0 | - | - | 19 | - |
| Canola | 54 | 27 | | 6.2 | 3.8 | 3.5 | 6 | - |
| English walnut | 23 | 55 | | 11.0 | - | - | 11 | - |
| **OTHER FOODS** | | | | | | | | - |
| Cow milk fat | 35 | 2 | | 1 | - | - | 62 | 8ozs=32 |
| Human milk fat | 42 | 7 | | 0.7 | 0.6 | 0.3 | 50 | |
| Chicken fat | 49 | 17 | | 1.0 | - | - | 33 | - |
| Egg yolk | 36 | 11 | | 0.2 | - | - | 53 | 1m=222. |
| Coconut oil | 10 | 2 | | - | - | - | 88 | - |
| Palm oil | 43 | 9 | | 0.3 | - | - | 48 | - |
| Beef, lean | 44 | 4 | | - | - | - | 39 | 81 |
| Chicken, white | 35 | 19 | | 4 | - | - | 29 | 73 |
| Lard | 53 | 10 | | 1.0 | - | - | 36 | 1T=15 |

(from Gruger et al. Fatty acid composition of Oils from 21 species of marine fish, freshwater fish and shellfish. J Am Oil Chemists society vol 41 Oct '64. & USDA Handbook, Washington, D.C.Govt Print Office, 1987 #8-15)

## Cholesterol Lowering Diet

Foods can be broken down into 3 main categories:

**1) Carbohydrates**
**2) Fats**
**3) Proteins**

We get all our calories from these 3 food components. Each gram of carbohydrate or protein yields 4 calories (Kcal) in the body. A gram of fat yields 9 calories. Ideally, each food component should comprise the following calorie percentage in our diet for the maintenance of good health:

**Carbohydrates 70%**–The 2 basic carbohydrates types are complex and simple.

*Complex Carbohydrates* are unrefined, unprocessed and as close to the whole natural state as possible. These should comprise 60% of your total calorie intake. Whole oats, whole wheat, whole rye, millet, bulgar, barley, legumes (beans such as pinto, lentil, black, navy, Lima, split peas), fresh vegetables, brown rice, whole white potato, sweet potatoes, and whole fresh fruit are sources of complex carbohydrates.

*Simple Carbohydrates* are refined, processed, sweetened foods which do not resemble their whole original state. They should comprise no more than 10% of our calories. "Simple" foods include sugar, corn syrup, white flour, doughnuts, pastries, cookies and food products that use the term **"wheat"** without the word "**whole**" in front of it. These foods are devoid of both the bran and germ of the whole grain. Other examples include soda pop, caffeinated beverages, white rice, cereals made with sugar or white flour, honey, and even fruit juice. Pasta made from durum semolina is commonly thought of as a complex carbohydrate, but it is actually refined white flour.

Simple carbohydrates raise your blood sugar levels quickly and cause your body to secrete large amounts of insulin. This results in increased amounts of fats being stored. Simple carbohydrates thus exacerbate diabetes, hypoglycemia, obesity, chronic yeast infections, high blood cholesterol, and high fats.

**Fats 20%**–Average Americans get 37% of their calories from fats. There are 2 basic types of fat in the diet, unsaturated and saturated.

*Unsaturated fats* include essential fatty acids–fats which are essential for health and survival. They are used to regulate the immune system, control blood pressure, and keep triglyceride and cholesterol levels down. Found in foods such as whole grains, nuts, seeds, oils, and fish, unsaturated fats should comprise 15% of our caloric intake. Much of our current unsaturated fats come from omega 6 oils such as corn, cottonseed, safflower and sunflower oils. We should actually try to balance these out with more omega 3 oils such as flax, soy, fish, and canola oils. In addition we could benefit from more oils from rice and olives.

*Saturated fats* are fats which tend to clog our arteries by raising cholesterol and fat in the blood. They worsen diabetes, irritate inflammatory states (bursitis, arthritis, tendonitis), aggravate asthma, and raise blood pressure. The main sources of saturated fats are dairy products, red meats, and certain processed foods. Foods with high saturated fat contents are lean beef (50% fat), cheese (60-80% fat), fried chicken (60% fat), chips (55% fat), and baked goods such as croissants, scones, doughnuts, cookies and various creamy dressings and sauces (40-90% fat). Eggs are 55% fat. They should be eaten boiled or poached rather than fried or scrambled. Avoid margarine, palm, cottonseed, and coconut oils. Read labels carefully.

**Protein 10%**–Most Americans eat far too much protein. This leads to allergies, increased risk of cancer, heart disease, osteoporosis, and other problems. Environmentally our planet can not do well if we continue to overeat protein. In some individuals, it may be necessary to increase protein levels especially if there is a problem with blood sugar.

# ANGINA PECTORIS

- When the coronary arterial system is unable to supply the oxygenated blood that is needed for cardiac work, angina pectoris occurs.
- Usually manifesting after periods of exercise or excitement, this syndrome is characterized by increased heart rate and blood pressure which precedes a sense of discomfort, pressure or pain.
- Coronary atherosclerosis is an almost invariable condition found in patients who suffer fatal attacks of angina. Patchy myocardial fibrosis is also almost always present.

## I. Etiology

Any increased demand for oxygen due to increased heart rate, increased systolic tension, or contractility in the context of advanced atherosclerotic lesions in the coronary arteries can cause the onset of angina.

## II. Signs and Symptoms

Symptoms can be very varied. Anginal pain can range from slightly noticeable pressures or aches to sudden, intense precordial crushing sensations. While it usually is felt beneath the sternum, radiating into the left shoulder and down the inside of the arm, it may also shoot straight through to the back and into the throat, the jaws, and the teeth. It may, occasionally, radiate down the right arm. The pain and pressure of angina may be felt in the upper and lower abdomen as well. It is often described as a constricting sensation around the chest and **may often be confused with heartburn or other digestive disturbances.**

## III. Treatment

**1) Treat the underlying cause which is usually atherosclerosis.**

**2) Magnesium**–500mg/day (check ionic magnesium or sublingual smear, see Mg & CVD). Can use slow release magnesium, Mag-Lo-Plex by Omnivite.

**3) Co-enzyme Q10**

STUDY–Kamikawa, T. *Effects of coenzyme Q10 on exercise tolerance in chronic stable angina.* Am. J. Cardiol.56:247,1985. ABSTRACT–10 men and women with stable angina received in random order 150mg CoQ10 daily or placebo. After 4 weeks, subjects on CoQ10 experienced a 53% reduction in the frequency of anginal episodes. Treadmill tolerance time increased by about 20% and ST depression was delayed by 50%.

**4) Taurine**

**5) Bromelain**–500mg (2100mcu) 3x/day

**6) L-Carnitine**–500mg t.i.d.

**7) Vitamin E**–400iu 3x/day

**8) Aspirin**–A few years ago a study compared aspirin and a placebo taken every other day. It was found that a marked and statistically significant reduction in the incidence of fatal and nonfatal MI's occurred in the aspirin group. What wasn't noted in the study was that the incidence of strokes, sudden death, and other cardiovascular events were higher in the aspirin group than in the placebo. **As a result, the total death rate was identical between the 2 groups!!**

**9) Omega 3 fatty acids**–super EPA has 500mg EPA/DHA 6-8caps per day.

STUDY–Saynor, R., Verel D. *Eskimos and their diets.* Letter. Lancet 1:1335, 1983. ABSTRACT–150 patients with angina pectoris and normal volunteers were supplemented with fish oils (MAXEPA) for up to 3 years. Long term pts were able to reduce nitrate therapy and exhibited increased exercise tolerance while taking the supplements. TG's which fell sharply during the 1st few weeks remained low. Total cholesterol was significantly lower and HDL cholesterol was significantly higher. Bleeding time increased when the daily dose was 3.6gms of EPA per day but not when it was 1.8g per day.

## Notes

---

# HYPERTENSION

- Hypertension is an asymptomatic condition wherein a patient's blood pressure measured greater than 140/90 on two separate occasions. Usually, a somewhat higher value is allowed for patients who are more than 60 years old.
- There are two categories of hypertension: essential hypertension, in which the specific causal factor is unknown, and secondary hypertension which can be traced to various agents or conditions.
- Essential hypertension constitutes 92-94% of all hypertension. The next two most common causes of hypertension are from oral contraceptive use and renal parenchymal disease.

## I. Epidemiology

Hypertension is found almost exclusively in developed countries and, while environmental, stress and genetic factors undoubtedly play their roles, the standard western diet is strongly linked to essential hypertension. Essential hypertension is virtually nonexistent in undeveloped areas. There, increased blood pressure is not related to advancing age. But when people from these "primitive" societies move into industrialized areas and adopt "civilized" diets (low fiber, high protein, fat, sugar and salt), the incidence of hypertension increases dramatically among them.

Hypertensives are prone to disabling or fatal strokes, myocardial infarctions, cerebral hemorrhaging and renal failures. In diagnosing hypertension, primary attention is generally paid to the diastolic pressure. However, high systolic pressure is closely associated with increased cardiovascular disease and, in males, with normal diastolic pressure but elevated systolic pressure (>158mm Hg) the cardiovascular mortality rate is 2.5x greater than in men with normal (<130mm Hg) systolic pressures.

Hypertension is twice as common in blacks (37%) than whites (18%) in the U.S. However, when isolated diastolic or systolic hypertension is included, more than 50% of both blacks and whites over the age of 65 have hypertension.

## II. Etiology

While it is generally agreed that essential hypertension has no single cause, the following are etiological factors:

1) **Excess sodium**–in U.S. the average intake is 5.5 gms per day (see sodium under minerals)
2) **Decreased potassium**–Modern Americans consume only about 2gms per day in comparison to hunters and gatherers thousands of years ago who ate 8-10gms per day (see *The K Factor*, George Webb, M.D. & *The High Blood Pressure Solution: Natural Prevention and cure with the K Factor,* Richard D. Moore, M.D., Ph.D.). Their $K^+$ to $Na^+$ ratio was at least 8 to 1 compared to today in which the ratio is reversed $Na^+$ to $K^+$ 2 to 1.
3) **Deficiency of fiber**–Americans currently only consume 12gms per day. Ideally 35-50gms of fiber should be eaten each day (paleolithically 100-150gm fiber was eaten).
4) **Excess sucrose** (see John Yutkin, *Sweet and Dangerous*)
5) **Food sensitivities**–when other more obvious causes have not been found to be causative

factors, food sensitivities should be evaluated, especially in someone who is relatively young. Diastolic blood pressure can rise as much as 18 points after a food allergen has been eaten (see William Philpott, *Victory over Diabetes*). Consider caffeine sensitivity

6) **Hypothyroidism or hyperthyroidism**

7) **Deficiency of EFA**

8) **Obesity**

9) **Deficiency of calcium and/or magnesium**

10) **Cadmium toxicity**–Acid rain increases lead, cadmium, and aluminum. Preeclamptic women may have higher levels of cadmium than normotensives.

11) **Lead toxicity**

STUDY–Harlan, W. *Blood lead and BP Relationship in the adolescent and adult US population* JAMA 253(4):530-34,1985 ABSTRACT–Lead levels that were previously thought safe were found to be associated with increased blood pressure.

12) **Smoking-**may deplete magnesium stores as well as directly vasoconstrict.

13) **Vitamin E toxicity**–See Wilfrid Shute, M.D.: *Vitamin E for Ailing & Healthy Hearts*

## III. Diagnosis

Generally, there are no discernible symptoms unless the blood pressure goes very high. Some symptoms or signs patients may experience are dizziness, headaches, fatigue, and injection of the conjunctiva. Recommended diagnostic procedures are:

1) Take the patient's blood pressure with arm level and on left. Having patient's arm down can elevate blood pressure 18 points. Also have patient take Bp at home with good cuff.

2) Fantus test–measures urinary chloride. This is a useful test for evaluating the consumption of sodium in the diet.

3) Hair analysis for lead and cadmium.

4) Measure ionic magnesium or .(see magnesium chapter).

5) Intracellular Diagnostics Inc. (800)874-4804, measures intracellular potassium and magnesium through a sublingual smear.

6) Test and evaluate thyroid function.

## IV. Treatment

1) **Decrease sodium and increase potassium**–It has been found that as the extracellular level of potassium increases, the sodium-ATP pump is activated which causes a decrease in intracellular sodium.

STUDY–Patki, PS. *Efficiency of potassium and magnesium in essential hypertension: A double-blind, placebo-controlled, crossover study.* Brit J Med 521-23; 301, 1990. ABSTRACT–37 adults with mild hypertension were treated with either 1) 2.5gms of K, 2) 2.5gms & 480mg mag or, 3) placebo for 8 wks. They then crossed over for another 8 wks. Results showed that K lowered systolic Bp an avg of 12pts and diastolic Bp of 16pts! The 8 wk period where magnesium was added to the K made no difference in Bp.

STUDY–Cappuccio, FP et al.. *Does potassium supplementation lower blood pressure? A meta-analysis of published trials.* J Hypertension 9:465-473,1991. ABSTRACT–A meta-analysis was performed on 19 clinical trials that examined the effect of K supplementation on all people and people with hypertension. In people with high Bp K suppl had the greatest effect lowering systolic Bp an avg of 8.2 pts and 4.5pts diastolically. In people who had normal Bp it only lowered Bp 5.9 and 3.4 pts respectively.

2) **Increase fiber**–As the level of fiber goes up blood pressure invariably goes down. In parts of the world where fiber intake is very high blood pressure tends to be very low.

3) **Decrease sucrose–**Sucrose can impair insulin function and can indirectly cause blood pressure to rise (Yutkin).

4) **Avoid caffeine**–A subset of the population may be sensitive to caffeine.

5) **Avoid alcohol**–Some people have a genetic hypersensitivity to alcohol which causes an increase in blood pressure.

6) **Decrease serum glucose**

STUDY–Salomaa, V.V., et al *Glucose tolerance and blood pressure: long term follow up in middle aged men* Brit Med J 302:493-6, 1990. ABSTRACT–1815 men were studied from 1974-86. In 1974, about half were normal and the other half had at least one risk factor for cardiovascular disease such as hypertension or glucose intolerance. Those who were hypertensive in 1986 had higher glucose levels in 1974. Glucose concentration in 1986 correlated with hypertension in 1986, even amongst those who were normotensive to begin with.

7) **Rule out food sensitivities**–consider hypoallergenic diet (see allergies) almost always will lower Bp 5-15 points diastolically within one week.

STUDY–Grant, C. *Food allergies and migraine*. Lancet p 966-69, May 5, 1979. ABSTRACT–15 migraine patients with diastolic blood pressure of 100mm Hg or greater followed a 5 day elimination diet consisting of lamb and pears. A reduction in diastolic blood pressure to 90 mm Hg or lower was noted in every patient. When offending foods were reintroduced, blood pressure rose again. Upon avoidance of the offending foods blood pressure's fell again to normal

8) **Calcium citrate**–1 gm/day–It may take up to 6 weeks to have an effect. One study showed 90 patients, ages 16-29, with mild hypertension had a median drop in their diastolic blood pressure of about 6 points.

9) **Magnesium**–The average American gets 180-250mg/day. (RDA is 300-350mg/day) at 400-800mg/day, watch for diarrhea. Magnesium acts as a natural calcium channel blocker. It prevents $Ca^+$ from entering the cell and causing vasal constriction. Magnesium is difficult to absorb. Consider special time release formulation (SloMag® or Omni-Mag-Lo-Plex® from Omnivite Nutrition.)

10) **EFA, linoleic acid, flax oil or fish oil**–1-5T/day or 3-6gms–It may take 4-8weeks, but it can decrease up to 10 points from the max EPA level. Some people may not be able to convert linolenic acid from flax oil into EPA & DHA. It may be an advantage to use fish oil in these cases.

11) **Cratagus solid extract–(Scientific Botanicals)1/2t 3x per day**

12) **Coenzyme Q10–100-300mg/day** Coenzyme Q10 is especially indicated where there are other cardiovascular complications. May take 8-16 weeks to work.

STUDY–Digiesi V, et al.. *Effect of coenzyme Q10 on essential arterial hypertension.* Curr Ther Res 47:841-845, 1990. ABSTRACT–18 patients with essential hypertension received 100mg/day of coenzyme Q10 or placebo, each for 10 wks. with a 2 wk washout period, in a double-blind crossover trial. Mean systolic Bp dropped by 10.6pts and diastolic Bp by 7.7pts.

STUDY–Digiesi V, et al.. *Coenzyme Q10 on essential hypertension.* Molec Aspects med 15(suppl):S257-63. ABSTRACT–26 patients with essential hypertension received 50mg 2x per day for 10 weeks. Mean systolic Bp decreased an avg of 18pts systolically and 12pts diastolically (98.1 to 86.1).

STUDY–Digiesi V, et al.. *Mechanism of action of Coenzyme Q10 in essential hypertension.* Curr Ther Res 51:668-672, 1992. ABSTRACT–10 patients with essential hypertension received 100mg/day of coenzyme Q 10 and their Bp fell 19.5mm/Hg and 13.5mm/Hg.

13) **Chelate cadmium or lead if necessary** (can use DMSA).

14) **Garlic**

STUDY–Petkov, V: *Plants with hypotensive, antiatheromatous and coronary dilating action* A J Chinese Med 7:197-236,1979. ABSTRACT–In humans garlic was found to lower systolic and diastolic blood pressure by 20-30 points and 10-20 points respectively.

15) **Treat thyroid condition**–Either high or low thyroid can cause hypertension.

# CONGESTIVE HEART FAILURE

- When a decrease in the myocardial contractile state is such that the heart cannot keep up with the body's needs, congestive heart failure occurs. There are many possible etiologies for this common syndrome.
- Initially, the reduced cardiac function may manifest only during times of exercise; but as the disease progresses, the heart's failure to provide the basic cardiac requirement may occur even at times of rest.
- When CHF is diagnosed and treated with conventional treatment the 10 year survival rate averages about 10-20%.
- The signs and symptoms associated with congestive heart failure are fatigue, shortness of breath, edema, intolerance to cold, tachycardia, cough, paroxysmal nocturnal dyspnea, and labored breathing

## I. Etiology

There are multiple etiologies for congestive heart failure. Those related to nutritional factors are:

- deficient myocardial calcium
- deficient intracellular magnesium (60% of people with heart disease are low)
- deficient intracellular potassium
- excess intracellular sodium
- deficient myocardial Coenzyme Q10

Consider Intracellular Diagnostics, Inc. for measuring intracellular $Na^+$, $K^+$, $Mg^{++}$ and $Ca^{++}$

## II. Treatment

1) **Calcium citrate**–1gm/day but must be careful not to deplete magnesium levels.

2) **Magnesium chloride or sulfate–500mg/day**–Consider oral slow release magnesium Mag-lo-plex, Omnivite Nut. Consider, in advanced cases, using IM, IV or combined as part of the "Myers' cocktail" 1x every week ( Myers' cocktail is a combination of vitamin B-12, B complex, B-5, B-6, calcium, magnesium and vitamin C that is an IV formulation put together by a Dr. John Myers, a physician whom Dr. Gaby took over for back in the early '80s). Up to 2-3gm magnesium sulfate can be used IV. Care should be used in people who have low blood pressure because it could further drop their blood pressure. Most people with heart disease are low in magnesium.

STUDY–Wester, P. & Dyckner, T. *Intracellular electrolytes in cardiac failure.* Act Med Scand. 707:33-36, 1986.
ABSTRACT–In congestive heart failure there is loss of magnesium (along with an elevation of intracellular sodium and reduction of intracellular potassium) due to the activation of the renin-angiotensin-aldosterone system. Because magnesium is necessary for the "sodium-potassium pump" its deficiency may add to the elevation of intracellular sodium and reduction of intracellular potassium.

3) **Potassium**–100-3,000mg/day preferably through diet

STUDY–as above–ABSTRACT–In congestive heart failure the activation of the renin-angiotensin-aldosterone system causes potassium losses, while the secondary hyperaldosteronism may give rise to low intracellular potassium through a direct permeability effect on the cell membrane. In addition, magnesium loss leads to further loss of intracellular potassium as magnesium is necessary for the sodium-potassium pump. In 297 patients with diuretic treatment for congestive heart failure, 42% had hypokalemia and 52% had depletion of muscle potassium.

4) **Coenzyme Q10**–100mg/day
**L-carnitine**–1000mg/day (divided doses)
**Taurine**–500mg t.i.d. (up to 4 gms/day) These are found to be 3x lower in the mycocardium of CHF patients (Alan Gaby states that many times patients can come directly off lasix and digitalis with the above treatment).

STUDY–Mortensen, S. *Long-term Coenzyme Q10 therapy: A major advance in the management of resistant myocardial failure.* Drugs Exp. Clin Res 11(8):581-93, 1985. ABSTRACT–12 patients with advanced congestive heart failure and an insufficient response to diuretics and digitalis received Coenzyme Q10 100mg daily and were followed for a mean period of 7 months. In 30 days 8/12 showed definite improvement, feeling less tired. Their general activity tolerance increased and dyspnea at rest disappeared. Heart rate fell; there was a significant decrease in atrial size and overall improved myocardial performance. Withdrawal of the supplement caused severe clinical relapse with improvement upon resumption.

STUDY–Langsjoen, P. *Effective and safe therapy with Coenzyme Q10 for cardiomyopathy.* Klin Wochenschr 66:583-590, 1988. ABSTRACT–88 patients with congestive heart failure due to cardiomyopathy received 100mg of Coenzyme Q10/day for periods ranging from 1-24 months. Responses were monitored by ejection fraction, cardiac output, and improvement in functional New York Heart Association classification. 75-85% of patients showed significant improvements in 2 monitored cardiac parameters. By functional classification, about 82% of those patients improved to lower classes. Blood levels of Coenzyme Q10 were below normal prior to treatment in a substantial % of patients.

5) **Vitamin E**–400-1200 IU/day of D alpha tocopherol (mixed tocopherols)

6) **Arginine**–1gm 3x per day Arginine is concentrated in the muscles and may be deficient in CHF.

8) **Testosterone or DHEA**–consider if levels are low

9) **Thyroid**

**NOTE**–Concerning idiopathic hypertrophic subaortic stenosis (IHSS), it has been found that IHSS may have hypothyroidism as a possible etiological factor. One study found that of 17 patients with documented hypothyroidism, 15 of them had IHSS. When they were treated with thyroid hormone the IHSS went away. These patients are often deficient in magnesium.

## Notes

---

# INTERMITTENT CLAUDICATION

- Peripheral atherosclerotic diseases are basically the aggregation of atheromatous plaques in the lower extremities. This cuts off the blood supply and, consequently, the transmission of oxygen to the muscles. The result is intermittent claudication, a deficient blood supply in an exercising muscle.
- It may be felt as a pain, ache, cramp or feeling of fatigue during any physical exertion.
- Signs and symptoms may occur in the feet, thighs, hips, or buttocks.

## I. Etiology

Atherosclerosis and the subsequent loss of blood flow cause intermittent claudication.

## II. Treatment

1) **Diet & exercise**(see atherosclerosis)–Start with minor exercise and work up.

2) **Vitamin E**–up to 2000iu/day–It may take months for this treatment to work. It is probably a good idea to start with a relatively low dose and increase gradually over a long time. After improvement is noted the dosage can be decreased.

3) **Vitamin C**–to bowel tolerance

4) **Inositol Hexaniacinate**–1gm 3x per day(has been used in Europe for over 30 years).

5) **Calcium pangamate**–50mg t.i.d.

6) **Ginkgo biloba**- 24% standardized extract may work best.

7) **Carnitine** 1 gm 3x per day

8) **Zinc picolinate**–30mg tid.

9) **Magnesium**–both orally and topically as epsom salts. Soak in concentrated epsom salt bath for 20-30minutes 2-4x per day daily until improved.

10) **EPA/DHA**–3-10gms 3x per day will decrease platelet stickiness and allow the blood to flow more freely.

11) Hydrotherapy

### Notes

---

# MITRAL VALVE PROLAPSE

- A bulging of one or more leaflets into the left atrium during systole so that a crisp systolic click is heard on auscultation is characteristic of mitral valve prolapse.
- 25% of patients with MVP have skeletal abnormalities such as joint laxity, high arched palate, scoliosis, funnel chest.
- MVP is present in 6% of the U.S. population.

## I. Etiology

There are indications that some cases of MVP may be related to a magnesium deficiency.

## II. Signs and Symptoms

While most patients have no signs or symptoms, some may experience palpitations, dyspnea, fatigue or non-anginal chest pain due to atrial or ventricular arrhythmias. There are rare occurrences of cerebral emboli, ventricular tachycardia and sudden death.

## III. Treatment

**1) Magnesium**–It has been found that, compared to matched controls, 42 mitral valve prolapse patients had lower mean red blood cell magnesium, but no significant difference in serum magnesium or serum ionized magnesium. Other studies have confirmed the same findings that 85% of people with MVP have magnesium deficiency. It is probably wise to monitor ionic or sublingual intracellular magnesium levels(see magnesium chapter).

STUDY–Fernandes JS, et al. *Therapeutic effect of a magnesium in patients suffering from mitral valvular prolapse and latent tetany.* Magnesium 5:175-81, 1986.

STUDY–Galland LD, et al.. *Magnesium deficiency in the pathogenesis of mitral valve prolapse.* Magnesium 5:165-74, 1986.

**2) L-carnitine**

STUDY–Trivellato, M., de Palo, E., Gatti, R., Parenti, Piazza. *Carnitine deficiency as the possible etiology of idiopathic MVP :case study with speculative annotation.* Texas Heart Inst J 1984;11:370. ABSTRACT-A 44 year old man with mitral valve prolapse and a history of palpitations, tachycardia, dyspnea, asthenia and recurrent anxiety of 5 years duration, unresponsive to various drugs, was studied. Free plasma and urinary carnitine were below normal. The patient was put on L-carnitine 1gm t.i.d. After 4 months patient became symptom free and heart rate had fallen from 115 to 70 beats/min. In 4 other random patients with mitral valve prolapse all were found to have low levels of plasma or urinary carnitine or both.

**3) Coenzyme Q 10–**

STUDY–Oda T & Hamamoto K, *Effect of coenzyme Q10 on the stress-induced decrease of cardiac performance in pedicatric patients with MVP* Jap Circ J 48:1387, 1984.

**4) Crataegus oxycantha**–May help strengthen the connective tissue of the heart and improve its contractile function.

# DIABETES MELLITUS

- Diabetes Mellitus (DM) is characterized by fasting hyperglycemia and glycosuria. The risks of developing atherosclerosis, microangiopathy, nephropathy, and neuropathy are greatly increased. Chronic infections–including urinary tract infections and yeast overgrowth–are common.
- 5.2% (13 million people) of the U.S. population has DM. Of these, 90% have non-insulin dependent diabetes mellitus (NIDDM) and remainder suffer from insulin dependent diabetes mellitus (IDDM). Nationally, there are over 6.5 million undiagnosed cases of DM. 17% of the population between the ages of 65-74 years old has DM. 40% of NIDDM require exogenous insulin to maintain normal blood glucose levels.
- Diabetes mellitus is currently the fourth leading cause of death by disease in the U. S. and the number of people afflicted is increasing at the rate of 6% annually. At this rate the number of people with diabetes will double every 15 years. In 1992 diabetes costs in the U.S. were estimated at $92 billion.
- The prevalence of Diabetes mellitus is particularly high in ethnic minorities in the U.S., such as Hispanic populations, Native Americans, and African-Americans. Hispanics have about a 2-fold increased incidence and Africans have about 1.3x the risk compared to the average population.

Clinical note–Pima Indians of Arizona have an extremely high rate of DM with about 55% of their population over the age of 35 having NIDDM. A closely related groups of Indians living in Maycoba, a remote village in northwestern Mexico, have been found to have DM rate of about 10%. They, on the average, weighed about 50lbs less. Their lifestyle is such that they are very active and eat a diet which has as its main staples beans, corn, and potatoes. Analysis shows that their diet is composed of 63% CHO, 23% fat and 13% protein, with a daily fiber intake of >50gms. Their diet contrasts to the high fat diet of the Pima Indians living in Arizona.

## I. Etiology

Strongly associated with Western lifestyle and diet, diabetes mellitus is a chronic metabolic disorder in which carbohydrates, fats and proteins are inadequately metabolized. While there is no distinct etiology for diabetes mellitus, the following are generally viewed as factors:

1) **Genetics**–It seems that genetic factors play a more dominant role in NIDDM than in IDDM. Studies of identical twins have shown that when one twin has NIDDM, the other one will have it almost 100% of the time. However, if one twin has IDDM, the other will have it only 50% of the time.

2) **Obesity**–90% of NIDDM sufferers are obese. With every 20% increase in body weight, the chance of becoming diabetic doubles.

**3) Autoimmunity**–Antibodies to all types of pancreatic cells are found in 75% of IDDM cases. Among normals only .5-2% have these antibodies. It is possible that antibodies to foods may find suitable binding sites to insulin receptors (see diagram ). Current evidence has led to the recent postulation that cow's milk protein may be the inciting antigen which triggers the production of autoantibodies to pancreatic islet cells.

**Possible Mechanisms of Insulin Insensitivity**

Insulin receptors, which are protein molecules embedded in the phopholipid bilayer, can become altered preventing normal insulin binding. As demonstrated below, a number of different antibodies can either bind to the receptor itself or else bind to the insulin itself both of which results in insulin insensitivity. Other substances found in foods such as lectins may also bind to insulin receptors making them unavailable for normal insulin binding. Lastly, as in IDDM antibodies may attack the beta cells of the pancreas itself severely diminishing the output of insulin.

Abnormal insulin receptor caused by xs TGs, trans-fatty acids, oxidized fatty acids or lectin binding.

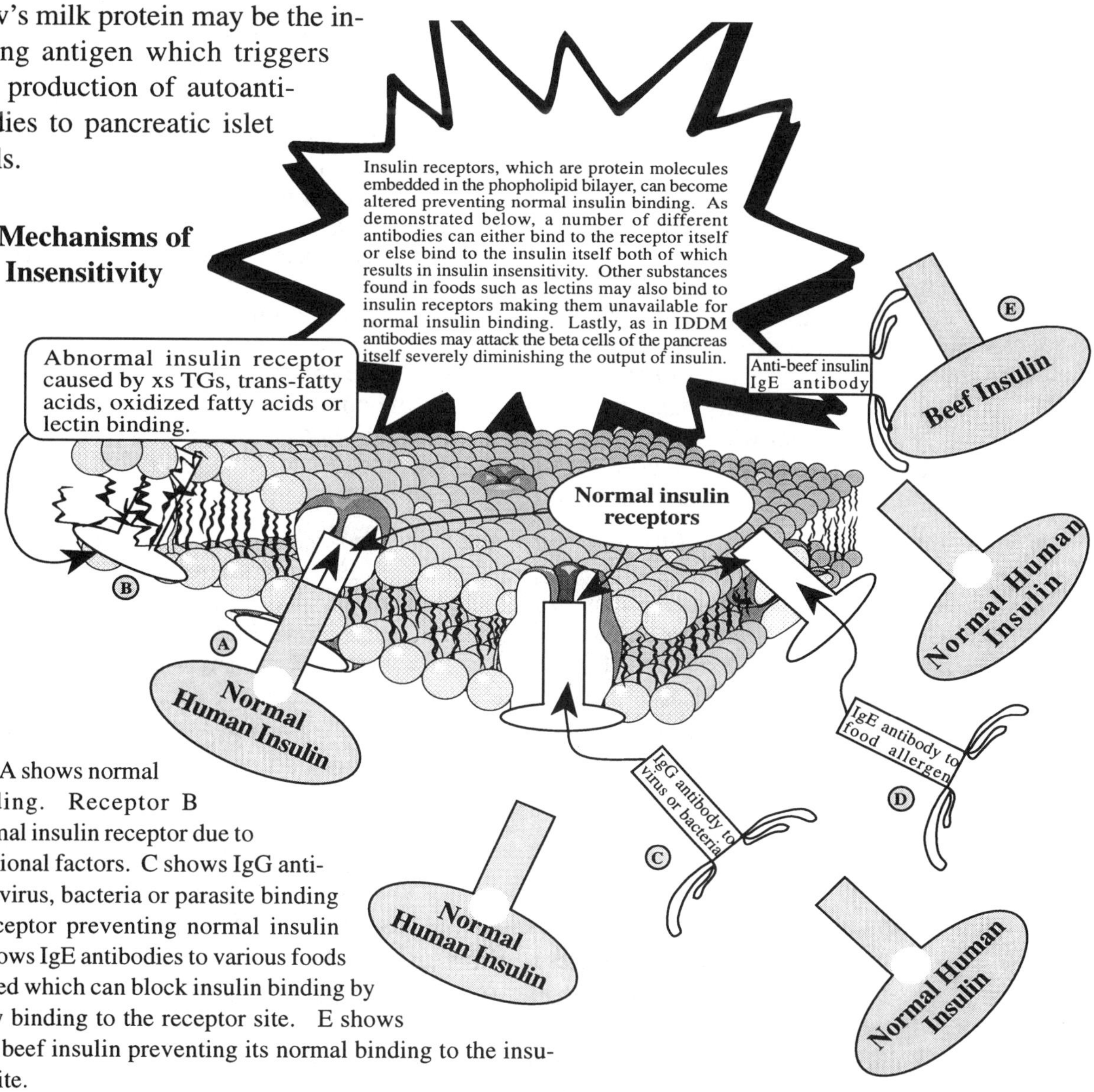

Receptor site A shows normal insulin binding. Receptor B shows abnormal insulin receptor due to various nutritional factors. C shows IgG antibody against virus, bacteria or parasite binding to insulin receptor preventing normal insulin binding. D shows IgE antibodies to various foods being produced which can block insulin binding by competitively binding to the receptor site. E shows antibodies to beef insulin preventing its normal binding to the insulin receptor site.

a) This represents the normal binding of endogenous insulin to the normal insulin receptor site (the diagram is schematic and normal insulin receptors are protein molecules that are embedded into the phospholipid cell membrane).

b) Various factors such as elevated triglycerides, trans fatty acids, and oxidized fat, food lectins can bind or in some way alter the normal insulin receptor preventing or diminishing the normal insulin binding. The net effect is a lack of insulin response.

c) Antibodies to bacteria, viruses or parasites can bind onto insulin receptors thus blocking the normal insulin response. In addition, lack of essential nutrients like chromium and EFAs can alter the insulin molecule preventing it from properly binding onto the insulin receptors.

d) An antibody to a food allergen, such as milk or wheat, can bind directly to the insulin receptors preventing the normal binding of insulin to the receptor site.

e) Insulin resistance: An allergy to beef insulin can occur, in a person who is taking exogenous beef insulin, resulting in antibodies being produced which can bind the beef insulin and prevent it from properly binding to its receptor sites. Switching to another source of insulin such as human or pork can correct the problem. Physicians need to be cognizant of this.

STUDY–Maclaren, N., Atkinson, M. *Is insulin-dependent diabetes mellitus environmentally induced?* NEJM vol 327:5, July 30, 1992. ABSTRACT–In this editorial it is noted that only one in every three pairs of identical twins affected by IDDM becomes concordant for the disease and that the incidence of IDDM is increasing. Along with the fact that certain viruses can stimulate the body to make autoantibodies to pancreatic cells and that numerous antibodies have been found against very specific tissues of the pancreas it seems certain that an environmental etiology is likely. In rat studies substitutions of various proteins markedly affect the frequency of diabetes. It is noted that an increased frequency of antibodies to cow's milk proteins in children with newly diagnosed IDDM parallels the frequency with which cow's milk is consumed worldwide. Lastly, in the review they mentioned that two of their patients in whom IDDM recently developed at one year of age had never had products containing cow's milk.

**Note**–In regard to this last item I must ask: 1) Whether the children were breast fed and, if so, did their mothers eat any dairy products? 2) Did the children consume any wheat products? I have noted that when there is a reaction to wheat, there is often a reaction to milk. Thus, milk-triggered autoantibodies could be present. In IDDM both wheat and milk allergy should be considered as a possibility of the autoimmune reaction.

STUDY–Hlasivoca, V. & Streda, M. *Glucose tolerance tests in patients with allergic respiratory disease.* Czechoslovakia Academy of Science. Prague Acta Allerg, 22:253-260, 1967. ABSTRACT–It was found that diabetics with food allergies commonly had hyperglycemic reactions.

STUDY–Goldstein, S. et al: *Hormone receptors.* Endocr Res Commun, 2(4&5):367-376, 1975. ABSTRACT–Using radio-isotope-labeled insulin and glucagon, Goldstein was able to show that cell membranes of mature diabetics were less capable of binding both insulin and glucagon to their receptor sites. He postulated that different immunoglobulins may be binding to receptor sites thus preventing their activation. **NOTE**–Autoimmune reactions can also occur. In these type reactions, antibodies to food, bacteria, parasites or viruses attack the pancreatic islet cells, thus preventing insulin production and/or release.

4) **Viral**–A higher onset of IDDM from October-March, the viral season, has been noted. It seems that, in some cases, the pancreas can suffer direct attack from a virus such as mumps, hepatitis, infectious mononucleosis, etc. Thus, viral infections may provide an etiological basis for some cases of diabetes mellitus. It should also be noted that there is an increased incidence of DM in colder climates–Finland 29.5 per 100,000 and 1.7 per 100,000 in Japan.

STUDY–Notkins Science June 15, 204:4398, 1979. ABSTRACT–A new virus specimen was obtained from a previously healthy 10 year old boy who was admitted to the National Naval Medical Center in a diabetic coma within 3 days after onset of symptoms of a flu-like illness. The boy died 7 days later and a postmortem exam showed destruction of ß-cells. Isolation of this virus into cultures of mouse, monkey, and human cells proved to be a variant of Coxsackie B4. Injection of this new virus into susceptible mice produced diabetes. The virus was then recovered from the diabetic mice.

5) **Toxins**–An N-nitroso derivative of glucosamine, Streptozotocin, is currently the preferred toxin for animal experiments which require destruction of β-cells. Experimentally it has been shown that N-nitroso compounds found in smoked and cured meats may cause beta-cell destruction in certain susceptible individuals and thus cause the onset of IDDM. Also, various medications–such as cortisone, BCP, inhalers, etc.–have been shown to elevate glucose levels. Certain vaccinations may also be implicated in DM, by triggering antibodies to β-cells.

### 6) Lack of fiber

STUDY–Rosman, M. *The effect of long term high fiber diets in diabetic outpatients*. S. AFR. MED J. 63(63):310-13,1983. ABSTRACT–10 patients were placed on a high fiber diet using readily available, low cost foodstuffs. Although only 3 people approached the projected dietary fiber intake, after 3 months significant correlations were found between the mean plasma glucose changes and serum triglyceride changes, and the dietary fiber increments.

STUDY–Philipson, H. *Dietary fiber in the diabetic diet.* Acta Med. Scand. 671:91-93,1983. ABSTRACT–It was found that diabetics were able to substantially reduce their insulin or oral hypoglycemic agents when placed on high fiber diets.

**7) Excess sucrose consumption**–Both sucrose and/or fructose consumption alone seem to alter insulin sensitivity and glycosylated hemoglobin. They should be avoided.

STUDY–Szanto, S., & Yudkin, J. *The effect of dietary sucrose on blood lipids, serum insulin, platelet adhesiveness and body weight in human volunteers.* Postgrad. Med. J. 45:602, 1969. ABSTRACT–The intake of a self-selected diet in which 60% of calories were from carbohydrate in the form of sucrose, as compared to starch, significantly increased fasting insulin and the insulin response to a GTT in 6 of 19 human volunteers.

STUDY–Reiser, S., Szepesi, B., Scogs *Report on the health aspects of sucrose consumption. Letter to the Editor.* Am. J. Clin. Nutr. ABSTRACT–Sucrose alone may be a very important etiologic factor in diabetes in the 10% of the population which is carbohydrate sensitive. In the rest of the population, sucrose still must be considered an important risk factor due to synergistic interactions with dietary cholesterol and triglycerides.

STUDY–Thorburn, Crapo, et al. *Long term effects of dietary fructose on CHO metabolism in NIDDM.* Metabolism 39:1;58-63, 1990. A comparison of fructose and glucose consumption was made where subjects ate 13% of their calories from each sugar. Over 3 months the study determined, 1) weekly fasting glucose levels and postprandial serum glucose and insulin levels after 4 sugar tolerance tests, 2) basal hepatic glucose production, and 3) hepatic and whole body insulin sensitivity during a hyperinsulinemic euglycemic clamp. Fructose feeding did not alter fasting glucose concentration, postprandial glucose and insulin responses to either glucose or fructose loads or to mixed meals. This study concluded that *substitution of sucrose by fructose for prolonged periods is unlikely to have adverse effects on glucose metabolism in diabetic subjects who are being treated with diet alone.* However, in some patients with high triglycerides, fructose caused fasting insulin to increase from 50-294! In all patients no change was seen in the glycosylated hemoglobin or insulin sensitivity.

**8) Excess iron** may stimulate the production of free radicals which can damage the beta cells of the pancreas, damage the insulin molecules that are secreted, or in some way effect the insulin receptors.

STUDY–Phelps, Chapman, Hall, Brand, and Mackinnon. *Prevalence of genetic hemochromatosis among diabetic patients.* Lancet 2:233-34, 1989. ABSTRACT–Among 418 patients attending a diabetic clinic, 21(5%) had persistently high serum ferritin levels and 5 of these had transferrin saturations consistently over 55%. Idiopathic hemochromatosis was confirmed by liver biopsy in 4 patients. The prevalence of unrecognized idiopathic hemochromatosis was 9.6 per 1000, compared to a general population prevalence of 4 per 1000. Note that heterozygous hemosiderosis affects up to 8-9% of the population.

STUDY–Cutler, P. *Deferoxamine therapy in high-ferritin diabetes.* Diabetes 38:1207-10, 1989. ABSTRACT–Serum ferritin levels were elevated in 9/18 poorly controlled NIDDM patients. None of the patients had a disorder known to cause iron storage. Serum iron and TIBC were normal in all cases. Because excess iron, as in hemochromatosis, is associated with diabetes and, because diabetes has been shown to improve after lowering the total body iron load through repeat venesection, all 9 patients with high serum ferritin and 7 of 9 with normal ferritin were treated with the iron chelating agent deferoxamine (10mg/kg IV in 500ml ringer's lactate given over 2 hours, 2x/wk). The number of treatments ranged from 9-26 (mean=16). Treatments were stopped when ferritin became normal and patients were maintained without hypoglycemia agents. **Of 9 patients with high serum ferritin, 8 had an improvement in blood sugar, which was frequently dramatic and occurred even though insulin or oral hypoglycemic agents were discontinued in all 8 patients.** Serum cholesterol, triglycerides, and hemoglobin A1c levels also improved considerably in these patients. In all 7 patients with normal serum ferritin, and in 1 with high serum ferritin, treatment with deferoxamine failed to improve diabetic control. This study demonstrates that idiopathic iron overload is an important etiologic factor in as many as 50% of patients with poorly controlled diabetes. That percentage is likely to be somewhat lower in other clinics, since Dr. Cutler, who practices orthomolecular medicine, presumably eliminated other nutritional causes of poor diabetic control.

## II. Signs and Symptoms

- While most patients with recent onset DM have no overt signs and symptoms, excess urination, excessive hunger, fatigue, weight loss, vaginal itching, visual changes and poor wound healing are classic indicators. These signs and symptoms are usually associated with advanced DM and may take many years to develop.
- **Skin tags**–It has been found, **mostly in males, that large, multiple, hyper-pigmented, lateral skin tags are associated with DM.** In one study, 500 consecutive hospital admissions were tested for DM. Of these, 62 patients tested positive. 47 of the 500 patients showed skin tags. Of this 47 it was found that 34 had DM. 7 of these were completely unaware of their diabetic conditions. Another study showed that 90% of patients with skin tags, both males and females, had abnormal GTTs.
- Chronic candida infections are also indicative of diabetes mellitus.

## III. Diagnosis

**1) Signs and symptoms**–Most people who become more insulin insensitive and whose fasting and postprandial blood sugar starts to rise have no or very few symptoms.

**2) Fasting blood glucose**–As recommended by the ADA, as of July 1997, any fasting blood glucose 8hrs or more of greater than 126mg/dl on two different occasions is diagnostic of DM. **Be aware of ingestion of vitamin C supplements as this may falsely elevate serum glucose.** The NDDG on the top of the next page has established different criteria.

**3) Glucose insulin tolerance test (OGITT)**

STUDY–Kraft, J. *Detection of DM, in situ (occult diabetes).* Laboratory Medicine, Vol.6 #2, p10-22, Feb 1975. ABSTRACT–3650 patients suspected of having DM had glucose-insulin tolerance tests run. 1713 had normal GTT curves according to the criteria of the AM. Diabetes Assoc. Of these 1713 so-called normal curves, only 568 (33%) had normal insulin tolerance tests. 862 (50%) showed patterns of latent diabetes, 240 (14%) were in the borderline range, and 43 (3%) were low insulin. **67% of the GTTs that were judged normal were found to be latent diabetic when the insulin tolerance test was taken into consideration.**

Normal values for insulin-fasting 0-30units:

- 2nd and 3rd hour total– < 50 units
- 2nd and 3rd hour total– 50-100units = borderline high
- 2nd and 3rd hour total– > 100units = latent diabetes

Currently there are no officially established criteria for insulin levels during the OGITT. However this test I believe is invaluable for assessing the nature and the degree of the diabetes or impaired glucose tolerance. Some physicians draw insulin levels every hour and then plot the area under the insulin levels. The bottom line is if there is an elevated glucose level along with a higher than average insulin level it is safe to conclude that there is IGT and measures should be sought to bring the levels down concomitantly with glucose levels.

**National Diabetes Data Group Criteria for diagnosis of DM**
serum (mg/100ml)

| OGTT | Normal | Dx of DM | Dx of Gest. DM |
|---|---|---|---|
| Fasting | 70-115 | >140 | >105 |
| 30-90min | <200 | >200 | >190 |
| 2 hour | <140 | >200 | >165 |

***NOTE**–As of July 1997, the American Diabetes Association has recommended that a glucose valve of 200mg/dl at 2 hrs during the OGTT diagnostic of DM if it occurs on two separate tests. Glucose values of 140-199mg/dl are now termed "impaired glucose tolerance."

Diagnosis has been permitted by the NDDGC in any one of the following ways:

a) Sufficient classical symptoms of DM (e.g. polydipsia, polyuria, ketonuria, and weight loss) **plus** either an unequivocal elevation of the fasting blood glucose level or an elevation of the non-fasting blood glucose (random) level greater than 200mg/100ml.
b) Fasting blood glucose greater than 126mg/dl on more than one test.
*c) Two different glucose readings, at least one hour apart, higher than 200 during the OGITT
d) 1 hour postprandial–above 180mg/dl is a criteria, but needs confirmation by other tests.

**Gestational Diabetes Diagnostic Criteria**

**Screening during pregnancy**–A 50gm oral glucose challenge (does not have to be fasting) at 24-28weeks gestation is recommended for all pregnant women. A serum glucose of ≥ 140mg/dl after one hour is an indication for further testing. Criteria for the diagnosis of DM during pregnancy utilizes a 100gm challenge of glucose instead of 75gms. A normal diet that contains at least 150gms of CHO needs to be consumed for 3 days prior to the test to make for valid interpretation. During normal pregnancy, fasting glucose levels are normally lower than in non-pregnant women. At 1-2 hours postprandial (after eating a meal with a moderate amount of carbohydrates), glucose should normally be <120mg/dl and rarely goes over 140mg/dl unless there is a problem.

Criteria for Gestational Diabetes Mellitus

| Fasting | ≥105mg/dl |
|---|---|
| 1 hour | ≥190mg/dl |
| 2 hour | ≥165mg/dl |
| 3 hour | ≥145 |

**NOTE on Gestational DM (GD)**–2-4% of all pregnant women develop GD, usually during the second or third trimester. Most often the diabetes that develops occurs because of insulin resistance. GD increases fetal morbidity so it is very important to identify women who develop it. In 90% of women who develop GD, their glucose tolerance returns to normal following delivery. However, 40-60% will develop NIDDM within 5-15 years! Women who have given birth to babies weighing more than 9 lbs, who are obese, or have a strong family history of DM are at greater risk for developing GD.

STUDY–Stout, Robert W. "*The relationship of Abnormal Circulating Insulin Levels to Atherosclerosis.* Atherosclerosis, 27:1, 1-13, 1977. ABSTRACT–It was found that the greater the levels of insulin, the greater the damage to blood vessel walls. Thus, controlling insulin levels is a very important aspect in the treatment of DM.

4) **Glycosylated hemoglobins**–This is an excellent method of monitoring the long-term efficacy of a treatment. Ideally, the value should be below 7.5% (dependent on lab).

**NOTE**–Both hemolytic and megaloblastic anemia produce falsely low glycosylated hemoglobin because red blood cells have a shortened life span. Increases in glycosylated hemoglobin take 2-3 weeks of elevated glucose in blood, while decreases take 4 weeks with a sustained decrease in average blood glucose. It should be noted that the glycosylated hemoglobin may be directly toxic to cells in higher concentrations.

5) **Hair analysis for minerals and heavy metals**–especially chromium, selenium, zinc, copper, magnesium, calcium, manganese, and vanadium.

6) **Check thyroid levels**

7) **Fructosamine**–gives a measure of short-term (1-3wks) glucose control in diabetics. This test can be administered in the physician's office and is extremely useful for evaluating short term glucose control, e.g. if you are administering a therapeutic diet.

8) **Protein bound glucose**–evaluates glucose avg. for the previous 2-3 days.

Robert Bradley, M.D., President of the Joslin Diabetes Center states, "Large vessel diseases of the heart, legs, and brain are the endpoints which account for the largest part of the overall mortality and morbidity due to DM. This alone is a strong argument for early diagnosis and control of blood glucose relative to macrovascular complications."

**Impaired glucose tolerance (IGT)**–People who have elevated glucose levels in their blood but, not high enough to be called diabetics, have what is termed Impaired glucose tolerance. IGT effects about 11% of the U.S. population. About 25% of people with IGT eventually develop DM. We could probably refer to these people as borderline diabetics. They do not have the same increased risk of developing microvascular sequelae, but they do have increased risk for CVD.

## IV. Treatment

1) **Increase complex carbohydrates to 60-70% of caloric intake; decrease fat to 20%.**

STUDY–Chait, A. *Dietary management of DM.* Contemp. Nutr. (2),Feb,1984. ABSTRACT–Diets proportionally high in carbohydrates have been shown to improve blood glucose control by enhancing insulin sensitivity, provided adequate insulin is present.

2) **Decrease sucrose and other simple carbohydrates.** It should be noted that all simple sugars, including fructose, should be markedly lowered. Fructose is now being touted as "good" food for diabetics because of its **lack of insulin stimulation.** This is unfortunate because fructose eventually gets converted into sugar and a number of studies have shown that there are long-term deleterious effects of fructose consumption.

STUDY–Beck-Neilsin, Pedersen, Lendskov. *Impaired cellular insulin binding and sensitivity induced by high-fructose feeding in normal subjects.* Am.J. Clin. Nut. 33:273. ABSTRACT–Normal human volunteers were fed their usual diets plus **1000 cal/day of fructose** for one week. There was a **significant reduction of both insulin binding to isolated monocytes and insulin sensitivity.** In contrast, 1000 cal of glucose under the same conditions did not significantly change insulin binding or sensitivity.

STUDY–Hallfrisch, J. et al. *The effects of fructose on blood lipid levels.* AJCN 43:151-59, 1986. ABSTRACT–12 men with a hyperinsulinemic response to sucrose loading and suitable controls were each alternately fed a diet with either 15% fructose or 15% starch. Fructose caused a general increase in both the total serum cholesterol and in the LDL cholesterol in most subjects in both groups, while triglycerides rose significantly only in the hyperinsulinemic group.

**NOTE**–In acute loading studies a synergism between glucose and fructose with regard to insulin secretion exists. Neither glucose nor fructose, when given as the sole monosaccharide, stimulates insulin secretion as potently as glucose and fructose combined.

**3) Increase consumption of foods with low glycemic indexes, especially legumes.** Legumes in the morning have been shown to have an extremely beneficial effect on blood glucose. In fact, legumes seem to keep the blood glucose at a fairly low level for almost 4-6 hours.

**4) Treat food sensitivities.**

STUDY–Pots, J., Lange, M. *Avoidance provocative food testing in assessing diabetes responsiveness.* Diabetes, vol 26, suppl. #234, 1977 & Diabetes 29, 6, 1980. ABSTRACT–Potts, working on IDDM (adult-onset) patients, found that 2/3 of these were able to discontinue insulin with good control of their blood glucose following withdrawal from their maladaptive reactive substances. The remaining 1/3 were able to reduce their insulin requirements by an average of 70%.

STUDY–Philpott & Kalita, *Victory Over Diabetes, a Bio-ecologic triumph.* Keats Pub, Inc., 1983 CASE–Carl, a 15 year old boy diagnosed as a juvenile-onset diabetic by two physicians, was receiving insulin to control his blood sugar. He had other signs and symptoms such as weakness, headaches, irritability, depression, and lethargy. Individual foods were tested for maladaptive reaction and it was found that wheat, oats, and milk produced hyperglycemic reactions above 230mg/dl. In addition, a 30 minute test exposure to auto exhaust produced a shift in blood glucose from 90 to over 180. When placed on a hypoallergenic diet, his blood glucose stayed in the normal range and his signs and symptoms cleared.

CASE–A 38 year-old who had been diagnosed as a chronic schizophrenic for 15 years was tested and found to have hyperglycemic reactions, all of which were over 200, to 6 foods. The highest reaction was to cane sugar. This person when tested for maple syrup and honey showed only a rise at one hour of 135 and 110 respectively.

**5) Increase omega-3 fatty acids.** These fats provide many benefits that relieve cardiovascular complications. They reduce triglycerides in the blood and improve the ability of insulin to bind onto receptor sites. Omega-3 fatty acids should be used with caution as there have been several short term studies showing that omega-3 fatty acids may actually impair glucose tolerance. Consider complete fatty acid analysis with BodyBio (609) 825-8338

STUDY–Vessby B & Boberg, M. *Dietary supplementation with n-3 fatty acids may impair glucose homeostasis in patients with NIDDM.* J Intern Med. 228:165-171, 1990. ABSTRACT–14 patients with NIDDM were randomly assigned to receive 10g/day of fish oil in the form of MaxEPA or placebo (olive oil), in a double-blind cross-over trial. Each supplementation period lasted 8 weeks before switching. There was a statistically significant difference between the two groups with glucose concentrations going up in the MaxEPA treated group and down in the olive oil supplemented group.

STUDY–Horwitz, N. *Fish oil decontrols diabetics.* Med Tribune 1;13, July 8, 1987. ABSTRACT–In this review article it was noted that in a small group of NIDDM patients 8gms/day given over a period of 8wks significantly lowered both cholesterol and triglycerides by 11% and 33% respectively. However, both fasting glucose and postprandial glucose levels went up significantly. In another study 5.5gms/day of fish oil over 4 weeks resulted in a decreased secretion of insulin and also a rise in fasting and postprandial blood glucose.

**NOTE**–My personal feeling is that if the studies were carried out for a longer period of time there would be an overall improvement in glucose control and that less insulin would be required to keep down blood sugars. In general, fats tend to slow down the rate of absorption of glucose and therefore tend to be favorable toward post prandial glucose levels.

**6) Chromium (GTF)**–200mcg/day

STUDY–Martinez, O.B. et al. *Dietary chromium and effect of chromium supplementation on glucose tolerance of elderly Canadian women.* Nutr. Res. 5:609-20, 1985. ABSTRACT–A double-blind study–85 elderly women ages 59-83, 62% of whom were on medications that could effect glucose metabolism, were divided into "high risk" and "low risk" categories on the basis of a 2 hour GTT and received either trivalent chromium or placebo. After 10 weeks there was no significant difference between the experimental subjects and controls except for a small but significant improvement after a GTT in the high risk, non-medicated group. This sub-group was found to have a significantly lower median chromium intake compared to the experimental low risk non-medicated group. This suggests that suboptimal chromium status may account for the difference. Because it appears that drugs may have obscured this effect in the medicated subjects, the researchers suggest that future studies omit medicated subjects.

STUDY–Liu, V. Abernathy, R. *Chromium and insulin in young subjects with normal glucose tolerance.* Am. J. Clin. Nut. 25(4):661-67,1982. ABSTRACT–20 normal college students were found to have an inverse relationship between peak glucose and chromium levels. It was also found that the amount of insulin required for the lower serum glucose levels was lower in the students who had the highest chromium levels.

**7) Brewer's yeast**–1 tablespoon tid (also contains glutathione)

STUDY–Mertz, W., Schwarz, K. *Chromium(III) and the glucose tolerance factor.* Arch. Biochemical Biophys. *85:292*-5, 1959.

STUDY–Offenbacher, E., Stunyer, F. *Beneficial effect of chromium-rich yeast on glucose tolerance and blood lipids in elderly patients.* Diabetes 29:919-25,1980. ABSTRACT–24 elderly patients, including 8 NIDDM patients, randomly received either 9gms of brewer's yeast which was rich in chromium or the equivalent amount of chromium-poor tortula yeast. After 8 weeks, glucose tolerance, insulin sensitivity and total lipids improved only in the group receiving the brewer's yeast.

**8) Fiber**–up to 80gms/day. Excellent sources of fiber are **guar gum** (5g/meal)**, pectin** (10g/meal)**, and oat bran** (1 cup oats provides 9gms fiber). Diabetics ingesting 14-26 grams of guar per day needed less insulin and had less glysuria.

**9) Avoid coffee**

STUDY–Tuomilehto, J., et al. *Coffee consumption as a trigger for IDDM in childhood.* Brit Med Journal 300:642-3, March 1990. ABSTRACT–Finland has the highest incidence of IDDM in the world. The incidence has increased during recent years as has the consumption of coffee. In data derived from the Diabetes Epidem. Research International Study Group regarding coffee consumption, there was an association between the annual average national coffee consumption per person and the age standardized incidence of IDDM. Countries with the highest coffee consumption per capita had the highest incidence of IDDM. Caffeine, the most widely used psychotropic agent, could be a risk factor in utero of IDDM. Its half-life is prolonged in pregnancy and is known to cross the placenta into the fetus. Pregnant women who consume large amounts of coffee have increased risk for spontaneous abortions, premature deliveries and giving birth to infants with low birth weight.

**10) Vitamin B-6–**Pyridoxine is especially beneficial for treating diabetic neuropathy. It should be noted that xanthurenic acid is often elevated in diabetics. In addition, B-6 inhibits platelet aggregation and prevents thromboxane release. It also inhibits clotting by blocking the clotting activity of thrombin. 100mg in humans can block platelet function for up to 52 hours.

STUDY–Davis, R., Calder, J. and Curnow, D. *Serum pyridoxal and folate concentrations in diabetics.* Pathology, April 151-156, 1976. ABSTRACT–518 patients with diabetes had serum levels of pyridoxal measured. It was found that 25% were B-6 deficient. This deficiency was unrelated to the patients' diets or to whether they were taking insulin or other anti-diabetic medications. It was postulated that diabetics may have a higher than average requirement for B-6.

STUDY–Jones, Charles, and Gonzalez. *pyridoxine deficiency: A new factor in diabetic neuropathy.* J of Am Podiatry Assoc, Sept. 646-653, 1978. ABSTRACT—10 IDDM patients who had signs and symptoms of peripheral neuropathy were found to excrete more xanthurenic acid than did the diabetics without neuropathy. Each was given 50mg B-6 tid. for 6 weeks. Xanthurenic acid excretion became normal and the signs and symptoms of peripheral neuropathy became normal in **all** the patients. In addition, every patient remarked that their eyes felt better.

STUDY–Kotake, Y. & Murakami, E. *A possible diabetogenic role for tryptophan metabolites and effects of xanthurenic acid on insulin.* Am J Clinical Nut. July; 826-29, 1971. ABSTRACT–It was found that people deficient in B-6 had certain abnormalities in their tryptophan metabolism (see tryptophan metabolism). They developed excess xanthurenic acid which has the ability to bind onto insulin making it inactive.

11) **Zinc picolinate**–30mg/day. Zinc is involved in the synthesis, secretion and utilization of insulin. It is concentrated in the pancreas and may protect pancreatic beta cells. Zinc itself has "insulin-like" activity. Diabetics require zinc supplementation because they tend to hyperexcrete zinc. Laboratory tests have shown that glucose tolerance has been increased in hyperglycemic mice through zinc supplementation.

12) **Vitamin E**–400 IU/day. Diabetic patients have tocopherol deficiencies which cause increased free-radical damage. Vitamin E, as an antioxidant, may help prevent diabetic complications. It also increases HDL-cholesterol levels and aids in fatty acid metabolism.

STUDY–Vogelsang, A. *Vitamin E in the treatment of DM.* Ann. N.Y. Acad. Sci 393, 1982. ABSTRACT–**Warning**–Vitamin E may reduce the insulin requirement. Diabetics on insulin should be started on 100 IU or less daily. The dosages should be raised slowly with corresponding adjustments of the insulin dose.

STUDY–Ozden, et al. *The effect of Vitamin E on glycosylated hemoglobin levels in diabetic rats: a preliminary report.* Diabetic Research, 12:123-124, 1989. ABSTRACT–Intraperitoneal injections of 500mg/kg and 1000mg/kg vitamin E every 3-4 days were given to respective groups for 21 days. On day 25, significantly lower glycosylated hemoglobin levels were found in the high vitamin E group.

13) **Garlic**–decreases platelet aggregation and is useful in preventing the microangiopathy associated with diabetes. It has also been shown to lower blood glucose levels.

14) **Magnesium**–500mg/day. Diabetics show significantly lowered magnesium levels, especially those who suffer severe retinopathy. The lack of magnesium seems to increase the risk of cardiovascular disease. Magnesium is a cofactor in glycolysis and an important cell regulator. Evidence shows that magnesium may prevent retinopathy, increase HDL levels, decrease platelet aggregation, and prolong clotting time.

15) **Vitamin C**–2gm/day increasing to 2-4grams/day. Vitamin C decreases levels of sorbitol in red blood cells. In the 1970's Dr. Mann of Vanderbuilt University theorized that vitamin C and glucose have the same transport mechanism because they are so structurally similar. As a result, excess glucose can inhibit vitamin C transport into cells and may produce localized scurvy. The end organ pathologies of diabetes look very similar to that of scurvy. It may be that a chronic Vitamin C deficiency leads to the microangiopathy of DM.

STUDY–Friend, Time. USA Today, Life Section, Sept. 18, 1990. ABSTRACT–When measured against controls, people with certain types of cataracts had reduced levels of vitamin C in their blood. Follow up on this study showed that a daily dose of 800mg vitamin C was required to raise a person's blood vitamin C level enough to result in a lower level of cataract formation.

16) **Vitamin D**–Recent studies show that vitamin D may stimulate insulin production 500% in animals. This was a study done at Oregon Health Sciences University in 1993-4.

17) **Fenugreek seeds**

STUDY–Sharm, R. et al. European J of Clin Nut. 44:301-6, 1990. ABSTRACT–Defatted fenugreek seed powder (100mg divided into 2 equal doses) was placed in the diet of 10 IDDM patients between the ages of 12-37 years old for two 10 day periods to see the effect on blood glucose and serum lipid profiles. The fenugreek diet significantly reduced fasting blood sugar and improved glucose tolerance while there was a 54% reduction in daily urinary glucose excretion. Cholesterol LDL, VLDL cholesterol and triglycerides were significantly reduced. HDL stayed the same.

18) **Bioflavonoids–quercetin 500mg/day.** Quercetin inhibits aldose reductase and thus prevents glucose from converting to sorbitol. This is important with regard to cataract formation. Quercetin also stabilizes cell membranes and acts as an antioxidant.

### 19) Gymnema sylvestre

STUDY–Shanmugasundaram, et al. *Possible regeneration of the islets of Langerhans in streptozotocin-diabetic rats given Gymnema sylvestre leaf extracts.* J of Ethnopharmacology 30: 265-279, 1990. ABSTRACT–Two water soluble extracts, GS3 and GS4, were given to IDDM diabetic rats. After 60 days the fasting glucose levels returned to normal. Both components were shown to double the number of ß-cells. During the study insulin levels rose to near normal.

### 20) Niacin and/or niacinamide–250mg-1500mg should be given, especially at the early onset of IDDM.

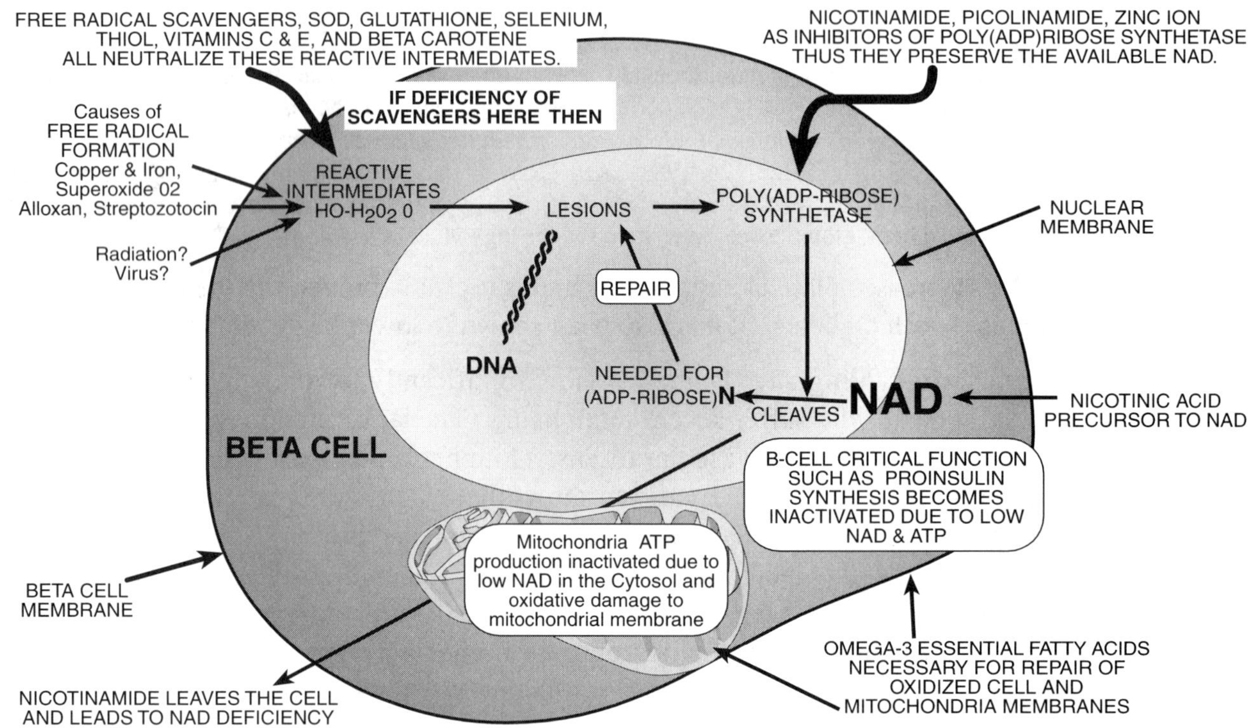


*The importance of oxidative injury as a cause of impaired mitochondrial oxidation in diabetes by John P. Cleary, MD.*

STUDY–Cleary, J. *Vitamin B-3 in the treatment of DM: case reports and review of the literature*, J of Nut Med. 1:217-25, 1990. ABSTRACT–Nicotinamide may have a protective ß-cell effect in IDDM while niacin may help with insulin resistance in NIDDM. ß-cell injury may be associated with low NAD and ATP levels resulting in oxidative injury and organ failure. NAD levels are known to be low in diabetics. In the 40s niacinamide was used to reduce insulin requirements in the treatment of DM. In IDDM niacinamide is used to inhibit poly (ADP-ribose) synthetase, which would normally catalyze the loss of NAD in the ß-cells and subsequent loss of insulin production. Consider 100-200mg niacinamide at the onset of IDDM.

STUDY–Cleary, J. *The importance of oxidative injury as a cause of impaired mitochondrial oxidation in diabetes.* J Orthomolec Med. 3:164-74, 1988. ABSTRACT–Evidence is presented that diabetes is associated with reduced intracellular levels of NAD which contribute to the organ damage seen in this condition. Experimental diabetes induced by chemical alkylating agents causes a reduction of NAD levels in the pancreas which leads to metabolic failure and cell death. Treatment with niacin or niacinamide prevented experimental diabetes. 6 cases are presented in which improvement of diabetes followed treatment with niacin and other vitamins.

STUDY–Vague, P., Viallettes, B., Lassman-Vague,V., Vaillo, J. *Nicotinamide may extend remission phase in IDDM.* Lancet 1:619-20, 1987. ABSTRACT–In newly diagnosed IDDM functional beta cells can be protected by halting the autoimmune process through the regeneration of beta cells or by increasing their resistance to destruction. In animal studies high dose B-3 prevented induction of diabetes by alloxan or streptozotocin, improved the condition of partly pancreatectomized diabetic rats, and prevented or delayed the onset of autoimmune diabetes. B-3 restored normal intracellular levels of NAD in pancreatic islets, thereby preventing beta cell damage and improving regeneration. In the present study, a double-blind trial, 16 IDDM received B-3 (n=7; 3g/day) or placebo (n=9) one week after the start of insulin therapy. Insulin was discontinued in 6 (85.7%) patients taking B-3 compared to 5 (55.6%) patients taking placebo ($p<0.05$). Though complete remission for more than 2 years rarely occurs in IDDM, 3 patients treated with B-3 for 18 months remained in remission for more than 2 years. These results suggest that B-3 reduces destruction of beta cells and enhances their regeneration; thereby extending remission time.

21) **Thyroid**–There have been studies done with IDDM patients showing that they have difficulty converting T4 to T3. Transport of glucose across cell membranes becomes impaired when the thyroid hormone is deficient.

22) **Vanadium(Vanadyl sulfate)**–15-50mg/day has "insulin-like" activity and improves glucose tolerance. It also prevents zinc loss from pancreas.

23) **Biotin**–May require up to 16mg/day. Biotin helps as a cofactor for glucokinase, an enzyme that breaks down glucose into metabolic substrates for energy production. If glucokinase is inactive, the patient can develop DM.

24) **Vaccinium myrtillus**–has long been used as a folk remedy in the treatment of diabetes. It increases capillary integrity and improves venous tone. It is specifically effective in the treatment of macular degeneration and cataracts. It has potent antioxidant properties.

## Additional notes:

*Somogyi phenomenon*– This phenomenon may occur in IDDM individuals who present with increasing morning glucose levels in spite of increasing insulin doses. These patients are experiencing middle of night hypoglycemia with a hyper counterregulatory response due to cortisol, growth hormone, glucagon, and catecholamines. This effect can be seen in hypoglycemic people. I first witnessed this phenomenon in a patient, a 16 year old male who had been experiencing dizziness, on whom I was doing a glucose tolerance test. His blood glucose peaked after one hour at around 170mg/dl. His glucose dropped over the next hour to about 100mg/dl. At the 4th hour of the test his blood glucose went up to 169 after hovering around 90mg/dl for 3 hours. His blood glucose was immediately tested again and his glucose measured 172. The patient experienced feelings of fatigue and dizziness at this time. The significance of this phenomenon is that if it goes unrecognized, excessive insulin will be given which can lead to many problems.

*Dawn phenomenon*–Another strange reaction that may occur but is more rare than the Somogyi effect is the Dawn phenomenon. Between the hours of 4-9A.M. there is a decreased sensitivity to insulin, due to a surge in growth hormone. Both the Somogyi Effect and Dawn Phenomenon can be diagnosed by having the patient monitor their own blood glucose at 3-4A.M. (Lots of fun!)

*Syndrome X*–this refers to marked insulin resistance, hypertension, increased LDL, increased triglycerides, obesity (with a characteristic intra-abdominal fat deposition), and cardiovascular disorders such as MI and stroke. The characteristic high waist to hip ratio is strongly associated with CVD. This conglomeration of conditions has been linked to increased levels of stress and is sometimes referred to as "civilization syndrome" where stress leads to further bad habits such as smoking, drinking, overeating and "couch potato" phenomenon. This condition may respond better to a higher fat diet with most of the fat calories coming from omega 3 fatty acids and small amounts coming from saturated fats. Certainly coping strategies such as meditation, exercise, and diet management are essential to treat this all too common syndrome. Exercise has been found to increase insulin receptors.

## Glycemic Index of Foods (using white bread as standard 100 score)

| Food with highest glycemic Index | Gly I. | Foods with intermediate glycemic index | | Foods with lowest glycemic index | |
|---|---|---|---|---|---|
| Maltose | 152 | Rice, polished, boiled 15 min | 79 | Lima beans | 50 |
| Glucose | 138 | Oatmeal cookies | 78 | Peas, green, dried | 50 |
| Honey | 126 | Potato chips | 77 | Peas, Chick (Garbanzo) | 49 |
| Rice, instant boiled 6 min | 121 | Yam | 74 | Rye kernels | 47 |
| Cornflakes | 121 | Peaches, canned | 74 | Milk, Skim (1% fat) | 46 |
| Potato, instant | 120 | Buckwheat | 74 | Peas, Black-eyed | 46 |
| Puffed wheat | 110 | All Bran | 74 | Spaghetti, white boiled 5min | 45 |
| Broad Beans (Fava beans) | 109 | Potato, sweet | 70 | Apple juice | 45 |
| Millet | 103 | Orange, juice | 69 | Milk, low fat (2% fat) | 45 |
| Bread, whole wheat | 100 | Grapefruit, juice | 68 | Whole milk (4% fat) | 44 |
| Bread, white | 100 | Spaghetti, white boiled 15min | 67 | Beans, kidney dried | 43 |
| Tortilla, corn | 100 | Pineapple, juice | 66 | Beans, Black | 43 |
| Corn chips | 99 | Rice, instant boiled 1 min | 65 | Peaches | 40 |
| Potato, mashed | 98 | Rice, parboiled boiled 25min | 65 | Sausage | 39 |
| Wheat, Shredded | 97 | Peas, green frozen | 65 | Lentils, red dried | 36 |
| Muesli | 96 | Bulgar | 65 | Plum | 34 |
| Rye, crispbread | 95 | Wheat kernels | 63 | Barley, pearled | 33 |
| Carrots, cooked | 92 | Pears, canned | 63 | Fructose | 26 |
| Apricots, canned | 91 | Grapes | 62 | Soybeans, canned | 22 |
| Apricots, dried | 91 | Spaghetti, brown boiled 15min | 61 | Soybeans, dried | 20 |
| Oats, porridge | 89 | Beans, baked canned | 60 | Peanuts | 15 |
| Raisins | 88 | Orange | 59 | Red meats-------low | |
| Banana (depends how ripe) | 84 | Pears | 58 | Fish-------low | |
| Sucrose | 83 | Lactose | 57 | Poultry----low | |
| Rice, brown | 81 | Ice Cream (depends on fat %) | 52 | | |
| Potato, boiled | 80 | Apple | 52 | | |
| Potato, baked | ? | Yogurt | 52 | | |
| Corn, sweet | 80 | Tomato soup | 52 | | |

In the past glucose was the standard 100 used, but has now been replaced by white bread as the standard.

**Note on the glycemic index (GI)**

The use of the glycemic index has been controversial mainly because it is cumbersome and somewhat complicated to use for the average diabetic person. Certainly it has important clinical relevance and can be used as a tool to provide information concerning foods which may elevate blood sugar. By looking at the glycemic index table one can see that certain foods increase blood sugar greater than others that don't seem particularly healthy. For example potatoes, which have always been thought of as a healthy complex carbohydrate, has a glycemic index of 98 (for mashed potatoes). Other foods such as ice cream are as low as 52. There are a number of complicating factors that play a role in the glycemic index including the form that a food is in (raw, cooked, ripeness) and how much fat, protein, fiber or other compounds in a food, These components all play a role in the glycemic index of the food.

For the diabetic, one can not just look at the glycemic index for foods to determine whether the food is good or not. Certain high fat foods, such as ice cream, may have a low glycemic index but they contain lots of saturated fat which, over the long term, will lead to more problems with insulin insensitivity and cardiovascular disease.

In clinical trials where diabetic patients reduced their GI 12 points down to 40% they had a significant drop in their cholesterol and triglycerides.

STUDY–Wolever TM, Nguyen PM, Chiasson JL, et al. Determinants of diet glycemic index calculated retrospectively from diet records of 342 individuals with NIDDM. Am J Clin Nut 9:1265-69, 1994.

STUDY–Miller JCB. Importance of Glycemic index in DM. Am J Clin Nut 59(suppl):747-752S, 1994. ABSTRACT–A meta-analysis of 11 published GI studies revealed that when GI was lowered from 66 down to between 38-54 over a period of 2-12 weeks, glycosylated HgB dropped by 9%, fructosamine by 8%, urinary C peptide by 20%, and day long blood glucose by 16%. Cholesterol fell by 6% and TGs by 9% on the average. In addition overall insulin production was significantly lowered in these NIDDM patients.

Consuming a very high carbohydrate diet (up to 80% of the total calories), has shown improvements in insulin sensitivity, which may be as a result of the high levels of fiber. Initially people put on high carbohydrate diets show an increase in the level of TGs in the blood and a worsening of the glycemic control. This effect reverses itself after a continuation of the diet.

Because of the concern that certain people may react adversely to high carbohydrate diets, an alternative diet has been proposed. In this alternative diet some of the carbohydrate is replaced by monounsaturated fats. In one study, a diet of 40% CHO, 38% as fat (21% monounsaturated), and 22% as protein resulted in lower levels of LDL, 24 hour urinary excretion of glucose, fasting TGs, and mean profile glucose levels. Fructosamine, fasting glucose, LDL and HDL remained the same however.

STUDY–Campbell LV, et al. The high-monounsaturated fat diet as a practical alternative for NIDDM. Diabetes Care. 17:177-182, 1994.

STUDY–Garg A, et al. The high-monounsaturated fat diet as a practical alternative for NIDDM. Diabetes Care. 17:177-182, 1994.

A number of researchers have now advocated a change from a high carbohydrate diet to one that is considerably higher in fats, especially monounsaturated fats(Garg A, Parillo M, Bonanome AGrundy, SM). Certainly there is room for biochemical individuality and there may be a number of circumstances where the high monounsaturated fat diet has its advantages. However, I think it is important to look at more specifically the types of carbohydrate that are being advocated for high carbohydrate diets. I have repeatedly advocated the use of complex carbohydrates in many conditions but I believe that this term is being thrown around too loosely. Recently in a book advocating a lower carbohydrate intake they made mention that they used to eat a high carbohydrate diet and as an example of their breakfast they consumed Grapenuts. Grapenuts is not a complex carbohydrate! It is made out of white flour. Other foods often advocated as complex carbohydrates include pasta, which is also a food made out of white flour and is *not* a complex carbohydrate. Furthermore, other foods that are considered complex carbohydrates such as whole wheat bread are only relatively more complex than say white bread. Looking at their glycemic index shows that they are virtually identical as far as their effect on blood glucose. What I recommend in terms of complex carbohydrate is more like what a cave-person would naturally eat. Instead of bread, eating of the cooked whole wheat kernels would be more what I would recommend. Whole oats rather than the rolled oats is another example. As you can see from the glycemic index table, wheat kernels have a glycemic index of only 63. Rye kernels have a glycemic index of only 47. Other complex carbohydrates that would be especially valuable would be the legume family of foods which consistently have very low glycemic indices.

From what we have seen from our evolutionary history, it seems obvious that an increase in omega 3 fatty acids would be beneficial for the diabetic person. A diet which is higher in omega 3 fatty acids and monounsaturated fatty acids to balance the remaining omega 6 fatty acids would certainly be helpful to lower triglycerides, increase HDL and generally reduce the risk of cardiovascular sequelae that is 3-4x higher in the diabetic than normals. The % fat could therefore vary anywhere from 15% to 35% of calories.

## Table on Insulin action for both Human and Animal Forms

| Insulin | Onset (Hr) | Peak (hr) | Effective duriation (Hr) | Maximum Duration (Hr) |
|---|---|---|---|---|
| **Human** | | | | |
| Regular | 0.5-1.0 | 2-3 | 3-6 | 4-6 |
| NPH | 2-4 | 4-10 | 10-16 | 14-18 |
| Lente | 3-4 | 4-12 | 12-18 | 16-20 |
| Ultralente | 6-10 | None | 18-20 | 20-30 |
| **Animal (beef or pork)** | | | | |
| Regular | 0.5-2.0 | 3-4 | 4-6 | 6-8 |
| NPH | 4-6 | 8-14 | 16-20 | 20-24 |
| Lente | 4-6 | 8-14 | 16-20 | 20-24 |
| Ultralente | 8-14 | minimal | 24-36 | 24-36 |

## Notes

# HYPOGLYCEMIA

- Hypoglycemia–an abnormally low blood glucose level which causes symptoms such as fatigue, weakness, palpitations, hunger, headaches, confusion, and marked personality changes–is not a particular disease but rather the result of other conditions.
- The two types of hypoglycemia are:
  1) **primary hypoglycemia**–due to the over production of insulin (insulinoma).
  2) **secondary hypoglycemia**–usually caused by diet, nutritional deficiency, **alcohol,** or food sensitivities. This type is relatively common.

## I. Etiology

Hypoglycemia is usually due to lack of fiber in the diet and the consumption of large amounts of simple carbohydrates. Food sensitivities may also play a large role in the onset of hypoglycemia.

## II. Signs and Symptoms

Common hypoglycemic symptoms are fatigue, shakiness, headache–especially in early morning or between meals–foggy mind, depression, crying spells, fits of anger, and profuse perspiration.

## III. Diagnosis

1) Signs and symptoms
2) Check adrenal function via **orthostatic hypotension test**
3) **6 hour GTT:** The following criteria indicate a diagnosis of hypoglycemia:
   a) any blood glucose below 60mg/Dl while fasting or during test
   b) any blood glucose drop of more than 50mg during any one hour.
   c) if blood glucose never rises above 50% of the fasting level during GTT.
   d) if the blood glucose falls 20% below the fasting level.
   e) if symptoms develop along with a drop in the blood glucose during GTT.
4) Child picture test–In this test, the child should write his name or draw a picture. He/she should be given glucose and continually write or draw as the glucose is metabolized. Notc any changes or reactions.

## IV. Treatment

1) **Treatment similar to DM.** Feed plenty of complex (low glycemic) carbohydrates(fiber).

2) **Increase the frequency of feedings**. This is not always necessary but it is important that meals are not missed.

3) **Avoid alcohol**. Increased hydrochloric acid via alcohol may cause excess release of gut secretagogues which augment ß-cell responsiveness to glucose changes, leading to excess insulin release.

4) **Chromium supplementation**–liquid chromium 400mcg 3-4x per day(Biotics)

5) **Vitamin C**–3gms/day

6) **Pantothenic acid**–500mg/day

7) **Niacinamide**–1gm/day

8) **Consider food sensitivities**–see *Victory Over Diabetes* by William Philpott, MD

## Notes

---

# ALLERGIES (Sensitivities or intolerances)

- Allergies, hypersensitive immunological reactions to specific substances, can be classified in two types: delayed or immediate hypersensitive reactions. Both types may be cyclical or fixed.
- When chronic symptoms are present and no discernible explanation can be found, begin searching for allergies.
- It is estimated that 60% of the U.S. population has symptoms associated with food reactions. It should be noted that the term *food allergy* denotes an immunological reaction involving antibody response. It is more appropriate to use the terms food sensitivity, intolerance, or reaction.
- Genetic predisposition may be the most prevalent cause of allergies. It has been found that if both parents are allergic, then 67% of offspring will be allergic. If one parent is allergic, then allergies will occur in 33% of the children.
- Boys with blue eyes and blond hair have the highest allergic tendencies.

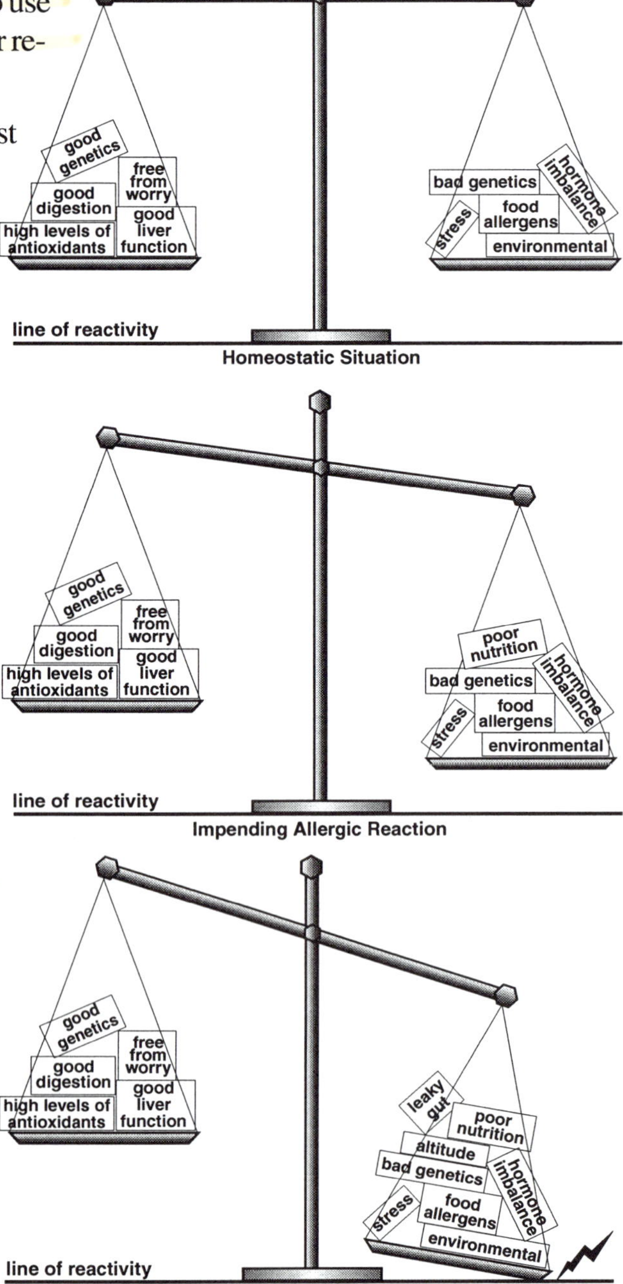


## I. Etiology

While no specific cause or causes for the onset of allergic reactions is known, the following may contribute to the development of allergies and food sensitivities:

1) **Early exposure to allergenic foods in utero.**
2) **Early exposure to highly allergenic foods as an infant.**
3) **Poor digestion of foods** with an absorption of macromolecules to which the body becomes sensitized.
4) **Frequent exposure to the same foods** in the same family in various forms.
5) **Decreased mucosal secretory IgA.**
6) **Decreased adrenal function** (may be caused by various factors including stress).
7) **Increased exposure to various environmental toxins** (chemical pollution in air, water, and food) and allergens. This increases the body's sensitivity to other allergens.

## II. Signs and Symptoms

In **children**, look for the following symptoms:

1) Denies' lines
2) Allergic shiners
3) Salute sign and chronic sinus drainage.
4) Bed wetting
5) Bruxism
6) Stomach aches or abdominal pain
7) Headaches
8) Chronic ear infections
9) Chronic tonsillitis or hypertrophied tonsils
10) Eczema or other chronic dermatitis, hives
11) Alternating constipation and diarrhea.
12) Foul smelling breath, feet, perspiration, or stools
13) Food cravings
14) Trouble concentrating
15) Hyperactivity and erratic behavior, Tourette syndrome
16) Asthma
17) Aphthous Stomatitis
18) Fatigue–(from organochlorides)

Symptoms indicating allergies or sensitivities in **adults** are:

1) Joint pain
2) Gall bladder pain
3) Ulcerative Colitis and Crohn's disease
4) Digestive problems, alternating constipation and diarrhea, stomach ulcers, duodenal ulcers, gluten sensitive enteropathy, mucus in stools, inability to go for long periods without eating.
5) Any number of chronic infections such as urinary tract infections, prostatitis, bronchitis, vaginitis, sinusitis, etc.
6) Hypertension
7) Low back pain or upper back pain, especially panniculofibrositis or fibrositis.
8) Hypoglycemia or hyperglycemia
9) Migraines
10) Skin conditions such as eczema, psoriasis, hives, and acne.
11) Autoimmune diseases such as systemic lupus erythramatosis (SLE), scleroderma, Sjogren's, rheumatoid arthritis, multiple sclerosis, etc.
12) Fluid retention and weight gain, especially in women before their period.
13) Thrombophlebitis
14) Meniere's disease
15) Withdrawal symptoms upon session of food (HAs, fatigue, joint pan, irritability).
16) Obesity

## III. Diagnosis

**1) Provocative testing**–By far the most accurate method of testing for food sensitivities or allergies is avoidance and reintroduction. This can be done via various methods:

**a) Fasting**–This can be done either via water fast or juice fast (juices can be either fruit or vegetable-I prefer apple or pear). The water fast is more difficult to get patient compliance and I believe is best monitored in an in-patient facility. It is my experience that people tolerate a juice fast much more readily, but care must be taken to select juices to which the person is not sensitive to.

**b) Elemental diets**–This involves using a synthetic formula that has all of the necessary nutrients for survival. This is especially useful in very severe sensitivity conditions such as ulcerative colitis and Crohn's disease. I like the formulation ENFOOD® [Dr. Gislison (604)270-8474], which is not too bad tasting and of higher quality ingredients than some of the more commercially available formulations. The more commercially available Tolerex®or Vivonex®T.E.N. [ Sandoz Nutrition (800) 777-8103] also uses free amino acids for its protein source. The drawbacks to these formulas are that they are expensive, usually taste awful, and contain artificial ingredients to which a person could react to. The advantage is that almost all people can tolerate them and are able to maintain weight, (this is especially important in growing children and patients who are of low body weight. Other alternatives include hydrolyzed protein products such as Medipro® (Thorne Research (800)228-1966), or Ultraclear® (800)692-9400. These formulations are usually broken down into tripeptides and for the most part are well tolerated . They are usually quite acceptable in taste and cheaper than the elemental formulations. The disadvantage is that they don't have as many calories and supplementary calories need to be added to prevent weight loss if someone is to subsist on these products for long periods of time (> three weeks).

**c) Hypoallergenic diets**–(see p.302-303). The types of food that a person eats on a hypoallergenic diet should be determined by his or her normal diet–whether they are omnivorous, vegetarian, lacto-ovovegetarian, vegan, macrobiotic, or other. The diet should consist of foods the person does not normally eat and which they know they aren't reactive to. Also, the availability of certain foods will determine what can be eaten. Finally, the time of year, location, and what a person's ancestry is should be taken into consideration. Ideally the hypoallergenic diet should be set up so that items in the same food families(pgs 309-311) are **not eaten twice** during the same week (unless they are very weak allergenic foods). If they are eaten the same week, they should be eaten at least 3 days apart

**d) Elimination of one or more food items**–This is a simple technique that involves analyzing the patient's diet diary to see what foods are most frequently eaten. If any food is eaten more than a few times in a week, then the food should be eliminated for one or two weeks. The eliminated foods should be brought back to the diet one at a time. The first reintroduction should be in a small portion. This will show how sensitive the person is to that food. If there is no reaction, the food should be eaten again after 2-3 days without eating it again. This is what I refer to as the "party day." The food being tested should be eaten liberally throughout the day. In this manner the food can be thoroughly evaluated for the degree of sensitivity. If a reaction to the food occurs, especially during the first introduction, it should be avoided for at least 3-6 weeks. Often if a food is a likely allergen, the patient will crave it and will usually be eating it daily several times per day. Patients frequently will complain that they simply can not go more than a few days without eating the food. Conversely, foods that are strongly disliked (especially with children) will often be reactive. It is wise to pay close attention to both cravings and dislikes.

These are a few of the simple techniques that can be employed for the diagnosis as well as treatment of food sensitivities. For most people I prefer the hypoallergenic diet with the reintroduction of foods in a sequential order (see hypoallergenic diets on pgs. 302-303). Foods should be reintroduced one at a time so that they may be evaluated separately. A period of one to 2 weeks avoidence is usually sufficient time to clear food allergens and then evaluate food reactions upon reintroduction. Occasionally it may take as long as 4-8 weeks to notice a change in symptoms, e.g. avoidence of solenacae and arthritis. Also a persons symptoms may not change with avoidence, but they might get significantly worse during reintroduction of the food they were avoiding. This is commonly referred to as the hypersensitive period. Below are additional diagnostic tests which may be employed to evaluate food sensitivities:

2) **Cytotoxic testing**–While the cost of this is moderate, it tends to have many false positives. The results depend largely on subjective observation. However, cytotoxic testing can pick up obscure sensitivities that might otherwise go undetected.

3) **RAST or ELISA testing**–These may not correlate well with real symptoms. While they are convenient to run, they are usually expensive, although in the last 5 years they have come down in cost quite significantly. Blood samples tend to be very stable and antibody detection is not adversely affected by transport of the specimen. Some find this testing to be quite useful.

4) **Electrodiagnosis e.g. Vega, Voll, Intero**–These tests measure subtle sensitivities and may be difficult to verify. Some physicians swear by these tests. The results can be variable. Electrodiagnostic tests are low cost, fairly easy to run, and the results immediate.

5) **Blood typing–**Although not an allergy measurement, it can identitify lectin incompatabilities that other tests may not uncover.

6) **Kinesiology**–Some physicians can work this method quite effectively. The accuracy of the tests depends largely on the skill of the practitioner. Kinesiology is low cost and fairly simple to do.

7) **"Food Intolerance"** This is a more esoteric test that some physicans claim works great. The results are difficult to reproduce and there is no clear mechanism why it works.

8) **DIMSOFT**–This test is not available yet. James Breneman, M.D. has researched the technique of using patches with DMSO. The advantage is that it evaluates many of the different antibodies IgG, IgM, IgG4, IgE, etc.

9) **Comprehensive digestive and stool analysis–**Meridian Labs, Diagnostechs, Great Smokies, and National Biotech.

10) **Secretory Intestinal IgA-** normally there should be high amounts of total sIgA

11) **Intestinal permeability**–Great Smokies or Diagnostechs involves giving fixed amount of 2 simple sugars–lactulose and mannitol. Lactulose has a low permeability. If it appears in the urine in significant amounts, then there is an increase in permeability. Mannitol, on the other hand, is freely absorbable and should appear readily in the urine. If it does not, then there is malabsorption.

STUDY–Annon. *Gastrointiestinal permabiltiy in Food-Allergic children* Nutrition Reviews 43(8): 233-9, 1985. ABSTRACT–Children with allergies were studied and found to have significantly increased intestinal permeability.

12) **Bowel transit time–** take 6 charcoal after evening meal and see how long it takes to have all of the black disappear from the stools. Ideally should be mostly gone by the next day. Black in the stools more than 2 days later is an indication of a delayed transit.

13) **Gastric pH via Heidelberg or Gastro-test-**(see page 18 for description)

14) **Urinary indican–** evaluates fermentation of aromatic amino acids such as tryptophan. Tryptophan, tyrosine and DLPA. These amino acids are acted upon by bacteria which converts the amino acids into indoles. These indoles get absorbed from the large intestine and then travel to the liver to be further metabolized into indican. Once indican is formed it then goes back into the blood where it then gets excreted in the urine.

15) **Chymex–**is used to evaluate maldigestion (see page 20).

16) **Adrenal evaluation–**Adrenal Stress Index Diagnostechs checks salivary cortisol on four separate occasions during a 24 hour period. DHEA levels are also measured.

17) **Microclot test**–measures fermentation in the GI tract and presence of endotoxins. This procedure involves drawing blood and mixing it with a lipoplysaccharide. After incubating for a period of 24 hours a number of microclots will form depending upon how well the liver is clearing endotoxins or how many endotxoins are being produced in the GI tract (Juhlin L & Shelley W *Microclot generation (MCG) test in disease.* ACTA Med Scand. 210:305-307, 1981).

18) **Thyroid-Basal Body Temperatures or Thyroid panel include TSH.**

## IV. Treatment

1) **Start with 3 basic options:**
   a) fasting
   b) elemental diet– ENFOOD® produced by Dr. Gislason in Vancouver, B.C. Canada (604) 270-8474. Tolerex or Vivonex will also work (available from Sandoz Nutrition).
   c) small trial elimination (see hypoallergenic diets).
   d) hypoallergenic diet–Go at least 7 days without suspected food sensitivities or allergies then introduce one food at a time. Introduce a small amount first followed by a larger amount 3 days later. Do not introduce a second time if there is a first time reaction.

2) **Decrease bowel transit time–** Consider bentonite clay, psyllium powder, HCL, magnesium or herbal bitters (see detox chapter on p.485). By decreasing bowel transit time there is less opportunity to absorb allergens from the gut.

3) **Improve digestion–** Eat slowly, chew food well, consider HCL and other digestive enzymes if symptoms are more severe. Food components, if they are broken down more completely, will have less of a chance to cause a reaction in the body.

4) **Improve bowel flora-**balancing gut flora will often decrease reactions toward foods.

5) **Improve resistance to environmental allergens and foods**: Consider some type filtration system or air purifier to reduce body burden of allergens.

6) **Antioxidants** will strengthen cell walls, preventing the release of chemotoxic substances. They will also prevent macromolecules from being absorbed as they tend to decrease intestinal permeability.

a) Vitamin E strengthens cells membranes, has cell membrane tightening properties and stimulates anti-inflammatory activity.

STUDY–Kamimura, M. *Anti-inflammatory activity of vitamin E* J Vitaminology 18(4): 204-9, 1972. ABSTRACT–Volunteers infected with histamine showed far less swelling around the infection site when pretreated with vitamin E for 5-7 days.

b) Selenium–involved in the synthesis of glutathione in the liver

c) Vitamin C acts as a natural antihistaminewith doses greater than 6-8gms.

d) Vitamin A–especially if skin or intestines are involved

e) Quercetin, hesperidin, catechin–all decrease degranulation of mast cells, inhibit lipoxygenase, phospholipase, and phosphodiesterase. Catechin inhibits histamine decarboxylase, the enzyme responsible for the conversion of histidine to histamine.

STUDY–Wendt. *The use of flavonoids as inhibitors of histidine decarboxylase in gastric disease*: Experimental and clinical studies. Naunyn-Schmiedeberg's Arch. Pharm (suppl) 313:238, 1980. ABSTRACT–Patients with urticaria and food allergies who received catechin prior to administration of food antigens were protected from an increase in histamine in the gastric mucosa in response to the antigens.

f) Essential Fatty Acids

7) **Support adrenal function**–Stress management, vitamin C, pantothenic acid and glandulars can all have positive effects on the adrenals. It is also important that the patient engages in physical activity and has some exposure to a natural environment (trees, water, mountains, negative ions, etc.).

Below is my favorite recipe for waffles in treating the allergically sensitive individual. If there are sensitivities to soy or corn these flours can be left out of the recipe. If some one has a total grain sensitivity the brown rice and corn flours can be substituted with another flour such as amaranth, buckwheat, or Teff.

***DR.MARZ WHEATLESS, GLUTENLESS & DAIRYLESS WAFFLES***

**ingredients**:

| | |
|---|---|
| 2/3 c Quinoa flour | *2 eggs yolks (Optional) |
| 2/3 c Brown Rice flour | 2 c soy or rice milk |
| 2/3 c Soy flour | 1 T vanilla |
| 1/3 c corn meal | 1/8 c canola oil or saffl oil |
| 1/2 t salt | 2 egg whites whipped (optional ) |
| chopped walnuts (optional) | 2t non AL bake powder |

**Directions**-Mix the dry ingredients well. Ideally they can be sifted. In another bowl beat 2 egg yolks, the soy milk, oil and the vanilla with a whisk or beater. Gradually mix in the dry ingredients. Lastly blend in the whipped egg whites and walnuts. Lightly oil up the waffle iron. Make sure the waffle iron is hot before you put the batter on! Top with fruit and maple syrup. Other types of milks that may be used are coconut, almond, cashew, walnut or other low allergy type drink. Access to a Vita-mix® food processor (800)848-2348 may be extremely helpful in making a wide variety of nut-milks.

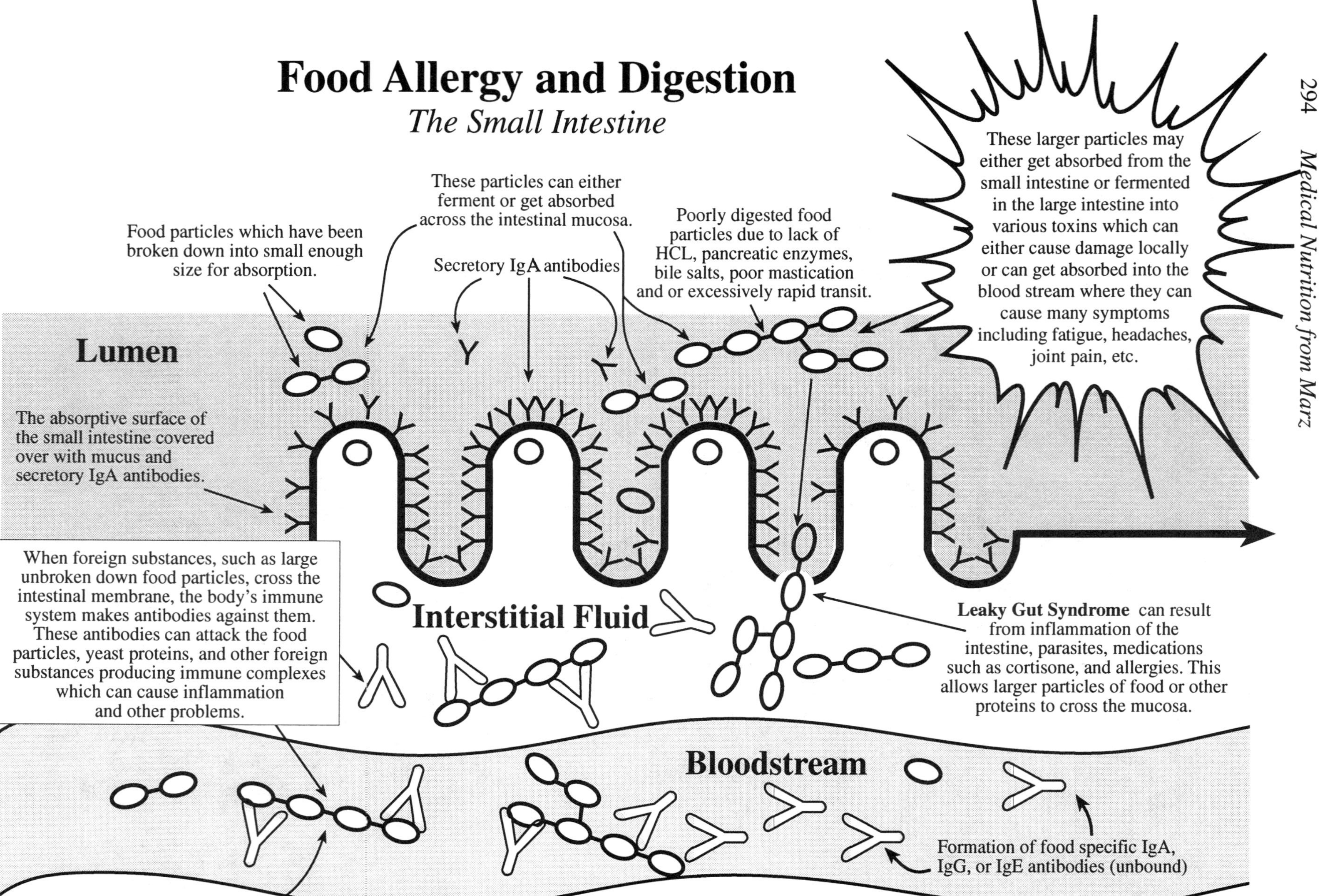
Food Allergy and Digestion
The Small Intestine
Food particles which have been broken down into small enough size for absorption.
These particles can either ferment or get absorbed across the intestinal mucosa.
Secretory IgA antibodies
Poorly digested food particles due to lack of HCL, pancreatic enzymes, bile salts, poor mastication and or excessively rapid transit.
These larger particles may either get absorbed from the small intestine or fermented in the large intestine into various toxins which can either cause damage locally or can get absorbed into the blood stream where they can cause many symptoms including fatigue, headaches, joint pain, etc.
Lumen
The absorptive surface of the small intestine covered over with mucus and secretory IgA antibodies.
When foreign substances, such as large unbroken down food particles, cross the intestinal membrane, the body's immune system makes antibodies against them. These antibodies can attack the food particles, yeast proteins, and other foreign substances producing immune complexes which can cause inflammation and other problems.
Interstitial Fluid
Leaky Gut Syndrome can result from inflammation of the intestine, parasites, medications such as cortisone, and allergies. This allows larger particles of food or other proteins to cross the mucosa.
Bloodstream
Formation of food specific IgA, IgG, or IgE antibodies (unbound)
Food-Immune Complexes
Composed of food-specific IgA, IgG and/or IgE antibodies, if not cleared from circulation, may deposit in tissues and initiate a host of allergic responses.
adapted from Nutritional Dietetics; Percival & Yevka

## Food Allergies and Mast cell reactions

Allergy reactions mediated by mast cells occur everywhere in the body. Mast cells line the entire digestive tract, all the mucus membranes of the mouth, throat, nose and lungs, along blood vessels and in the skin. When an allergen is encountered, antibodies get produced which then bind to the outside of the mast cells. Mast cells, that have antibodies attached to them become "sensitized." Mast cells that have become sensitized to foods, pollens or other chemicals, can react by degranulating and releasing histamine, leukotrienes, SRSA, serotonin and various other inflammatory mediators. In addition, the arachidonic acid, which makes up the cell membrane of the mast cells, gets used as substrate for further production of inflammatory leukotrienes. In the case of a blood vessel it reacts by dilating, thus forming a hive. In the head it can trigger migraine headaches. In the gastrointestinal tract it can cause an increased permeability as evidenced by the leaky gut phenomenon. Such reactions specifically depend upon sensitized mast cells and how easily they degranulate. Furthermore the level of arachidonic acid in the cell membranes of the mast cells also determines the level of added inflammation that can be mediated by 4 series leukotrienes.

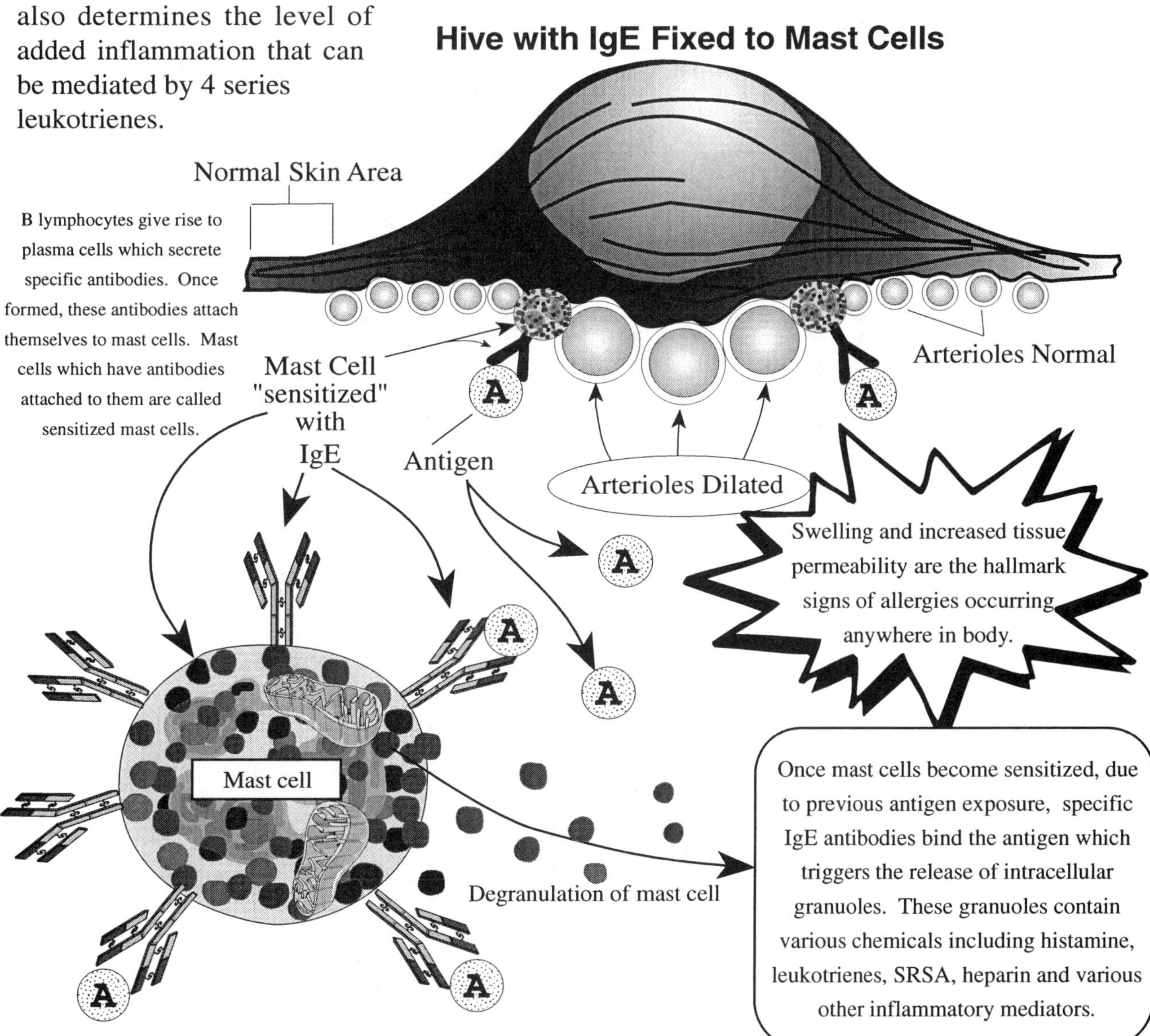

## Reactions to Foods and Their Timing

Below is a table adapted from Basics of Food Allergies, by Dr. James Breneman, that correlates allergic reactions with common offenders along with the frequency of the time interval between when the food is eaten and when the symptoms start to appear. One can see that some reactions such as heartburn may occur very shortly after eating a particular food offender and other reactions may not present for days. These reactions can be very difficult to assess and often go incorrectly diagnosed. Unless there is some suspicion and some type of thorough evaluation, such reactions can be ascribed to many things other than the real cause.

| | 30 min | 60 min | 2 hrs | 3 hrs | 6 hrs | 12 hrs | 24 hrs | 36 hrs | 48 hrs | 72 hrs | 96 hrs |
|---|---|---|---|---|---|---|---|---|---|---|---|
| Heartburn | *** | **** | *** | *** | * | coffee, wine, tomato sauce, citrus, beer, banana, apple | | | | | |
| Rhinorrhea | * | **** | *** | ** | ** | * | milk, cheese, wheat, corn, MSG, wine, beer, chocolate | | | | |
| Abdominal Cramps | ** | *** | *** | *** | **** | *** | * | milk, cheese, gluten, nuts, apples, coffee, pork | | | |
| Headaches | * | ** | *** | **** | *** | ** | coffee, cola, chocolate, nuts, MSG, foods containing tyramin, sucrose, simple sugars | | | | |
| Fatigue | *** | ** | * | ** | *** | **** | **** | simple sugars, milk, cheese, chocolate, wheat | | | |
| Gallbladder | * | *** | **** | *** | *** | | | egg, milk, onion, chicken, beef | | | |
| Colic | | | | | | | | pork | | | |
| Urticaria | * | *** | * | | | | | fish, shrimp, egg, peanut, chocolate | | | |
| Delayed Urticaria | egg, soy, corn | | | | *** | **** | **** | | | | |
| Migraine | | ** | * | | *** | **** | *** | chocolate, coffee, soy, corn nuts, cola, MSG | | | |
| Enuresis | | | | * | *** | ** | * | simple sugars, pop, milk, corn, egg, wheat | | | |
| Edema | | | | | * | ** | **** | ** | * | milk, dairy | |
| Seisures | | | | | * | ** | **** | ** | * | | |
| Diarrhea | * | ** | ** | ** | ** | *** | **** | *** | chocolate, eggs, dairy, wheat | | |
| Mental Confusion | * | ** | | | * | ** | **** | ** | * | | |
| Skeletal Cramps | | | | | | * | ** | *** | *** | **** | * |
| Aphthous Ulcers | gluten, citrus, sugars, apples, chocolate | | | | | * | ** | *** | *** | **** | *** |
| Joint Pains | wheat, coffee, meat, many foods | | | | | * | ** | *** | **** | * | |
| Gout | meat | | | | * | * | ** | *** | *** | *** | |
| | 30 min | 60 min | 2 hrs | 3 hrs | 6 hrs | 12 hrs | 24 hrs | 36 hrs | 48 | 72 hrs | 96 hrs |

**Note**–The foods listed across from the symptom or pathological condition are some of the more common causes of them. Certainly they are not the only foods or substances that can trigger such reactions as many environmental pollutants or toxic exposures can also trigger the same symptoms. The number of *'s displayed across from each of the pathologies represents the frequency with which the symptoms may appear after eating that food. Again this can be very variable in individuals and this table should just be used as a guide.

# Food Sources of Sulfites

**Alcoholic &non-alcoholic Drinks**: Wine, beer, cocktail mixes, wine coolers, most distilled liquors (sulfites are only required to be listed if they are found in concentrations of over 10ppm or greater). Drinks containing sugar and or corn syrup, dried citrus fruit beverage mixes, all canned, bottled or frozen fruit juices.

**Baked Goods**: Bread with dough conditioners, cookies, crackers, crepes, mixes with dried fruits or vegetables, pie crust, pizza crust, quiche crust, soft pretzels, tortillas and tortilla shells, waffles.

**Condiments**:
Horseradish, onion and pickle relishes, pickles, olives, salad dressing mixes, wine vinegar.

**Junk Foods:**
Frostings; all canned or packaged frosting mixes, puddings, fillings: fruit fillings, flavored and unflavored gelatin, pectin, jelling agents, hard candies: all clear hard candy, refined sugar: all sugars including brown, white, powdered an raw, dried fruit snacks, potato chips, tortilla chips, filled crackers and trail mixes.

**Dairy Product Analogs:**
All processed "cheese foods" containing filled milk (skim milk enriched in fat content by addition of vegetable oils).

**Dried Vegetables and fruits**: Chives, parsley, herbs, and spices, processed fruits, all dried fruit, including raisins, prunes, canned, bottled or frozen fruit, maraschino cherries, glazed fruit.

**Fish and Shellfish (Fresh and frozen):**
Shrimp, scallops, clams, lobster, crab, dried cod and salmon.

**Grain Products and Pasta**: Cornstarch, modified food starch, spinach pasta, gravies, hominy, breading, batters, noodle rice mixes.

**Fruits (fresh & dried):**
All dried fruits, grapes, fresh cut potatoes (as delivered to restaurants). Sulfur dioxide is used as fungicide on grapes.

**Jams and Jellies:**
All

**Nuts and Nut Products:**
Shredded coconut

**Plant protein products:**
Soy protein products including tofu, textured vegetable protein, and infant formula.

*Information compiled by Judith Campbell. Sources*

*1. "Sulfites: FDA Limits Uses, Broadens Labeling" (FDA Consumer, October 1986).*

*2."Guide to Sulfited Foods" (Center for Science in the Public Interest).*

# Introduction to Solid Foods

The introduction to solid foods in the infant has changed dramatically over the years. Most likely thousands of years ago the introduction of solid foods was something that mom did quite naturally. There were probably many factors that influenced her decision of when and what foods to introduce first but probably she relied on her intuition. Certainly she picked up some cues from the baby such as the baby cutting a few teeth, or the baby looking very interested in the food that the parents were eating and grabbing and crying out for such food. Over the years our spinal tumor the brain has come to alter what we knew intuitively years ago. At the turn of the century 99% of all moms, in the U.S., were breast feeding. By the 1950's and 60's this percentage dropped to about 20% of moms. This is certainly unfortunate since this change has led to an increase in morbidity and mortality in infancy especially concerning the development of food allergies. Bottle fed infants have about twice the rate of diarrhea as compared to breast fed ones. This irritation to the gastrointestinal tract causes an increase in the permeability of the intestines and, depending upon the type of foods that are being ingested, can trigger the body adversely react.

If there is a strong family history of food allergies or sensitivities it makes more sense to wait as long as possible before starting solid foods. It is best to first introduce low allergen foods' one at a time and gradually work up to the higher allergen foods. Introducing pureed fresh fruit is a good introduction to solid foods because of the ease of digestion. Ideally you should add foods' one at a time and wait 2-3 days before introducing a new food. Following fruits, steamed vegetables should be added into the diet next. Any adverse reaction should be monitored for and then reevaluated again in a week to confirm the food's reactivity. If an infant reacts to a food a second time, it should then be eliminated for 4-6 weeks before trying it again.

Mark Percival, D.C., N.D. in his handy little book, "Infant Nutrition" 2nd edition 1997, does a nice job going into details on how to prepare foods to maximize nutrients using whole foods including pits, seeds and skins of foods. By pureeing or liquefying all food parts, using a Vitamix® food processor (800)848-2348 or other comparable food processor, the infant can maximize their intake of all the nutrients found in foods. He also goes into detail on introducing solid foods and being aware of food reactions. This book is a valuable little addition to the science of food introduction for the infant. [Order # (800)348-1549].

There is considerable debate over supplementation of certain nutrients, specifically iron, zinc and Vitamin D in exclusively breast fed infants. Generally speaking iron is stored in the liver of the infant for an indefinite period. Most infants are probably iron replete until the age of 6 months. Past 6 months iron supplies steadily decline to very low levels unless foods with iron are consumed by the infant. Even though human milk is a rather poor source of iron, its absorption rate is much higher (50%) than that of iron-fortified formulas (4%) and cow's milk (10%). More recent studies have shown that iron from human milk may be absorbed up to 80-90%! It may be that the infant's body does not want to have high levels of iron since this might compromise their immune system. At higher levels iron has been found to inhibit the immune system and even promotes the growth of pathogenic bacteria. It is known that bottle fed infants have a higher rate of intestinal pathologies, including enterocolitis.

Zinc, like iron, is a mineral that has a greater absorptive rate in human milk than cow's milk or formula. It is believed that in human milk the zinc binds onto carriers such as picolinate, citric acid and certain proteins. Furthermore the level of zinc in human milk is very dependent upon the mom's intake. I thus strongly recommend for lactating mom's to supplement zinc (25-50mg/day).

## Schedule for the introduction of solid food in the allergic infant

**6-8 months (Wait until infant is very interested in solid foods or when first teeth are coming in).**

Iron containing foods that are low allergy foods to start infant on

| Highest Fe Levels | Moderate/high Fe | Medium (1.1-1.4) | Significant (from 1.0 to 0.3mg/serv) | |
|---|---|---|---|---|
| Swiss chard | Kale | Collard greens | Endive | Banana |
| Dulse | Pumpkin seeds | Beet greens | Green beans | Rasperries |
| Mustard greens | Spinach | Figs | Parsley | Blackberries |
| Dandelion greens | Broccoli | Raisins | Kelp | Apple sauce |
| Leeks | Pumpkin | Lambs quarters | Leaf lettuce | Mung bean sprout |
| Apricots | Peas | Prunes | Blueberries | Artichoke (Jerus.) |

**9-12 months**

Iron containing foods that are more complex allergy foods to follow the 6-8 month foods

| Highest Fe Levels for all of these foods listed | | | These are safe foods with low Fe & Zn | |
|---|---|---|---|---|
| Molasses, black | Lima beans | Pinto beans | Peaches | Pears |
| Amaranth | Potato, baked white | | Grapes | Cherries |
| | | | Carrots | Squash, all types |
| | | | Cauliflower | Cabbage |
| | | | Papaya | Pineapple |

**9-12 months** (Infant should be active and the need for foods high in zinc are critical for immunity).

Zinc containing foods that are relatively easy to digest but becoming more complex

| Highest Zn Levels | Moderate/high Zn | Medium | Significant |
|---|---|---|---|
| Colostrum | Mustard greens | Quinoa | |
| Swiss chard | Kidney beans | Human milk | |
| Lima beans | Peas, dried | | |
| Potato, white | Leeks | | |

**12-15 months** (Infant should be very active and cutting molars).

Foods containing significant amounts of protein

| Highest % protein | Moderate/high Pro | Medium % protein | Significant to low levels protein |
|---|---|---|---|
| Mung bean sprout | Quinoa | Spinach | White rice |
| Tofu | Amaranth | Kale | Corn |
| Lentils | Buckwheat | Broccoli | |
| Split peas | Garbonzo beans | Brussel Sprouts | |
| Pumpkin seeds | Potato, white | Teff | |
| Goats milk | Soy milks | Chicken (high) | |
| Tuna & fish small | | | |

**15-18 months** (Infant should be very active, cutting molars and be more able to chew).

Foods containing significant amounts of more complex protein

| Highest % protein | Moderate/high Pro | Medium % protein |
|---|---|---|
| Fish larger amts. | Oatmeal | Barley |
| Meats, red (high) | | |

**18-24 months** (These foods are the most difficult to digest and should be tried cautiously).

| | | |
|---|---|---|
| Egg | Rye | Wheat |
| Yogurt (cow's) | Yeast | |
| Cashew butter | Walnuts | |

# LOFFLER -WRIGHT INFANT FORMULA

Ingredients:

1 quart whole soy milk Eden Soy Extra (fortified)
1 cup carrot juice
2 teaspoons cod liver oil (Carlson Labs) or 1 gm pure DHA –Pure Encapsulations
1 teaspoon flax oil
2 capsules borage oil (240 mg GLA per capsule)
3 Tablespoons pure maple syrup
1 Tablespoon barley green or spirulina (optional for formula but need source of vitamin B-12; can use HydroxyFolate from Scientific Botanicals (2 drops per day=400mcg B-12 and 400mcg folate)
1 Tablespoon molasses
L-Carnitine 500mg (use especially in premature infants)
Can add vitamin K drops (Scientific botanicals, 1 drop = 21/2 mg phytonadione)

This formula should be made up daily. Since it oxidizes rapidly it is best to store in an airtight container in the refrigerator. Only make up a day supply. This formula can be made frozen in which case it can be stored up to one month or so.

The following modifications can be made in the formulation:

If the infant is sensitive to soy can use Almond milk. It should be noted that the almond milk does not have the same protein content of soy and if the infant is going to be solely on this formula a protein powder should be added to the formulation. In addition, Borage or Evening Primrose oil can be added as a source of gamma linolenic acid. Human milk has significant amounts of GLA and may be required for the synthesis of certain hormones.

Other modifications can be made to the formula if the infant is premature or has poor or delayed muscle development. In particular **carnitine** is critical for the oxidation of fatty acids. Human milk contains 50-100nmol/ml compared to soy based formulas who only have 4nmol/ml. Newborns have a very limited ability to synthesize carnitine, especially premature ones.

Another modification that can be made in the formula is the addition of DHA (Docosahexaenoic acid) is very critical for visual acuity and brain development. Infants fed formulas that were devoid of these essential fatty acids showed significantly slower brain development and less visual acuity than infants and toddlers who had these essential oils. These oils are found in significant amounts in breast milk, but depends upon Mom's intake of omega 3 fatty acids. Many countries in Europe and Asia require DHA be added to infant formulas. The FDA is currently considering this ingredient to be required in infant formulas in the U.S. but there is strong opposition by infant formula manufacturers.

2 excellent references concerning infant care and feeding.

*The Baby Book: Everything You Need to Know About Your Baby–From Birth to Age Two* by William Sears, MD, and Martha Sears, RN, Little, Brown and Company, New York, 1993.
Infant Nutrition" 2nd edition Mark Percival, D.C., N.D.,1997

## Comparison of LWM Milk (p.300) with Colostrum, Mature Human Milk, and ProSobee with RDAs

amounts listed are found in 1000cc (1 liter) of milk

| | Type | Kcal | Pro gm | fat gm | linoleic mg | linolenic & DHA mg | GLA mg | lactose | B carotene mg | vit A RE | vit D mg | vit E TE | vit K mg | vit C mg | vit B-1 mg | vit B-2 mg | vit B-3 mg | vit B-5 mg | vit B-6 mg | vit B 12 mg | Folate mg | Ca mg | Mg | Fe mg | Zn mg | I mg | Sel mcg | Na mg | K mg |
|---|---|---|---|---|---|---|---|---|---|---|---|---|---|---|---|---|---|---|---|---|---|---|---|---|---|---|---|---|---|
| | colo-strum | 580 | 23 | 29 | 1150 | 2100 | ? | 55 | 1.11 | 719 | --- | 13 | 2 | 44 | .15 | .25 | .7 | 1.8 | .12 | 2 mg | -- | 267 | 34 | .45 | 5.6 | 12 | --- | 450 | 740 |
| | mature human milk | 700 | 9 | 42gm 54% | 1300 | 600 & 630 | 100 | 73 gm | .23 | 470 RE | .4 mcg | 3.2 mg | 2 | 40 mg | .16 mg | .35 mg | 2 mg | 2.3 mg | .28 mg | .26 mg | 52 | 280 mg | 30 mg | .4 mg | 1.7 mg | 70 | 20 | 150 | 580 |
| | LWM milk | 910 | 39 | 26 | 800 | 3600 & 450 | 480 | -- | 1391 | 4000 | 62 | 3.0 | ? 2.5 mg | 55 | .9 | .6 | 7.8 | .47 | 1.56 | 6.0 | 68 | 780 | 268 | 9.4 | 3.9 | ? | ? | 380 | 3400 |
| | ProSobee | 640 | 19 | 34 | lots | small amts | -- | -- | ---- | 47 | 9.6 | 13 | 50 | 77 | .5 | .58 | 6.4 | 3.2 | .38 | 1.9 | .1 | 620 | 72 | 11.5 | 7.7 | 96 | 18 | 256 | 768 |
| RDA | 0.5-1.0 | | 13 | | | | | | | 375 | 7.5 | 3.0 | 5 | 30 | .3 | .4 | 5 | none ~.3 | .3 | .3 | 25 | 400 | 40 | 6 | 5 | 40 | 10 | ~ 500 | -- |
| Child | 1-3 | | 16 | | | | | | | 375 | 10 | 6 | 15 | 40 | .7 | .8 | 9 | | 1 | .7 | 50 | 800 | 80 | 10 | 10 | 70 | 20 | | |
| | 4-6 | | 24 | | | | | | | 500 | 10 | 7 | 20 | 45 | .9 | 1.1 | 12 | | 1.1 | 1.0 | 75 | 800 | 120 | 10 | 10 | 90 | 20 | | |

Newborns feed every 2-4 hours and ingest 12-24 ounces of milk at each feeding. The first fews days of human milk is colostrum, which is a thicker and has some specialized nutrients such as secretory IgA, GLA, DHA, and carnitine. The fat content of human milk is considerably higher than cow's milk which has much more calcium and phosphorus. It should be noted that newborn calves walk immediately whereas human newborns take many months to walk. Instead they have a very high requirement for essential fatty acids particularly omega 3 fatty acids such as DHA. This DHA level in human milk is dependant upon the level of ingestion by mom (see p.538).

**HYPOALLERGENIC DIET VEGETARIAN** **NAME:**________________

| MONDAY | TUESDAY | WEDNESDAY | THURSDAY | FRIDAY | SATURDAY | SUNDAY |
|---|---|---|---|---|---|---|
| Watermelon | Pears | Pineapple or Papaya | Peaches or Plums | Kiwi Fruit | Strawberries or Raspberries | Blueberries or Figs |
| | | ••••••••• drink plenty of water | | ••••••••• | | |
| Sweet Potato (baked) and Pecans | Cream of Brown Rice and Brown Rice Syrup | Steamed Squash and carrots and Lentils | Rice Cakes and Cashew Butter | Buckwheat, Peas, Onions and Toasted Sesame Oil | Oatmeal and Banana | Spli Pea Soup and Vegetables: steamed zucchini, acorn squash, green beans, etc. |
| | | ••••••••• drink plenty of water | | ••••••••• | | |
| Quinoa and Steamed Broccoli | Mixed Salad Greens with Kidney Beans and Lemon | Amaranth and Zucchini | Beets and Spinach | Millet and Steamed Spinach | Beans of choice: black beans, pintos, red, etc. & Wild Rice | Brown Rice, Steamed Peas & Toasted Sesame Oil |

SPECIAL INSTRUCTIONS;

1: Use only SEA SALT as a spice.

2: Drink only spring, filtered or distilled water.

3: Use only fresh vegetables and fruits, ideally organic. Frozen is next best.

4: If you must switch meals around it is best to switch the entire day.

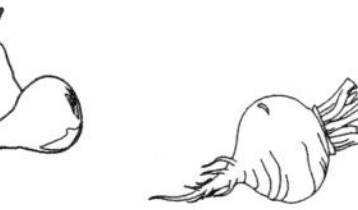

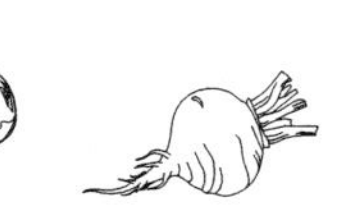

Notes: During the 2nd or 3rd week you may start the vegetable broth from Paavo Airola's book *How to Get Well*. This broth can be altered somewhat to suit the individual. Care must still be taken to observe possible allergens being used for the broth.

**HYPOALLERGENIC DIET OMNIVOROUS** NAME:__________

| MONDAY | TUESDAY | WEDNESDAY | THURSDAY | FRIDAY | SATURDAY | SUNDAY |
|---|---|---|---|---|---|---|
| Watermelon | Pears | Pineapple or Papaya | Peaches or Plums | Kiwi Fruit | Strawberries or Raspberries | Blueberries or Figs |
| | | drink plenty of water | | | | |
| Sweet Potato (baked) and Pecans | Cream of Brown Rice and Brown Rice Syrup | Steamed Squash and Lentils | Rice Cakes and Almond Butter | Buckwheat, Peas, Cashews, and Toasted Sesame Oil (sauté buckwheat groats and cashews in sesame oil for 5-10 min. add peas then steam with 2x as much water for 10 min. - do not stir while steaming - turn over & serve) | Oatmeal and Banana | Tuna and Carrots |
| | | drink plenty of water | | | | |
| Salmon and Steamed Broccoli | Cod and Asparagus (if wild game such as elk, deer or buffalo is available can substitute for fish) | Lamb and Zuchini | Baked Halibut and Spinach | Flounder and Steamed Spinach | Chicken and Wild Rice | Shrimp, Brown Rice, Steamed Peas & Toasted Sesame Oil |

SPECIAL INSTRUCTIONS;

1: Use only SEA SALT as a spice.

2: Drink only spring, filtered or distilled water.

3: Use only fresh vegetables and fruits, ideally organic. Frozen is next best.

4: If you must switch meals around it is best to switch the entire day.

Notes:

The following food lists, from pages 304-311, have been arranged alphabetically as well as by food families. The first list of foods is listed by family. The second list of foods, starting on page 306, lists individual foods aphabetically with a number preceding it. This number corresponds to the list of food families that begins below. In constructing a Rotary Diversified Diet these lists are essential in avoiding eating foods from the same family group in a repetative way. The listing below was adapted from *Coping with Your Allergies* by Natalie Golos and Francis Golos, Simon and Schuster, 1979. The original information was taken from *Clinical Ecology* by Lawrence D. Dickey, 1976, "The Rotary Diet and Taxonomy" pgs. 122-148.

## Food Families Numerical list 1

1 Algae
- agar-agar
- carrageenan (Irish Moss)
- *dulse
- kelp (seaweed)

2 Fungi
- baker's yeast "Red Star"
- brewer's or
  - nutritional yeast
- mold (in certain cheeses)
  - citric acid (Aspergilus)
- morel
- mushroom
- puffball
- truffle

3 Horsetail Family
- *shavegrass (horsetail)

4 Cycad Family
- Florida arrowroot

5 Conifer Family
- *juniper (gin)
- pine nut

6 Grass Family
- barley
  - malt
  - maltose
- bamboo shoots
- corn (mature)
  - corn meal
  - corn oil
  - cornstarch
  - corn syrup
  - hominy grits
  - popcorn
- Kamut
- lemon grass
  - citronella
- millet
- oat
  - oatmeal
- rice
  - rice flour
- rye
- spelt
- sorghum grain
  - syrup
- sugarcane
  - cane sugar
  - molasses
  - raw sugar
- sweet corn

grass family continued
- triticale
- wheat
  - bran
  - bulgar
  - flour
    - gluten
    - graham
    - patent
    - whole wheat
  - wheat germ
- wild rice

7 Sedge Family
- Chinese water chestnut
- chufa (groundnut)

8 Palm Family
- coconut
  - coconut meal
  - coconut oil
- date
  - date sugar
- palm cabbage
- sago starch

9 Arum Family
- ceriman
- dasheen
  - arrowroot
- taro
  - poi
- malanga
- yautia

10 Pineapple Family
- pineapple

11 Lily Family
- *Aloe vera*
- asparagus
- chives
- garlic
- leek
- onion
- ramp
- *sarsaparilla
- shallot
- yucca (soap plant)

12 Amaryllis Family
- agave
  - mescal, pulque, tequila

13 Tacca Family
- Fiji arrowroot

14 Yam Family
- Chinese potato (yam)
- ñame (yampi)

15 Iris Family
- orris root (scent)
- saffron *(Crocus)*

16 Banana Family
- arrowroot
- banana
- plantain

17 Ginger Family
- cardamon
- East Indian arrowroot
- ginger
- turmeric

18 Canna Family
- Queensland arrowroot

19 Arrowroot Family
- arrowroot

20 Orchid Family
- vanilla

21 Pepper Family
- peppercorn
  - black pepper
  - white pepper

22 Walnut Family
- black walnut
- butternut
- English walnut
- heartnut
- hickory nut
- pecan

23 Birch Family
- filbert (hazelnut)
- birch oil (wintergreen)
  - (some wintergreen flavor is methylsalicylate)

24a Eragrostis
- Teff *(gluten free)*

24 Beech Family
- chestnut
- chinquapin

25 Mulberry Family
- breadfruit
- fig
- *hop
- mulberry

26 Protea Family
- macadamia

27 Buckwheat Family
- buckwheat *(gluten free)*
- garden sorrel
- rhubarb
- sea grape

28 Goosefoot Family
- quinoa *(gluten free)*
- beet
- chard
- lamb's-quarters
- spinach
- sugar beet
- tampala

29 Carpetweed Family
- New Zealand spinach

30 Purslane Family
- amaranth *(gluten free)*
- pigweed (purslane)

31 Buttercup Family
- *goldenseal

32 Custard-Apple Family
- *Annona* species
- custard-apple
- papaw (pawpaw)

33 Nutmeg Family
- nutmeg
  - mace

34 Laurel Family
- avocado
- bay leaf
- cassia bark
- cinnamon
- *sassafras
  - filé (powdered leaves)

35 Poppy Family
- poppyseed

36 Mustard Family
- broccoli
- Brussels sprouts
- cabbage
- cardoon
- cauliflower
- Chinese cabbage
- collards
- colza shoots
- couve tronchuda
- curly cress
- horseradish
- kale
- kohlrabi
- mustard greens
- mustard seed
- radish
- rape
- rutabaga (swede)
- turnip
- puland cress
- watercress

37 Caper Family
- caper

38 Bixa Family
- annatto (yellow dye)

39 Saxifrage Family
- currant
- gooseberry

40 Rose Family
- a. *pomes*
  - applecider
    - vinegar
    - pectin
  - crabapple
  - loquat
  - pear
  - quince
  - *rosehips
- b. *stone fruits*
  - almond
  - apricot
  - cherry
  - peach (nectarine)
  - plum (prune)
  - sloe
- c. *berries*
  - blackberry
  - boysenberry
  - dewberry
  - loganberry
  - longberry
  - youngberry
  - *raspberry (leaf)
    - black raspberry
    - red raspberry
    - purple raspberry
  - *strawberry (leaf)
    - wineberry
- d. *herb*
  - burnet (cucumber flavor)

41 Legume Family
*alfalfa (sprouts)
beans
fava
lima
mung (sprouts)
navy
string (kidney)
black-eyed pea
(cowpea)
*carob
carob syrup
chickpea (garbanzo)
*fenugreek
gum acacia
gum tragacanth
jicama
kudzu
lentil
*licorice
pea
peanut
peanut oil
*red clover
*senna
soybean
lecithin
soy flour
soy grits
soy milk
soy oil
tamarind
tonka bean
coumarin
42 Oxalis Family
carambola
oxalis
43 Nasturtium Family
nasturtium
44 Flax Family
*flaxseed
45 Rue (Citrus) Family
citron
grapefruit
kumquat
lemon
lime
murcot
orange
pummelo
tangelo
tangerine
46 Malpighia Family
acerola (Barbados cherry)
47 Spurge Family
cassava or yuca
cassava meal
tapioca (Brazilian
arrowroot)
castor bean
castor oil
48 Cashew Family
cashew
mango
pistachio
poison ivy
poison oak
poison sumac
49 Holly Family
maté (yerba maté)
50 Maple Family
maple sugar
maple syrup
51 Soapberry Family
litchi (lychee)
52 Grape Family
grape
brandy
champagne
cream of tartar
dried "currant"
raisin
wine
wine vinegar
muscadine
53 Linden Family
*basswood (linden)
54 Mallow Family
*althea root
cottonseed oil
*hibiscus (roselle)
okra
55 Sterculia Family
*chocolate (cacao)
*cocoa
cocoa butter
cola nut
56 Dillenia Family
Chinese gooseberry
(kiwi berry)
57 Tea Family
*tea
58 Passion Flower Family
granadilla (passion fruit)
59 Papaya Family
papaya
60 Cactus Family
prickly pear
61 Pomegranate Family
pomegranate
grenadine
62 Sapucaya Family
Brazil nut
sapucaya nut
(paradise nut)
63 Myrtle Family
allspice
clove
*eucalyptus
guava
64 Ginseng Family
*American ginseng
*Chinese ginseng
65 Carrot Family
angelica
anise
caraway
carrot
carrot syrup
celeriac (celery root)
*seed & leaf
chervil
coriander
cumin
dill
dill seed
*fennel
finocchio
Florence fennel
*gotu kola
*lovage
*parsley
parsnip
sweet cicely
66 Heath Family
*bearberry
*blueberry
cranberry
*huckleberry
67 Sapodilla Family
chicle (chewing gum)
68 Ebony Family
American persimmon
kaki (Japanese persimmon)
69 Olive Family
olive (green or ripe)
olive oil
70 Morning-Glory Family
sweet potato
71 Borage Family
(Herbs)
borage
*comfrey (leaf & root)
72 Verbena Family
*lemon verbena
73 Mint Family
apple mint
basil
bergamot
*catnip
*chia seed
clary
*dittany
*horehound
*hyssop
lavender
*lemon balm
marjoram
oregano
*pennyroyal
*peppermint
rosemary
sage
*spearmint
summer savory
thyme
winter savory
74 Potato Family (solanaceae)
eggplant
ground cherry
pepino
(melon pear)
pepper (Capsicum)
bell, sweet
cayenne
chili
paprika
pimiento
potato
tobacco
tomatillo
tomato
tree tomato
75 Pedalium Family
sesame seed
sesame oil
tahini
76 Madder Family
*woodruff
77 Honeysuckle Family
elderberry
elderberry flowers
78 Valerian Family
corn salad (fetticus)
79 Gourd Family
chayote
Chinese preserving
melon
cucumber
gherkin
loofah (*Luffa*)
(vegetable sponge)
muskmelons
cantaloupe
casaba
crenshaw
honeydew
Persian melon
pumpkin
pumpkin seed &
meal
squashes
acorn
buttercup
butternut
Boston marrow
caserta
cocozelle
crookneck &
straightneck
cushaw
golden nugget
Hummard varieties
pattypan
turban
vegetable spaghetti
zucchini
watermelon
80 Composite Family
*boneset
*burdock root
cardoon
chamomile
*chicory
coltsfoot
costmary
dandelion
endive
escarole
globe artichoke
*goldenrod
Jerusalem artichoke
artichoke flour
lettuce
celtuce
pyrethrum
romaine
safflower oil
salsify (oyster plant)
santolina (herb)
scolymus
(Spanish oyster plant)
scorzonera
(black salsify)
southernwood
sunflower
sunflower seed,
meal, & oil
tansy (herb)
tarragon (herb)
witloof chicory
(French endive)
wormwood
(absinthe)
*yarrow

**ANIMAL FAMILIES**

81 *Mollusks*
Gastropods
abalone
snail
Cephalopod
squid
Pelecypods
clam
cockly
mussel
oyster
scallop
82 *Crustaceans*
crab
crayfish
lobster
prawn
shrimp
83 ***Fishes (saltwater)***
84 Herring Family
menhaden
pilchard (sardine)
sea herring
85 Anchovy Family
anchovy
86 Eel Family
American eel
87 Codfish Family
cod (scrod)
cusk
haddock
hake
pollack
88 Sea Catfish Family
ocean catfish
89 Mullet Family
mullet
90 Silverside Family
silverside (whitebait)
91 Sea Bass Family
grouper
sea bass
92 Tilefish Family
tilefish
93 Bluefish Family
bluefish
94 Jack Family
amberjack
pompano
yellow jack
95 Dolphin Family
dolphin

96 Croaker Family
croaker
drum
sea trout
silver perch
spot
weakfish (spotted sea trout)

97 Porgy Family
northern scup (porgy)

98 Mackerel Family
albacore
bonito
mackerel
skipjack
tuna

99 Marlin Family
marlin
sailfish

100 Swordfish Family
swordfish

101 Harvestfish Family
butterfish
harvestfish

102 Scorpionfish Family
rosefish (ocean perch)

103 Flouder Family
dab
flounder
halibut
plaice
sole
turbot

***104 Fishes (freshwater)***

104 Sturgeon Family
sturgeon (caviar)

105 Herring Family
shad (roe)

106 Salmon Family
salmon species
trout species

107 Whitefish Family
whitefish

108 Smelt Family
smelt

109 Pike Family
muskellunge
pickerel
pike

110 Sucker Family
buffalofish
sucker

111 Minnow Family
carp
chub

112 Catfish Family
catfish species

113 Bass Family
white perch
yellow bass

114 Sunfish Family
black bass species
sunfish species
pumpkinseed
crappie

115 Perch Family
sauger
walleye
yellow perch

116 Croaker Family
freshwater drum

***117 Amphibians***

117 Frog Family
frog (frogs legs)

118 Reptiles

119 Snake Family
rattlesnake

120 Turtle Family
terrapin
turtle species

121 Duck Family
duck
eggs
goose
eggs

122 Dove Family
dove
pigeon (squab)

123 Grouse Family
ruffed grouse (partridge)

124 Pheasant Family
chicken
eggs
peafowl
pheasant
quail

125 Guinea Fowl Family
guinea fowl
eggs

126 Turkey Family
turkey
eggs

***127 Mammals***

128 Opossum Family
opossum

129 Hare Family
rabbit

130 Squirrel Family
squirrel

131 Whale Family
whale

132 Bear Family
bear

133 Horse Family
horse

134 Swine Family
hog (pork)
bacon
ham
lard
pork gelatin
sausage
scrapple

135 Deer Family
caribou
deer (venison)
elk
moose
reindeer

136 Pronghorn Family
antelope

137 Bovine Family
beef cattle
beef
beef by-products
gelatin
oleomargarine
rennin (rennet)
sausage casings
suet
milk products
butter
cheese
ice cream
lactose
spray dried milk
yogurt
veal
buffalo (bison)
goat (kid)
cheese
ice cream
milk
sheep (domestic)
lamb
mutton
Rocky Mountain sheep

## Food Families Listed Alphabetically

Below is an alphabetized list of foods with the number next to the foods corresponding to food family to which that food belongs to (see Food Families pages 304-306).

## Food List Alphabetically list 2

**A**

81 abalone
80 absinthe
41 acacia (gum)
46 acerola
79 acorn squash
1 agar agar
12 agave
98 albacore
41 alfalfa
1 Algae
63 allspice
40b almond
11 *Aloe vera*
54 althea root
28 amaranth
12 Amaryllis Family
94 amberjack
86 American eel
117 Amphibians
85 anchovy
65 angelica
65 anise
38 annatto
138 antelope
40a apple
73 apple mint
40b apricot
47 arrowroot, Brazilian (tapioca)
9 arrowroot (*Colocasia*)
17 arrowroot, East Indian
19 Arrowroot Family
13 arrowroot, Fiji
4 arrowroot, Florida
19 arrowroot (*Maranta* starch)
16 arrowroot (*Musa*)
18 arrowroot, Queensland
80 artichoke flour
9 Arum Family
11 asparagus
2 *Aspergillus*
34 avocado

**B**

2 baker's yeast
6 bamboo shoots
16 banana
16 Banana Family
46 Barbados cherry
6 barley
73 basil
114 bass (black)
113 bass (yellow)
53 basswood
34 bay leaf
41 bean
132 bear
66 bearberry
24 Beech Family
137 beef
28 beet
74 bell pepper
73 bergamot
23 Birch Family
121 birds
38 Bixa Family
114 black bass
40c blackberry
41 black-eyed peas
21 black pepper
80 black salsify
22 black walnut
66 blueberry
93 bluefish
80 boneset
98 bonito
79 Boston marrow
71 borage
71 Borage Family
40c boysenberry
137 Bovine Family
6 bran
52 brandy
47 Brazilian arrowroot
62 Brazil nut
25 breadfruit
2 brewer's yeast
36 broccoli
36 Brussels sprouts
27 buckwheat
27 Buckwheat Family
6 bulgur
80 burdock root
40 burnet
31 Buttercup Family
79 buttercup squash
101 butterfish
22 butternut
79 butternut squash

**C**

36 cabbage
55 cacao
60 Cactus Family
6 cane sugar
18 Canna Family
79 cantaloupe
37 caper
37 Caper Family
74 *Capsicum*
42 carambola
65 caraway seed
17 cardamon
80 cardoon
135 caribou
41 carob
111 carp
29 Carpetweed Family
1 carrageen
65 carrot
65 Carrot Family
79 casaba melon
79 caserta squash
48 cashew
48 Cashew Family
47 cassava
34 cassia bark
47 castor bean
47 castor oil
88 catfish (ocean)
112 catfish species
73 catnip
36 cauliflower
104 caviar
74 cayenne pepper
65 celeriac
65 celery
80 celtuce
9 ceriman
80 chamomile
52 champagne
28 chard
79 chayote
40b cherry
65 chervil
24 chestnut
73 chia seed
124 chicken
41 chickpea
67 chicle
80 chicory
74 chili pepper
36 Chinese cabbage
56 Chinese gooseberry
14 Chinese potato
79 Chinese preserving melon
7 Chinese water chestnut
24 chinquapi
11 chives
55 chocolate
111 chub
7 chufa
40a cider
34 cinnamon
1 citric acid
45 citron
6 citronella
45 citrus Family
81 clam
73 clary
63 clove
41 clover
55 cocoa
55 cocoa butter
8 coconut
79 cocozelle
87 cod (scrod)
76 coffee
55 cola nut
36 collards
80 coltsfoot
36 colza shoots
71 comfrey
80 Composite Family
5 Conifer Family
65 coriander
6 corn
78 corn-salad
80 costmary
54 cottonseed oil
41 coumarin
36 couve tronchuda
41 cowpea
82 crab
40a crabapple
66 cranberry
114 crappie
82 crayfish
52 cream of tartar
79 Crenshaw melon
96 croaker
79 crookneck squash
79 cucumber
65 cumin
36 curly cress
39 currant
79 cushaw squash
87 cusk
32 custard-apple
32 Custard-Apple Family
4 Cycad Family

**D**

103 dab
80 dandelion
9 dasheen
8 date
8 date sugar
135 deer
40c dewberry
65 dill
56 Dillenia Family
73 dittany
95 dolphi
122 dove
52 dried "currant"
96 drum (saltwater)
116 drum (freshwater)
121 duck
1 dulse

**E**

17 East Indian arrowroot
68 Ebony Family
74 eggplant
77 elderberry
135 elk
80 endive
22 English walnut
80 escarole
63 eucalyptus

**F**

41 fava bean
65 fennel
41 fenugreek
78 fetticus
25 fig
13 Fiji arrowroot
23 filbert
34 filé
65 finocchio
104 Fishes (freshwater)
83 Fishes (saltwater)
44 Flax Family
44 flaxseed
65 Florence fennel
4 Florida arrowroot
103 flounder
80 French endive
116 freshwater drum
117 frog (frogs legs)
2 fungi

**G**

41 garbanzo
27 garden sorrel
11 garlic
79 gherkin
5 gin
17 ginger
17 Ginger Family
64 ginseng
64 Ginseng Family
80 globe artichoke
6 gluten flour
137 goat
79 golden nugget squash
80 goldenrod
31 golden seal
121 goose
39 gooseberry
28 Goosefoot Family
65 gotu kola
79 Gourd Family
6 graham flour
58 granadilla
52 grape
52 Grape Family
45 grapefruit
6 Grass Family
61 grenadine
6 grits
74 ground cherry
7 groundnut
91 grouper
123 grouse (ruffed)
63 guava
125 guinea fowl
41 gum acacia
41 gum tragacanth

**H**

87 haddock
87 hake
103 halibut
101 harvest fish
23 hazelnut
22 heartnut
66 Heath Family
54 hibiscus
22 hickory nut
134 hog
49 Holly Family
6 hominy
79 honeydew
77 Honeysuckle Family
25 hop
73 horehound
133 horse
36 horseradish
3 horsetail
3 Horsetail Family

79 Hubbard squash
66 huckleberry
73 hyssop

**I**

15 Iris Family
1 Irish moss

**J**

68 Japanese persimmon
80 Jerusalem artichoke
41 jicama
5 juniper

**K**

68 kaki
36 kale
6 kamut
1 kelp
41 kidney bean
56 kiwi berry
36 kohlrabi
45 kumquat

**L**

137 lamb
28 lamb's-quarters
34 Laurel Family
73 lavender
41 lecithin
11 leek
41 Legume Family
45 lemon
73 lemon balm
6 lemon grass
72 lemon verbena
41 lentil
80 lettuce
41 licorice
11 Lily Family
41 lima bean
45 lime
53 linden
53 Linden Family
51 litchi
82 lobster
40c loganberry
40c longberry
79 loofah
40a loquat
65 lovage
79 *Luffa*
51 lychee

**M**

26 macadamia
33 mace
98 mackerel
76 Madder Family
9 malanga
54 Mallow Family
46 Malpighia Family
6 malt
6 maltose
127 Mammals
48 mango
50 Maple Family
50 Maple products
19 *Maranta* starch
73 marjoram
99 marlin
49 maté
84 menhaden
12 mescal
6 millet
73 Mint Family
6 molasses
2 mold
135 moose
2 morel
70 Morning-Glory Family
25 mulberry
25 Mulberry Family
89 mullet
41 mung bean
45 murcot
52 muscadine
2 mushroom
109 muskellunge
79 muskmelon
81 mussel
36 Mustard Family
36 mustard greens
36 mustard seed
137 mutton
63 Myrtle Family

**N**

14 ñame
43 nasturtium
43 Nasturtium Family
41 navy bean
40b nectarine
29 New Zealand spinach

## Biological Classification of Foods (plant & animal)

Below begins the biological classification of plants and then starting on page 311 begins the biological classification of animals. Between the solid lines represents allergically identical foods. Between the dotted lines represents foods still in the same family but a different subgrouping. In some cases foods may be tolerated in different subgroups between the dotted lines.

## Biological Classification of Plants

**GRASS/GRAINS**
- bamboo shoots

. . . . . . . .

- barley
  - malt
  - maltose
- rye
- wheat
  - brans
  - bulgur
  - farina
  - flour
    - gluten
    - graham
    - patent
    - semolina
    - whole wheat
  - wheat germ oil
- triticale
- **spelt**
- **kamut**

. . . . . . . .

- oats/oatmeal

. . . . . . . .

- rice
  - rice flour

. . . . . . . .

- wild rice

. . . . . . . .

- millet
- sugar cane
  - molasses
  - raw sugar
- sorghum
  - grain
  - syrup
- corn
  - hominy grits
  - corn oil
  - cornmeal
  - corn sugar sweetener
  - syrup, high fructose
- corn syrup
  - dextrose
  - vitamin C (some)
  - popcorn

- macadamia nut

-----

**LEGUMES**
- alfalfa
- bean
  - bush
  - garbanzo
  - jack
  - kidney
  - navy
  - pinto
  - string

. . . . . . . .

- bean
  - broad
  - tonk
  - windsor

. . . . . . . .

- carob
- clover
- coumarin
- cowpea
- fenugreek
- flaxseed
- gum acacia
- gum tragacanth
- lentil
- licorice
- lima bean
- mung (sprout)
- pea (sweet/green)

-----

- pea
  - black-eyed
  - chick
  - split

. . . . . . . .

- peanut
- pigeon pea
- soybean
  - flour
  - grits
  - lecithin
  - milk
  - oil
  - tofu
- tamarind

- hickory
- pecan
- walnut
- black
- English
- white (butternut)

-----

- purslane
  - pigweed
- **amaranth**

-----

- **buckwheat**
- garden sorrel
- rhubarb

-----

- beets (beet sugar)
- Swiss chard

. . . . . . . .

- lamb's quarters
- **quinoa**
- spinach
- tampala

-----

**POTATO** (nightshade)
- eggplant
- ground cherry
- pepper
  - garden-green/bell
    - sweet/red
  - ceyenne
  - chili
  - paprika
  - pimento
- potato (white Irish)
- tomato tobacco

-----

**ROSE FAMILY**

**BERRY**
- blackberry
- boysenberry
- dewberry
- loganberry
- youngberry
- raspberry
- rose hips
- strawberry
- wineberry

-----

- litchi nut (lychee)

-----

**APPLE**
- butter
- cider
- pectin
- vinegar
- cranapple
- loquat
- pear
- quince

-----

**PLUM**
- almond
- apricot
- cherry
- peach
  - nectarine
- plum or prune
- Brazil nut

-----

- currant
- gooseberry

-----

- arrowroot

-----

- comfrey

-----

**CITRUS**
- angostura
- citron
- grapefruit
- kumquat
- lemon
- lime
- mandarin orange
  - tangerine
- orange

-----

- Barbados cherry (acerola)

-----

- cassava (meal)
- tapioca
  - (Brazilian arrowroot)
- yucca

-----

- Chinese water chestnut

-----

- filbert
- hazelnut
- oil or birch

-----

**GOURDS**
- Chinese preserving melon
- cucumber

. . . . . . . .

- melon
  - cantaloupe
  - casaba
  - crenshaw
  - honeydew
  - musk
  - Persian
  - Spanish

. . . . . . . .

- Indian gherkin

. . . . . . . .

- pumpkin
  - seeds/meal
- summer squash
  - crookneck, yellow
  - pattypan
  - vegetable spaghetti
  - zucchini

. . . . . . . .

- large pumpkin
- winter squash
  - acorn
  - butternut
  - hubbard
  - turban

. . . . . . . .

- watermelon

-----

- grape
  - cream of tartar
  - raisin
  - muscadine
  - slip-skin
  - vinegar (wine)
  - wine (brandy, champagne)

-----

- pineapple

-----

**Mint**
apple mint
basil
bergamot
chia seed
Clary
Chinese artichoke
horehound
horse mint
hyssop
lavender
lemon balm
marjoram
oregano
pennyroyal
peppermint
rosemary
sage
savory
spearmint
thyme
water mint

---

sesame
oil
seeds
tahini
butter

---

**PALM**
coconut
oil
meal
sago palm
starch (vitamin C)
date palm
dates
sugar
palm cabbage

---

Breadfruit
fig
hop
mulberry

---

beechnut
chestnut

---

sugar maple
maple sugar
maple syrup
sugar maple
maple sugar
maple syrup

---

**HEATH**
bearberry
blueberry
cranberry
wintergreen

---

yam
American
Chinese
Indian
tropical
name

---

sweet potato

---

Chinese
water chestnut

---

beachnut
chestnut

---

cocoa
chocolate
cola nut

---

Coffee

---

allspice
clove
eucalyptus
guava

---

nutmeg
mace

---

Ginseng
American
Asian

---

grape
cream of tartar
raisin
muscadine
slip-skin
vinegar (wine)
wine (brandy,
champagne)

---

persimmon
American
Oriental

---

Tea
- - - - - - - - - - - - -
passion fruit

---

**Olive**
green
olive oil
ripe

---

East Indian arrowroot
curcuma

---

WestIndian arrowroot
maranta

---

vanilla

---

black pepper

---

Ginger
tumeric
cardamon

---

saffron
orris root

---

Florida arrowroot
(zamia)

---

Fiji arrowroot
(tacca)

---

taro
poi
malanga (Arrowroot)

---

Chinese lotus

---

sarsaparilla

---

honey

---

cassava (meal)
tapioca
(Brazilian arrowroot)
yucca

---

caper

---

pomegranate

---

Brazil nut

---

chicle

---

juniper (gin)
pine nut

---

kiwi berry
(Chinese gooseberry)

---

banana
plantain
arrowroot (musa)

---

papaya

---

cottonseed
meal
oil
okra

---

**MUSTARD**
broccoli
brussel sprouts
cabbage
cauliflower
celery cabbage
collards
kale
kohlrabi
- - - - - - - - - - - - -
Chinese cabbage
horseradish
mustard
greens
seed
radish
rutabaga
turnip
watercress

---

**LILY**
aloe
asparagus
chives
garlic
leek
onion
ramp
shallot
yucca

---

agar
cheese mold
yeast
brewers
bakers
mushrooms
truffle

---

cactus pear (prickly)

---

**CARROT**
angelica
anise
caraway
carrot
celeriac
celery
chervil
coriander
cumin
dill
fennel
parsley
parsnip

---

avocado
bay leaf
cinnamon
sassafras (file)

---

**LETTUCE**
absinthe
artichoke
common
Jerusalem
burdock
cardoon
chamomile
chicory
coltsfoot
costmary
dandelion
endive
escarole
golden rod
lettuce
romaine
safflower
sunflower
salisfy (oyster plant)
santolina
scolymus
(Spanish oyster)
scozzonera (black)
salsify
southernwood
tansy
tarragon
vermouth

---

New Zealand spinach

---

elderberry

## Animal kingdom

Sea & bay scallops

oyster

clam
butter, pismo
geoduck
quahog
soft shell
mussel

abalone
green, pink & red

edible snail

North American squid

octopus

shrimp
brown & pink
grooved
prawn

lobster
Am. & European

crab
European
dungeness & blue

honeybee (honey)

shark

beluga
sturgeon (caviar)

N. Am. paddlefish

tarpon

herring
Atlantic, Pacific
(sardines are 1/2 grown herrings)

menhaden
shad

anchovy

**Salmon**
Atlantic
caho, dog
king, pink
sockeye
trout
brook, brown
lake, rainbow

lake whitefish

common smelt

muskellunge
northern pike
pickerel

buffalo
bigmouth & black
sucker

carp
chub

catfish
yellow bullhead

conger eel

Atlantic cod (scrod)
cusk, haddock
pollack, tomcod
silver hake

mullet
gray, striped
silver
silver sides
white bait

barracuda

bass
Black sea, striped
Oriental spotted

brown, red grouper
red hind, rockfish
speckled hing
white perch

red snapper

tilefish

grunt
gray, common, yellow

bass (black)
large & small mouth
spotted
bluegill
longear sunfish
pumpkinseed

pike
yellow perch
walleye

bluefish

amberjack
jack mackerel
pompano

dolphin

Atlantic croaker
freshwater drumfish
king whiting
silver perch
weakfish

porgy (scup)

albacore
Atlantic bonito
bluefish tuna
Chile bonito
mackerel
Atlantic
frigate
king
Spanish
skipjack tuna

marlin
sailfish

swordfish

butterfish
harvestfish

dab
flounder

halibut

sole
turbot

ocean perch
rosefish

sea robin
sea tag

puffer

American edible bullfrog
European edible bullfrog

African buffalo
American bison
brahman
**domestic cattle (beef)**
butter
cheese
cow's milk
gelatin
liver
other organs
veal
goat
cheese
goat's milk
sheep
lamb
mutton

snapping turtle

diamondback terrapin
green turtle

American elk
European red deer

caribou, moose
reindeer
white-tailed deer

giraffe

antelope

eastern & western diamondback rattler

American alligator

mallard duck
egg
greylag goose
egg

partridge (ruffed grouse)
prairie chicken

peacock
egg

domestic chicken
Cornish hen
egg
liver
domestic pheasant
Indian pheasant
peafowl
quail

domestic duck
egg
domestic goose
egg

guinea fowl

turkey
egg

dove
pigeon (squab)

opossum

Belgian hare
domestic rabbit
eastern cottontail
jackrabbit
snowshoe rabbit
western cottontail

domestic guinea pig

prairie dog

squirrel
fox
gray
red
woodchuck

beaver

whale

porpoise

dolphin

wolf

bear
black
brown
grizzly
polar

raccoon

lion
tiger

walrus

sea lion

common seal

elephant

horse

pig (pork)
bacon
gelatin
ham
lard

hippopotamus

camel
llama

# HYPERACTIVITY

- Attention deficit disorder (ADD) encompasses a wide range of similar disorders, e.g. hyperactive child syndrome, minimal brain damage, minimal brain dysfunction, minor cerebral dysfunction.
- Learning disability–the child displays a developmentally inappropriate brief attention span and poor concentration for mental and chronological age.
- Each year over 12 million arrests of children are made for alleged delinquent acts other than traffic offenses. Of this group, over 2.5 million are formally arrested and referred to the nation's juvenile courts. It costs over $10 billion per year to handle these juvenile offenders!
- 3 separate disorders are viewed:
  1) Attention deficit disorder with hyperactivity
  2) Attention deficit disorder without hyperactivity
  3) Attention deficit disorder residual

## Attention Deficit Disorder with Hyperactivity

- By conservative estimates, 3% of school age children are affected
- Boys are affected ten times as often as girls
- Onset often occurs as early as age 3, but diagnosis is not made until child is in school

## I. Signs and Symptoms

1) Hyperactivity
2) Perceptual motor impairment
3) Emotional liability
4) General coordination deficit
5) Disorders of attention such as short attention span, distractibility, lack of perseverance, failure to finish things, listening problems, poor concentration.
6) Impulsiveness
7) Disorders of memory and thinking
8) Specific learning disabilities
9) Equivocal neurological signs and electroencephalographic irregularities

## II. Etiology

**1) Food additive sensitivities**– "Feingold hypothesis"–Benjamin Feingold, M.D. estimated that 40-50% of hyperactive children are sensitive to artificial food colors, flavors, and preservatives as well as naturally occurring salicylates and phenolic compounds. His claims were based on over 1,200 cases in which food additives were linked to learning and behavior disorders. He presented his findings to the AMA in 1973. Researchers focused on only 10 of the food dyes versus the 3,000 additives with which Feingold was concerned. A negative correlation was found and the National Advisory Committee on Hyperkinesis and Food Additives to the USA Nutrition Foundation in 1980 filed a negative report about the role of food additives and hyperactivity.

Most of the research refuting Feingold's hypothesis comes from C. Keith Conner's book, Food Additives and Hyperactive Children. Rippere has reviewed much of the work done by Conner and has placed criticism in 6 areas:

a) The placebo used was a chocolate cookie. Conner even admits in a follow-up two years later that 21% of the mothers mentioned that chocolate adversely affected their children's behavior.
b) Only 26 mgs worth of additives were used compared with 76.5mg average and 150 mg 90th percentile.
c) The dose interval was relatively long.
d) Conner used the cytotoxic test for determining allergies. This test has many false positives and negatives.
e) Evaluation was not done on a daily basis and the evaluations were very subjective.
f) Conner consistently minimizes and discounts findings which support Feingold's findings.

STUDY–Swanson & Kinsbourne. *Food dyes impair performance of children on laboratory learning task.* Science 207:1485-7, 1980. ABSTRACT–20 Hyperactive children were given varying amounts of food dyes–26mgs, 75mgs, 100mgs, and 150mgs. It was found that at 26mgs of food coloring there was no change in the children's behavior, but at the higher doses 17 of 20 kids had significant impairment of learning performance.

STUDY–Egger. *Controlled Trial of Oligoantigenic Treatment in the Hyperkinetic Syndrome.* Lancet 1:540-5, 1985. ABSTRACT–62 of 76 overactive children treated with an oligoantigenic diet improved. 21 of these achieved a normal range of behavior. 28 of the improved children completed a double-blind crossover placebo-controlled trial in which suspicious foods were reintroduced. Symptoms worsened much more often on the suspicious foods as compared to the placebo. Of the 48 foods incriminated, artificial colors and preservatives were the most common provoking substances.

**2) Food allergy/sensitivities**

STUDY–Swain. *Salicylates, oligoantigenic diets, and behavior.* Letter to the editor. Lancet, July 6, 1985, 41-2. ABSTRACT–86 of 140 children with behavioral disorders experienced significant improvement with a modified elimination and challenge protocol. 64 of these 86 kids reacted to a double-blind challenge with salicylates but not to the placebo.

STUDY–McGovern. Int J. of Biosocial Res. 4:40-2, 1983. ABSTRACT–13 hyperkinetic kids and 13 controls were challenged with 20 different food and inhalant allergenic extracts, 20 phenolic food components and traditional antigens. They were observed for behavioral changes consistent with hyperactivity. Acetyl salicylate was the phenolic compound provoking the greatest frequency of responses (80%), while from foods, sugar, corn, beef and egg were the next most common offenders at 30%.

**3) Hypoglycemia**–75% of criminals were hyperactive children and more than 50% have abnormal GTT's. Hypoglycemia can stimulate increased catecholamine secretion.

STUDY–Langseth & Dowd; *Glucose tolerance and hyperkinesis.* Food Cosmet. Toxicol. 16:129-33, 1978. ABSTRACT- 261 hyperactive kids were given 5-hour GTT's. 74% of these kids had abnormal curves. The predominant curve was a flat one.

**4) Nutrient deficiencies**–Many nutrient deficiencies can cause impaired CNS function. Iron is the most common nutrient deficiency in American children. Most research has been done with vitamin B-6, vitamin B-3, and calcium.

STUDY–Brenner. *The effects of megadoses of selected B-complex vitamins on children with hyperkinesis: Controlled studies with long term follow up.* J Learning Disabil. 15:258,1982. ABSTRACT–100 children were given megadoses of various B-complex vitamins or placebo. 15% responded to B-6 and 8% to B-1 and 3% to B-3.

5) **Lead toxicity**–It has been estimated that the human body can tolerate about 1mg of lead without suffering from toxic side effects. In an urban environment the average person ingests, with solid foods, 1mg/wk. Another .1mg/wk comes from beverages. The World Health Organization estimates only 10% of the lead ingested is actually absorbed. Typical airborne inhalation of lead in an urban environment is about .2mg/day. Researchers have demonstrated that children absorb and retain much higher amounts of lead than adults.

6) **Abnormal lighting**–TV and fluorescent lighting

**Foods containing artificial colors and flavors and safe alternatives**

| Foods to Avoid | Permitted Foods |
|---|---|
| **Cereals**–all cereals with artificial colors or flavors and all instant breakfast preparations | Any cereals that do not contain artificial colors or flavors, dry or cooked |
| **Bakery Goods**–all manufactured cakes, cookies, pastries, sweet rolls, doughnuts, pie crusts, frozen baked goods and packaged baking mixes | Most bakery products must be prepared at home. All commercial breads except egg bread and whole wheat. |
| **Luncheon Meats**–bologna, salami, franks, sausages, meat loaf, bacon, ham and pork | all fresh meats |
| **Poultry**–all barbequed types, turkey with prepared basting (called self basting), poultry with prepared stuffing. | all fresh poultry except stuffed |
| **Desserts**–manufactured ice creams, unless the label specifies no synthetic colorings or flavoring. This also applies to sherbet, ices, gelatins, junkets, puddings, all powdered puddings, desert mixes and flavored yogurt. | Homemade ice cream without artificial coloring or flavoring, gelatins made from pure gelatins with any permitted natural fruit or fruit juices, tapioca, homemade custards, puddings and plain yogurt., |
| **Candies**–all manufactured types, soft or hard. | Homemade candies without almonds. |
| **Beverages**–cider, wine, beer, diet drinkd, all instant breakfast drinks, all quick mix powdered drinks, tea–hot or cold,prepared chocolate milk. | Grapefruit, pineapple, pear nectar, guava nectar, homemade lemonade or limeade from fresh lemons or limes, 7-up, milk. |
| **Miscellaneous items**-oleomargarine, colored butter, mustard. | All cooking oils and fats, sweet butter without added color or flavor, mustard prepared at home with pure powdered distilled vinegar. |

## III. Treatment

1) **Avoid all salicylates, phenolic compounds and additives**–The following foods contain natural salicylates:

a) Fruits–almonds, apples, apricots, cherries, currants, nectarines, peaches, plums and prunes

b) Berries–blackberries, boysenberries, gooseberries, raspberries, strawberries

c) Grapes and raisins or any product made with grapes–wine, wine vinegar, jellies, foods containing fruit juice sweeteners

d) Oranges (**note**–grapefruit, lemon and lime are permitted)

**2) Hypoallergenic diet**

**3) Avoid sucrose and other simple carbohydrates**

**4) Avoid lead**–Check via hair analysis. Check pipes, food sources, water, etc. Hard water is protective against lead leaching.

**chelate**–Vitamin C–3gms/day, pectin (apples), alginate (seaweed) methionine, cysteine and cystine–foods such as beans, eggs, onions, and garlic

**5) Vitamin supplementation**

**a) Niacinamide**–1-3gms/day

STUDY–Hoffer.. *Vitamin B-3 dependent child.* Schizophrenia 3:107-113, 1971. ABSTRACT–33 children under age 13 with disturbed behavior were placed on nicotinamide with doses from 1.5 to 6gms daily along with 3gms ascorbic acid (rarely tranquilizers or antidepressants also). All recovered and then had their nicotinamide tablets switched to placebo tablets. Only 1 out of 33 kids failed to respond to B-3 therapy. All of the kids that responded to the B-3 relapsed upon substitution with placebo, then improved again upon restarting the B-3.

**b) Vitamin B-6**–20-30mg/kg/day-If patients have low serum serotonin levels, this treatment may be beneficial.

STUDY–Coleman. *A preliminary study of the effect of B-6 administration in a subgroup of hyperkinetic children: a double-blind crossover comparison with methylphenidate.* J Biol. Psych. 14(5):741-51, 1979. ABSTRACT–6 hyperactive children with low serum serotonin levels were given B-6. The B-6 increased serotonin levels and was more effective than Ritalin in decreasing hyperkinesis. The effect continued into the placebo period whereas the Ritalin effect did not.

**c) Calcium**

**d) Magnesium**–especially consider this if the patient is constipated

**e) EFA**–2-4 teaspoon/day–Males have a much higher requirement for EFA than females. Check for other allergies such as asthma and eczema.

STUDY–Colquhoun and Bunday. *A lack of EFA as a possible cause of hyperactivity in children.* Med Hypotheses. 7:673-9, 1981. ABSTRACT–5 hyperactive children received EPO 1-1.5gms 2x/day with very positive results.

**6) Avoid television and fluorescent lights**

yeah - right!

## Notes

# ASTHMA

- Asthma is characterized by recurrent attacks of dyspnea, cough, and expectoration of tenacious mucoid sputum. There are over 12 million people with asthma in the U.S. and from 1982-1992 the incidence has gone up 42%.
- Prolonged expiration phase with generalized wheezing and musical rales
- Eosinophilia, with increased serum IgE
- Asthma most commonly occurs in children with a 2:1 male:female ratio

## I. Etiology

**Intrinsic Asthma** is associated with a bronchial reaction that is due to physical irritants such as chemicals, cold, exercise, infection, agents that activate the alternate complement pathway, and emotional upset.

**Extrinsic Asthma**–Atopic asthma is associated with an immunologically mediated condition with a characteristic increase in serum IgE.

**Major factors**

1) Hypersensitivity of the bronchial airways
2) Release of inflammatory mediators from mast cells
3) Decreased Beta adrenergic stimulation - Adrenal glands play a major role in asthma since they release the hormones cortisol and epinephrine. Cortisol and epinephrine are considered to be prime stimulators of Beta-receptors. During asthmatic attacks there may be a relative deficiency of these 2 hormones.
4) Imbalance of cyclic nucleotides - Cyclic guanosine monophosphate (cGMP) levels in asthmatics block Beta-2 receptors and prevent dilation of bronchioles. In addition, cyclic adenosine monophosphate (cAMP) levels, which normally cause dilation of the bronchioles (see diagram in eczema), are usually depressed in asthmatics.
5) Leukotriene A4 production via lipoxygenase pathway (see diagram on following page).

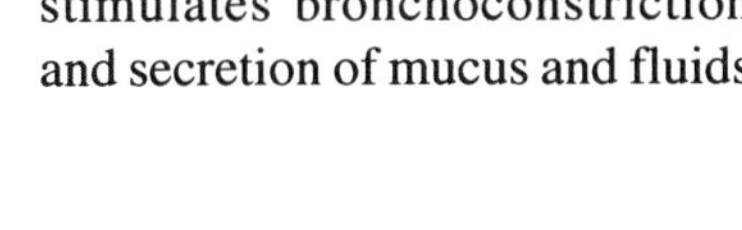

Leukotrienes of the 4 series stimulates bronchoconstriction and secretion of mucus and fluids

Cross section of bronchiole showing marked narrowing of air passage

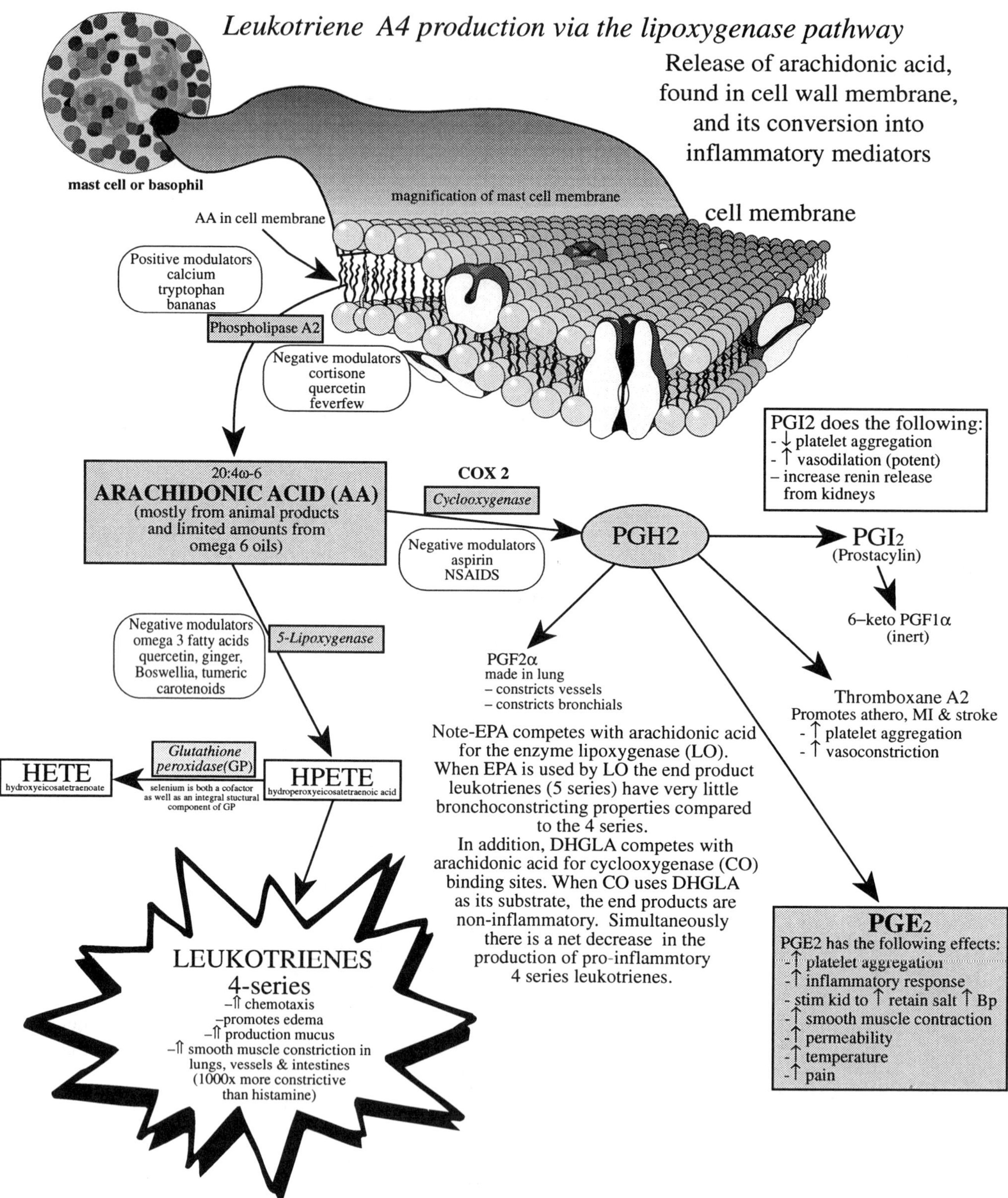


STUDY–Clark, William, et al. *Omega 3 fatty acid dietary supplementation in SLE* Kidney International, Vol 36:653-60, 1989. ABSTRACT–Omega 3 fatty acid supplementation of daily doses of 6gms and 18 gms. This supplementation resulted in a 16-20% reduction in platelet arachidonic acid incorporation. Neutrophil leukotriene B4 release was reduced 78-42% by the respective low and high doses.

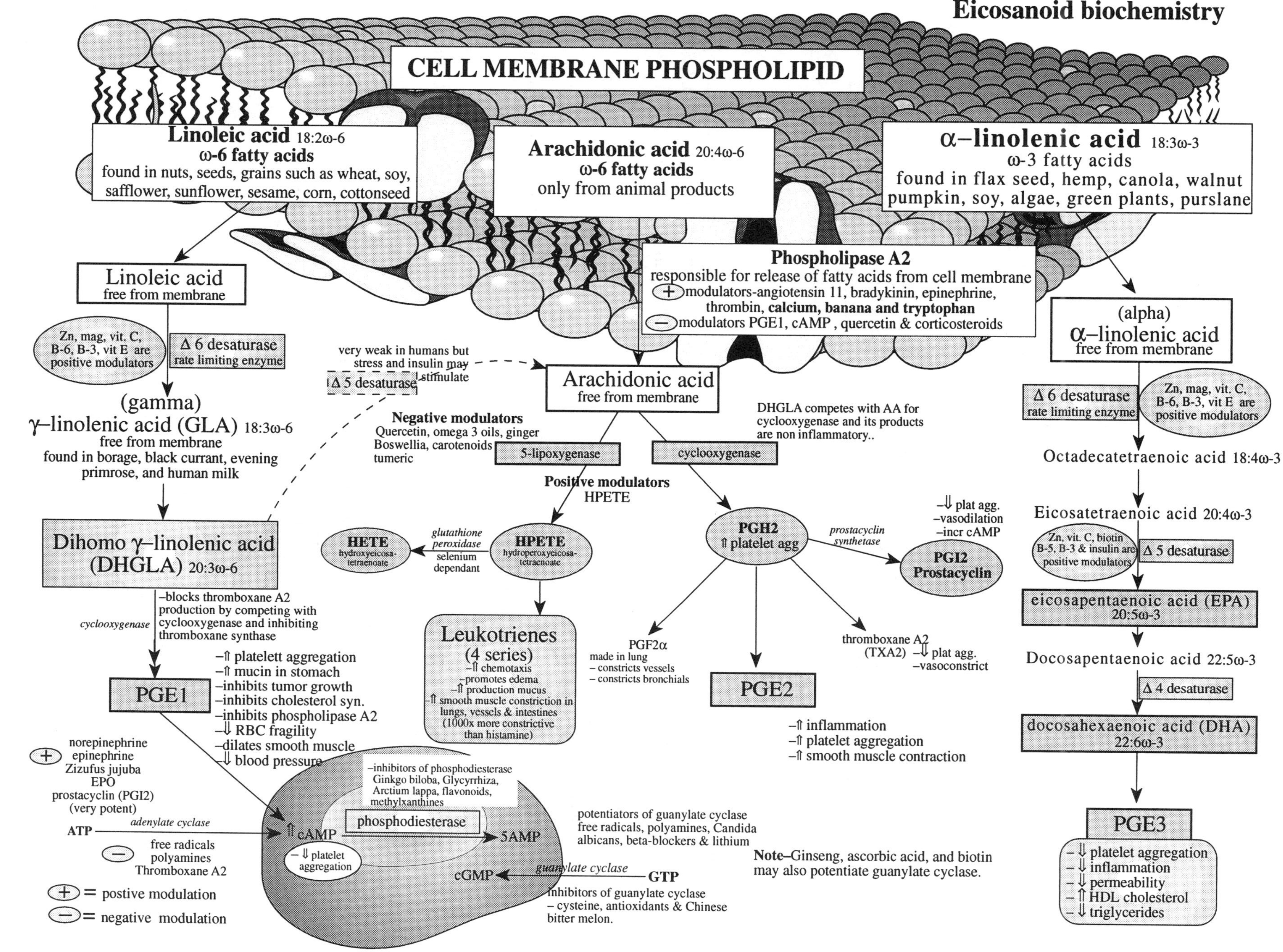
Eicosanoid biochemistry
CELL MEMBRANE PHOSPHOLIPID
Linoleic acid 18:2ω-6
ω-6 fatty acids
found in nuts, seeds, grains such as wheat, soy, safflower, sunflower, sesame, corn, cottonseed
Arachidonic acid 20:4ω-6
ω-6 fatty acids
only from animal products
α–linolenic acid 18:3ω-3
ω-3 fatty acids
found in flax seed, hemp, canola, walnut pumpkin, soy, algae, green plants, purslane
Phospholipase A2
responsible for release of fatty acids from cell membrane
+ modulators-angiotensin 11, bradykinin, epinephrine, thrombin, calcium, banana and tryptophan
– modulators PGE1, cAMP , quercetin & corticosteroids
Linoleic acid
free from membrane
Zn, mag, vit. C, B-6, B-3, vit E are positive modulators
Δ 6 desaturase
rate limiting enzyme
(gamma)
γ–linolenic acid (GLA) 18:3ω-6
free from membrane
found in borage, black currant, evening primrose, and human milk
Dihomo γ–linolenic acid (DHGLA) 20:3ω-6
very weak in humans but stress and insulin may stimulate
Δ 5 desaturase
Arachidonic acid
free from membrane
Negative modulators
Quercetin, omega 3 oils, ginger Boswellia, carotenoids tumeric
5-lipoxygenase
cyclooxygenase
DHGLA competes with AA for cyclooxygenase and its products are non inflammatory..
Positive modulators
HPETE
HETE
hydroxyeicosa-tetraenoate
glutathione peroxidase
selenium dependant
HPETE
hydroperoxyeicosa-tetraenoate
Leukotrienes
(4 series)
–⇑ chemotaxis
–promotes edema
–⇑ production mucus
–⇑ smooth muscle constriction in lungs, vessels & intestines (1000x more constrictive than histamine)
PGH2
⇑ platelet agg
prostacyclin synthetase
–⇓ plat agg.
–vasodilation
–incr cAMP
PGI2
Prostacyclin
PGF2α
made in lung
– constricts vessels
– constricts bronchials
PGE2
thromboxane A2 (TXA2)
–⇓ plat agg.
–vasoconstrict
–⇑ inflammation
–⇑ platelet aggregation
–⇑ smooth muscle contraction
–blocks thromboxane A2 production by competing with cyclooxygenase and inhibiting thromboxane synthase
cyclooxygenase
PGE1
–⇑ platelett aggregation
–⇑ mucin in stomach
–inhibits tumor growth
–inhibits cholesterol syn.
–inhibits phospholipase A2
–⇓ RBC fragility
–dilates smooth muscle
–⇓ blood pressure
+ norepinephrine epinephrine Zizufus jujuba EPO prostacyclin (PGI2) (very potent)
ATP
adenylate cyclase
– free radicals polyamines Thromboxane A2
+ = postive modulation
– = negative modulation
–inhibitors of phosphodiesterase Ginkgo biloba, Glycyrrhiza, Arctium lappa, flavonoids, methylxanthines
⇑ cAMP
phosphodiesterase
5AMP
– ⇓ platelet aggregation
cGMP
guanylate cyclase
GTP
potentiators of guanylate cyclase free radicals, polyamines, Candida albicans, beta-blockers & lithium
inhibitors of guanylate cyclase – cysteine, antioxidants & Chinese bitter melon.
Note–Ginseng, ascorbic acid, and biotin may also potentiate guanylate cyclase.
(alpha)
α–linolenic acid
free from membrane
Δ 6 desaturase
rate limiting enzyme
Zn, mag, vit. C, B-6, B-3, vit E are positive modulators
Octadecatetraenoic acid 18:4ω-3
Eicosatetraenoic acid 20:4ω-3
Zn, vit. C, biotin B-5, B-3 & insulin are positive modulators
Δ 5 desaturase
eicosapentaenoic acid (EPA) 20:5ω-3
Docosapentaenoic acid 22:5ω-3
Δ 4 desaturase
docosahexaenoic acid (DHA) 22:6ω-3
PGE3
– ⇓ platelet aggregation
– ⇓ inflammation
– ⇓ permeability
– ⇑ HDL cholesterol
– ⇓ triglycerides

## II. Signs and Symptoms

There is a wide variation in the signs and symptoms of asthma. Some asthmatics have symptoms all the time while others have asymptomatic periods, followed by severe exacerbations. Mild symptoms may include slight coughing followed by minor wheezing. Sometimes symptoms start with some coughing and progress into severe coughing, often accompanied by extreme difficulty in breathing. In children a sensation over the anterior neck or upper chest is an early sign of an impending attack. Often, a certain stressor–such as exercise, breathing cold air or some noxious agent–may initiate the onset of an attack. Over a long period of time asthma can wear out the body's adrenal and immune functions and cause a person to be very fatigued and susceptible to various infections.

## III. Diagnosis

Diagnosis can usually be made upon patient examination. Often an elevated eosinophil count is found although the asthma may not necessarily be mediated by an IgE mechanism. $FEV_1$ can be useful in evaluating the intensity of an attack. Staging is done according to percent of $FEV_1$:

Mild = 50-80%
Moderate = 50% of normal
Severe = 25% of normal
Going to see one's maker = 10% or less

> NOTE–Sometimes chronic mild bronchitis is actually a form of asthma if properly evaluated. The hallmark sign is a hyperreactivebronchoconstrictive response to many stimuli, with the severity of the asthma linked to the degree of inflammation present.

## IV. Treatment

1) **Eliminate food allergies**–Immediate sensitivity reactions are usually caused by (in decreasing order), eggs, fish, shellfish, nuts, and peanuts.

Delayed sensitivity reactions are caused by (in decreasing order) milk, chocolate, wheat, citrus, and food colorings (tartrazine), but really any and all foods can cause or add to the allergic burden.

STUDY–Rowe & Young. *Bronchial asthma due to food allergy alone in 95 patients*. JAMA 1959:169,1958. ABSTRACT–50 children and 45 adults were treated solely by eliminating allergenic foods from their diet. The typical patient had recurrent attacks every 2-6 weeks with total relief in the summer. Patients in this study often did not give a history suggestive of food allergy. Negative skin tests to foods were present in 48% of food sensitive patients. In this study, these patients all responded well within 1-4 weeks. Diagnosis depended on a trial diet which eliminated cereal grains, milk, egg, chocolate, fish, and other less commonly consumed foods. Recurrent head and bronchial colds particularly from autumn to late spring, were also relieved by food elimination. Of 173 patients over the age of 55, food allergy alone appeared to be the cause in 40%. **Inhalants were about equally important in this age group.**

> **Note**–Generally, the younger an asthma patient, the more the allergen will be foods. The older a patient, the more the allergen will be related to inhalants.

**2) Diet**

a) Decrease consumption of foods with arachidonic acid (red meats and dairy products). Amino acids are the major substrate for lipoxygenase which results in increased levels of leukotrienes. It should be noted that safflower, sunflower, and other oils contain high levels of linoleic acid and small amounts can get converted to arachidonic acid (via Δ 5 desaturase in the presence of stress) after their conversion to DHGLA.

b) Increase consumption of foods containing flavonoids and carotenes. Both inhibit the action of lipoxygenase. Yellow vegetables and other leafy vegetables contain abundant amounts of these important nutrients.

c) Increase consumption of EPA and linolenic acid sources such as flax oil, canola oil, walnuts, cold water fish, herring, sardines, and salmon. EPA selectively inhibits lipoxygenase by binding onto the enzyme and forming the "5" series of leukotrienes which have little broncho-constricting properties.

d) Onions and grape skins contain quercetin which has the effect of stabilizing mast cells, inhibiting lipoxygenase, and increasing cAMP levels.

e) Avoid excessive calcium sources and bananas as these potentiate phospholipase.

f) Vegan diet

STUDY–Lindahl *Vegan diet regimen with reduced medication in the treatment of bronchial asthma* J. Asthma 22:45-55,1985. ABSTRACT–25 patients were treated with a pure vegan diet which prohibited meat, fish, eggs, dairy products, coffee, ordinary tea, chocolate, sugar, salt, tap water, apples, citrus, soybeans and peas. Grains and potatoes were either very restricted or eliminated. 71% improved within 4 months and 92% improved by one year.

**3) Eliminate environmental allergies**–Eliminate rugs, wall hangings, cats, feather pillows and clean air filters for heating and cooling systems. Use environmentally sound cleaning solutions ["LIVOS PLANT CHEMISTRY", Santa Fe, NM (505):988-1911]. Wet mop walls, floors, ceilings and use special high quality vacuum ("Rainbow" or "Princess"). Consider using an ionizer and/or ozone generator. Consider a formaldehyde bomb or shots.

STUDY–Spurlock, B., Daily, Thomas, *Toothpaste-Induced bronchospasm* NEJM, 323(26): 1845-46, Dec 27 1990 ABSTRACT–A 21 yr old woman on theophylline, a beta antagonist, and an inhaled steroid product switched toothpastes and found dramatic relief of her symptoms. When rechallenged, her wheezing returned in 10 minutes. The only difference between the two toothpastes was that they had different artificial flavorings.

**4) Vitamin B-12 shots**–1000mcg/day IM. Give the shots daily for 4-7 days

I first learned about this therapy from Jonathan Wright in 1984. In my experience, it has never failed to help young children, at least to some extent. Sometimes the effects are dramatic.

STUDY–Simon. *Vitamin B-12 therapy in allergy and chronic dermatosis*. J. Allergy 2:183-5,1951. ABSTRACT–18/20 patients improved following IM injections of B-12 1000mcg once weekly for 4 weeks.

STUDY–Simon. *Sulfite-sensitive asthma* Res Instit of Scripps Clinic Scientific Report 39:57-58,1982-83. ABSTRACT–Vitamin B-12 was more effective than pharmacologic agents in blocking asthmatic reactions and was effective over a longer period of time, when given prior to a sulfite challenge.

**5) Vitamin B-6**–50mg 2x/day

STUDY–Collip et al. *Pyridonine treatment of childhood bronchial asthma.* Ann. Allergy 35:93-7, 1975. ABSTRACT–76 asthmatic children who received B-6 200mg daily demonstrated significant symptoms improvement and a reduction in dosage of bronchodilators and cortisone required to relieve symptoms.

STUDY–Reynolds, Anatta. *Depressed plasma pyridoxal phosphate conc in adult asthmatics*. Am. J. Clin. Nutr. 41:684-8, 1985. ABSTRACT–7 patients and 6 controls received 50mg 2x daily. Both plasma and red blood cell pyridoxal phosphate levels only increased significantly in the controls. All asthmatics reported a dramatic decrease in the frequency, duration, and severity of asthmatic attacks and wheezing ceased in about one week.

6) **EPA**–3gms/day

7) **Flax oil**–1-2 Tablespoon/day

8) **Quercetin**–500mg 1/2hour before meals. Thorne Res. now offers an inhalent form.

9) **B Carotene**–100,000iu/day

10) **Selenium**–250-400mcg/day

11) **Vitamin E**–800iu/day

12) **Avoid tryptophan which is converted to serotonin, a bronchoconstrictor**

13) **Vitamin C**–1-2gms/day

STUDY–Clemetson. *Histamine and ascorbic acid in human blood.* J. Nutr. 110(4):662-68,1980. ABSTRACT–When 11 normals with either low vitamin C levels or high blood histamine levels were given ascorbic acid 1gm for 3 days, blood histamine levels fell in all 11 subjects.

14) **Magnesium**–400mg/day Can use IV magnesium in acute asthmatic conditions and works very well. Also consider compounding pharmacy MgCl with glutathione in nebulizer.

STUDY–Brunner et al. *Effect of parenteral magnesium on pulmonary function, plasma cAMP, and histamine in bronchial asthma.* J. Asthma 22:3-11,1985. ABSTRACT–Parenterally administrated magnesium significantly improved pulmonary function of asthmatic patients. The degree of improvement was positively correlated with serum magnesium levels.

15) **Staphage Lysate**–(Delmart Labs) This should used with caution as can cause anaphylac tic or severe allergenic reaction.

16) **Ephedra**

17) **Lobelia**

18) **N-acetyl cysteine** has the effect of a mucolytic agent and also acts as an antioxidant. Mucomist® (NAC as a nebulizer approved for treatment of cystic fibrosis).

19) **Gingko biloba** has very strong phosphodiesterase inhibitor.

20) **HCL**–Start with vinegar and work your way up by 5 grains at a time

STUDY–Bray. *The hypochlorhydria of asthma of childhood.* Quart. J. Med. 24:181-97,1931. ABSTRACT–80% of 200 asthmatic children had sub-normal levels of gastric acidity.

21) **Molybdenum IV** stimulates sulfite metabolism. However, it is not very effective orally (try molybdenum picolinate–1mg).

## Notes

# BRONCHITIS

- Can be chronic or acute
- Bacterial or viral origin must be ruled out

## I. Etiology

- Viral, bacterial, or allergic

## II. Treatment

1) **Avoid allergens**–First, try milk and milk products. Second, try grains, especially wheat. Chronic bronchitis may respond within the first few days of the food avoidence. A short fast, followed by a hypoallergenic diet, can also be beneficial.

2) **Enhance immune function**

a) **Vitamin C**–2gms 4x/day

STUDY–Bucca & Caterina, et al. *Effects of vitamin C on histamine bronchial responsiveness of patients with allergic rhinitis.* Annals of Allergy 65:311-14, Oct. 1990. ABSTRACT–16 patients, with seasonal allergic rhinitis without history of asthma, off their normal medications were given 2 grams of vitamin C or placebo in a double-blind cross-over study. 44% of the patients were found to have reduced FEV1. The vitamin C supplemented group was found to have a significant increase in FEV1. It appears that vitamin C stimulates a non-enzymatic histamine degradation.

b) **Vitamin A**– 25,000iu 2x/day

c) **Zinc picolinate**–30mg 2x/day

d) **Vitamin B-6**–50mg 2x/day

e) **Vitamin E**–400iu 2x/day–has been shown in one study to be effective in improving antibody response to influenza virus.

f) **Quercetin-**1gm 3-4x per day (effective against parainfluenza virus).

g) **N-acetyl cysteine-**has mucolytic activity and can be used when a lot of phlegm is present.

3) **Heat or cool** depending upon the condition. If the patient is on the cool side and presents with a thick white moss on their tongue, they need drying heating herbs. If their tongue has a thick yellow coat they need cooling and drying herbs. Do not give these patients heat producing herbs only.

a) **Ginger-**generally a warming herb with some antibacterial properties

b) **Cayenne-**a heating herb

c) **Garlic-**a heating herb with antibacteria and antiviral properties

d) **Warm drinks**–I often recommend for a cough where the patient is on the cool side a warming drink that is prepared by grating frozen ginger(about 1-2 thumb size chunks) into hot water and adding raw honey and lemon. Have them first take a hot bath and then drink several cups of this while dressing warmly. They can also prepare a tincture of Lobelia, Echinacea, Zingiber, and Glycyrrhiza in equal parts and have them drink 35 drops in hot water 4-5 times per day.

4) **Consider IV nutrients or IM Echinacae Pascotox (IM or IV Echinacae)** Available from Germany through Merrit Pharmaceuticals.

# EMPHYSEMA

- Damage of the epithelial tissue of the lungs with loss of elasticity

## I. Treatment

Work to improve the elasticity of the tissues and improve diffusion of oxygen across damaged epithelial tissue.

1) **Lecithin**–1200mg 3x/day–improves the surfactant of the lungs

2) **Vitamin E**–400iu 3x/day

3) **Vitamin A**–50,000iu/day

4) **Zinc picolinate**–30mg 2x/day

5) **Vitamin C**–3gms/day

6) **Flax oil**–2 Tablespoons/day

**NOTE**–Rule out cadmium toxicity and allergy.

STUDY–Rowe. *Food allergy: its role in emphysema & chronic bronchitis.* Dis. Chest 48:609, 1965 .

### Notes

# ANEMIA

- Anemia is a condition where there is a deficiency of the size and/or the number of red blood cells. It can also be caused by a lack of hemoglobin. Fragile RBC's (possibly showing elevated bilirubin) or chronic blood loss are some etiologies.
- The most important nutritional factors are iron, folate, and vitamin B-12, although vitamin B-6, vitamin C, copper, and other heavy metals may also be involved.

# IRON DEFICIENCY ANEMIA

## I. Etiology

Iron deficient anemia is by far the most common form and effects 10-20% of the world population. There are three primary causes of this condition.

1) Chronic blood loss, i.e. from a bleeding ulcer, hemorrhoids, malignancy, parasites, menorrhagia, hereditary telangiectasia, etc.
2) Faulty iron intake or absorption
3) Increased iron requirement for growth of blood volume, which occurs in infancy, puberty, pregnancy and lactation.

**NOTE**–Another cause is from the defective release of iron into the plasma from iron stores. This occurs in chronic inflammation and other chronic disorders (not true iron deficiency anemia).

## II. Signs and Symptoms

Fatigue, although popularly thought to be an early symptom of iron deficiency anemia, has not been correlated with decreased hemoglobin levels. **Fatigue, weakness, anorexia and pica may be due to tissue depletion of iron-containing enzymes and not to decreased levels of blood hemoglobin.**

As the iron deficiency becomes more severe, epithelial tissues are effected, especially the tongue, nails, mouth and stomach. Fingernails become thin, flat, and even spoon shaped. Koilonychia, spooning of the fingernails, can develop in latter stages. Mouth changes include atrophy of the tongue papillae, burning and redness, and, in severe cases, a completely smooth and waxy appearance. Angular stomatitis and paleness of the conjunctiva may also be seen. In rare instances severe iron deficiency can cause esophageal webs in the upper aspect of the esophagus (Plummer-Vinson Syndrome), and can be a cause of achalasia.

## III. Diagnosis

- Serum ferritin is the most sensitive parameter of iron status. It falls only when there is true iron deficiency. However during hepatocellular injury, acute infection or inflammatory reaction it can be falsely elevated.
- Hemoglobin concentration is relatively an unreliable indicator as **some iron replete women have low hemoglobin.** Always check % transferrin saturation or ferritin
- Signs and symptoms
- Microcytic and hypochromic RBC's

## IV. Treatment

1) **Treat the underlying cause**. If iron deficiency based on ferritin & MCV then give foods with high iron (see table pg 331).

2) **Ferrous sulfate**–100mg/day of elemental iron. (I use liquid Fe drops from Levine) Make sure it is taken on an empty stomach to maximize absorption if the patient can tolerate it. If not then give with foods along with vitamin C. Prescription iron can be given as combined with certain proteins to minimize irritation to GI tract.

3) **Vitamin C**–1gm/day buffered–helps keep Fe reduced and greatly aids in the absorption of iron. Take along with iron supplement several times during the day.

> **NOTE**-Response to this therapy usually takes 1-3weeks with an **increase in RBC's being the first change.** Hemoglobin levels are next to rise, and epithelial changes are last. Fe therapy should continue for 6-12 months, even after hemoglobin levels return to normal. This allows iron reserves to be repleted (check ferritin). I like to see ferritin levels in females at least 30ng/ml and in males 40ng/ml .

4) **Liver extract (Phytopharmica or Cardiovascular Research)**–3-9 capsules per day in divided doses along with vitamin C. The liver extract from Phytopharmica has 2.5mg iron per capsule. Can also give liver extract IM (LiB from Merrit) or as straight iron sulfate if someone has extreme nausea or they have a digestive disorder that might hamper their absorption or tolerance to the iron orally.

5) **Increase dietary sources of Iron** (see list of iron containing foods on page 331).

If Fe stores are depleted then absorption is:
- 35% if from heme sources (animal)
- 8% if from non-heme sources (grains and vegetable source)

If Fe stores are repleted then absorption is:
- 15% if from heme sources
- 3% if from non heme sources

Note-Iron in the heme form is better absorbed but there is another factor referred to as MPF (Meat, Poultry and Fish) that also seems to enhance absorption of iron.

**NOTE**–Both EDTA and tea with meals can each reduce Fe absorption by 50%.

### Summary of Anemias

| Macrocytic or megaloblastic | Microcytic |
|---|---|
| Vitamin B-12 | Iron |
| Folate | Vitamin B-6 |
| | Copper |
| | thiamin |

# SUMMARY OF IRON ABSORPTION AND METABOLISM

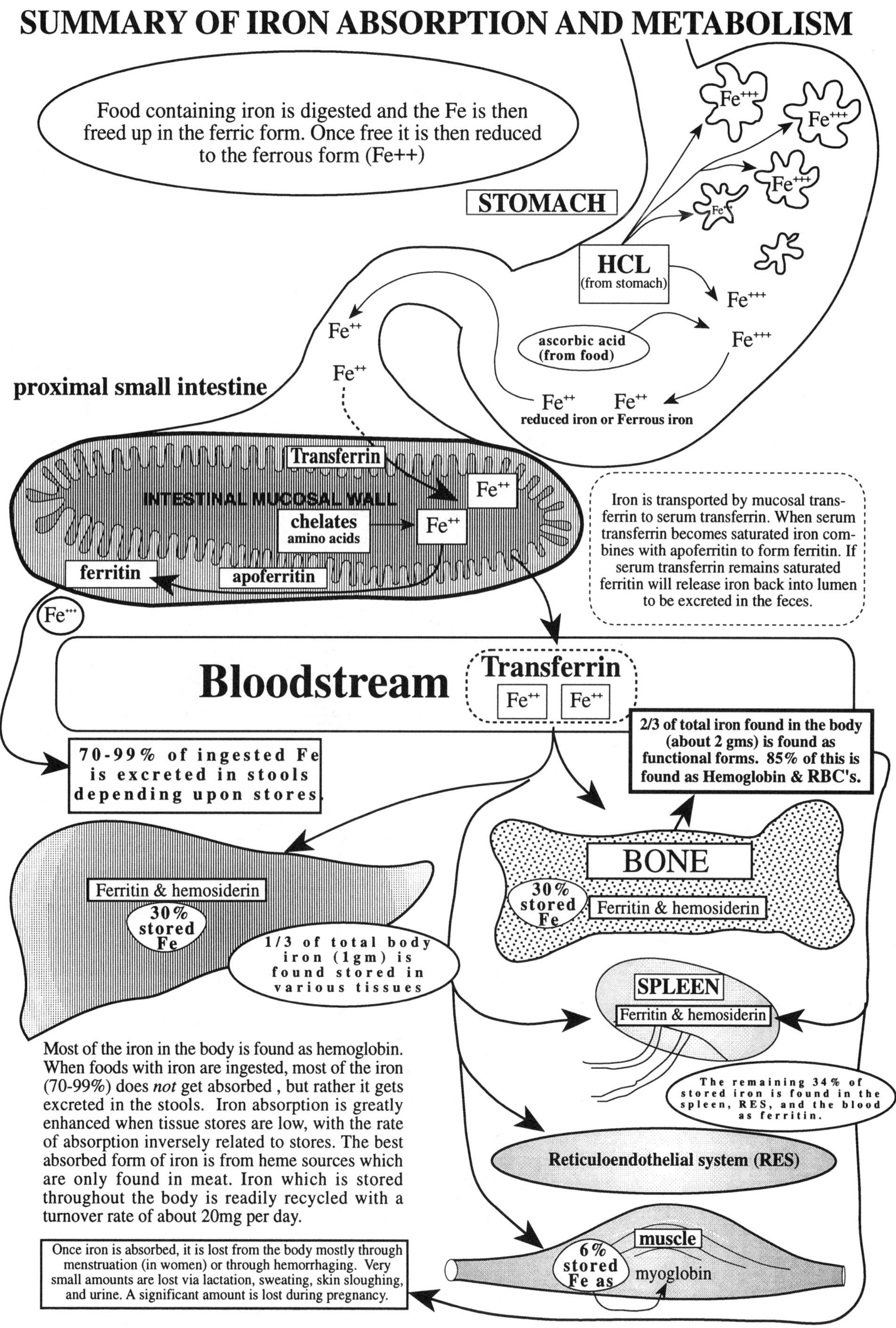

# FOLATE DEFICIENCY ANEMIA

## I. Etiology

1) Dietary deficiency
2) Increased requirements
   - Cirrhosis
   - Pregnancy
   - Infancy
3) Congenital folate malabsorption
4) Drug induced folate malabsorption
5) Gluten sensitive enteropathy

## II. Signs and Symptoms

Weakness, tiredness, dyspnea, sore tongue, diarrhea, irritability and forgetfulness, anorexia, dizziness, headache, palpitations, hypersegmented neutrophils, megaloblastic and macrocytic RBC's, fever, weight loss, glossitis, abnormal liver function tests.

## III. Diagnosis

1) First, differentiate folate deficiency from B-12 anemia.
2) Very low serum folate and low B-12 are characteristic of folate deficiency.
3) FIGLU (foraminoglutamic acid) excretion is increased in folate deficiency. B-12 also results in increased excretion of FIGLU, but to a lesser extent.
4) Hypersegmented neutrophils is an early sign of folate deficiency although it is not specific to folate deficiency as vitamin B12 can also show hypersegmented neutrophils. It is more common to folate deficiency.

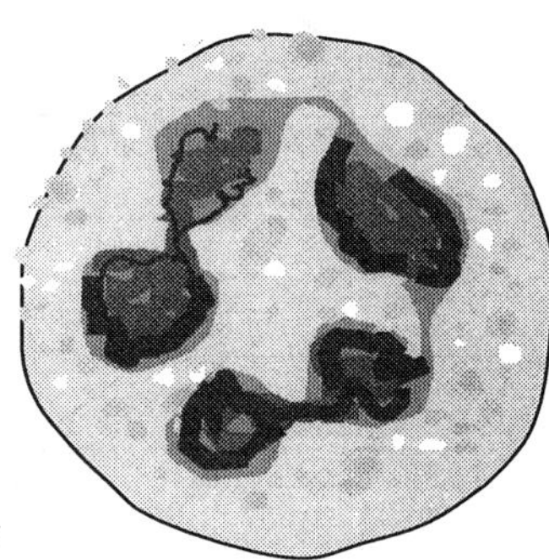

*Hypersegmented Neutrophil*

## IV. Treatment

1) **Folate**–1-5mg/day–Symptomatic treatment usually is apparent before the hematologic values are back to normal.

2) **Eat foods with lots folate**–Liver, asparagus, dried beans, brewer's yeast, spinach, wheat bran, dark green leafy vegetables, whole wheat bread. Since heat destabilizes folate, it is good to eat foods as raw as possible.

3) **Correct the underlying condition** such as Celiac disease.

4) **Vitamin C**–Macrocytic anemia of scurvy may produce a relative folate deficiency since vitamin C is required to convert folic acid into folinic acid.

# VITAMIN B-12 DEFICIENCY ANEMIA/PERNICIOUS ANEMIA

- Vitamin B-12 deficiency is usually caused by a decreased absorption from the intestines. There are many causes of malabsorption including surgical resection of the terminal ileum, parasites, ulcerative colitis, Crohn's disease, allergies and lactose intolerance to name a few. Congenital abnormalities of the ileum can also cause malabsorption.
- Deficiency of intake is seen in starvation states and also in strict vegans who do not eat any animal products.
- A specific a lack of Intrinsic Factor is the cause of pernicious anemia (PA). This is considered an autoimmune condition and usually there are auto antibodies to the parietal cells or to intrinsic facter itself.
- PA presents a similar picture as folate deficiency anemia, but, in addition, certain neurological symptoms are present.

## I. Etiology

1) Vitamin B-12 dietary deficiency, which is uncommon except in strict vegans, may cause pernicious anemia. An excellent review was presented in 9/91 issue of East West Journal.
2) Lack of intrinsic factor (usually autoimmune antibodies to IF)
3) Functionally abnormal intrinsic factor
4) Deficiency of HCl
5) Tapeworms
6) Diseases affecting the ileum (e.g. Crohn's, Irritable Bowel Syndrome, Celiac disease).
7) Abnormal bacterial flora

## II. Signs and Symptoms

- Most notably, neurological symptoms develop, such as paresthesia, especially numbness and tingling in the hands and feet; decreased senses of vibration and position. Also noted are poor muscle coordination, poor memory and hallucinations. If left untreated for long enough, the symptoms will become permanent.

## III. Diagnosis

1) **Methylmalonic acid (MMA) in serum**- is the most sensitive test to determine low tissue levels of vitamin B-12. High levels of MMA indicate vitamin B-12 deficiency.
2) **Radio immune assay for serum B-12**-has a wide reference range (150-900pg/ml) and sometimes will pick up cobalamin analogs that do not have any B-12 activity. Thus the test is not very qualitative.
3) **Schilling urinary excretion test**–An oral dose of radioactive B-12 is given. Urinary excretion is measured. If there is no urinary excretion, then B-12 is not getting absorbed. The same test is repeated, giving the intrinsic factor orally. If there is still no urinary output then there is no pernicious anemia. The Schilling test can identify if there is no **IF** or if there is a malabsorption syndrome going on.
4) **Antibodies in serum to intrinsic factor**- This confirms pernicious anemia diagnosis.

## IV. Treatment

1) **Vitamin B-12**–IM 1000mcg/day for 1 week–normally it only requires about 3mcg/day to prevent pernicious anemia.

2) **Eat foods with B-12**–animal foods, brewers yeast., blue green algae (see list on p.221)

3) **Treat the underlying cause**–parasites, diarrhea, IBD, abnormal gut bacteria, etc.

# VITAMIN B-6 RESPONSIVE ANEMIA

- Severe hypochromic, microcytic anemia in the presence of high serum iron and tissue levels.
- Inherited sex linked anemia
- The synthesis of heme is impaired because vitamin B-6 is required for the formation of D-aminolevulinic acid (ALA)
- Iron builds up in the mitochondria of immature RBC's, which are then called sideroblasts. Symptoms of iron overload and anemia develop due to vitamin B-6 deficiency.

## I. Treatment

1) **Vitamin B-6**–100mg 3x/day–Patients respond in varying degrees. P5P may also work.

2) **Eat foods with B-6**–whole grain cereals and breads, vegetables, meats, and liver.

# COPPER DEFICIENCY ANEMIA

- Copper is required for proper formation of hemoglobin.
- When copper is deficient, iron can not be released from its storage sites. The protein ceruloplasmin is the essential copper containing substance.

# SICKLE CELL ANEMIA

- Try to strengthen the cell wall membranes.

## I. Treatment

1) **Zinc** increases the oxygen carrying capacity of both normal and sickle shaped RBC's.

2) **Vitamin E**–450iu's/day for 6-35 weeks–decreases the number of irreversibly sickled cells.

3) **Selenium-200-400mcg per day**

4) **Bioflavonoids2-6gms per day**

5) **Vitamin C**-2-6 gms per day

# Best Food Sources of Iron

| Food item | amount | mg Fe | % absorb | Food item | amount | mg Fe | % absorb |
|---|---|---|---|---|---|---|---|
| Beef liver | 3 oz | 7.5 | 30.0 | Cocoa powder | 2 T | 1.5 | |
| Tofu | 1/2 c | 6.7 | | Peas cooked | 1/2 c | 1.5 | |
| Black strap molasses | 1 T | 5.0 | | Collard greens | 1 c cook | 1.5 | |
| Amaranth, cooked | 1 oz=2/3 c | 4.0 | | Beet greens | 1/2 c | 1.4 | |
| Oysters | 1 oz | 3.8 | | Brewers yeast | 1 T | 1.4 | |
| Lentils, cooked | 1/2 c | 3.3 | | Quinoa, cooked | 1 oz=2/3 c | 1.3 | |
| Swiss chard | 1 c | 3.2 | | Teff, cooked | 1 oz=2/3 c | 1.3 | |
| Ground beef | 3 oz | 3.0 | | Figs | 1/4 c | 1.3 | |
| Roast beef | 3 oz | 3.0 | | Sunflower seeds | 1/8 c | 1.3 | |
| Dulse, dried | 1/16 c=2 gm | 3.0 | | Raisins | 1/4 c | 1.3 | |
| Lima beans | 1/2 c | 2.9 | | Beans, green cook | 1/2 c | 1.2 | |
| Iron fortified formula | 8 oz | 2.9 | | Millet, cooked | 1oz=2/3 c | 1.2 | |
| Beef ground | 3 oz | 2.8 | | Shredded wheat | 1 biscuit | 1.2 | |
| Potato, baked | 1 med | 2.8 | | Whole wheat bread | 1 slice | 1.2 | 7.5 |
| Mustard greens | 1 c | 2.7 | | Lambs quarters | 1/2 c | 1.2 | |
| Wheat germ toasted | 1/4 c | 2.5 | | Prunes | 1/4 c | 1.1 | |
| Soy beans | 1/2 c | 2.5 | 5.2 | Endive or Escarole | 1 c | 1.0 | |
| Garbonzo beans, cook | 1/2 c | 2.4 | | Cod | 3 oz | 1.0 | |
| Rice white enriched | 1 c | 2.3 | 1.0 | Turkey white | 3 oz | 1.0 | |
| Pinto Beans, cooked | 1/2 c | 2.2 | | Egg | 1 large | 1.0 | |
| Kidney beans | 1/2 c dried | 2.2 | | Parsley, chopped | 1/4 c | 0.9 | |
| Turkey dark meat | 3 oz | 2.0 | 30.0 | Rye, cooked flakes | 1 oz=2/3 c | 0.9 | |
| Leeks | 1 c cooked | 2.0 | | Kelp, dried | 1/16 c=2 gm | 0.8 | |
| Dandelion greens | 1 c cooked | 1.9 | | Oats, cooked | 1 oz=2/3 c | 0.8 | |
| Apricots | 1/4 c | 1.8 | | Corn | 1/2 c 4 oz | 0.8 | 2.5 |
| Cornflakes | 1 c | 1.8 | | Frankfurter | 1 lg | 0.8 | |
| Kale | 1 c cook | 1.8 | | Peanuts | 1/4 c | 0.8 | |
| Pumpkin or squash | 2T seeds | 1.8 | | Cashew butter | 1 T | 0.8 | |
| Black beans | 1/2 c | 1.7 | 3.6 | Buckwheat, cooked | 1 oz=2/3 c | 0.7 | |
| Infant cereal | 1 T | 1.7 | | Rice | 1 oz dry | 0.7 | |
| Infant cereal rice | 1 T | 1.7 | | Pork chop | 1 med | 0.7 | |
| Spinach raw chopped | 1 c | 1.7 | 3.5 | Leaf lettuce | 1 c loose | 0.6 | 7.8 |
| Broccoli raw | 1 stalk 1/2 c | 1.7 | | Almond butter | 1 T | 0.6 | |
| Almonds chopped | 1/4 c | 1.6 | | Blueberries | 1/2 c | 0.5 | |
| Tuna | 3 oz | 1.6 | | Banana | 1 med | 0.4 | |
| Pumpkin canned | 1/2 c | 1.6 | | Raspberries | 1/2 c | 0.4 | |

# OSTEOPOROSIS

- Osteoporosis is the most common metabolic bone disease in U.S.
- Not a problem of the bone matrix, osteoporosis is a decrease in formation relative to resorption.
- After age 40 skeletal mass begins to decline in both men and women, but more rapidly in women. 40% of women in America will experience spontaneous fractures by age 70.
- Bone loss is most severe in vertebral bodies, metacarpals, femoral head and neck, and distal radius.
- Obese people have decreased bone loss due to increased weight bearing and (in women), increased estrogen storage.

** 500mg/day is the average Calcium turnover

STUDY–Albanese, Edelson, Lorenze. *Problems of bone health in the elderly*, New York State Journal of Medicine

ABSTRACT–In 2197 healthy women, aged 15 to 97, bone density, as measured by X-ray densitometry, was found to peak at ages 35 to 45, and then to decline steadily. In 936 healthy men, peak bone density occurred at 45 years of age and fell slowly thereafter. Bone loss reversal was radiographically evident in 24 to 36 months in 12 women 78-86 years old following ingestion of 700-800mg of supplemental calcium daily. Significant improvement was found in shorter term studies in women 42 to 63 years old when calcium, with and without estrogen, was given.

## I. Risk Factors

### 1) Congenital

Female
Premature graying of hair
(50% gray by age 40)
Caucasian, Asian
Family history of osteoporosis
Slight of build

### 2) Lifestyle

Sedentary work and leisure habits; immobilization due to sickness or injury
Smoking, Alcohol; >2 ounces per day; Coffee; consumption of >5 cups per day
High protein diet (typical of U.S. diet)
High sodium intake (typical of U.S. diet)
Nulliparity

### 3) Adult health

Presence or history of compression or stress fracture
Presence or history of gum disease or excessive tooth decay
Amenorrhea; natural or surgical
Liver, kidney or thyroid disease
Chronic use of medications; corticosteroids, antiepileptic drugs, cholesterol lowering drugs, estrogen blocking drugs, methotrexate
Rheumatoid arthritis
Chronic obstructive pulmonary disease
Renal disease

**4) Endocrine:**

Cushing's syndrome
Hyperparathyroidism
Hypergonadism
Acromegaly
Hyperthyroidism
Diabetes mellitus (metabolic acidosis)
Hyperadrenocorticoids

**5) Hereditary diseases**

Marfan's syndrome
Ehlers-Danlose syndrome
Turner's syndrome
Mucopolysaccharidosis
Pseudohypoparathyroidism
Thalassemia
Christmas disease
*Increased protein=increased acid ash
Osteogenesis imperfecta
Homocysteinuria
Klinefelter's syndrome
Gaucher's disease
Sickle cell anemia
Hemophelia
Iron overload (hemochromotosis)
Ulcerative colitis, Crohn's disease, Celiac disease

**Vitamin D Synthesis**

**NOTE**–1,25 dihydroxy vitamin D is produced in the kidneys in response to low serum calcium from the secretion of PTH. It's function is to stimulate the active transport of calcium from the intestines and to resorb calcium from the bones. **Elderly people with osteoporosis generally have lower levels of** 1,25 **dihydroxy vitamin D than normal,** indicating a **decreased ability of their kidney's to hydroxylate** 25 **hydroxycholecalciferol.**

STUDY–Gallagher. *Intestinal calcium absorption and serum vitamin D metabolites in normal subjects and osteoporotic patients.* J Clin Invest 1979;64:729. ABSTRACT–In 27 osteoporotic patients, mean serum levels of 25-OH-Vitamin D were not significantly different than that of controls. However, **levels of 1,25 dihydroxy**

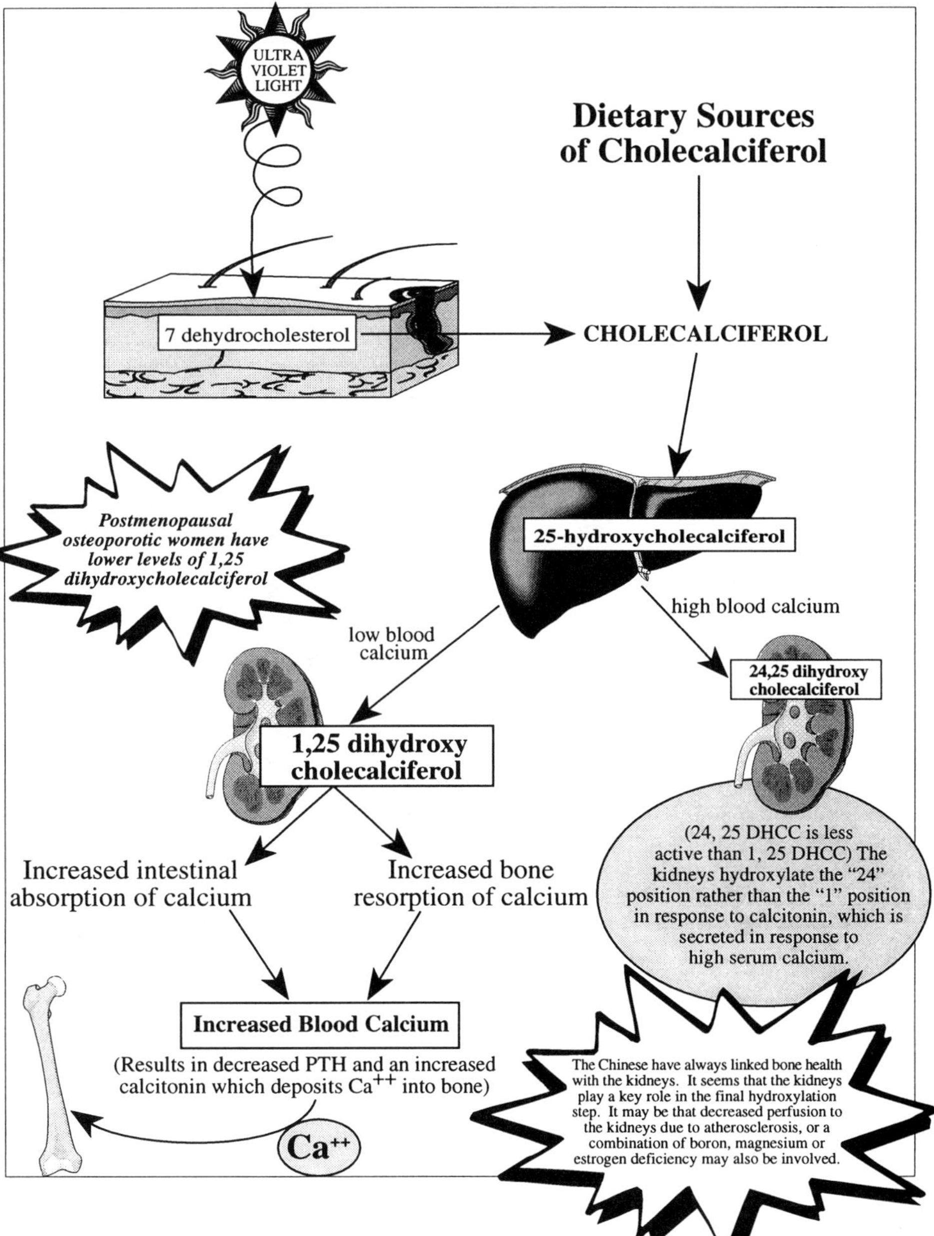

**Vitamin D were significantly lower in the osteoporotic patients** than in controls. Regression analysis showed that most of the decrease in calcium absorption found in these 27 patients could be attributed to lower 1,25 dihydroxy Vitamin D levels. However, differences in levels of this Vitamin D metabolite could not entirely explain differences in calcium absorption. Apparently, some other factor was also involved. In 20 of 24 osteoporotic individuals taking 0.4 mcg of **1,25 dihydroxy Vitamin D (Calcitriol)** per day, there was a **significant increase in calcium absorption.** These data suggest that many o**lder individuals with osteoporosis have a primary defect in their ability to convert 25-hydroxy Vitamin D to 1,25 dihydroxy Vitamin D.**

STUDY–Tsai. *Impaired Vitamin D metabolism in women: possible role in pathogenesis of senile osteoporosis.* J. Clin.Invest. 73:1668-1672, 1984. ABSTRACT–The level of 25-hydroxy vitamin D was not found to decrease with age but 1,25 dihydroxy vitamin D was lower in elderly women, both with and without hip fractures, than it was in normal premenopausal women and normal women within 20 years of menopause. Infusion with a tropic agent for the converting enzyme (bovine parathyroid fragment 1-34) resulted in a higher increase in **1,25 dihydroxy vitamin D** for the younger women than for the other groups and the **least increase for the elderly women with hip fractures**, suggesting that an **age-related decrease in the kidney's ability to synthesize 1,25 dihydroxy vitamin D is a contributing factor to the development of senile osteoporosis.**

## II. Signs and Symptoms

Generally there are no symptoms associated with osteoporosis, but there are indirect signs and symptoms concerning problems with calcium metabolism. Periodontal disease, nocturnal leg cramps, osteoarthritic changes in the joints, poor nail growth, backaches, and decreased height are common signs and symptoms that may be related to osteoporosis. Vertebral compression fractures may be painless, but can be associated with decreased height and can be seen on radiographs.

**NOTE**–The first apparent changes on x-rays appear in the femoral neck, vertebral bodies, metacarpals, and distal radius.

## III. Diagnosis

X-rays (later stages)–very insensitive, will not show bone lose until 30-50% lost

**Bone densiometry**–

- *Radiographic absorptiometry*–density is measured via comparison of bone versus referenced aluminum wedge on standard x-ray film. This technique typically measures the metacarpals.
- *Single photon absorptiometry (SPA)*–can only measure sites of the appendicular skeleton, sites that are predominantly cortical bone (e.g.distal radius, calcaneus). This technology is being supercede by single x-ray asorptiometry (SXA).
- *Dual photon absorptiometry (DPA)*–DPA has the ability to measure the proximal femur, vertebrae, and/or the forearm. This technology has been replaced by DEXA.
- *Dual energy x-ray absorptiometry (DEXA)*–composite advantages of: low x-ray exposure, high accuracy, high reproducibility, ability to measure lumbar spine, proximal femur, forearm.
- *Quantitative computed tomography (QCT)*–has the ability to measure vertebral cancellous bone separate from cortical bone. Poorer precision and markedly higher x-ray exposure (as compared with DEXA).

**Urine studies**

bone loss measurements include:

24 hour calcium
hydroxyproline
Type 1 collagen (cross-links)
Pyridinoline
Deoxypyridinoline

**Vitamin K levels**–Meridian Valley Labs can check
**Hair analysis**-look for elevated lead levels which has been linked to osteoporosis & caries.
**Signs and symptoms**
**Heidelberg (HCL evaluation)**
**Urinary pH** (should be more alkaline to decrease calcium excretion)

## IV. Etiology

**1) Diet high in acid ash**

a) inactivates PTH (remember PTH increases 1,25 dihydroxy vitamin D)

b) Increases excretion of calcium in urine (calcium pulled from the bones to buffer the acid pH of the serum)

STUDY–Barzel, U.S. *Acid loading and osteoporosis.* J Am Geriatrics Soc. September p.613, 1982. ABSTRACT–meats, high protein foods, whole grains which yield an acid ash, all increase calcium excretion.

**2) Diet high in protein**–has been shown in controlled studies using protein supplements. The evidence is less strong in mixed diets with a moderately high protein level. Considering that homocystinuria is a risk factor and is much more common than what has previously been thought, higher levels of protein, particularly animal proteins in which there is a lot of methionine which can be metabolized into homocysteine in genetically susceptible individuals

STUDIES–Johnson, Alcantara, Linkswiler. *Effect of level of protein intake on urinary and fecal calcium and calcium retention of young adult males*, J. Nutr. 100:1425, 1970.

• Walker & Linkswiler. *Calcium retention in the adult human male as affected by protein intake,* J. Nutr. 102:1297,1972.

• Anand & Linkswiler. *Effect of protein intake on calcium balance of young men given 500mg of calcium daily.* J. Nutr.104:695, 1974.

• Linkswiler, Joyce, and Anand. *Calcium retention of young adult males as affected by level of protein and of calcium intake,* Trans.N.Y. Acad. Sci 36:333, 1974.

ABSTRACT–In a series of 4 carefully controlled human metabolic studies, the influence of protein intake (47, 95, and 142gms daily) on urinary calcium, calcium retention, and calcium absorption was assessed in 33 men between the ages of 18 and 23 years. Dietary calcium was provided at levels of 500, 800, and 1400mg daily, and in each study protein intake varied while calcium intake remained constant. The studies were 45 to 55 days in length, and the period of observation at any level of protein intake was at least 15 days. **Positive calcium balance occurred when 47gms of protein was consumed regardless of the calcium intake.** Intakes of 800 & **1400mg Calcium caused no higher retention than an intake of 500mgs.** On the other hand, protein intake of **142gms resulted in markedly negative calcium balances at ALL calcium intake levels.**

**3) High phosphorus diet** (see phosphorus p.108 and also table p.338)

**4) Reduced calcium consumption**–average consumption ~500mg/day in the U.S.

**5) Coffee, alcohol, smoking**–Caffeine increases urinary calcium excretion. Alcohol and smoking have been shown to decrease bone mass.

STUDY–Hollingbery, P.W., et al. *Effect of dietary caffeine and aspirin on urinary calcium and hydroxyproline excretion in pre and postmenopausal women.* Fed Proc. 44:1149, 1985. ABSTRACT–31 women ingested decaffeinated coffee to which caffeine had been added at different times. 3 hours later, urinary calcium excretion increased significantly, but only in women taking estrogen, suggesting that caffeine ingestion may offset the beneficial effect of estrogen on calcium metabolism.

STUDY–Massey, L.K., Berg TA. *The effect of dietary caffeine on urinary excretion of Calcium, Magnesium, Phosphorus, Sodium, Potassium, Chloride, and Zinc in healthy males.* Nutr. Res 5:1281-84, 1985. ABSTRACT–15 males drank decaffeinated coffee to which 0, 150, or 300mg caffeine had been added. Total urinary 3 hour excretion of calcium, magnesium, sodium, and chloride, increased significantly after caffeine intake, while zinc, phosphorus, creatinine, and volume were unchanged.

**6) Inactivity**

**7) Low gastric pH** (hypochlorhydria and achlorhydria)

STUDY–Hunt, J.N., Johnson, C. *Relation between gastric secretion of acid and urinary excretion of calcium after oral supplementation of calcium.* Dig Dis Sci 28(5):417-21, 1983. ABSTRACT–12 subjects were given either 1500mg of calcium carbonate or calcium citrate. Urinary calcium excretion was measured as well as gastric pH. Subjects with normal levels of HCL seemed to absorb both forms of the calcium. Subjects who were achlorhydric absorbed the calcium citrate significantly better.

**8) Estrogen deficiency**

**9) Aluminum toxicity**

## V. Treatment

**1) Decrease protein consumption** down to 1gm/3.8lbs)

**2) Increase pH of blood** (see acid-base p.339) A more acid ash increases calcium excretion.

STUDY–Metz, JA, Anderson, JB, Gallagher, PN JR. *Intakes of calcium, phosphorus, and protein and physical activity are related to radial bone mass in adult women.* AM J Clin Nutr 1993;58:537-42. Allen, LH, Oddoye EA, Margen L. *Protein-induced hypercalciuria.* AM J Clin Nutr 1979;32:741-9. Spencer HJ, et. al.. *Affect of a high protein (meat) intake on calcium metabolism in man.* Am J Nutr. 1978;37:453-6

**3) Bring calcium/phosphorus** 2:1 **or** 1:1 (see Calcium/Phosphorus table p.338)

**4) Supplement highly absorbable calcium** such as calcium-citrate–400mg-800mg–or citrate malate. In addition the patient should eat foods rich in Calcium (see handout) for a total intake of 800-1200mg. It should be noted that calcium citrate is only about 18% calcium which means that you can only have a limited amount of actual elemental calcium in each capsule or tablet. The percentage of calcium absorbed from the more absorbable calcium forms, even though it may be higher, does not make up for the low percentage of actual elemental calcium. In other words I recommend doing some form of mixed calcium (the more expensive low percent and the cheaper high percent calcium forms).

**5) Magnesium**–400-600mg–regulates PTH secretion & tissue sensitivity)

STUDY–Cohen & Kitzes *Infrared spectroscopy and magnesium content of bone mineral in osteoporotic women.* Israel J. Med. Sci. 17:1123-5, 1981. ABSTRACT–16 of 19 **Osteoporotic pts. had lower than normal trabecular bone magnesium content** (by infrared spectrophotometry) and clinical magnesium deficiency (based on Thoren's magnesium load test)

**6) Increase physical activity**–1hr. 3x/week–This has been shown to actually increase bone mass in postmenopausal women.

**7) Stop smoking & cut back on alcohol and coffee**

**8) Vitamin K1 (phytonadione)**–1mg/day. Vitamin K is involved with the synthesis of osteocalcin, a protein containing gamma carboxyglutamic acid which is involved in the mineralization of bone (formation of hydroxyapatite crystals). Calcium is attracted to and binds with gamma-carboxyglutamic acid. Vitamin K deficiency is quite high in patients with gastrointestinal disorders.

**Test via prothrombin anti-antigen or serum vitamin K assay.**

STUDY–Hart, J.P., Hearer, M.J., Klenerrman, L., Shearer, M.J., Caterall, A., et al. *Electrochemical detection of depressed circulating levels of vitamin K in osteoporosis.* J Clin Endocrinol Metab 60:1268-69, 1985. ABSTRACT–16 patients with osteoporosis were found to have mean serum vitamin K concentrations only 35% of aged matched controls.

STUDY–Knapen, M.H.J., Hamulyak, K., Vermeer, C.. *The effect of vitamin K suppl on circulating osteocalcin and urinary calcium excretion* Annals of Internal Medicine 111:1001-5, 1989. ABSTRACT–In postmenopausal women, osteocalcin levels were 50% that of premenopausal women. Vitamin K induced increased serum immunoreactive osteocalcin concentration; normalization of HAB capacity of serum immunoreactive osteocalcin.

STUDY–Tomita, A. *Post menopausal osteoporosis calcium study with vitamin K2.* Clin Endocrinol(Japan) 19:731-736,1971. ABSTRACT–Osteoporotic patients treated with vitamin K suppl reduced urinary Calcium loss by 18-50%.

**9) Vitamin D3 (cholecalciferol)**–400-1000iu/day

STUDY–Norden. *A prospective trial of the effect of Vitamin D supplementation on metacarpal bone loss in elderly women.* Am. J. Clin. Nut. 42(3):470-74, 1985. ABSTRACT-109 women randomly selected elderly women (ages 65-74) received orally either Vitamin D2 15,000iu weekly or placebo. After 2 years, Vitamin D significantly reduced the rate of cortical bone loss as measured by hand radiographs (p less than 0.01)

**10) Vitamin A**–20,000iu/day–is involved in bone matrix formation by osteoblasts.

**11) Folic acid**–5mg–Folate is a coenzyme in the conversion of homocysteine to methionine (see chapter on cardiovascular disease & folate supplementation references).

STUDY–Brattstriom *Folic acid responsive postmenopausal homocysteinemia.* Metabolism 34(11):1073-7,1985. ABSTRACT–5mg folate daily for 4 weeks substantially reduced homocysteine concentrations (p less than 0.01) both before a methionine load and afterwards (despite the fact that subjects had normal levels of serum and RBC folate) in normal men and pre- and postmenopausal women, suggesting that **folic acid may have a prophylactic action against postmenopausal osteoporosis** if moderate homocysteinemia promotes its development (homocysteine which is increased in postmenopausal women, interferes with collagen cross-linking leading to defective bone matrix and osteoporosis.

**12) Boron**–2mg–is involved in the hydroxylation of 17 ßeta-estradiol and 1,25DH vitamin D.

STUDY–Nielsen, F.H., Hunt, C.D., Mullen, L.M., Hunt, J.R. *Effect of dietary boron mineral, estrogen, and testosterone metabolism in postmenopausal women.* FASEBJ 1:394-397, 1987. ABSTRACT–Postmenopausal women were fed a standard diet for 119 days consisting of 0.25mg boron. Supplementing this diet with 3mg boron reduced urinary calcium excretion by 44% and markedly increased serum concentrations of the estrogenic hormone, 17ß-estradiol. The increased levels of 17ß-estradiol were the same as in women receiving estrogen therapy.

**13) Silica**–1mg/day–has been found to be important in the matrix of bone.

**14) Manganese**–stimulates the production of mucopolysaccharides (bone's organic matrix).

**15) Zinc**–20-40mg/day–has been found to be important in the matrix of bone.

**16) Copper**–1-3mg/day-is involved in lysyl oxidase in cross linking of collagen.

**17) Omnivite** (Omnivite Nutrition Inc)**., Osteoprime forte** (Metagenics or Phytopharmica)or other bone formula which contains substantial amounts of vitamins K, D, A, minerals calcium, magnesium, boron, silica, manganese as base formula. Currently there are some uncontrolled and unpublished studies showing Omnivite can reverse bone lose.

## Additional notes on osteoporosis:

STUDY–Albanese. *Effects of Calcium and micronutrients on bone loss of pre-and postmenopausal women.* Paper presented at Am. Med. Assoc. meeting, Jan.1981. ABSTRACT–12 healthy women, ages 39-65, whose usual daily diets contained 200-425mg of Calcium took a supplement containing 600mg of Calcium and "all known micronutrients" at RDA levels. 11 healthy women with comparable diets took 700-800mg of Calcium per day without the additional nutrients. Periodic x-ray measurements showed that, within 9-11 months, the **rate of bone density increase was 2-3x greater in the women receiving the Calcium plus micronutrients than in those taking the Calcium alone.**

STUDY–Recker, R. *Calcium absorption and achlorhydria.* NEJM 313(2)70-73, 1985. ABSTRACT–9 normal fasting patients were compared to 11 achlorhydric patients. The normal pH subjects absorption was similar for both forms of calcium. In the achlorhydric patients, **calcium citrate was absorbed an average of 10x that of the carbonate form**.

STUDY–Harvey, J.A., Zobitz, M.M., Pak, C.Y.C. *Dose dependency of calcium absorption: a comparison of calcium carbonate and calcium citrate* J Bone Min Res 3(3): 253-8, 1988. ABSTRACT–**It was found that a 500mg dose of calcium citrate resulted in a greater amount of absorption than a 2000mg load of calcium carbonate.** The authors suggest that just prescribing higher amounts of the carbonate form doesn't necessarily increase the total amount of calcium absorbed.

STUDY–Nicar, M.J., Pak, C.Y.C. *Calcium bioavailability from calcium carbonate and calcium citrate.* J Clin Enodocrin Met 61:2 391-3, 1985. ABSTRACT–Calcium citrate was found to be better absorbed in all patients including normochlorhydrics.

STUDY–Schuett, S., Knowles, J. *A comparison of calcium absorption from calcium citrate versus calcium $H_2(PO4)_2$ by two methods* Am J Clin Nut 45:4; 863, 1987.

**Note-**It seems that recent evidence shows that certain flavonoids from soy and synthetic analogs called ipriflavones show great promise concerning bone growth stimulation (see *Osteoporosis Solution* in Bibliography)

**Citric acid** promotes GI absorption by opening up epithelial tight junctions, enhancing the paracellular shunt pathway of calcium transport. It also helps inhibit calcium oxalate crystallization and possible renal or urinary calculi due to high dose calcium.

### Best Food Sources of Calcium

| Food | amount | mg | mg Phos | Food | amount | mg | mg Phos |
|---|---|---|---|---|---|---|---|
| Cheese, Gruyere | 3 oz | 860 | 450 | Ice cream, vanilla | 1 cup | 176 | 125 |
| Cheese, mozzarella | 3 oz | 621 | 405 | Edensoy, extra fortified | 1 cup | 167 | 120 |
| Cheese, cheddar | 3 oz | 612 | 405 | Cheese, cottage 2% | 1 cup | 155 | 525 |
| Cheese, American | 3 oz | 525 | 405 | Dandelion, greens cooked | 1/2 cup | 147 | 44 |
| Turnip greens, cooked | 1 cup | 492 | 100 | Molasses, black strap | 1 T | 137 | 15 |
| Torula yeast | 1 oz | 490 | 2000 | Soy flour, full fat | 1/2 cup | 132 | 280 |
| Lambs quarters, cooked | 1 cup | 400 | 100 | Rice Drink, Pacific, fortified | 1 cup | 120 | 80 |
| Sardines, with bones | 3 oz | 372 | 424 | Mustard greens, cooked | 1 cup | 104 | 60 |
| Collard greens, cooked | 1 cup | 357 | 50 | Almonds | 1/4 cup | 92 | 250 |
| Rhubarb, cooked | 1 cup | 348 | 55 | Beans, baked | 1/2 cup | 64 | 180 |
| Yogurt | 1 cup | 345 | 99 | Filberts | 1/4 cup | 60 | 90 |
| Milk, skim & 2% | 1 cup | 300 | 240 | Orange | 1 med | 52 | 25 |
| Spinach, cooked | 1 cup | 276 | 65 | Halibut | 3 oz | 51 | 200 |
| Oatmeal, fortified | 1 cup | 208 | 178 | Kale, cooked | 1 cup | 47 | 18 |
| Rice Drink, Westbrae, fort. | 1 cup | 200 | 80 | Spinach, fresh | 1 cup | 44 | 15 |
| Salmon, canned w/bones | 3 1/2 oz | 185 | 400 | Tahini, toasted sesame paste | 2T=15gms | 42 | 240 |
| Tofu, firm (about 2/3 cup) | 6.1oz | 190 | 170 | Garbonzo beans, chick peas | 1/2 c cook | 40 | 138 |
| Broccoli, cooked | 1 cup | 180 | 120 | Sesame seeds (varies) | 3T=24gms | 33 | 160 |

**Non-dairy Sources of Calcium are shaded in the above table.**

## ACID AND ALKALINE ASH OF ELECTED FOODS

Alkaline ash forming foods (the higher the number the more alkaline the food)

*Generally speaking, in the treatment of osteoporosis, you want your blood to be more alkaline. The more acidic your blood the greater the loss of calcium in your urine.*

| Food | Measure | Effect | |
|---|---|---|---|
| Molasses | 2 t | 60.0 | most alkaline |
| Beans | 1/8 c | 42.0 | ***Best*** |
| Raisins | 1/3 c | 34.0 | |
| Figs, dried | 1 1/2 | 33.0 | |
| Beet greens | 1 c | 27.0 | |
| Spinach | 1 c | 18.0 | |
| Yeast, brewers | 1 c | 17.1 | |
| Almonds | 12 nuts | 12.0 | |
| Carrots | 1 large | 11.0 | |
| Soy flour | 2 T | 9.5 | |
| Celery | 2 stalks | 7.8 | |
| Grapefruit juice | 1/2 c | 7.0 | |
| Sweet Potato | 1 medium | 6.7 | |
| Beans, baked | 1/2 c | 6.0 | |
| Peas, dried | 2T | 6.0 | |
| Tomato | 1 small | 5.6 | |
| Strawberry | 12 medium | 5.5 | |
| Banana | 1 small | 5.6 | |
| Mushrooms | 7 medium | 4.0 | |
| Apple | 1 large | 3.7 | |
| Milk, whole | 1 c | 2.3 | |
| Buttermilk | 1 c | 2.2 | |
| Onions | 1 medium | 1.5 | *worst* |
| Squash, summer | 1 c | 1.0 | least alkaline |

Acid ash forming foods (the higher the number the more acid the food)

| Food | Measure | Effect | |
|---|---|---|---|
| Wheat germ | 2 T | 20.0 | most acidic |
| Lentil, dried | 2 T | 16.0 | *worst* |
| Macoroni or Spaghetti | 1/4 c | 14.0 | |
| Chicken | 4 oz | 14.0 | |
| Eggs | 1 medium | 11.0 | |
| Beef, steak | 4 oz | 11.0 | |
| Beef, liver | 4 oz | 11.0 | |
| Lamb chops | 2 small chops | 9.7 | |
| Cod fish | 4 oz | 9.4 | |
| Walnuts, English | 12 medium nuts | 7.8 | |
| Buckwheat flour | 2 T | 7.1 | |
| Rice, brown | 3 T | 5.7 | |
| Cheese, cheddar | 1 cube | 5.0 | |
| Cheese, cottage | 1/8 c | 4.5 | |
| Peanuts | 16 nuts | 3.9 | |
| Bread, whole wheat | 2 slice | 3.6 | |
| Honey | 1 T | 1.1 | ***Best*** |
| Butter | 1 T | 0.0 | least acidic |

# PERIODONTAL DISEASE

- Inflammation of gingiva &/or periodontium
- Can be systemic or local
- Can cause alveolar bone loss which is non-inflammatory
- Men have a higher incidence than women

**Prevalence** (in U.S.) 15% at age 10
38% at age 20
46% at age 35
54% at age 50

## I. Etiology

1) **Environment of gingival sulcus (depth)**
2) **Bacterial factors**–Numerous compounds that are very detrimental to the host defense mechanisms are produced by bacterial plaque. Among these compounds are: endotoxins and exotoxins; free radicals and collagen-destroying enzymes; leukotoxins, bacteria, antigens, and toxic compounds.
3) **Polymorphonuclear leukocyte function** is the primary defense against microbial overgrowth. PMN function is depressed in patients with diabetes, Crohn's disease, Chediak-Higashi.
4) **Complement Activation**
5) **IgE and mast cell function**–A major factor in periodontal disease, mast cell degranulation, results in the release of inflammatory mediators, such as histamine, leukotrienes, prostaglandins, kinins, etc. It is an indication of allergy.
6) **Amalgam restoration**–Mercury released from amalgams depletes free radical scavengers, glutathione peroxidases, SOD, etc. Mercury is also a catalyst for free radical damage
7) **Structure and integrity of collagen matrix of periodontium and gingiva**–The rate of diffusion from the oral cavity and the permeability of inflammatory mediators, destructive enzymes, bacteria and their by-products is determined by the status of the collagen matrix of the periodontium.
8) **Occlusion problems**–Obviously, if teeth are missing, bruxism, malocclusion or tongue thrusting is present, abnormal strain will be put on the teeth and surrounding tissues, setting the stage for progression of periodontal disease.

## II. Therapeutic Considerations

1) Decrease wound healing time
2) Improve membrane & collagen integrity
3) Decrease inflammation & free radical damage
4) Enhance immune status, especially PMN'S
5) Increase salivation

## III. Treatment

1) **Vitamin C**–3-5gms/day
   a) maintains membrane & collagen integrity
   b) decreases wound healing time
   c) decreases free radical damage
   d) improves PMN function

STUDY–Stephens & Snyderman. *Cyclic nucleotides regulate the morphologic alterations required for chemotaxis in monocytes*. J Immunology 128:1192-7, 1982. ABSTRACT–In patients with Chediak-Higashi syndrome, an autosomal recessive trait presents in which patient's **PMN's have compromised chemotaxis and phagocytosis.** This syndrome **responds** remarkably well to **Vitamin C supplementation.**

2) **Decrease sucrose consumption**–sucrose increases plaque formation and decreases PMN chemotaxis.

3) **Zinc picolinate**–30mg/day orally and 5% solution as a mouth wash 2x/day–Periodontal disease is inversely related to zinc status and directly related to copper status. Copper is a free radical cofactor. Zinc is marginally deficient in many of the elderly.

   **Zinc functions**:
   a) stabilizes membranes
   b) antioxidant activity
   c) inhibits plaque growth
   d) decreases mast cell degranulation
   e) increases PMN chemotaxis & phagocytosis
   f) decreases wound healing time

4) **Vitamin E**–400-800iu/day
   a) antioxidant activity
   b) decreases wound healing time
   c) decreases membrane permeability

5) **Selenium**–400mcg/day–acts as an antioxidant and is synergistic with vitamin E.

6) **Co-enzyme Q10**–150mg/day–involved in mitochondral oxidative phosphorylation and is an effective antioxidant.

STUDY–Folkers & Yamamura. *Biomedical and clinical aspects of Coenzyme Q*. North Holland Biomedical Press, Amsterdam, 1977. 294-311. ABSTRACT–70% of 332 patients with periodontal disease responded favorably to supplementation.

7) **Folate**–2mg/day and mouth wash with 1/2oz 0.1% sol. 2x/day. Folate has been shown to bind onto plaque derived endotoxin. Epithelial cells of the cervix and the oral cavity appear to undergo the same changes associated with folate deficiency. **Its use is particularly indicated for pregnant women and for oral contraceptive users.**

8) **Quercetin**–500mg 3x/day–prevents mast cell degranulation by stabilizing cell membranes.

9) **Avoid flossing with petrochemicals (waxed dental floss)**. Consider using botanicals and other nutrients in dental floss. Consider making mouth wash.

## NOTES

# RHEUMATOID ARTHRITIS (RA)

- RA is a chronic syndrome characterized by nonspecific, usually symmetric inflammation of the peripheral joints. It can progress resulting in the destruction of the articular and periarticular structures.
- RA affects ~1% of the U.S. population. Females are afflicted at 2-3 times the rate of males. The age of onset is variable, usually beginning between the ages of 25- 50 years.
- 94% of all arthritis patients have tried "quack" therapies.

## I. Etiology

Generally RA is considered an autoimmune condition. Possible contributing factors are:

1) Food sensitivities
2) Heavy metal toxicity
3) High fat diet
4) Hypothyroidism
5) Free radical damage
6) Nugleema amoeba

## II. Signs and Symptoms

The onset may be abrupt, with simultaneous inflammation in multiple joints, or insidious, with progressive joint involvement. Tenderness in affected joints with synovial thickening is most common. Symmetrical involvement of MP and PIP joints, feet, wrists, elbows, and ankles is typical. Stiffness from prolonged inactivity is common. Deformities such as ulnar deviation of hands and fingers are typical.

## III. Diagnosis

The American Rheumatism Association has established the following criteria for the diagnosis of RA:

1) Morning stiffness
2) Pain on motion or tenderness in at least 1 joint
3) Swelling of soft tissues, not bony overgrowth alone, in at least one joint
4) Swelling of at least 1 other joint (any interval free of joint symptoms between the 2 joint involvements may not be more than 3 months).
5) Symmetric joint swelling with simultaneous involvement of the same joint on both sides of the body.
6) Subcutaneous nodules over bony prominences on the extensor surfaces or in juxta-articular regions.
7) X-ray changes typical of RA (must include bony decalcification localized to, or greatest around, involved joints).
8) Positive agglutination test–Demonstration of the rheumatoid factor by any method which in 2 labs has been positive in not greater than 5% of controls.
9) Poor mucin precipitate from synovial fluid (with shreds and cloudy solution). An inflammatory synovial effusion with 2000 WBC/ml.

10) Characteristic histologic changes in synovial membrane with 3 or more of the following: marked infiltration of chronic inflammatory cells (lymphocytes or plasma cells predominating), with tendency to form "lymphoid nodules," deposition of compact fibrin either on surface or interstitially.
11) Characteristic histologic changes in nodules showing granulomatous foci with central zones of cell necrosis, surrounded by a palisade of proliferated mononuclear cells, peripheral fibrosis and chronic inflammatory cell infiltration.

**Definite RA** = 5 or more of the above criteria. In 1-5 the joint signs or symptoms must be continuous for at least 6 weeks.

**Probable RA** = 3 of the above criteria; at least 1 of criteria 1-5. Signs or symptoms must be continuous for at least 6 weeks.

## IV. Treatment

**1) Decrease fats to 20% of calories**–Saturated fats, because of their arachidonic acid content, promote the production of $PGE_2$ and pro-inflammatory mediators.

STUDY–Lucas, C. & Power, L. *Dietary fat aggravates active RA.* Clin. Res. 29(4):754A, 1981 & JAMA 4/9/82. ABSTRACT–6 patients, 2 of which were obese, were treated for RA with a low calorie, fat free weight control formula or diet. The 2 obese patients remained symptom free for 9-14 months and the other 4 patients also experienced a remission in symptoms. Within 24-72 hours of introducing vegetable oil, animal fat, cheese, safflower oil, beef, coconut oil or other foods with a high proportion of calories from fat, they experienced exacerbations of symptoms, i.e. joint swelling, morning stiffness, and tenderness.

STUDY–Skoldstam, L. *Fasting and vegan diet in RA.* Scand. J. Rheumatol. 15(2):219-21, 1987 ABSTRACT–20 patients were placed on a vegan diet following a 7-10 day fast. Also excluded or used sparingly were refined sugar, corn flour, salt, strong spices, alcohol, tea, and coffee. After 4 months, 12 patients reported some improvement, 5 reported no change, and 3 felt worse. Most felt less pain and were better able to function, although there were no changes in objective measures such as grip strength and joint tenderness.

**2) Avoid food sensitivities**

STUDY–Panush, R. *Food-induced allergic arthritis.* Arthritis Rheum. 29(2):220-226, 1986. ABSTRACT–52 year old white female with an 11 year history of joint pain, tenderness, swelling and stiffness fulfilled the criteria for active RA and achieved only fair results from NSAID's. She was placed on a baseline diet for 6 days, a 3 day mineral water fast and vanilla flavored Vivonex. **There were no notable responses to 52 placebo challenges, but she responded with symptomatic deterioration and worsening of ESR and other peak responses to cow's milk challenge on 4 separate occasions.** While there was no elevation of IgE antibodies to foods, there was a mild elevation of IgG and **large amounts of $IgG_4$ anti-milk antibodies.**

STUDY–Hicklin, J. *The effect of diet in RA* . Clin. Allergy 10:463, 1980 ABSTRACT–22 patients, 15 of which were seronegative, followed allergen exclusion diets. 20 subjectively improved, and 19 reported that certain foods would repeatedly exacerbate arthritic symptoms. **Improvement occurred an average of 10 days after the correct exclusions** with a maximum of 18 days. **Reactions to provocation varied from 2 hours to 2 weeks. Grains were by far the most common allergen.** Symptom evoking foods were: grains (14 patients), milk (4), nuts (8), beef (4), eggs (5), and 1 each for chicken, fish, potato, onion, and liver.

STUDY–Skoldstam, L. *Effects of fasting and lactovegetarian diet on RA.* Scand J. Rheum. 8:249-55, 1979. ABSTRACT– Of 26 patients with classical RA (all on NSAIDs), 16 were placed on a diet of fruit and vegetable juices and herbal tea for 7-10 days (1 stopped after 2 days) while the other 10 were controls. Most of the 15 experimental patients **felt better by day 5-6.** At the end of the first diet, 10 reported reduction in pain and stiffness. 5/15 showed objective improvement defined as a greater than 10% decrease in the SED rate with concomitant decrease in joint tenderness, while only 1 of the controls improved. A subsequent lactovegetarian diet was ineffective for all but 1 patient..

STUDY–Seignalet J.. *Diet, fasting and RA..* Lancet. 339:68-69, 1992. ABSTRACT– 46 adults with RA were placed on a diet that consisted of raw foods, while avoiding grains and dairy products. The study lasted for between 1-3 years. 36 patients had significant improvement in painful joints, swollen joints, morning stiffness, SED rate and other parameters. Among the 36 people who had positive benefits, 17 were clearly improved and 19 were in complete remission for 1-5 years. 8 of these 19 pts stopped all medications and no relapse was noted. Improvements were noted in 32 of the 36 responders before the end of the 3rd month. Improvement was progressive and often rapid. 7 of the people that had positive results had all of their symptoms return when they abandoned their diet, but again improved when they resumed their diet.

**3) Vegetarian or Vegan diet**–1.8gms/day (9 caps standard fish oil or 31/2 caps of Super EPA)

STUDY–Nenonen M, et al.. *Effects of uncooked vegan food- "living food"- on RA, a 3 month controlled and randomized study.* AJCN 56:762, 1992. ABSTRACT–40 patients with RA were randomly assigned to receive an uncooked vegan diet or a control diet for 3 months. After this period pts on the vegan diets reported relief of stiffness, joint welling and general well being. When the vegan eating group switched back to their normal omnivorous diet most all of the symptoms became worse.

STUDY–Kjeldsen-Kragh J et al.. *Controlled trial of fasting and one year vegetarian diet in the treatment of RA.* Lancet 338:899-902, 1991. ABSTRACT–27 pts with RA were put on a 7-10 partial fast in which they were allowed to consume vegetable broth various spices and teas, and juices made from potato, parsley, beets, carrots, beets and celery (There was a control group of 26 pts that ate a standard diet with no restrictions). After the partial fast the treatment group introduced one food every 2 days. If the food provoked symptoms, it was removed from the diet and then retested in 7 days. If the food again provoked symptoms, it was then not permitted in the diet. During the first 31/2 months gluten, meat, fish, eggs, dairy products, refined sugar, citrus fruit, preservatives, coffee, tea, alcohol, salt, and strong spices were avoided. Both dairy and gluten were returned to the diet after 31/2 months if they did not provoke symptoms. After 4 weeks the tx group showed a significant improvement in the number of tender joints, Ritchie's articular index, number of swollen joints, pain scored, duration of morning stiffness, grip strength, SED rate, C-reactive protein, WBC count, and a health assessment questionnaire score. In the control group only the pain scored improved significantly. The improvements were still noted in the treatment group one year later.

STUDY–Kjeldsen-Kragh J et al.. *Vegetarian diet for patients with RA-status 2 years after introduction of the diet..* Clin Rheumatol 13:475-82, 1994. ABSTRACT–The above study was followed up and it was found that if the people who responded to the vegetarian diet continued for another year their symptoms remained improved.

**4) Omega 3 fatty acids**–1.8gms-9.1gms per day (6 caps of standard MAXEPA)

STUDY–Kremer, J. *Effect of manipulation of dietary fatty acids on clinical manifestations of RA.* Lancet 1:184-87, 1985. ABSTRACT–17 patients were placed on a high PUFA, low saturated fat diet and supplemented with 10 caps of Max EPA/day, while 20 controls received a typical American diet and placebo caps. **After 12 weeks, the EPA group had significantly less morning stiffness compared to a worsening in the control group**. Joints were also less tender and Hgb improved. A rapid deterioration with increased pain and stiffness was seen in treated patients compared to controls upon cessation of the experimental diet.

STUDY–Kremer, J et. al., . *Fish-oil supplementation in active RA: A double-blinded controlled cross-over study.* Annals of Int Med 106, 497-507, 1987.

STUDY–Das UN. *Beneficial effect of EPA & DHA in the management of SLE and its relationship to the cytokine network.* Prostaglandins, Leukotrienes, EFAs 51:207-213, 1994. ABSTRACT–10 pts with SLE received capsules of 300mg EPA/DHA, 1080IU vitamin A, and 153IU of vitamin D per day for between 3 months and 3 years (median 1 year). All patients had previously been evaluated for GLA, EPA and DHA levels prior to study and were found to be low. Pts. showed improvement biochemically and clinically. All medications were discontinued and pts remained symptom free for up to 3 years.

STUDY–Geusens P et Al.Long-term effect of *Omega 3 fatty acid suppl in active RA. A 12 month, double-blind, controlled study..* Arthritis Rheum Jun 37:824-9, 1994. ABSTRACT–90 pts with active RA were divided into 3 groups; one receiving 2.6gms omega 3 oil (fish), another 1.3 gms omega 3 & 3gms olive oil, and lastly 6 gms of olive oil in a double blind randomized study for 12 months. The 2.6 gms of fish oil group had the most significant improvement and was able to reduce their arthritic medications the most.

**5) Zinc**–750mg zinc sulfate or 90mg zinc picolinate–It was found that, on the average, RA patients have lower serum and intracellular zinc levels. In one unpublished study in Poona, India, half of 18 RA patients were given 50mg of elemental zinc (as zinc sulfate) 3x/day and the other half a placebo. The zinc treated group showed significant improvement in joint swelling, joint tenderness, morning stiffness, onset of fatigue, general condition of the patient and 50 foot walking time. A similar response was observed in the placebo group when they were given zinc. Patients were able to cut back their NSAID by half.

STUDY–Simkin, P. *Oral zinc sulfate in RA.* Lancet 2:539, 1976 ABSTRACT–12/24 treatment resistant patients received 50mg zinc 3x daily for 12 weeks while the rest received placebo. The remaining 24 patients received zinc for 12 more weeks along with the initially supplemented group. There were significant improvements in joint swelling, morning stiffness, walking time and subjective symptoms during the first part of the study with continuing impressive improvement in the second part in both groups.

6) **Antioxidants–Vitamin E**–1000iu/day & **Selenium** 200-400mcg per day–acts as an anti-inflammatory by altering leukotriene production.

7) **EPO or Borage oil**–1gm 4x/day–this treatment takes 4-12 weeks and the patient should not be on NSAID because of the effect of inhibiting PGE1 formation which acts as an anti-inflammatory.

STUDY–Hansen, T. *Treatment of RA with Prostaglandin E1 precursors cis-linoleic acid and GLA.* Scand. J. Rheum. 12:85, 1983 ABSTRACT–When combined with cofactors zinc, vitamin C, B-3, B-6, and EPO was as effective as conventional treatment for 20 patients switched to it from NSAID.

STUDY– Leventhal LJ, et al. *Treatment of RA with GLA.* Annal Intern Med. 119:867-873, 1993. ABSTRACT–37 pts with RA were randomly assigned to receive 1.4gms per day of GLA from borage oil or placebo (cottonseed oil). This was a double-blind trial that lasted 24 weeks. The GLA treated group had significant reduction in signs and symptoms of disease activity whereas pts receiving the placebo showed no change in symptoms. GLA reduced the number of tender joints by 36% and tender joint score by 45%. All pts were allowed to continue with their NSAIDS during the study.

8) **Avoid iron**–Iron is found in elevated amounts in the synovial fluid of RA sufferers compared to normals, and was significantly reduced in serum. If an RA patient is anemic, iron supplementation is often contraindicated. However if patient has low ferritin levels and very anemic (low HCT and HgB) then certainly consider giving at least a liver extract. Remember that ferritin is usually going to be falsely elevated in a patient who has active RA.

9) **Copper salicylate**–64mg 2x/day–may form complexes which serve as selective antioxidants.

STUDY–Hangarter, W. *Copper salicylate in RA and rheumatism-like degenerative disease.* Med Welt. 31:1625, 1980. ABSTRACT–60mg 2x/day was compared with salicylic acid and copper acetate in equal doses in patients with RA. The copper salicylate was more effective than either salicylic acid or copper acetate and produced reduction in morning stiffness, increased joint mobility, and reduced need for other drugs.

10) **Glycosaminoglycans found in Perna canaliculus (green lipped mussel extract)**–350mg 3x/day

STUDY–Gibson, R. *Perna canaliculus in the reaction of arthritis.* Practitioner 224:955-60, Sept.. 1980 also in another study in Lancet 1:439, 1981. ABSTRACT–Perna canaliculus (green-lipped mussel), a rich source of glycosaminoglycans, benefited in the treatment of RA. The 1980 study was a double blind study of 25 pts average age 57 years with RA who had failed to respond to NSAIDS. Pts randomly received either placebo or 1gm of Perna c. After 3 months 67% of treated pts vs 30% of placebo pts responded. Following this the placebo treated pts were then switched to the Perna c. and 60% of these people responded favorably.

STUDY–DOUBLE BLIND-El-Ghobarey, A. Quart. J. Med. 47:385, 1978. ABSTRACT–28 patients on NSAIDs were supplemented with **perna canaliculus 350mg 3x/day daily or placebo for 6 months with significant benefit to the experimental group as compared to controls.**

11) **Bromelain**–Acute flare-ups–1000mg of 2800 mcu (milk clotting units) 4x/day. Maintenance – 500mg 3x/day.

STUDY–Cohen, Goldman. *Bromelain Therapy in RA.* Pennsyl. Med. J. 67:27-30, June, 1964. ABSTRACT–25 patients with stages 2 or 3 RA were on small maintenance doses of steroids and they received 20-40mg of bromelain 3-4x/day. It was found, after 13 weeks, that 28% had excellent results, 45% had good results, 14% had fair results, and 14% had poor results.

12) **Curcumin**–has potent antiinflammatory effects especially for acute inflammation. It has been found to be equal or even more potent than cortisone and phenylbutazone in acute inflammation. It has long been used in Ayurvedic medicine both locally and internally to treat inflammation as well as in Chinese medicine in the treatment of shoulder inflammation.

STUDY–Srimal R & Dhawan B. *Pharmacology of diferuloyl methane (curcumin), an NSAID agent.* J Pharm Pharmacol 25, 447-52, 1973.

13) **Ginger**–inhibits prostaglandin and leukotriene synthesis as well as acting as an antioxidant. It also inhibits platelet aggregation and may thus enhance circulation. It contains proteases similar to bromelain which have antiinflammatory effects. (1 oz fresh ginger)

STUDY–Srivastava KC and Mustafa T. *Ginger in rheumatism and musculoskeletal disorders.* Med Hypothesis 39:342-348, 1992 ABSTRACT–28 patients with RA and 18 with OA and 10 with muscular discomfort were treated with 1-4gms of powdered ginger for periods of 3months to 21/2 years. There was significant improvement in many of the patients, but especially in the patients that just had muscular pain.

14) **Sea Cucumber**–500mg 4x/day

STUDY–Hazelton RA.(senior lecturer in medicine (rheumatology, U of Queensland, Australia.. *C-cure in RA: A six month placebo controlled trial, Unpublished manuscript, 1988.* ABSTRACT–34 pts with RA received either C-Cure (Pacif. Pharm., LTd, Australia).1 capsule 2x per day or placebo. No difference was seen in grip strength between the 2 groups. After 18-24 weeks, the articular index was significantly lower and the grip strength significantly higher in the experimental group.

15) **Pantothenic acid**–500mg 4x/day

16) **Quercetin**–500mg tid before meals–inhibits leukotriene formation, effective at stabilizing cell membranes, has antioxidant activity, and inhibits allergies.

17) **Treat hypothyroid**

18) **Treat heavy metal toxicity or other environmental sensitivities**

19) **Avoid NSAID**–they increase permeability of the intestinal mucosa and can worsen the actual joint tissue

20) **Treat parasites**–There have been reported cases of amoebas triggering off severe RA. Treatment involves the use of Flagyl 2gms per day on 2 consecutive days during the week. Take in divided doses with food and each week for 6 weeks (i.e., 2 days per week for 6 weeks). The 2 gm dose per day is for a person weighing 150lbs and different weight people should adjust the dose accordingly. Flagyl has a great deal of toxicity so I recommend taking Silymarin 80% standardized extract 400mg per day during the treatment protocol. Avoid alcohol or any other liver toxic substances while doing the treatment.

21) **Bee venom therapy–contact the American Apitherapy Society (802)436-2708**

# OSTEOARTHRITIS (OA)

- OA is a degenerative joint disease, also called "old age" or wear and tear arthritis.
- X-ray studies in the U.S. and Great Britain reveal that almost 50% of the adult population has OA. Men and women are equally affected, but males generally get it earlier.
- OA first appears asymptomatically at age 20 and by age 40 almost all people have some pathologic changes of weight bearing joints.
- OA occurs in almost all vertebrates, including animals supported in the water. In 2 mammals that hang upside down, bats and sloths, OA changes are not seen.

## I. Etiology

Generally, the etiology is unknown but prolonged overuse is thought to aid in its development. It is interesting that pneumatic hammer drillers and long-distance running champions have no increase in OA compared with age and sex matched controls.

Other factors include:

1) Nutrient deficiencies
2) Food sensitivities
3) HCL deficiency–It was found in one study that OA women had 3x greater incidence of both achlorhydria and hypochlorhydria than normals.

## II. Signs and Symptoms

Tenderness and crepitus of joints progressing to limiting the range of motion. Heberden's nodes, along with joint enlargement and a decrease in joint space, appear on X-rays.

## III. Diagnosis

Signs and symptoms, and X-rays.

## IV. Treatment

1) **Avoid Solanaceae foods**–eggplant, tomato, green pepper, potato, paprika, cayenne, tobacco

**NOTE**–It may take 4-6 weeks to clear out all of the solanacean compounds from the body.

2) **Niacinamide**–800mg 3x/day (Wilner Labs in NY)–Monitor liver enzymes. If the patient is suffering from nausea, liver enzymes are elevated. However, 10% of the population may have elevated liver enzymes without experiencing nausea.
3) **Vitamin B-6**–100mg 3x/day–This treatment is especially effective for menopausal or rheumatic-type arthritis
4) **Vitamin E**–400-800iu/day
5) **Selenium**–200mcg/day

6) **Cod liver oil**–2-4 T/day

7) **Glycosaminoglycans** (green lipped muscle extract)

8) **Vitamin C**–1-2gms/day

9) **Pantothenic acid**-200-1500mg/day

10) **Boron**

STUDY–Traver, R.L., et al. *Boron and Arthritis: The results of a Double Blind Pilot Study.* J of Nut Med 1:127-32, 1990. ABSTRACT–20 patients were studied in a double blind trial comparing 6mg/day boron with a placebo. Of the 10 patients on boron, 5 improved. Only 1 of 10 in the placebo group improved. The boron had a significant benefit for those patients with severe osteoarthritis. The 6 mg boron was administered in 2 tablets containing 25mg borax (sodium tetraborate decahydrate). The experiment was carried over an 8 week period. There were no side effects.

11) **Yucca saponin extract** (Desert Pride Herbal Food Tabs)

STUDY–Bingham, R. *Yucca saponin in the management of arthritis.* J. Applied Nutr. 27:45-50, 1975. ABSTRACT–149 arthritis patients were studied, of which 58.9% were found to have OA. Compared to placebo, from 1 week to 15 months, 61% of the yucca extract patients noted less swelling, pain and stiffness as compared to 22% of Placebo. There was a lot of variability in the time of onset of improvement.

12) **Glucosamine sulfate–**500 mg, 3x/day

STUDY–Vas AL, *Double-blind clinical evaluation of the relative efficacy of ibuprofen and glucosamine sulfate in the management of OA of the knee in out-patients.* Curr Med Res Opin 8, 145-49, 1982. ABSTRACT–In this double-blind study 40 pts. with osteoarthritis of one knee received glucosamine sulfate 500mg tid or Motrin 1.2gms/day in an eight-week double-blind study. The group that received the Motrin was significantly better at 2 wks., by about 3.8wks. both groups were doing about the same, and finally at 5-6wks. the group receiving the glucosamine sulfate was significantly better than the Motrin group. Physicians were 3 times more likely to rate the glucosamine sulfate group as having a "good overall response compared to the Motrin group.

STUDY–Tapadinhas MJ, et al. *Oral glucosamine sulfate in the management of arthrosis: report on a multi-centre open investigation in Portugal.* Pharmicatherapeutica 3, 157-168, 1982. ABSTRACT–1,208 pts. with arthrosis received 1.5gms glucosamine sulfate for an average of 50 days. 95% of physicians rated the efficacy as good (59%) or sufficient. Improvement lasted for 6-12 wks. after the treatment was discontinued.

13) **S-Adenosyl-L-methionine–**(SAMe) is now available over-the-counter in the U.S.

STUDY–Konig H, et al.. *Magnetic Resonance tomography of finger polyarthritis: Morphology and cartilage signals after ademetionine therapy.* . Aktuelle Radiol 5, 36-40, 1995. ABSTRACT–This was a double-blinded study on 14 pts. with OA of the hands. MRI showed an actually increased cartilage in the affected joints.

STUDY–Konig H, et al. *A longo-term (2 years) clinical trial with SAMe for the treatment of OA.* Am J Med 83(suppl 5A), 89-94, 1987. ABSTRACT–97 pts. with OA of the knee, hip and spine were treated with 600mg of SAMe for the 1st 2 weeks and then 400mg for the remaining 102 weeks. This long term study involved 10 different practitioners at 10 different clinics. Clinical improvement (morning stiffness, pain at rest, and pain on movement) was noted after the first few weeks of therapy and continued up until the end of the study. Note only were there no side effects, but symptoms of depression that some of the patients experienced improved significantly.

STUDY–Berger R , Nowak H. *A new medical approach to the treatment of OA: Report of an open phase IV study with ademetionine (Gumbaral).* Am J Med 83(suppl 5A), 84-88, 1987. ABSTRACT–This was an open non-controlled trial involving 20,641 pts. with OA of the knee, hip and spine. The pts. were given 1200mg SAMe the first week, 800mg the second week, and 400mg the third week. No other anti-inflammatory drugs were permitted to be used. 71% of pts. described the efficacy as very good or good, 21% said moderate and 9% said poor. Over 95% of pts. tolerated SAMe well.

14) **Arthrivite® –**This is a combination formula of niacinamide, glucosamine sulfate, boron, selenium, B-6, and Vitamin E to simplify the long-term treatment of osteoarthritis (available through Omnivite Nutrition, Inc. 1-800-424-OMNI).

# GOUT (ARTHRITIS)

- Gout is one of the oldest diseases in recorded medical history. It is an inherited disorder in which an abnormal purine metabolism results in elevated levels of uric acid in the blood. When the uric acid reaches a critical level it precipitates as crystals into the joints, especially in the big toe, feet and knees. The crystals can also precipitate out in the kidneys resulting in uric acid kidney stones.

- Clinical findings show that the disease usually occurs after the age of 35.

## I. Etiology

Gout is a recurrent acute inflammatory arthritis of the peripheral joints that occurs due to the precipitation and deposition of monosodium urate crystals. When uric acid goes above 7.0mg/dL, the plasma becomes supersaturated and the likelihood of precipitation becomes significantly higher. A deficiency of hypoxanthine-guanine phosphoribosyltransferase or overactivity of phosphoribosylpyrophosphate synthetase are possible etiological factors. The latter enzyme is related to the formation of kidney stones. Overindulgence of rich foods, along with the consumption of alcohol, which both blocks urate secretion of renal tubules and increases the formation of lactic acid, are common precipitating factors. About 1/3 of urate is excreted in the feces and 2/3 is excreted in the urine. Normal 24 hour uric acid excretion is between 400-900mg and on a low purine diet excretion decreases to 300-600mg indicating that diet may only contribute at most 600mg per day. This, however, is disputable and certainly diet may play a major role in the treatment of gout. All people who have high uric acid levels don't experience gouty arthritis symptoms and all people with gout don't have high levels of uric acid.

## II. Signs & Symptoms

Acute gouty arthritis can occur suddenly without any warning signs. It can be precipitated by trauma, overindulgence in food or alcohol classically. Surgery, fatigue, emotional stress, infections, or vascular insufficiency may also precipitate the condition. Pain often first occurs at night and becomes progressively more severe and debilitating. The affected joints usually become red, swollen, hot and exquisitely tender to touch. The overlying skin becomes shiny red or purplish with signs of infection. The MP joint of the big toe is the most often affected joint. The first attack usually affects a single joint, but later attacks can affect multiple joints. Fever, tachycardia chills, and malaise may also occur. The first few attacks usually last only a few days but later attacks can persist for weeks with joint deformity occurring if the person has many attacks. Often, urate deposits called tophi can appear in the walls of bursae and tendon sheaths as well as the pinna of the ear.

## III. Diagnosis

Signs and symptoms along with history are usually sufficient to make the diagnosis. A lab uric acid above 7.0mg/dL is strong circumstantial evidence. 30% of patients having an acute gouty arthritic attach have normal serum uric acid levels. In the past administration of colchicine was used as a trial and if the response was dramatic, then the diagnosis was clear. 10% of gout patients have positive rheumatoid factor. Heberdon's nodes at the DIP joints may often accumulate tophi. The external ears also tend to accumulate tophi.

## IV. Clinical considerations

There is a question as to how much effect dietary restriction of purine containing foods has on overall uric acid production, since drugs like allopurinol have powerful effects at decreasing its production . Certainly everything that can be done to decrease its production should be done dietarily. Probenecid or sulfinpyrazone decreases the blood uric acid level by increasing urinary excretion of uric acid. Plenty of liquid should be used with drugs so that the uric acid does not crystallize in the kidneys forming stones.

Everything that was talked about with RA should be done to reduce the levels of inflammatory leukotrienes such as eliminating animal products which contain arachidonic acid.

## V. Treatment

Conventional treatment uses colchicine–1mg orally every 2 hours–until a response is obtained or until diarrhea or vomiting occurs. Very severe attacks may require from 4-7 mg in a 48 hour period. No more than 7mg should be taken in 48 hours. In the elderly it is important to treat the resulting diarrhea to prevent electrolyte imbalance.
Allopurinol–200-600mg/day in divided doses can be used to block synthesis of uric acid. NSAIDs or prednisolone tebutate 10-50mg can also be used effectively.

1) **Drink lots of fluids and eliminate alcohol–**It is best to try and dilute the contents of the blood so that the uric acid has less chance of precipitating out of the blood.

2) **Short juice fast followed by diet very low in purines–**This diet will eliminate out many precipitating toxins.

3) **Cherry juice–**Eating 8oz of fresh or canned cherries has been shown to decrease levels of uric acid. Other berries because of their anthocyanidin content, such as blackberries, blueberries, Hawthorn berries, and others may have significant antiinflammatory effects

STUDY–Blau LW. Cherry diet in the control of gout & arthritis. Texas Rep Biolog Med 8:309-11, 1950.

4) **Weight loss with low fat and low protein diet and high levels of fiber**–Overall goal is to lose weight over long term.

5) **Eliminate homogenized milk**–may be a source of xanthine oxidase which can increase levels of uric acid

6) **Potato juice raw–** 4-6oz every hour–may increase the excretion of uric acid

7) **Quercetin–**1gm 3x per day-may inhibit uric acid production and inhibits leukotriene formation.

8) **Bromelain and curcumin–**Antiinflammatory actions

9) **Folate**–25mg 3x per day in acute situations may inhibit xanthene oxidase when given together with vitamin C.

10) **Lithium carbonate**-200mg 3x per day-can be used with essential oils safflower or flax seed oil to reduce the risk of toxicity (Jonathan Wright).

**Foods containing purines**

| Foods with high levels of purines 100-1000mg/100g of food | | Foods with moderate levels of purines 9-100mg/100g of food | |
|---|---|---|---|
| Anchovies | Mackerel | Fish | Asparagus |
| Bouillon | Meat extracts | Poultry | Beans, dried |
| Brains | Mincemeat | Meat | Lentils |
| Broth | Mussels | Shellfish | Mushrooms |
| Consomme | Partridge | | Peas, dried |
| Goose | Roe | | Spinach |
| Gravy | Sardines | | |
| Heart | Scallops | | |
| Herring | Sweetbreads | | |
| Kidney | Yeast, baker's/ brewer's | | |

| Foods containing small amounts of purine(< 9mg per 100g food) | | | |
|---|---|---|---|
| Bread & crackers | Custard | Macaroni products | Relishes |
| Butter or margarine | Eggs | Noodles | Rennet desserts |
| Cereals/related products | Fats | Nuts | Rice |
| Cheese | Fruit | Oils | Salt |
| Chocolate | Gelatin Dessert | Olives | Sugar and sweets |
| Coffee | Herbs | Pickles | Tea |
| Condiments | Ice cream | Popcorn | Vegetables (not above) |
| Cornbread | Milk | Puddings | Vinegar |
| Cream | | | White sauce |

**11) Bee venom therapy**–can also be used topically

**12) Apis homeopathic–**

## Notes

# BURSITIS

- Bursitis is defined as inflammation of a bursa, either chronic or acute
- Bursitis most commonly appears in the shoulder (subacromial or subdeltoid)

## I. Etiology

Overuse of joint with a lack of essential nutrients.

## II. Signs and Symptoms

Pain, swelling, and point tenderness to the affected bursa.

## III. Treatment

1) **Short fruit and vegetable fast**–This decreases the amount of saturated fats which provides less substrate to make PGE2.
2) **Pineapples and bromelain**
3) **Vitamin B-12**–IM 1000mcg/day for 1 week
4) **Vitamin C and bioflavonoids**
5) **EFA**
6) **Topical DMSO and bromelain**
7) **Vitamin E**–400-800iu/day

## Notes

# CARPEL TUNNEL SYNDROME (CTS)

- CTS is defined as peripheral neuropathy in the hands resulting from compression of the median nerve in the volar aspect of the wrist between the longitudinal tendons of the forearm.
- CTS is more common in females than males.

## I.Etiology

Median nerve compression due to trauma, overuse, hypothyroidism, arthritis

## II. Diagnosis

1) Signs and symptoms
2) Positive Tinel sign
3) Phalen's test
4) Finger bending test
5) Nerve conduction

## III.Treatment

**1) Vitamin B-6**–100mg 3x/day–P5P may also be effective.

STUDY–Ellis. *Clinical results of a cross over treatment with B-6 and placebo of the carpal tunnel syndrome* Am. J. Clin. Nutr. 32:2040-6, 1979 ABSTRACT–A patient with severe CTS and a significant deficiency of B-6 as determined by EGOT activity was studied. Patient was treated with 2mg/day for 11 weeks, then 100mg/day for 12 weeks, then placebo for 9 weeks, and again B-6 100mg/day for 11weeks. 2mg/day reduced the EGOT activity deficiency, maintained the P5P levels at a deficiency and relieved most of the symptoms. 100mg/day caused EGOT to be at maximal activity, relieved the P5P deficiency levels, and all symptoms. Introduction of placebo caused reappearance of EGOT activity, P5P deficiency, and symptoms. Readministration of 100mg/day of B-6 eliminated the deficiencies and all of the symptoms.

**2) Bromelain**–500-1000mg tid of 2100mcu–This is best taken on an empty stomach.

**3) Topical Arnica oil, DMSO and hypericum**–Apply 3-4x per day These topical agents can be used for any type nerve pain or paresthesias.

**4) Biomechanics**–Consider splinting, bracing, ergonomic keyboards, making sure work space is suited to your special needs or requirements.

### Notes

---

# ESOPHAGITIS

- Esophagitis is any inflammation of the esophagus, either chronic or acute.
- Due to the irritating effects of gastroesophageal reflux disease (GERD), esophagitis usually occurs in the lower esophagus. This symptom is commonly known as "heart-burn." Foods, hormones, anatomy, obesity, scarring, allergies, bulimia and trauma can all lead to GERD and subsequent esophagitis.
- Various bacteria or viruses can cause esophagitis including Candida albicans, Helicobacter pylori, Cytomegalovirus, Herpes simplex virus, HIV, & Cryptosporidium
- Iron deficiency can lead to esophageal webs rarely (Plummer-Vinson syndrome).
- **Basal LES pressure is not decreased, but rather reflux is due to transient relaxations of the LES** (Lower Esophageal Sphincter).

## I. Etiology

*Acute esophagitis* can be caused by:

a) Ingestion of irritating agents, e.g. antifreeze or other corrosive compounds
b) Viral or bacterial inflammation
c) Trauma, such as intubation
d) Candida esophagitis (single most common cause of infection in esophagus in AIDS patients), other infectious agents: cytomegalovirus, Epstein–Barr and Herpes virus
e) Radiation, chemotherapeutic agents, NSAIDs, and aspirin
f) Zollinger Ellison Syndrome–excess secretion of gastrin and Crohn's disease

*Chronic esophagitis* can be caused by:

a) Hiatal hernia and hiatal hernia syndrome
b) Recurrent vomiting (bulimia, alcoholism)
c) Increased abdominal pressure (obesity, pregnancy, allergic bloating, eating too much or too quickly)
d) Decreased LES pressure due to foods or medications
e) Hormones–especially during pregnancy
f) recent studies indicate that the esophagus may, like the stomach, secrete bicarbonate
g) mixed connective tissue disorders such as scleroderma, SLE, and polymyositis

## II. Signs and Symptoms

Pain can be experienced immediately or shortly after eating. Generally the pain is felt in the epigastric or substernal area and has been described as a burning sensation. **The pain can radiate to the interscapular region, neck, and even down both arms. It must be differentiated from an MI which is generally made worse by motion**. Bending over or lying down makes esophagitis worse.

Other diagnostic criteria are esophageal brushings for Candida esophagitis, 95% sensitive and 87% specific.

## III. Therapeutic Considerations

1) Rule out bulimia, anorexia, hiatal hernia and hiatal hernia syndrome.

2) Eat slowly! Don't stuff your face too fast.
3) Avoid foods that aggravate the condition (direct irritants and foods which both lowers LES pressure and increase gastric acid secretion).

## IV. Treatment

**1) Relax while eating**

a) Have the patient sit down without getting up until the meal is complete.
b) Direct the patient to put utensils down between bites.
c) Count the number of chews.
d) Prohibit TV, reading, or other distracting activities during meals. Avoid excessive chatter which distracts from thorough chewing.

**2) Eat small meals with low fat content**. High fat foods tend to stay in the stomach. This increases intra-abdominal pressure and also decreases LES pressure.

**3) Avoid foods that commonly aggravate esophagitis**

a) Coffee decreases LES pressure and increases acid secretion

STUDY–Dennish and Castel. *On the genesis of Heartburn.* Am. J. Dig. Dis. 18:391,1973. ABSTRACT–Coffee at a dosage of 1-2 cups decreased LES pressure slightly and greatly stimulated HCL secretion.

b) Chocolate–Decreases LES pressure
c) Tomato–Decreases LES pressure
d) Milk–Delays gastric emptying and stimulates acid secretion (allergy mediated)

STUDY–Forget and Arends. *Cow's milk protein allergy and gastroesophageal reflux.* Eur. J Pediatr. 144:298,1985.

e) Alcohol

STUDY–Hogen *Ethanol induced acute esophageal sphincter motor dysfunction.* J. Appl. Physiol 32:755,1972. ABSTRACT–Alcohol was found to relax the LES and decrease peristaltic force.

f) medications such as NSAID, aspirin etc

**4) Increased fiber decreases intra-abdominal pressure by softening stools.** Fiber also increases positive peristalsis which prevents stagnation and keeps stools from becoming hard and dry.

**5) Avoid Nicotine**–A major factor in decreasing LES pressure

**6) Choline**–Has been used even in pregnancy to increase LES pressure. I have also used lecithin in the form of phosphatidyl choline.

**7) Pantothenic acid**–1gm bid and thiamin 500mg/day

**8) Manganese (citrate)**–50mg/day

**9) HCL**–Dr. Wright is a strong believer of HCL therapy (see Healing with Nutrition). Probably a good idea to check Heidelberg first.

**CLINICAL NOTE**–Severe untreated esophagitis may lead to *Barrett's esophagus* in which the squamous mucosa of the lower esophagus is replaced by gastric-like columnar epithelium. These cellular changes may lead to adenocarcinoma. The prevalence of adenocarcinoma in Barrett's esophagus is about 10%, which is 40x the rate of the general population. Surgical treatment has a poor prognosis. One study showed that of the patients with surgically treatable cancer only 27% survived the first year and 10% survived 5 years.

## NOTES

# PEPTIC ULCERS (duodenal and gastric)

## DUODENAL ULCERS (DU)

- 10% of the population has a DU at some point, although this figure is declining.
- DU are 5x more common than gastric ulcers
- Males have 5x as many DU than females.
- **1/2 to 2/3rds of DU sufferers secrete more acid than normal** (2x as many parietal cells compared to normals)
- Females, age 40-50, and males, age 20-30, are the most common DU sufferers.
- DU occurs most often in people with type O blood

## GASTRIC ULCERS (GU)

- GU generally occur later in life (50-60 years)
- **80% of people with GU have reduced acid**
- GU's are more common in people with type A blood

## I. General Considerations

Both duodenal and gastric ulcers are similar in nature. Pain is experienced 30-60 minutes after eating. Nocturnal pain is common. Symptoms are chronic and periodic. Always consider the possibility of bacterial flora imbalance in either condition. **Never assume anything concerning this condition.**

## II. Diagnosis

Occult blood
X-rays
Endoscopy
Heidelberg (gastric telemetry)
Anti-Helicobacter (Campylobacter) pylori antibodies–IgG & IgA antibodies had a sensi tivity of 100% and 94% and a specificity of 86% and 76% respectively for H. pylori.
Oral zinc taste test, white blood cell zinc, finger nail exam and vertical lines forehead
Intestinal permeability mannitol and lactulose

STUDY-Hollander, Vadhiem, Brettholtz, et al. *Increase intestinal permeabilty in patients with Crohn's disease and their relatives.* Ann Intern Med 105:883-5, 1986. ABSTRACT–It was determined that Crohn's patients had increased permeability compared to normals. It was also postulated that there may be the same phenomenon in other GI diseases such as stomach and duodenal ulcers.

## III. Etiology

### 1) Drugs

a) Smoking decreases bicarbonate and decreases gastric emptying time.

STUDY–Person, Ahlbom & Hellers. *Inflammatory bowel disease and tobacco smoke–a case control study* Gut 31:1377-81, 1990. ABSTRACT–A case control study was carried out in Stockholm, Sweden between 1984-87 to evaluate the association of childhood cigarette smoking and exposure to environmental tobacco smoke and the subsequent development of irritable bowel disease. Over 500 patients were evaluated and it was found that there was a significant increase risk of developing Crohn's disease later in life if the child was exposed to secondary cigarette smoke.

b) Aspirin increases membrane permeability and is irritating.
c) Caffeine and alcohol both stimulate acid secretion
d) NSAID
e) Xanthine oxidase
f) Chlorine

**2) Decreased production of protective substances lining the stomach (PGE1 synthesis)** (Cytotek® is a prescription drug that is a synthetic analog of PGE1 used to prevent stomach ulcers in patients taking antiinflammatory drugs that may cause ulcers).

**3) Allergies**

**4) Abnormal bacterial flora** *(Helicobacter pylori)* produces urease. This converts urea present in the stomach, producing localized ammonia and bicarbonate. It migrates into the mucosa where it inhibits mucus secreting cells. It also produces protease and lipase which digest the mucus layer.

**5) Poor nutritional status especially of zinc, vitamin A, glutamine, EFA and vitamin E.**

## IV. Treatment

**1) Avoid drugs which exacerbate condition**–NSAID, aspirin, alcohol, caffeine.

**2) Increase production of protective substances in stomach.**

**a) Zinc picolinate**–30mg/day–increases mucin production.

**b) EFA's,** both linoleic acid and GLA–1-2 T safflower oil & 4-6 caps black currant oil. PGE1 inhibits acid secretion and increases mucosal cell resistance to injury.

**3) Avoid allergens,** especially milk, and other irritants such as black pepper and coffee.

STUDY–Ippoliti. *The effect milk on patients with duodenal ulcers.* Br. Med. J 293:666,1986 ABSTRACT–65 patients with duodenal ulcers being treated with cimetidine were given either normal hospital diet or milk diet. The milk diet was 25% worse.

STUDY–Siegal. *GI ulcer-Arthus reaction!* Ann Allergy 32:127,1974. ABSTRACT–98% of patients with radiographic evidence of peptic ulcers had coexisting lower and upper respiratory infections.

**4) Increasing dietary fiber delays gastric emptying time.**

STUDY–Rydning, Berstad, Aadland & Odegaard. *Prophylactic effects of dietary fiber in duodenal ulcer disease.* Lancet 2:736-9,1982.

STUDY–Rydning & Berstad. *Fiber diet and antacids in the short term treatment of duodenal ulcer.* Scand. J. Gastroenterol. 20(9):1078-82,1985. ABSTRACT–80 patients were treated with 1 low dose antacid 4x/day. In addition they were randomly divided to receive a fiber rich and a fiber poor diet. A very slightly increased rate of healing was seen in the fiber rich diet.

**5) Supplements**

**a) Catechin** (bioflavonoid)–1gm 5x/day–decreases histamine levels.

**b) Cabbage (raw juice)**–1 liter/day. It appears that glutamine is the specific active ingredient. One study has shown it to be effective alone (may stimulate mucin production).

c) **Zinc picolinate**–90mg/day

STUDY–Frommer. *The healing of gastric ulcers by zinc sulfate.* Med J. Aust. 2:793, 1975. ABSTRACT–Double blind study involving 15 patients with gastric ulcers who were treated randomly with either zinc or placebo. After 3 weeks, the absolute reduction in size of the ulcer crater was 3x as great in the treated group. Zinc reduced pain markedly within 4 days in some patients. There were no side effects and pretreatment zinc levels were normal.

d) **Bismuth citrate salts** form a glycoprotein-bismuth complex which acts as a local diffusion barrier to gastric acid. It does not decrease acid production by the stomach. Conventional treatment for H. pylori involves the use of bismuth, amoxicillin and metronidazole for 7 days. Serologic assays showed a marked reduction in the triple antibiotic group compared to controls (80% cure rate). In 1998 the most updated conventional treatment protocol involved the treatment for H. Pylori with Biaxin, Prilosac and Bismuth.

STUDY–McKenna, Humphreys, Dooley, Bourke, et al. *Campylobacter pyloritis and histological gastritis in duodenal ulcer: a controlled prospective randomized trial.* Gastroenterology 92:1528; 1987. ABSTRACT–64 patients with endoscopically proven duodenal ulcers were randomized to receive either cimetidine (H-2 receptor antagonist) or 120mg equivalents of bismuth salts qid for 6 weeks. In this blind & controlled study it was found that 93% of the patients who entered the study had Campylobacter pylori present. Healing rates for cimetidine and bismuth were similar, but the bismuth showed a decreased incidence of Campylobacter pyloritis from 94% to 52%. There was no change in the cimetidine treatment group. **Recurrence rate in the bismuth treated group was lower.**

e) **Vitamin A**–20,000iu 3x/day

f) **Vitamin C** (buffered)–1gm 3x/day

g) **Deglycyrrhizinated licorice root**–250mg 3x/day–stimulates mucus formation and secretion

STUDY–*A comparison between cimetidine and CAVED S in the treatment of gastric ulceration and subsequent maintenance therapy.* Gut 23:545, 1982. ABSTRACT–In a comparison with cimetidine it was found that Glycyrrhiza was equally effective (88% healing rate in 12 weeks).

STUDY–*Comparative study of carbenoloxone and cimetidine in the management of duodenal ulcer.* Acta Gastroent. Bel. 46;459, 1983. ABSTRACT–It was found that DGL was as effective as cimetidine, but without the undesirable side effects of cimetidine.

h) **Various botanicals:** Ulmus fulva–1/2 tsp after meals, Comfrey, Aloe vera, unripe plantain banana. (Comfrey should only be used for short periods of time because of the pyrrolizidine alkaloids which have been associated with liver disease).

i) **Hydrastis canadensis & Berberis aquafolium–**may be used in the treatment of Helicobacter pylori.

j) **Glutamine–1**gm every 4-6hrs

k) **Digestive enzymes**

l) **Peptic ulcer cocktail–**if you want to avoid swallowing pills or taking vitamins the following can be made into a drink:

- Glutamine powder
- Cabbage juice
- Carrot juice (beta carotene)
- Wild purslane (vitamin E)
- Swiss Chard (zinc)
- Cod liver oil and borage oil (vitamin A & PGE1 precursor)

The treatment plan for this cocktail is to sip this drink throughout the day so you have localized epithelial contact along with a fresh supply of nutrients.

## Notes

# CELIAC DISEASE
# (Gluten-sensitive Enteropathy or Non-tropical Sprue)

- Gluten-sensitive enteropathy is characterized by chronic intestinal malabsorption caused by an **intolerance to gluten.**
- It typically involves the small intestine (the **proximal part** is most severely effected). This results in flattened intestinal villi, lymphocytic infiltration, and hypertrophy.
- Bulky, pale, frothy, foul smelling, greasy stools with increased fecal fat are indicative of celiac disease, however, people with CD may be **asymptomatic**.
- Weight loss and signs of multiple vitamin and mineral deficiencies are common. In children, growth is often stunted with loss of bone density in adults common.
- Celiac disease usually presents in the **first 3 years of life** (usually when solid foods are first introduced), and may reappear again with the **average age of onset being 35-40 years.**

## I. Epidemiology

HLA-B8 antigens have been found in 90% of celiac patients. Most frequently found in northern and central Europe and in northwest India, the highest rate occurs in **southwest Ireland** (1:300 as compared to the U.S., 1:2500). In these areas people have only been eating wheat products for the last 3,000 years, which is a relatively short period of time since wheat agriculture started about 9,000 years ago in the Middle East. People with a longer history of eating wheat products have a considerably lower incidence of celiac disease.

A recent study (Catassi, C., et al., *High prevalence of undiagnosed coeliac disease in 5,280 Italian students screened by anti-gliadin antibodies.* Acta Pediatr 84, 672-76, 1995) found that in asymptomatic students the rate was as high as 1:200.

## II. Etiology

1) **Gluten stimulates a T-cell dysfunction which increases the permeability of the intestinal mucosa.** This increased permeability allows other grain and milk proteins to cross the intestinal mucosa, initiating an antigen-antibody response. It should be noted that gluten, which is found in **the endosperm moiety** of a number of grains, is comprised of 2 main components, glutenin and gliadin. The fraction that stimulates this T-cell dysfunction is **gliadin**.

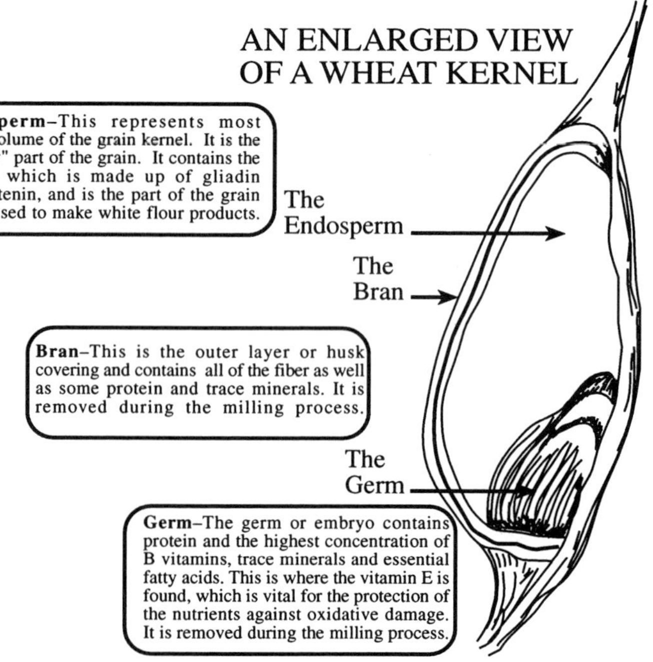

2) **Cow's milk, early introduction**–It is thought that the early introduction of cow's milk along with grains may sensitize babies to gluten. Breast fed infants have a lower incidence of celiac disease. This may be as a result of delayed feeding of solid foods or an enhanced mucosal barrier.

3) **Genetics**–It is thought that the gene for breaking down the N-pyrrolidone peptides is missing.

4) **Viral** (adenovirus type 12 may predispose to onset of the disease near the time of the infection. The adenovirus type 12 produces a protein that is very similar to the gliadin molecule. However, studies to date do not show much of a pattern in isolated cases.

## III. Pathology

Severe cases are characterized by severe inflammation, total villus atrophy, and crypt hyperplasia. Mild cases are characterized by lymphocytes infiltrating the epithelial lining. These intraepithelial T lymphocytes are characterized by an increased proportion of $\gamma/\delta$ receptors. Activated T lymphocytes release cytokines that amplify the immune response and recruit other inflammatory cells. The lamina propria of the villi is therefore expanded with lymphocytes, plasma cells and mast cells as well as eosinophils and neutrophils. In particular, eosinophils and mast cells both are involved in the early gliadin induced reactions of the small intestine. The surface area of the villi is greatly reduced and also the mucosal enzymes are also proportionally lowered. A secondary pancreatic insufficiency may develop because of a diminished cholescystokinin and secretin response of the small bowel mucosa.

Patients with celiac disease have more antigliadin spot forming cells in the gut mucosa compared to normals. Mostly found are IgA secreting cells. It should be noted that people deficient in IgA can still develop celiac disease. This indicates that antibodies are not the main cause of the enteropathy.

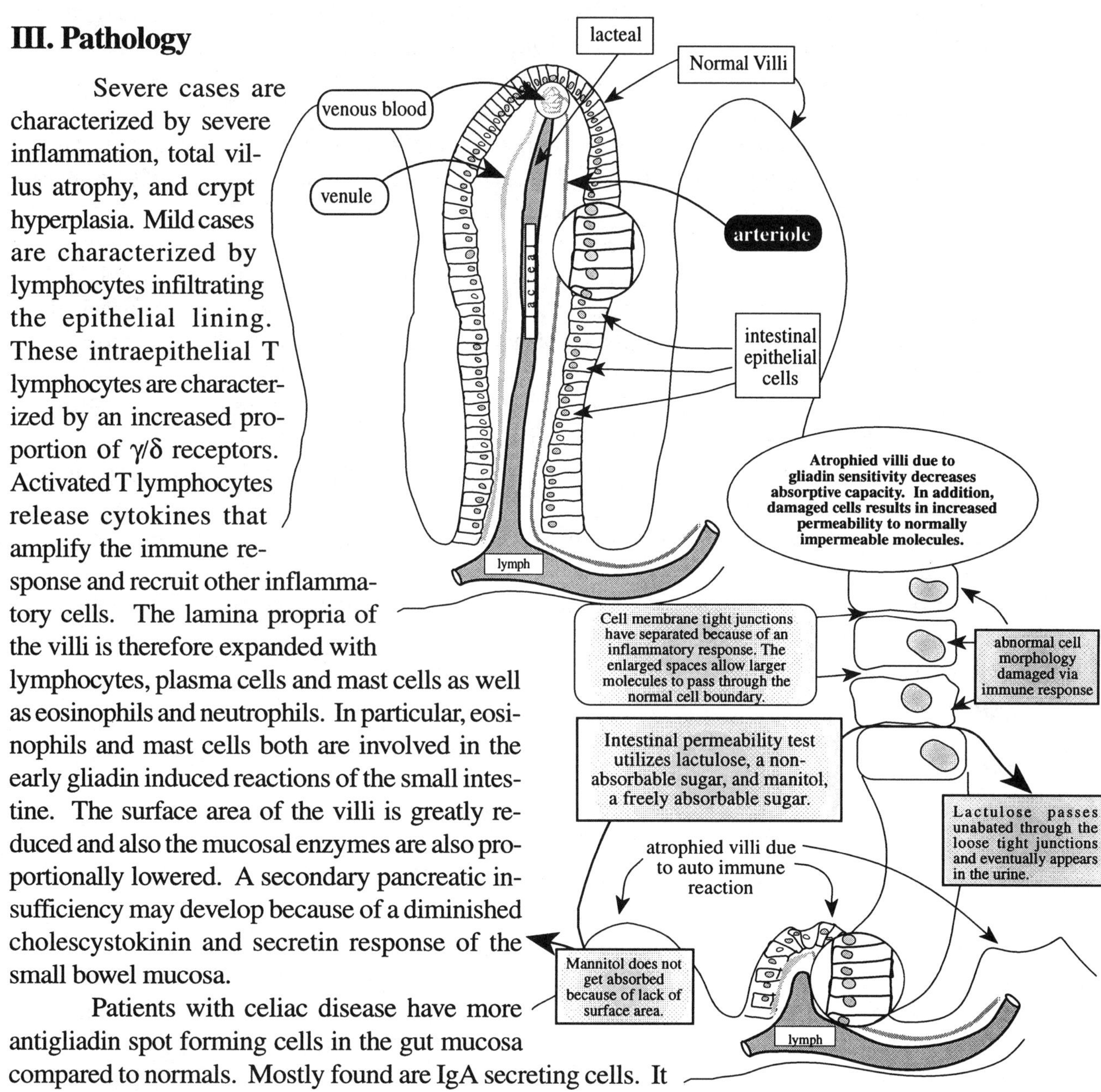

IgM and IgA antibodies, as well as high intraepithelial lymphocyte (IEL) levels, may be early markers for celiac disease. One study (Arranz and Ferguson; I*ntestinal antibody pattern of celiac disease: Occurrence in pts with normal jejunal biopsy history.* Gastroenterology 104:1263, 1993) found that 38 out of 41 patients with normal jejunal biopsy had altered IEL enteropathy and active celiac disease.

## IV. Signs and Symptoms

Celiac disease usually manifests in the first few years of life (6 mo.-3 yrs) when the infant starts eating solid food. Classically, patients suffer chronic diarrhea, projectile vomiting, bloated abdomens, cramping and growth failure. Stools are usually loose, foul smelling, frothy, gray, greasy, and floating. There may be up to 15 bowel movements per day. *It should be noted that some patients may present with constipation.* Often alternating constipation and diarrhea are present and **it is not unusual for the patient to experience no abdominal pain**.

In adults symptoms may present as increased appetite, weight loss, weakness, and fatigue. There may be hematological abnormalities. Many other symptoms secondary to malabsorption may be apparent. Fatigue, muscle cramps, and weakness are common. In women the disease first occurs 10-15 years earlier, compared to men, when it manifests in adulthood.

Associated conditions include lymphocytic gastritis. These patients, when evaluated for H. pylori, come out negative. The small bowel has characteristic changes of celiac disease but may also show involvement of the stomach. Symptoms are similar to CD with diarrhea and malabsorption.

**Extraintestinal manifestations:**

a) **Bone derangements** may occur even in patients who never had symptoms of malabsorption. One study revealed that in 29 untreated CD patients, bone mineral density measured by dual photon bone densitometry showed significantly lower bone density compared to controls and treated CD patients.
b) **Lymphoma**–increased incidence in long standing CD patients.
c) **Adenocarcinoma**
d) **OB-GYN problems–**CD patients had increased incidence of spontaneous abortions and infertility. Amenorrhea is also common.
e) **Dermatitis herpetiformis**
f) **Type I Diabetes mellitus**

## V. Diagnosis

1) Stool analysis–Check for fats and undigested food particles.
2) D-Xylose load (either 1 hour blood or 5 hour urine) is not specific for Celiac disease but can be a helpful screening tool (93% sensitive and 47% specificity).
3) Jejunal biopsy–this gives a *definitive diagnosis* but doesn't pick up all cases, especially early or minor cases.
4) Diffusion in Gel, Enzyme-linked Immunosorbent Assay (DIG-ELISA)–IgA and IgG gliadin antibodies (IgG has a very high sensitivity at 100% and low specificity at 58%, and the IgA has a high specificity at 93% and a low sensitivity at 53%).
5) Intestinal permeability–**"Mannitol and Lactulose Test."** Mannitol is a freely permeable simple sugar, to the normal intestinal wall, which shows up in lower amounts in the urine when there has been damage to the intestinal villi and malabsorption. Lactulose is a non

permeable sugar that will appear in higher amounts in the urine if there is inflammation and a hyper-permeable state (if the tight junctions have been separated).

6) Endomysial antibody (EMA)–This IgG class of antibody is specific for celiac disease. It is almost always elevated in people with dermatitis herpetiformis.

## VI. Treatment

1) **Avoid all gluten**–wheat, barley, oats, rye, triticale. Rice, corn, buckwheat, and sometimes millet are often tolerated. Initially, however, they should be avoided. Other grains that might be tolerated later are quinoa and amaranth. Read labels very carefully. It should be noted that 30% respond in 3 days, 80% in one month, and 90% in 2 months. 10% respond only after 2-3 years of gluten avoidance. Sometimes cortisone is useful in such cases to stabilize the condition. It seems likely that there are other food sensitivities that are exacerbating the condition, probably related to "leaky gut syndrome," and lack of pancreatic and intestinal mucosal digestive enzymes.

2) **Avoid all milk products**–Since patients are often milk sensitive, it is a good idea to avoid milk products as well.

3) **Megavitamin and mineral supplementation**–Many nutrients, especially fat-soluble vitamins, can be deficient due to malabsorption. Important nutrients which may need supplementation are:
   - a) **Folic acid**–15mg–is especially effective because most is absorbed in the proximal small intestine, the area most effected by the disease.
   - b) **Vitamin B-12**–best given IM–1000mcg-3000mcg
   - c) **Calcium citrate**–3gms–is important in prevention of osteoporosis and muscle spasms.
   - d) **Fat soluble vitamins**
     - **Vitamin A-75,000iu**
     - **Vitamin D-3,000iu**
     - **Vitamin E-1000iu**
     - **Vitamin K-3mg**
   - e) **General high potency multivitamin and mineral supplement**

4) **Digestive enzymes**–especially bile salts, pancreatic enzymes, and HCl.

STUDY–Carroccio A, et al. *Pancreatic enzyme therapy in childhood celiac disease: A double-blind prospective randomized study.* Dig. Dis. Sci. 40, 2555-60, 1995. ABSTRACT–It was demonstrated that supplemental pancreatic enzymes improved the growth of children with controlled Celiac disease.

5) **Quercetin**–stabilizes mast cells and eosinophils to keep them from degranulating. Sodium cromolyn can also be used.

**Clinical Note**–Almost all patients with **dermatitis herpetiformis (DH)** have some mucosal lesions similar to that of celiac disease. DH is characterized by clusters of intensely itchy vesicles, papules and urticaria type lesions. They are sensitive to gluten 90% of the time, showing positive antibodies in almost all cases. However, people with celiac disease don't always have dermatitis herpetiformis.

## Notes

# APHTHOUS STOMATITIS (CANKER SORES)

- Canker sores are shallow, painful ulcers found alone or in clusters anywhere in the oral cavity. They range from 1-15mm in diameter.
- They usually clear up in 7-21 days, though they are often recurrent.
- Canker sores affect 20% of the population.

## I. Etiology

1) Food sensitivities
   a) Take note of hemoagglutination antibodies acting against the oral mucosa.
   b) IgE bearing lymphocytes are significantly increased in aphthous lesions.
   c) Mast cell degranulation plays an important role in the production of recurrent ulcers.

STUDY–Hay and Reade. *The use of elimination diet in the treatment of recurrent aphthous ulceration of the oral cavity.* Oral surg 57:504-7, 1984.

2) Stress
3) Nutrient deficiency

## II. Therapeutic Considerations

STUDY–Wray, Ferguson, McLennan, and Dagg. *Nutrient deficiencies in recurrent aphthae.* J Oral Path 7:418-23, 1978. ABSTRACT–It was found that of 330 patients with recurrent aphthous ulcers **14% were deficient in iron, folate or Vitamin B-12**, or a combination of these nutrients. When these deficiencies were corrected, the majority had complete remission.

STUDY–Ferguson, Bashu, Asquith, and Cooke. *Jejunal mucosal abnormalities in patients with recurrent aphthous ulceration.* Br Med J 1:11-3, 1975. ABSTRACT–Jejunal biopsy of 33 patients with RAS showed 8 to have the **villous atrophy typical of celiac disease** along with histological signs of immunological reactions to food allergens. The remaining patients also exhibited these types of signs, but to a lesser degree.

STUDY–Kowolik, Muir, & MacPhee. *Di-sodium cromoglycate in the treatment of recurrent aphthous ulcers.* Br. Dent. J. 144:384-9, 1978. ABSTRACT–Cromoglycate, an anti-allergy drug very similar in action to quercetin, was shown to increase the number of ulcer-free days and provide mild symptomatic relief.

**NOTE**–Two studies have shown that if you remove gluten from the diet of patients with celiac disease, complete remission of the recurrent aphthous stomatitis results.

## III. Treatment

**1) Eliminate allergies**–especially rule out gluten sensitivity. Some people are sensitive to sodium laural sulfate found in most toothpastes. Consider switching to one without it.

**2) Vitamin C**–1gm/day

**3) Zinc picolinate**–25mg/day

**4) Multivitamin & mineral supplements**

**5) Lactobacillus mouth rinse**–2-3x/day

**6) Zinc lozenges**

**7) Quercetin**

# TROPICAL SPRUE

- Chronic recurrent afebrile disease occurs most commonly in the tropics and subtropics (south of the Sahara desert is one exception).
- Manifestations are similar to non-tropical sprue with diarrhea and malabsorption.
- The intestinal mucosa alterations are **much less severe** than with celiac disease.

## I. Etiology

1) **Bacteria, viruses and parasites** are all possible factors
2) Nutrient deficiencies, especially **folate and B-12,** may decrease patient's resistance

## II. Signs and Symptoms

Presents with recurrent diarrhea, fatigue, weight loss, pallor, cheilosis, glossitis, weakness, edema, and many symptoms associated with other nutrient deficiencies.

## III. Diagnosis

1) Stool analysis
2) D-Xylose load
3) Vitamin B-12 and folate deficiency in serum (megaloblastic anemia)
4) Hypochlorhydria in 50% of cases

## IV. Treatment

1) **Tetracycline** and other broad spectrum antibiotics can result in clinical remission.
2) **Folate**–15-25mg/day
3) **Vitamin B-12**–1000-3000mcg IM/day–It has been found that many patients with tropical sprue have a lack of intrinsic factor or the receptors for B-12 absorption in the ileum.
4) **Protein**–100-150gms/day–Many patients are hypoalbuminemic and edematous. Give hydrolyzed protein so as to not induce allergies.
5) **Multivitamin/mineral supplementation**–cover multiple nutrient deficiency
6) **HCl**
7) **Lactobacillus acidophilus**

# GALL BLADDER DISEASE (CHOLELITHIASIS AND CHOLECYSTITIS )

- Cholelithiasis is the formation of stones in the gallbladder in the absence of infection and cholecystitis is actual inflammation of the gallbladder.
- In the U.S., 20% of people over age 65 have stones, and each year more than 500,000 undergo cholecystectomies.
- Gallstone problems affect women more frequently than men.
- In most cases of gall stones, there are no symptoms. In someone who has symptoms of gall bladder pain, concurrently with stones, there is no assurance that the stones have anything to do with the pain.

## I. Etiology

1) Obesity
2) Family history
3) Western diet–decreased fiber, increased refined carbohydrate, high fat intake

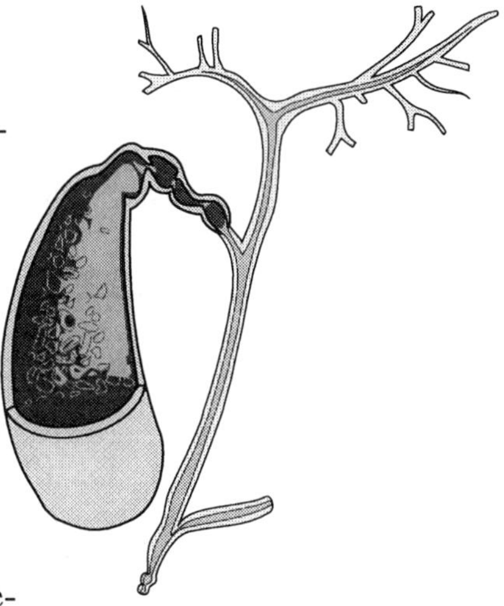

Supersaturation of cholesterol in the bile solution of the gall bladder is necessary for stones to form. People who fast often have supersaturated cholesterol; that is why extreme weight loss programs increase the possibility of gall stones and gall bladder attacks. In addition, stasis of bile within the gall bladder can trigger gall stone formation and biliary colic. Colic may be due to biliary duct spasm from irritation. Irritation can come from stasis or allergic swelling. Often times pain can persist even after cholecystectomy, indicating that the etiology of the pain is coming not from the gall bladder but rather from spasm of what is left of the duct system.

## II. Signs and Symptoms

- Most patients remain asymptomatic for long periods, frequently for life. Stones may traverse the cystic duct with or without symptoms.
- Transient cystic duct obstruction results in colicky pain, while persistent obstruction usually produces inflammation and acute cholecystitis.
- Most obstructive events are transient, producing biliary colic which can last several hours.
- Pain location varies, but most often occurs in the epigastrium or right upper quadrant, radiating to the right lower scapula. The typical pain is constant, progressively rising to a plateau and falling gradually. Nausea and vomiting are frequently associated with this pain along with gas. The Merck Manual p. 86, of the 16th ed. reports that symptoms of

fatty food dyspepsia are often misdiagnosed as gall bladder related when in actuality they are caused by peptic ulcer disease or functional distress (functional distress?!?).

- When a stone becomes lodged in the common bile duct and blocks off the normal secretion of bile salts into the small intestine the stools turn a pasty color.

## III. Diagnosis

1) Signs and symptoms
2) Ultrasound usually can't readily determine the size of the stones. Sensitivity is 98% and specificity (false positives) is about 90%.

## IV. Treatment

**1) Increase fiber** and avoid refined carbohydrates.

STUDY–*Report: How sugar can get you stoned?* New Scientist Vol. 14, March 21, 1985. ABSTRACT–Gallstone formation in young people was correlated with and increased intake of soft drinks and sweets as well as an increased energy or fat intake, suggesting that sugar may increase cholesterol synthesis by stimulating insulin secretion.

STUDY–Thorton, J. *Diet and gallstones: Effects of refined carbohydrates on bile cholesterol saturation and bile acid metabolism.* Gut 24:2-6, 1983. ABSTRACT–13 patients with radiolucent gallstones ate refined or unrefined carbohydrate diet for 6 weeks each, in random order. While the unrefined carbohydrate diet averaged 27gms of fiber, the refined carbohydrate diet averaged only 13 gms/day. The bile saturation index was higher in 12/13 during the refined carbohydrate period.

**2) Decrease animal fats and fats in general.**

**3) Allergies!!**–from "Basics of Food Allergy," James Breneman.

**4) Lecithin**–4-6gms/day–supplementation may normalize the abnormally low phospholipid to cholesterol ratio associated with cholesterol gallstones.

STUDY–Tuzhilin, Dreiling, Narodetskaha, Lukash. *The treatment of patients with gallstones by lecithin.* Am. J. Gastroenterol. (65):231, 1976. ABSTRACT–8 patients ages 38 to 58, with gallstones, took lecithin 100mg tid for 18-34 months. There were significant increases in bile phospholipid content and a significant decrease in bile cholesterol after lecithin treatment. In one individual, gallstones decreased in size and changed in shape. The stones of the other 7 were not affected by lecithin treatment.

**5) EFA**

STUDY–Bell, Doran. *Gallstone dissolution in man using an essential oil preparation.* Brit. Med J. 1:24, Jan 6, 1979. ABSTRACT– 23 patients took "Rowachol," an EFA preparation, for 6-12 months. 3 patients had complete, and 4 had partial, dissolution of gallstones.

**6) "Liver Flush"** The patient should prepare for the flush procedure by drinking lots of apple juice for 5 days and cutting fat consumption way down. As much fresh fruit as possible should be eaten. 2 days before the flush, the patient should take 500-800mg of magnesium and 30 drops Dioscorea tincture 3-4 per day.

On the day of the flush, the patient takes 2 t disodium phosphate in warm/hot water after lunch. Repeat the disodium phosphate two hours later. The patient should drink a big glass of grapefruit or other citrus juice for dinner (that's all). At bedtime the patient should drink 1/2 cup extra virgin olive oil along with 1/2 cup of lemon or grapefruit juice.

Following the olive oil, the patient should go to bed and lie on his/her right side with the right knee pulled up to the chest. If any cramping occurs for an extended period of time, another dose of Dioscorea can be taken. The next morning the patient should take 2 teaspoons of disodium phosphate in 2 ozs of hot water 1 hour before breakfast. This flush can be repeated in 2 weeks if necessary.

**7) Bile salts–Standard Process "Cholacol I & II"**

STUDY–Tooli, J., Jablonski, P., Watts, J. *Gallstone dissolution in man using cholic acid and lecithin.* Lancet (2):1124, 1975. ABSTRACT–Cholic acid 750mg/day and soybean lecithin 2250mg/day were given to 7 patients with radiolucent gallstones and 2 patients with radiolucent stones in the biliary tree. The treatment period was 6 months. In 2 patients the stones disappeared, in one the stones the lithogenic index of bile decreased during the treatment.

**8) Vitamin E**–400-800iu/day

**9) HCL and other digestive enzymes**

**10) Methionine**–In 1984 Frezza and colleagues discovered that intrahepatic cholestasis could be reversed in women by giving 800mg of SAM (S-adenosyl-methionine) per day. It has been useful in the treatment of cholestasis in pregnancy by inhibiting the action of estrogen. However, researchers are not exactly clear how it works.

STUDY–Breneman, J.C. *Allergy elimination diet-gallbladder diet.* Ann. Allergy 26:83-89, 1968. ABSTRACT–69 patients with either x-ray or surgical evidence of gallstones were placed on an elimination diet to determine if there were certain guilty foods not generally suspected of causing gallbladder symptoms. All 69 patients were free from all gallbladder symptoms while they were on the basic elimination diet. Gallbladder symptoms recurred in the following % of patients when each of the following foods were added back into the diet:

| Food | # of patients whose symptoms returned | % | Food | # of patients whose symptoms returned | % |
|---|---|---|---|---|---|
| Egg | 64 | 92.8% | Apple | 6 | 8.7% |
| Pork | 44 | 63.8% | Tomato | 6 | 6.0% |
| Onion | 36 | 52.0% | Peas | 4 | 5.8% |
| Fowl | 24 | 34.8% | Cabbage | 4 | 5.8% |
| Milk | 17 | 24.6% | Spices | 3 | 4.3% |
| Coffee | 15 | 21.7% | Peanut | 3 | 4.3% |
| Orange | 13 | 18.8% | Fish | 2 | 2.9% |
| Corn | 10 | 14.5% | Rye | 1 | 1.4% |
| Beans | 10 | 14.5% | Medications | 14 | 20.3% |
| Nuts | 10 | 14.5% | Other | 29 | 42.0% |

**11) Drug therapy**–Gallbladder calculi may sometimes be dissolved in vivo by giving bile acids orally for many months. The bile salt usually given is chenodiol 15mg/kg/day, which acts in part by reducing hepatic synthesis and biliary secretion of cholesterol. **Cholesterol saturation of bile is reduced** and cholesterol-containing stones may slowly dissolve. **Gallstones may dissolve completely in 30-40% of patients at this dose**, but recurrence of stones and colic after cessation of drug is usual. Urodeoxycholic acid (an investigational drug) may be used (10mg/kg/day) with similar clinical expectations, but without the diarrhea or disturbed liver function seen in occasional patients on the earlier drug.

**Treatment is contraindicated when:**

1) Stones are calcified, very large, or made up of bile pigment
2) During pregnancy
3) If liver disease is present
4) The gallbladder is nonfunctional
5) If patient is very obese

## Notes

---

# HEPATITIS

- Inflammation of the liver either chronic or acute. Can be caused by a number of different viruses including A, B, C, D, E varieties. It may also be caused by other non viral causes such as Tuberculosis, fungi (such as Actinomycosis, Histoplasmosis, Cryptococcosis, Candida albicans, Aspergillus), protozoa (Entamoeba histolytica, Leishmaniasis, Toxoplasmosis), Helminths, Spirochetes, medications, vitamins, environmental and food (Amanita mushrooms) toxins.

- Clinical findings show that the disease usually occurs after the age of 35.

## I. Etiology

Hepatitis A is generally caused by fecal contamination of water or food. Hepatitis B is transmitted by contaminated blood. Hepatitis C is transmitted usually through contaminated blood as well, usually through transfusions. It is believed that as high as 10% of people who are receiving blood transfusions develop hepatitis C.

## II. Signs & Symptoms

Signs and symptoms of hepatitis depend upon the type of hepatitis and whether it is active or chronic. Acute active hepatitis usually shows symptoms of nausea, vomiting, loss of appetite, fatigue, headaches and generally feeling very weak. The liver is often enlarged and tender (positive Murphy sign). When bilirubin levels are high there is usually jaundice throughout body with characteristic yellow sclera. The urine is dark yellow and liver enzymes may be very high.

## III. Diagnosis

The history can yield important information regarding diagnosis of hepatitis. Food born hepatitis A often occurs in small epidemics traced to a restaurant or other public frequented place of eating. Hepatitis B can often be traced to IV drug use, transfusion or other exposure to blood contaminants. In acute hepatitis liver enzymes SGOT & SGPT can often be quite high in the early stages. Urinary bile can give clues along with elevated bilirubin and decreased direct bilirubin. Blood tests for Hepatitis B antigen or antibodies are strong evidence but lack of does not totally exclude the possibility. Hepatitis C antibodies may take up to 12 months to become positive following exposure.

Hepatitis A usually resolves in 4-8 weeks, but with acupuncture, vitamins and botanicals symptoms and liver enzymes may return to normal in as little as 7-14 days. In hepatitis B and C the prognosis is much more uncertain. In the elderly mortality may reach as high as 10-15%. Hepatitis B can turn chronic in 5-10% of infections and hepatitis C up to 50%. Chronic hepatitis C may develop into cirrhosis in about 20% of chronic hepatitis C.

## IV. Clinical considerations

The Merck Manual states that, "...no special treatment required. Undue restrictions on diet or activity are without scientific basis. Vitamin supplements are not required." The conventional train of thought has probably lead to much suffering. There are many alternative treat-

## V. Treatment

Diet should be concentrated with fruits and vegetables because of their flavonoid compounds which will benefit the liver. Especially useful are soups with various green leafy vegetables. Avoiding alcohol, caffeine, coffee, black tea, cola and chocolate, and sugar are important to decrease the stress load on the liver.

1) **Silymarin-** standardized extract (70-80%) 400mg twice per day (1/4 teaspoon 2x/day Omnivite nutrition Inc). Can also use intravenously (IV from Apothecure pharmacy).

2) **High potency multivitamin and mineral supplement without iron**. The fat soluble vitamins are the most critical, especially if cirrhosis present (50% of patients have fat malabsorption). Vitamin K 5mg IM daily for 3 days is often given to rule out hypothrombinemia. Must be careful with vitamin A retinol and niacin because of liver toxicity.

3) **Multi antioxidant formula–Oxyquench** (Omnivite nutrition Inc.) 3 capsules per day

4) **Vitamin C (buffered)–** 2 gms 3x per day or more tolerated. **Bioflavonoids** (catechin)

5) **Green tea–**couple cups per day.

6) **DHEA** if levels are low in chronic hepatitis

7) **Glycyrrhiza**- solid extract 1/2 teaspoon 2x per day

8) **N-acetyl cysteine** 500mg 2x per day

9) **IV or IM weekly treatments of antiviral IV** multivitamin and minerals (Alan Gaby). Dr. Robert Cathcart has used very high levels of IV vitamin C 40-100mg per day in the treatment of hepatitis and has had great success. Can use Silymarin IV.

10) **Phyllanthus amarus–**200mg 3x per day (hepatitis B)

11) **Mushrooms-Shiitake, Reishi, Trametes versicolor (Coriolus)-**Extracts of Trametes, PSK and PSA, have been used to treat cancer, HIV, hepatitis and generally stimulate the immune system (*Medicinal Mushrooms: An Exploration of Tradition, Healing & Culture*, 2nd ed. Chris Hobbs, 1995)

12) **Tumaric or Curcumin**–has shown hepatoprotective effects against inflammatory conditions of the liver found in toxic exposure to carbontetrachloride and glucosamine. It tends to prevent liver enzymes from going really high. It also increases the flow and solubility of bile, so that it may protect against gall bladder stone formation.

13) **Taurine–**4 gms 3x per day (acute hepatitis)

14) **Protomorphagin therapy-Liver extract—**can be given IM or orally (Phytopharmica/Merit or Cardiovascular research). Also consider thymus extract.

# INFLAMMATORY BOWEL DISEASE

## CROHN'S DISEASE (regional enteritis)

- Intermittent bouts of diarrhea, low grade fever, and right lower quadrant pain are typical in Crohn's disease.
- Anorexia, weight loss, gas, and malaise may also be present.
- Crohn's disease affects the **submucosa and mucosa** of the small intestines and the colon. Classically, a patchy distribution and granulomatous inflammatory reaction shows a *cobblestone* appearance with ulcerations involving all layers of the mucosa and submucosa. For this reason fistulas of various organs are a common complication of the disease.
- General abdominal tenderness may be present, especially in the right lower quadrant, with signs of peritoneal inflammation.
- X-rays may reveal abnormalities in the terminal ileum.

In Crohn's disease any area from the mouth to the anus can be affected. In this example the ileum is effected by the inflammation. This is an area where vitamin B-12 is absorbed. Parenteral B-12 can be helpful for people with Crohn's disease.

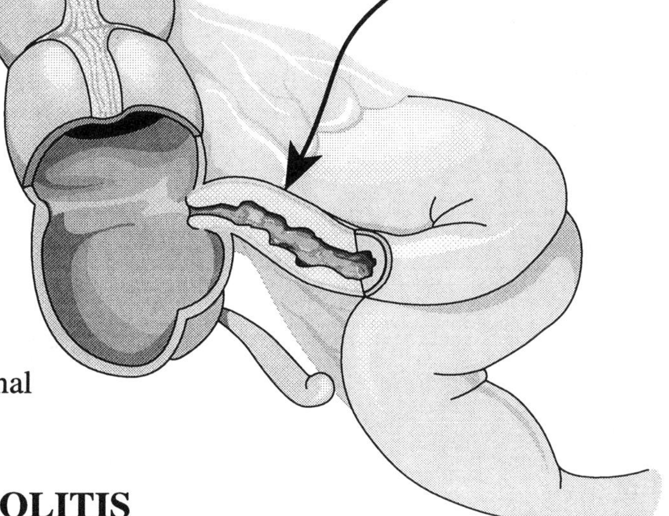

## ULCERATIVE COLITIS

- Bloody diarrhea with cramps in the lower abdomen is a sign of ulcerative colitis.
- Mild abdominal tenderness, weight loss and fever may also be present.
- **Rectal involvement is common.**
- Ulcerative colitis usually only affects the **mucosa and submucosa of the colon,** but sometimes affects the ileum as well.

## I. Epidemiology

- Both UC and CD share a common etiology. Ulcerative colitis is about three to four times more common than Crohn's disease, but the incidence of Crohn's is increasing.

- Inflammatory bowel disease is two to four times more common in whites
- IBD is four times more common in Jews than non-Jews.
- IBD attacks more than one family member 15-40% of the time

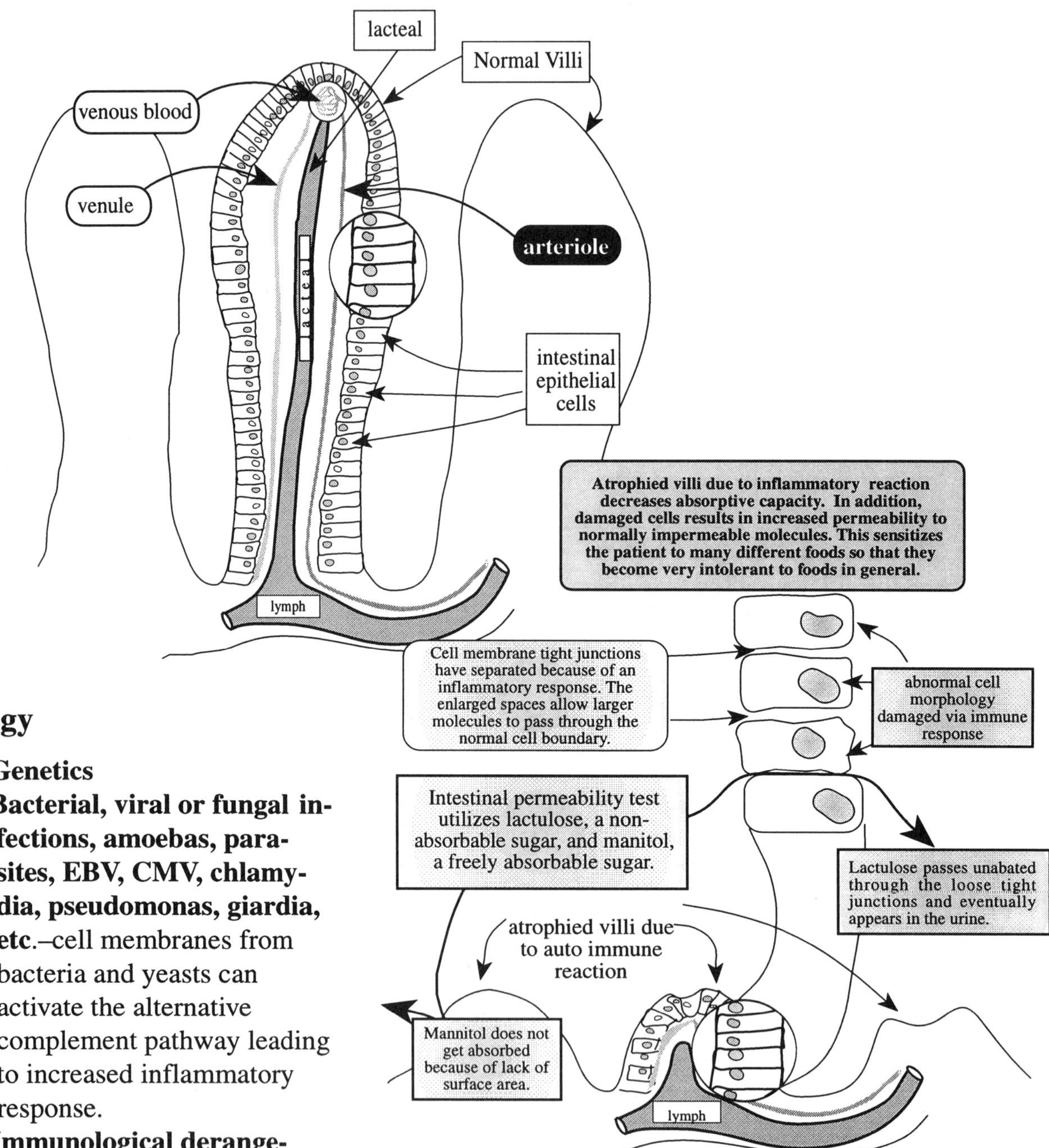


## II. Etiology

1) **Genetics**
2) **Bacterial, viral or fungal infections, amoebas, parasites, EBV, CMV, chlamydia, pseudomonas, giardia, etc.**–cell membranes from bacteria and yeasts can activate the alternative complement pathway leading to increased inflammatory response.
3) **Immunological derangements**
4) **Food allergy, sensitivity or lectin incompatibility**
5) **Refined foods, lack of fiber**
6) **Stress, especially with regard to UC**

## III. Diagnosis

Sigmoidoscopy and biopsy
Intestinal permeability
(mannitol and lactulose)
Stool analysis
- Ova Parasites
- Bacterial culture
- Butyrate–low levels indicate increased risk of cancer.
- Intestinal secretary IgA–Evaluates mucosal immunity against various toxins.

Food allergy testing
Blood typing
Gliadin antibodies
Heidelberg–low levels of HCL may increase the risk of developing abnormal bacteria including Helicobacter and candida.

Urinary indican–indicates putrefication, bowel stagnation or high intake of tryptophan.
SED rate
Albumin (3.0-3.5 target)–If the patient goes below this level, feeding becomes a real problem with regard to tolerance of solid foods.
Hematocrit and Hemoglobin
Weight
White blood cells

## Therapeutic Considerations

Virtually nonexistent in cultures consuming primitive diets, the incidence of Crohn's disease is on the increase in cultures which consume a western diet.

**NOTE**–Researchers in the National Coop Crohn's Disease Study observed 77 patients who received placebo therapy in a 17 week study. **20 of the patients with active bowel disease went into remission** after the 17 weeks. Of these 20 patients, 70% (14) remained in remission after 1 year and 45% (9) remained in remission after 2 years (about 12% of the original 77). In patients having **no previous history of steroid therapy, 41% achieved remission** after 17 weeks. In addition, 23% of this group continued in remission after 2 years as compared to 4% of the group with prior history of steroid therapy.

**Notes on cortisone and NSAID's.**

Increased permeability and an increase the number of food reactions were related to cortisone and NSAIDS.
An elemental diet is an excellent way to stabilize a patient with acute symptoms (see next page).

## IV. Treatment

The treatment of childhood Crohn's is difficult because the patient must consume enough calories and protein for proper growth. On the other hand, increasing the amount of protein tends to aggravate allergic sensitivities. It is important to monitor growth in a child with Crohn's as chronic colitis can have an effect on the absorption of many critical nutrients.

1) **Elemental diet**–This treatment has been especially effective in stabilizing acute situations. ENFOOD® produced by Dr. Gislason in Vancouver, B.C. Canada {(604) 270-8474} has a formula that is relatively palatable. In the U.S.*Tolerex* and *Vivonex T.E.N.*® (Sandoz) are less tasty elemental formulas, the later has added branched chain amino acids and glutamine to enhance its effectiveness. Prior to 1990 in the literature the current Tolerex was Vivonex. This formula can be added to other nutrients as mentioned below. It is best to add these nutrients a couple at a time to make sure there is no reaction to them.

STUDY–Teahon, Bjarnason, Pearson, Levi. *10 years experience with an elemental diet in the management of Crohn's disease* Gut, 1133-37, 1990. ABSTRACT–96 of 113 patients with acute Crohn's disease who were treated with an elemental diet at Northwick Park Hospital in Harrow Middlesex, UK between 77 and 88. The elemental diet was found to be a safe and successful treatment for acute Crohn's disease with remission rates comparable to those achieved with steroids.

STUDY–Giaffer MH et al. *Controlled trial comparing elemental and polymeric diet as primary therapy for active Crohn's disease.* Lancet 1;816-19, 1990. ABSTRACT–30 patients with active Crohn's received either Vivonex (elemental diet) or Fortison, a polymeric (protein-containing) diet. 75% of the patients on the elemental diet improved significantly compared to 36% of the patients on the polymeric diet (p=0.03) after 10 and 28 day assessments.

STUDY–Sanderson IR et al. *Remission induced by an elemental diet in small bowel Crohn's disease.* Arch Dis Child 62(2):123-27, 1987. ABSTRACT–15 children with active Crohn's randomly received either Flexical (elemental diet) or IM ACTH followed by oral prednisolone along with sulfasalazine. The elemental diet proved to equally effective in improving the condition according to a series of evaluations, including growth (which was actually greater in the elemental diet) over the course of 6 months.

2) **Decrease consumption of refined foods**–Initially must be very careful not to aggravate the condition so refined and easy to digest foods are important. As the person stabilizes, fiber and unrefined foods are important to continue the health of the colon.

STUDY–Brandes, Lorenz-Meyer. *Sugar free diet:A new perspective in the treated of Crohn's disease?* Z. Gastroenterol.19(1)1-12,1981..ABSTRACT–**80% of patients** on a low carbo diet which **excluded all refined sugar** had **symptomatic relief within 18 months**, while **40% of patients** on a high carbohydrate diet which was **high in refined sugar** had to discontinue the diet because of **flare-ups.**

STUDY–Grimes. *Refined carbohydrate, smooth muscle spasm & disease of the colon.* Lancet 1:395, 1976. ABSTRACT–Lack of fiber does not stimulate normal bowel function and, as a result, an intensification of the muscle spasm that normally occurs with bowel disease becomes worse.

STUDY–Heaton. *Treatment of Crohn's disease with an unrefined-carbo, fiber-rich diet.* Brit. Med J. 2:762-6,1979 ABSTRACT–32 Crohn's patients were treated with a **fiber rich unrefined carbohydrate diet** in addition to conventional management and followed for over 4 years. Their course was compared to 32 matched patients who received no dietary instructions. **Hospital admissions were significantly fewer and shorter** in the diet-treated patients (111 days versus 533 days). 5 controls required surgery whereas only one of the diet-treated patients required surgery.

3) **Avoid allergens**–Avoiding allergens or food sensitivities is essential part of the treatment. In addition there may be some lectin incompatibilities so doing specialized blood typing may be helpful.

STUDY–Jones. *Crohn's disease: Maintenance of remission by diet.* Lancet 2;177-180 July 27, 1985 ABSTRACT–20 patients with active disease received either an unrefined carbo fiber-rich diet or a diet which excluded specific foods to which a patient was intolerant (via provocative testing). **7 of 10 patients** on the **exclusion diet**

**remained in remission for 6 months** compared with 0 of 10 on the unrefined diet. In an uncontrolled study, an **exclusion diet allowed 51 of 77 patients to remain well on the diet alone for periods of up to 51 months, with an annual relapse rate of less than 10%.**

STUDY–Nutri Res Newsletter Oct., 1984. ABSTRACT–10 patients were given 0.75mg prednisone daily for 14 days, while 11 patients were given a protein free elemental diet. At the end of 4 weeks 8/10 steroid patients and 9/11 diet patients were in remission. At 3 months, one patient in each group was a treated failure.

STUDY–O'Maorain, et al. *Elemental diet in acute Crohn's disease.* Arch. Disease. Childhood 53:44, 1983. ABSTRACT–15 patients, aged 6-20, were followed for up to 3 years on a hypoallergenic elemental diet. The diet was associated with remissions in the 14 patients who tolerated it.

STUDY–Nanda, et al. *Food intolerance and the IBS.* Gut 30:1099-104, 1989. ABSTRACT–200 patients with IBS were treated with dietary exclusion for 3 weeks. Of the 189 who completed this study, 48.2% showed symptom improvement. Subsequent challenge with individual foods showed that 73 of 91 responders remained well on a modified diet during the follow-up period of about 15 months. Of the 98 patients who showed no improvement during the trial, only 3 were symptomatically well at the time of follow up. There was a wide range of food intolerance. The majority (50%) identified 2-5 foods that upset them. The foods most commonly incriminated were dairy (40.7%) & grains (39.4%).

STUDY–Frieri, Claus, Boris et al. *Preliminary investigation on humoral and cellular immune responses to selected food proteins in patients with Crohn's disease* Annals of Allergy 64, 345-51, 1990. ABSTRACT–11 Crohn's patients were studied and 7 were revealed to have positive skin test to milk, wheat and soy protein. 5 of these had both allergic symptoms and Crohn's disease and 4 had complaints of food allergy. 6 patients had elevated sIgG4 to several food proteins in spite of negative sIgE reactions. The antigen most frequently associated with elevated sIgG4 levels was egg protein and the highest sIgG4 levels to eggs and milk protein occurred in skin test negative patients.

4) **Vitamin A and Beta carotene**–Be careful with vitamin A as it can cause problems if there is liver involvement.

5) **Zinc picolinate**–30mg/day The picolinate form may get into the cells better.

6) **Folate**–drugs commonly used in the treated of colitis inhibit folate absorption and also act directly as antagonists (sulfasalazine specifically). Also, folate has been shown to possibly decrease diarrhea in some studies.

STUDY–Lashner. *Effect of Folate supplementation on the incidence of dysplasia and cancer in chronic UC* Gastroenterology 97:255-59, 1989. ABSTRACT–99 patients with chronic colitis for more than 7 years were examined. 35 patients with neoplasia were compared with 64 patients in whom dysplasia was never found. The purpose was to determine the effect of folate supplements on the rate of development of neoplasia. Folate supplementation at 1mg was associated with a 62% lower incidence of neoplasia compared with individuals not receiving supplements.

STUDY–Elsborg, Larsen. *Folate deficiency in chronic IBD.* Scand J. Gastroenterol. 14:1019-24, 1979. ABSTRACT–Of 216 patients with chronic IBD, low serum folate levels were found in 59% and low red blood cell levels in 26%. It is suggested that folate deficiency is of multiple origin; "inadequate diet," malabsorption and chronic drug induced low grade hemolysis.

STUDY–Hodges, et al. *Vitamin and iron intake in patients with Crohn's disease.* J AM Diet Associated. 84(1):52-8, 1984. ABSTRACT–Mean daily intake of folate was below RDA for 23 male and 24 female patients. Serum folate was low in 21% of males and 26% females.

7) **EFA's–particularly omega 3 oils**. Synthesis of lipoxygenase products and inflammatory leukotrienes are inhibited by these oils. For this reason it is a good idea to avoid saturated fats. There is some debate about omega 6 oils because, in animals, they can get converted into arachidonic acid (AA) via Δ5 desaturase. In humans this enzyme has very little activity so that very little DHGLA gets converted to arachidonic acid. It is possible that in times stress this enzyme becomes more active and thus converts more of omega 6 FA into AA.

In the acute phase it is necessary to keep the amount of fats down to a minimum to avoid the synthesis of PGE2. It has been found that elemental formulas with greater than 15% fat tend to decrease protein balance.

STUDY–Gainsborough, H. *Treatment of ulcerative colitis with cod-liver oil retention enema* Lancet June 10, 1939. ABSTRACT–6 cases of UC were treated with high calorie/low residue diet. The retention enemas were administered with cod liver oil and starch. Opium and/or morphine was also given if necessary to allow for retention of the enema. Early infections were given during the day. For longer term infections, enemas were given at night and, ideally, retained over night. The initial dose was 2oz and was increased by 2oz at a time to a maximum of 8oz in accordance with the patients' capability to retain the enema. When the ulcer appeared on radiography up to and past the splenic flexure, the foot of the bed was raised by one foot to facilitate the spread of the oil. 3 of the patients who had symptoms for up to 1.5 years showed marked improvement and were symptom free for 2 years after. One patient who had the condition for 12 years was well for 15 months, then relapsed, but got better again The 5th case remained mostly well, but the 6th patient eventually went on to require an ileostomy.

STUDY–Mochizuki, Trocki, Dominioni, et al. *Optimal lipid content for enteral diets following thermal injury.* JEPN 8:638-646, 1984. ABSTRACT–Rats were anesthetized and then burned and fed set diets with varying amounts of fats from 0% to 50%, mainly consisting of safflower oil. It was determined that total nitrogen balance was greatest at 15%. It was noted that in growing rats, EFA deficiency can occur in a very short period of time during acute stress. This deficiency can lead to death quickly.

**Note**–Many enteral formulas contain between 35-50% fat, usually not of the best quality.

8) **Glutamine**–3-12gms/day–a conditionally essential amino acid. Muscle contains about 14% glutamine and alanine. During severe stress or surgery these 2 amino acids make up 60% of released amino acids. The majority goes to the gut and the kidneys where it is used for fuel.

STUDY–Souba, Smith, Wilmore Glutamine metabolism by the intestinal tract JPEN 9:608-17, 1985.

9) **Arginine**–3gms per day.

STUDY–Siefter, Returra, Barbul et al. *Arginine: an essential amino acid for injured rats* Surgery 84:224-30, 1978. ABSTRACT–Supplementation of arginine to rat chow enhanced healing significantly in rats compared to control diets.

10) **Vitamin E**–800iu. A free radical scavenger with anti-inflammatory properties, vitamin E is also involved with increasing sIgA, which helps to protect mucosal lining from invading bacteria and other toxins.

11) **Quercetin** inhibits mast cell degranulation, decreases leukotriene synthesis (by blocking phospholipase A2 and lipoxygenase), and protects cell membranes via its antioxidant activity.

STUDY–Stefanini, Bazzocchi, Prati, Lanfranchi, Gasbarrini. *Efficacy of oral disodium cromoglycate in patients with IBS and positive skin tests to foods.* Lancet 1:207-8, 1986. ABSTRACT–28 patients were given disodium cromoglycate, which is useful for specific food allergies that are mediated through mast cells and basophils. These patients were skin pricked and then placed on an elimination diet along with 1.5gms/day of disodium cromoglycate for 8 weeks. 19 of these with "+" skin tests had successful remission while only 1 of 9 who had negative skin tests improved with the treatment.

STUDY–*Use of cromolyn in combined GI allergy* JAMA 242:1169, 1979.

STUDY–*Immune complexes containing food proteins in normal and atopic subjects after oral challenge and effect of sodium cromoglycate on antigen absorption.* Lancet June 16: 1270, 1969.

12) **Vitamin B-12**–IM-1000µg–every 2-3 weeks. Often damage to the ileum leads to malabsorption. Many patients with Crohn's feel much better with B-12.

13) **Vitamin C and selenium**. Vitamin C must be given as tolerated. This will vary from person to person. In the acute phase of the disease it is important not to irritate the intestinal mucosa, thus, large dose vitamin C may be contraindicated. Selenium can be given in doses up to 300mcg over an extended period of time.

**14) Lactobacillus acidophilus** re-establishes flora.

STUDY–Bennet & Brinkman *Treatment of UC by implantation of normal colonic flora* Lancet Jan, 21, 1989. ABSTRACT–JDB had continuously active, severe UC for 7 years confirmed endoscopically and histologically. The condition was refractory to standard management including steroids and sulphasalazine and every time daily prednisone dosage was reduced below 30mg severe symptoms (bloody diarrhea, cramping tenesmus, skin lesions and arthritis recurred. For the past 4 years symptoms had been controlled with 4.2gms of alpha tocopherylquinone and a low fat diet. When the tocopheryl was discontinued or reduced, symptoms returned within 1-2 days. With a protocol developed to sterilize the bowel before surgery, his flora was greatly reduced. The donor flora was introduced by large volume retention enemas. 1 wk later tocopheryls were discontinued without any recurrence of symptoms. It has now been 6 months since this implantation of normal flora and patient has been symptom free for the first time in 11 years without any medications. 3 months after the implantation, colonic biopsy revealed chronic inflammatory cells but no active inflammation.

**15) Magnesium-**Mag-lo-plex® slow release magnesium (Omnivite nutrition) is tolerated better than standard magnesium supplements that tend to cause diarrhea even at moderate doses . Low tissue levels of magnesium can perpetuate intestinal spasm. Conversely larger doses taken as a conventional magnesium supplement may induce further diarrhea. It may also be helpful to use magnesium intravenously 1-3gms 2-3 times per week to raise tissue magnesium levels without directly stimulating the GI tract and inducing further spasm.

STUDY–Galland, L. *Mag and IBD.* Magnesium 7:78-83, 1988. ABSTRACT–This review article discusses possible reasons for deficiency: 1) decreased intake from restrictive diet or anorexia; 2) formation of magnesium soaps from steatorrhea, and from general diarrhea; 3) magnesuria induced via steroids or surgery; 4) increased requirements for healing and for rapid cell turnover. Symptoms include muscle cramps, bone pain, delirium, acute tetany, fatigue, depression, cardiac abnormalities, impaired healing and colonic motility problems.

**16) N-Acetylated glucosamino sugars**–800mg t.i.d.–bipasses the rate limiting step in mucopolysaccharide synthesis by providing preformed N-acetylated glucosamines.

STUDY–*Decreased incorporation of 14c glucosamine relative to 3H-N-Acetyl glucosamine in the intestinal mucosa of patients with IBD* Am. J. Gastroent 78:19, 1983

**17) Glycyrrhiza** has anti-fungal and anti-inflammatory activity

**18) Digestive enzymes (pancreatic and HCL)**

Travacid (time release HCL) is used to acidify colon.

**19) Butyrate enema**–can do a series of these (available from Tyler). Can also take orally (Cardiovascular research & Probiologics).

STUDY–Breuer, R (associate professor of medicine, NW U Chicago). *Presentation at a Boston meeting of the american College of Gastroenterology* Med World News December, 1991. ABSTRACT–21 patients with left sided ulcerative colitis treated themselves with an enema of acetate, proprionate, and butyrate in a 100ml solution 2x per day while the control group of 20 patients used enemas with saline alone. After 6 weeks 10 of 17 patients in the treatment group had improved significantly compared to 6 of 20 in the controls. 2 of the treated patients had complete remission of all symptoms and a follow up after one year showed that some of the patients had no relapse.

STUDY–Harig JM et al. *Treatment of diversion colitis with short-chain fatty acid irrigation.* NEJM 320:23-28, 1989.

**20) Cod liver oil enema**–can also do a series of these combining with butyrate (see reference on page 380 under EFA tx).

**21) Seacure®**–This product is a hydrolyzed fish protein that is relatively hypoallergenic and may be especially useful in someone who has weight loss and difficulty tolerating any types of proteins.

## Factors that promote translocation across damaged mucosal barrier:

a) Changes in bacterial flora
b) Impaired host deficiency mechanisms
c) Trauma
d) Endotoxemia
e) Protein calorie malnutrition
f) Long term treatment with cortisone

Miscellaneous treatments for colitis–similar to treatments for Crohn's disease.

STUDY–Jewel & Truelove. *Circulating antibodies to cow's milk in Ulcerative colitis.* Gut 13:796,1972. ABSTRACT–IgG & IgM antibodies to cow's milk proteins were found to be increased in patients .

STUDY–Wright & Truelove. *A controlled therapeutic trial of various diets in ulcerative colitis.* Brit. Med J. 2:138, 1965. ABSTRACT–After 1 year, 10 of 13 patients on a dairy free diet had remained symptom free compared to 5 of 13 patients on a dummy controlled diet.

STUDY–Siegel. *Inflammatory bowel disease: Another possible facet of the allergic diathesis.* Ann. Allergy 47:92-94,1981. ABSTRACT–42 of 59 patients were judged to be possibly allergic with both respiratory and abdominal problems were treated( along with the other 59) with inhalant hyposensitization and a rotary diversified diet. Over 50 of these patients were considerably improved after treated.

## Notes

---

# DIARRHEA & PARASITES

- Diarrhea is not a disease, but a symptom.
- It is characterized by frequent liquid stools.
- There are 4 types of diarrhea:
  1) *Osmotic*–caused by the presence of active solutes. Examples of osmotic diarrhea include dumping syndrome, lactase deficiency, and rapidly ingested simple carbohydrates.
  2) *Secretory*–caused by bacterial exotoxins, viruses or parasites.
  3) *Exudative*–is associated with mucosal damage, which leads to an outpouring of mucus, blood, and plasma proteins. Exudative diarrhea is usually caused by radiation and ulcerative colitis.
  4) *Allergic*–this type of diarrhea is often intermittent and commonly alternates with constipation.

## I. Treatment

**Osmotic diarrhea**–The general concerns with osmotic diarrhea are removal of active solutes and the replacement of fluids and electrolytes.

1) Remove all simple carbohydrates (especially in children)
2) Make sure all solutes are being broken down so they may be absorbed
3) Supplement digestive and pancreatic enzymes
4) Eat cultured foods such as yogurt and kefir if the patient has no sensitivity– Lactobacillus acidophilus (from ages 1-7, L. bifidus)

STUDY–Lerebours, Ndam, Lavoine, Hellot, Antoine, et al. *Yogurt and fermented, then pasteurized milk effects of short term and long term ingestion on lactose absorption and mucosal lactase activity in lactase deficient subjects.* AJCN 49 p. 823-27, 1989 ABSTRACT–In 16 lactase deficient individuals, lactose digestion was enhanced by ingestion of yogurt. This beneficial effect was destroyed by pasteurization. Long term ingestion of yogurt **did not increase lactase activity** of the duodenal mucosa. The increase in lactose absorption associated with yogurt ingestion must therefore be primarily related to an intraluminal process.

5) Charcoal
6) Miso soup
7) Rice water & rice
8) Psyllium seed powder or bentonite clay
9) Pectin
10) Carob powder
11) Avoid coffee

**Secretory diarrhea**–Bring about a balanced bacterial flora by replacing lost beneficial bacteria and inhibiting the growth of harmful bacteria. Replace electrolytes.

1) Lactobacillus acidophilus contains antibacterial, antiviral, and antifungal properties. It also acidifies the colon. Use enterically coated L. acidophilus or give with meals.
2) Garlic inhibits the growth of yeast as well as other pathogens.
3) Hydrastis canadensis is an anti-bacterial used for the treatment of infectious processes.
4) Charcoal absorbs toxins.

**Note**–Parasites must be suspected if there is no improvement and the patient has a suspicious history. Investigate thoroughly because parasites can be difficult to diagnose.

**Parasitism** is a symbiotic relationship in which one animal, the host, is to some degree injured through the activities of the other animal, the parasite.

**Obligate parasites** cannot survive in any other manner (Microsporida is an intracellular obligate parasite (usually requires electron microscopy.

**Facultative parasites** may exist in a free living state or as a commensal which, if opportunity presents itself, may become parasitic.

**Commensalism**, "eating at the same table," denotes an association that is beneficial to one partner and at least not disadvantageous to the other.

When such associations are beneficial to both organisms, it is known as mutualism.

## 3 TYPES OF PARASITIC INFECTIONS

1) Protozoa (single cell organisms) constitute the most prevalent parasitic infections, infecting 10% of the world's population. **Pathogenic protozoa** include:
   a) Amoeba–*Entameba histolytica, Entameba polecki*
   b) Flagellates–*Giardia lamblia, Dientamoeba fragilis*
   c) Sporozoa–*Isospora belli, Cryptosporidium species, Blastocystis hominis*
   d) Ciliates–*Balantidium coli*

   **Commensal protozoa** include those which **may cause symptoms**–*Endolimax nana, Entameba coli, Iodamoeba butschllii, Trichomonas tenax, Chilomastix mesnili, Retortamonas intestinalis*

   Commensal protozoa **not known to be symptomatic** include *Trichomonas hominis, Enteromonas hominis, Entameba hartimani.*

2) Platyhelminthes (flat worms)
3) Nemathelminthes (round worms)

An Ova & Parasite test is required for the detection of certain pathogenic protozoa.

Other organisms that cause diarrhea E. coli usually related to contaminated ground beef. Here in the N.W. there were several outbreaks one was from "The Sizzler" restaurant and the other was from "Jack in the Box" restaurant where the meat was contaminated. Other organisms include Campylobacter upsaliensis, Yersinia enterocolitica 0:3 (associated with contaminated pig intestines), Legionella (has caused or triggered colitis conditions). Candida albicans also can cause diarrhea especially in the elderly hospitalized patient also Cytomegalovirus.

## Diagnosis of Parasites

1. a) Giardia antigen–97% sensitivity serum antigens
   b) Cryptosporidium–93% sensitivity
2. A purged stool sample has a much higher chance of identifying parasites
3. Stool culture will reveal abnormal bacterial flora (Need to special order Clostridium. difficile culture). C. difficile is an anaerobe which can result in infection especially after antibiotic therapy. It can produce several different toxins including cytotoxin B and enterotoxin A which results in pseudomembranous colitis.

I have treated *Giardia lamblia* with the following treatment:

1) A 5 day fast using dilute fruit juice (fresh pineapple).
2) Bromelain–4500mcu (550mg) caps-3 caps 3x per day
3) Oxyquinolin sulfate Kollesol (Luties)–5 tabs QID
4) Pancreatic enzyme

You can also use:

5) 10 clove garlic/day
6) Artemesia annua
7) Grapefruit seed extract–"Paracan"
8) Berberis aquafolium
9) Chinese herbal formulas (contact ITM)
10) Papayasan (Herb Pharm)
11) Oregano oil
12) Tea Tree oil

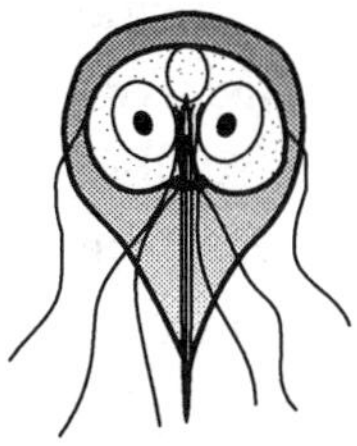

Giardia lamblia usually colonizes the duodenal area

Conventional treatment in Europe uses Tenatazol (not avail currently) or Flagyl.

*Cryptosporidium treatment*–has been treated with bovine colostrum as this organism occurs commonly in cattle.

*Clostridium difficile*–Convention therapy involves the use of vancomycin or Flagyl but treatment with Lactobacillus or Saccharomyces boulardii as an enema has been successful.

STUDY–Tvede M, Rask-Madsen J. *Bacteriotherapy for chronic relapsing Clostridium difficile diarrhea in 6 patients.* Lancet 1:1156-60, 1989.

STUDY–Seal DV, et al. *Treatment of relapsing Clostridium difficile diarrhea by administration of non-toxic strain.* Eur J Clin Microbiol Infect Dis 6:51-53, 1987.

STUDY–Kimmey MB et al. *Prevention of further recurrences of C. Diff. colitis with Saccharomyces boulardii.* Dig Dis Sci 35:897-901, 1990.

**Exudative diarrhea**–Try to remove the source of the irritation if possible. **Always rule out allergies** (this goes for any type of diarrhea). Heal the inflamed tissues. Check for excess permeability. Replace electrolytes.

1) Consider a short fast to avoid physically irritating the tissues
2) Consider a hypoallergenic diet (see handout)
3) *Ulmus fulvus*
4) *Symphytum officianale*
5) Vitamin C–1-2gms divided dose, buffered
6) Zinc picolinate–30mg/day
7) Vitamin A–25,000iu
8) Apple sauce

# CONSTIPATION

- Constipation is a subjective symptom where stools are too hard, too small, too infrequent, difficult to expel, or when the patient has a feeling of incomplete evacuation after the bowel movement is over. Other objective signs are fewer than 3-5 stools per week, more than 3 days without a stool, or if stools weigh less than 35gms. Average bowel transit time is 50-100 hours, and the average stool weight is 100gms, in the U.S.
- I consider a patient constipated if a day passes without a BM. Even if the patient has a BM every day, there still may be problems. Bowel transit time should be 17-30 hours. Usually I give 6 "00" caps of activated charcoal and see how long it takes for the black to appear and to go completely away. Various dyes, including beets, can also be used.

## I. Clinical Significance

Constipation may predispose the patient to the following:

1) Hemorrhoids
2) Diverticular disease
3) Bowel flora imbalance including PSC
4) Allergies
5) Colon cancer–**4 factors involved**:
   a) Increased toxin concentration against colon wall
   b) Increased time exposure to toxins
   c) Increased overall exposure to the number of different toxins (both ingested or synthesized in gut)
   d) physical trauma

## II. Diagnostic Procedures

1) Bowel Transit Time (BTT)
2) Stool butyrate–evaluate the types of bacteria and risk of CA
3) Urinary indican–this is an inexpensive test that gauges the degree of putrefaction
4) Microclot test (see handout) evaluates endotoxins in gut
5) Stool culture may find aberrant bacteria

## III. Treatment

**1) Increase fiber**–both water soluble and non-water soluble

**2) Consider allergies**, especially milk, when you see alternating constipation and diarrhea

**3) Hydration**–make sure the patient is drinking enough water (50-60 ozs/day)

**4) Psyllium powder,** and, if cholesterol is high, add other fibers such as pectin

**5) Vitamin B complex**–10mg/day multi-B complex orally for infants

**6) EFA**–consider if high triglycerides, blood pressure, dry skin, dermatitis, inflammation. EFA's will act both physically and through prostaglandin synthesis.

7) **Magnesium–**600-900mg/day
8) **Exercise**
9) **HCL** if hypochlorhydric
10) **Trace elements**
11) **Fruit**
12) **Herbs**
13) **Vitamin C**–3-10gms/day

**Note**–Megacolon can often be treated through diet and supplements, especially magnesium.

## Notes

---

# HEMORRHOIDS

- Hemorrhoids are abnormally swollen veins around the anus.
- Most hemorrhoids begin when the patient is in his/her mid 20's or 30's, but may not become noticeable until later.
- Over 50% of people over 50 years old have symptoms associated with hemorrhoids and up to 33% of the U.S. population have some form of hemorrhoids.

## I. Etiology

The causes of hemorrhoids are similar to those of varicose veins. Usually there is some genetic weakness of the veins with the addition of increased intra-abdominal pressure. This increased intra-abdominal pressure may be caused by delayed bowel transit time (constipation); lack of fiber, fluid, or exercise; pregnancy; excessive coughing, sneezing, vomiting, and heavy "grunt work." In addition, long periods of standing or sitting and portal hypertension due to cirrhosis can cause problems associated with hemorrhoids.

## II. Signs and Symptoms

Symptoms may include itching burning, pain, swelling and bleeding. Itching is usually due to trauma from irritating toilet paper. Parasites, yeast, and allergies can also cause itching. Bleeding is usually associated with internal hemorrhoids. External hemorrhoids may become thrombosed and bleed. Usually the thrombus heals and is replaced with connective tissue.

## III. Treatment

Treat the same way as constipation. Add herbs, astringents and supplements to strengthen the integrity of epithelial tissue.

1) **Kesey technique**
2) **Hamamelis virginiana**–As an astringent
3) **Vitamin E**–400iu-800iu/day
4) **Vitamin C**–2-3gms/day–Helps build up the connective tissue around the hemorrhoids
5) **Vitamin A**–25,000iu–Enhance the healing and integrity of the epithelial cells.
6) **Bioflavonoids**–1-3gms/day–Strengthens cell membranes.
7) **Flax oil**–Acts physically as a lubricant, builds up the mucosal membranes and enhances prostaglandin production.
8) **Psyllium seed powder**–Softens stool and increases the number of bowel movements.
9) **Flax seed powder**

# POLYSYSTEMIC CANDIDIASIS (PSC)

- The chronic overgrowth of Candida albicans is associated with many varied and difficult to assess symptoms.

## I. Etiology

1) Chronic over consumption of simple carbohydrates; rule out diabetes mellitus
2) Chronic broad spectrum antibiotic use
3) Chronic use of BCP and of estrogen hormones
4) Multiple cortisone use systemically
5) Bowel toxicity "stagnation"

**NOTE**–It is thought that many symptoms experienced by patients are caused by metabolites that Candida albicans produces in the body. Candida metabolizes sugar into acetaldehyde and alcohol. These substances can be produced in enough quantity to cause behavioral changes and even drunkenness.

## II. Signs and Symptoms

The symptoms of PSC are extremely varied and can mimic many other conditions, especially allergies. Some special symptoms seem to be more related to PSC than others.

1) Chronic vaginal candida infections
2) Chronic tinea pedis, tinea cruris, or fungal infections anywhere on the body
3) Digestive problems such as bloating, gas, fullness, especially after eating and/or especially after eating simple carbohydrate.
4) Symptoms aggravate on damp, muggy, humid days or in moldy homes or buildings
5) Heightened sensitivity to environmental chemicals such as perfumes, soaps, petrochemicals, household cleaners, insecticides, tobacco or other chemicals
6) Any number of food cravings, especially for wheat, sugar and other simple carbohydrates
7) Any number of allergic symptoms such as headaches, irritability, fatigue, muscle aches, abdominal symptoms, etc.

## III. Diagnosis

1) Signs and symptoms–Give the patient the Candida questionnaire from *The Yeast Connection*, William Crook, M.D. A trial of the anti-candida diet may also be useful.
2) Comprehensive stool analysis
3) Candida immune complexes and circulating antigen test (blood)
4) Intestinal permeability
5) Salivary Adrenal Test–measures cortisol (4 readings) and DHEA levels
6) Candida specific secretory IgA or overall intestinal sIgA
7) Allergy testing
8) Heidelberg or Gastro test
9) Consider CEBV

## IV. Treatment

1) **Anti-Candida diet**–Have the patient follow the diet strictly for 1 week, then gradually introduce new foods. Initially the patient should avoid almost all carbohydrates, especially pop, fruit juice and high glycemic index foods (see Diabetes Mellitus, pg. 282). I usually have patients eat a significant amount of meat (fish, poultry, red meat) the first week; grains only a couple of times, during this first week.

2) **Increase Dietary Fiber**–This should come primarily from vegetable sources. Psyllium, pectin, flax powder or other soluble fiber can also be added to the diet. This tends to stabilize blood sugars.

3) **Lactobacillus acidophilus**–1/2 tsp 3x/day; "Superdophilus" or "Myco-Gard" 2 caps 3x/day–Decreased pH in large intestine speeds transit time and competitively inhibits growth of candida.

STUDY–Kennedy, M. and Volz, P. *Ecology of Candida albicans gut colonization: Inhibition of Candida adhesion, colonization, and dissemination from the gastrointestinal tract by bacterial antagonism.* Infection & Immunology 49:654-663, 1985. ABSTRACT–Increased indigenous microflora reduced the mucosal association of C. albicans by forming a dense layer of bacteria in the mucus gut, out-competing yeast cells for adhesion sites, and producing inhibitor substances (possibly volatile fatty acids, secondary bile acids or both) that reduced C. albicans adhesion.

4) **Garlic**–3 caps 3x per day for 1-2 weeks-Raw garlic is probably the most effective at inhibiting yeast growth.

5) **Bentonite clay** binds to endotoxins. I use a product called Springgreen® 1 T 2x per day; which is a colloidal suspension of bentonite clay.

6) **Caprylic acid** promotes the growth of beneficial bacteria.

7) **Undecylenic acid,** an 11 carbon fatty acid, inhibits the growth of Candida albicans.

8) **Nystatin**–STARTING DOSE-1/8 teaspoon 3x/day. Gradually increase the dose by 1/8 teaspoon per dose every 1-2weeks. (1/8 t =500,000units)

   Nystatin was discovered by 2 women scientists, Rachel Brown, an organic chemist, and Elizabeth Lee Hazen, a mold researcher working for the New York State Department of Health. Hazen found many antifungal substances in the soil, but many of them were toxic. Finally, while vacationing, Hazen dug up a mold which "knocked out" other yeasts and molds without harming animals. Squibb and Sons met with Hazen and Brown and patented the new yeast fighting mold. They named it *"NY-State-in"* in honor of the New York State Dept. of Health. It was also agreed that royalties were to be put in a special Brown-Hazen scientific and educational fund.

**NOTE**–Use only the yellow powder by 1-800-Lederle or Biopharmaceuticals, Inc. (800) 543-7737 or 643-4322.

9) **HCl in the form of Travacid**–3 grain tablets start with 1 before each meal–Time release HCl has a stronger effect on the pH of the lower bowel. Often HCl will increase the number of bowel movements. Can check the pH of the stool to see if it is more on the alkaline side.

**10) Butyric acid–**The preferred metabolic substrate for colonic epithelial cells

STUDY–Cummings, J. *Short-Chain fatty acids in the human colon.* Gut 22: 763-779, 1981. ABSTRACT–It was found that 3 short chain fatty acids, butyrate, acetate, and propionate, compose a major solute fraction of fecal water. Basically they come from unabsorbed dietary carbohydrates which have been fermented. Of these three fatty acids, butyrate is the single biggest metabolite of fiber. It has been shown that several cell types in the colon used butyrate to help induce differentiation.

STUDY–Whitehead, R., Young, G., Bhatal, P. *Effects of short-chain fatty acids on a new human colon carcinoma cell line (LIM1215)* Gut 27:1457-63, 1986. ABSTRACT–A neoplastic cell line isolated from a 34 year old man with colon cancer was used to study the effects of various short and medium chain fatty acids on growth and differentiation. It was found that butyrate significantly inhibited the growth of these neoplastic cells.

**11) Antioxidants**–Flavonoids, Vitamins A, C, and E, Selenium

**12) Oregano oil (Biotics)**

**13) Tea tree oil**

**14) Diflucan** (fluconazole)–this tends to work more systemically.

**15) Ketoconizole** (Nizoral) or Itraconazole (Sporanox)–200mg 1x per day for 14-28 days (GABY)

**16) Diflucan** (fluconazole)–100mg 2x daily on 1st day en 100mg per day for 2-4weeks (Alan Gaby). This tends to work more systemically.

## Notes

---

# Yeast & Food Allergy and Digestion

## *The Small Intestine*

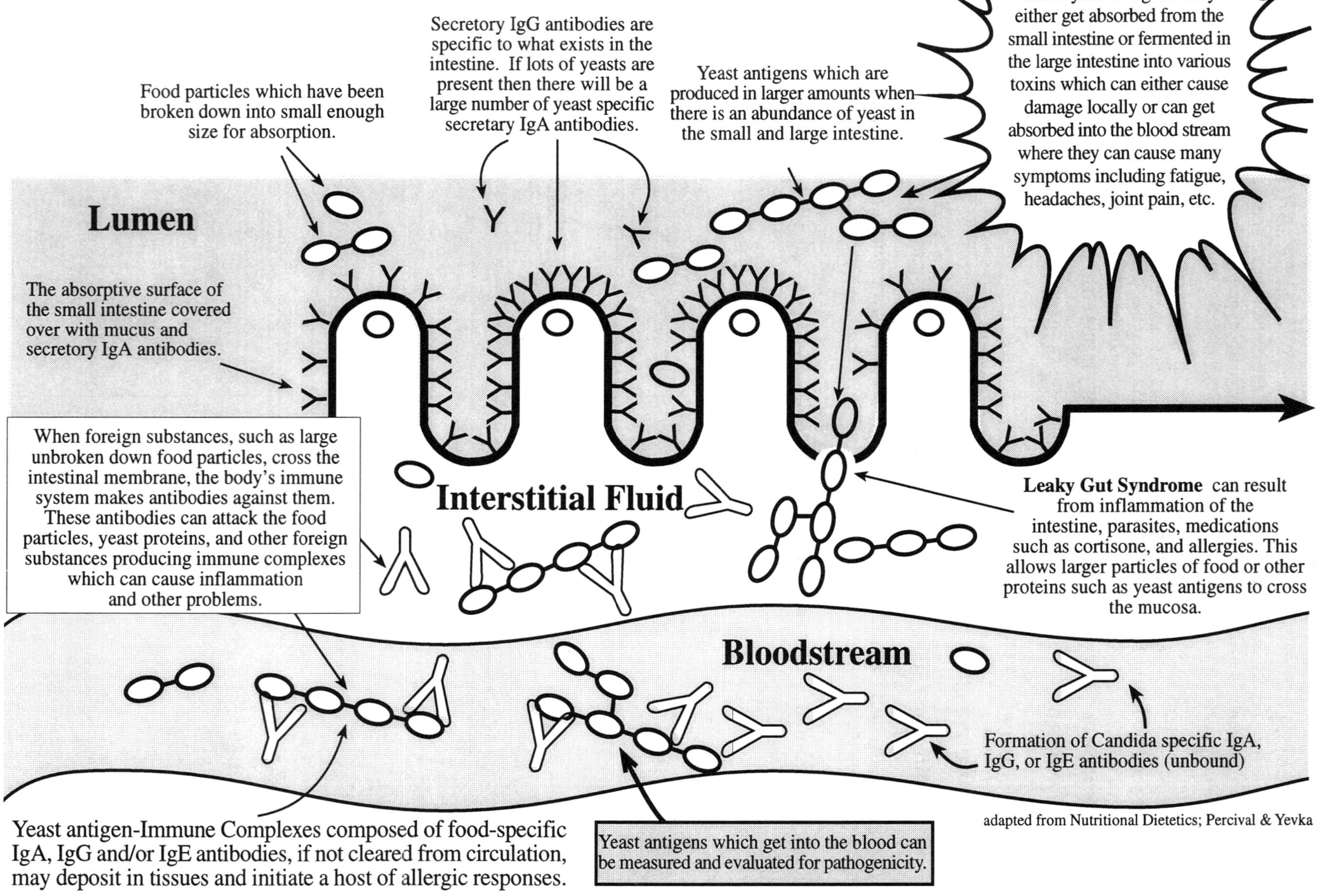

Food particles which have been broken down into small enough size for absorption.

Secretory IgG antibodies are specific to what exists in the intestine. If lots of yeasts are present then there will be a large number of yeast specific secretary IgA antibodies.

Yeast antigens which are produced in larger amounts when there is an abundance of yeast in the small and large intestine.

These yeast antigens may either get absorbed from the small intestine or fermented in the large intestine into various toxins which can either cause damage locally or can get absorbed into the blood stream where they can cause many symptoms including fatigue, headaches, joint pain, etc.

**Lumen**

The absorptive surface of the small intestine covered over with mucus and secretory IgA antibodies.

When foreign substances, such as large unbroken down food particles, cross the intestinal membrane, the body's immune system makes antibodies against them. These antibodies can attack the food particles, yeast proteins, and other foreign substances producing immune complexes which can cause inflammation and other problems.

**Interstitial Fluid**

**Leaky Gut Syndrome** can result from inflammation of the intestine, parasites, medications such as cortisone, and allergies. This allows larger particles of food or other proteins such as yeast antigens to cross the mucosa.

**Bloodstream**

Formation of Candida specific IgA, IgG, or IgE antibodies (unbound)

adapted from Nutritional Dietetics; Percival & Yevka

Yeast antigen-Immune Complexes composed of food-specific IgA, IgG and/or IgE antibodies, if not cleared from circulation, may deposit in tissues and initiate a host of allergic responses.

Yeast antigens which get into the blood can be measured and evaluated for pathogenicity.

## Anti-Candida Diet

**VEGETARIAN** - Enlarge this by 124% onto 8.5x14" paper

| MONDAY | TUESDAY | WEDNESDAY | THURSDAY | FRIDAY | SATURDAY | SUNDAY |
|---|---|---|---|---|---|---|
| Sweet Potato & Walnuts | Cream of Brown Rice & Pecans | Quinoa & Steamed Broccoli | Avocado & Rice Cakes | Amaranth & Zucchini with Chopped | Buckwheat, Peas & Toasted Sesame Oil | Oatmeal & Cashews |
| Beets & Spinach with fresh Lemon | Baked Acorn or Butter Nut Squash | Lentil Soup, Carrots, Broccoli & Celery | Rice Cakes & Cashew Butter | Sweet Potato & Walnuts | Pinto Beans & Brown Rice | Split Pea Soup & Vegetables |
| (if need a snack, eat more walnuts or carrots) | (if need a snack, eat more pecans or squash) | (if need a snack, eat sunflower seeds) | (if need a snack, eat cashews) | (if need a snack, eat almonds) | (if need a snack, eat filberts) | (if need a snack, eat more cashews or celery) |
| Quinoa & Steamed Cauliflower, Zucchini | Brown Rice & Eggplant Baked with Olive Oil | Millet & Asparagus | Split Pea Soup with Carrot & Celery | Baked Potato & Red Chard | Beans with Wild Rice | Brown Rice, Peas & Toasted Sesame Oil |

**Special Instructions:**
1) Use only sea salt as a spice
2) Drink only spring, distilled, or filtered water.
3) Use only fresh vegetables & fruits, ideally organic. Frozen is next best if not organic.
4) If you must switch meals around, it is best to switch the entire day in the week.
5) If still hungry after eating, eat more of the foods (or snacks listed) before the next meal.

## Anti-Candida Diet

**OMNIVORE** - Enlarge this by 124% onto 8.5x14" paper

| MONDAY | TUESDAY | WEDNESDAY | THURSDAY | FRIDAY | SATURDAY | SUNDAY |
|---|---|---|---|---|---|---|
| Sweet Potato & Walnuts | Cream of Brown Rice & Pecans | Quinoa & Steamed Broccoli | Poached Eggs & Rice Cakes | Amaranth & Zucchini with Chopped Almonds | Buckwheat, Peas & Toasted Sesame Oil | Oatmeal & Cashews |
| Tuna & Carrots | Baked Acorn or Butter Nut Squash | Lentil Soup, Carrots, Broccoli & Celery | Rice Cakes & Cashew Butter | Tuna & Carrots | Pinto Beans & Brown Rice | Baked Chicken & Steamed Vegetables |
| (if need a snack, eat more walnuts or carrots) | (if need a snack, eat more pecans or squash) | (if need a snack, eat sunflower seeds) | (if need a snack, eat cashews) | (if need a snack, eat almonds) | (if need a snack, eat filberts) | (if need a snack, eat more cashews or celery) |
| Salmon & Steamed Cauliflower | Poached Eggs & Rice Cakes | Cod & Asparagus | Red Snapper & Eggplant Baked with Olive Oil | Millet & Steamed Spinach | Chicken with Wild Rice | Brown Rice, Peas & Toasted Sesame Oil |

**Special Instructions:**
1) Use only sea salt as a spice
2) Drink only spring, distilled, or filtered water.
3) Use only fresh vegetables & fruits, ideally organic. Frozen is next best if not organic.
4) If you must switch meals around, it is best to switch the entire day in the week.
5) If still hungry after eating, eat more of the foods (or snacks listed) before the next meal.

## CANDIDA QUESTIONNAIRE

| SECTION A: HISTORY | POINT SCORE |
|---|---|
| 1. Have you taken antibiotics an average of 2 times per year or more for the last 3 years? | 20 |
| 2. Have you taken tetracyclines (Sumycin, Panmycin, Vibramycin, Minocin, etc.) or other antibiotics for acne for 1 month (or longer)? | 35 |
| 3. Have you, at any time in your life, taken other "broad spectrum" antibiotics for respiratory, urinary or other infections (for 2 months or longer, or in shorter courses 4 or more times in a 1-year period? | 35 |
| 4. Have you taken a broad spectrum antibiotic drug—even a single course? | 6 |
| 5. Have you, at any time in your life, been bothered by persistent prostatitis, vaginitis or other problems affecting your reproductive organs? | 25 |
| 6. Have you been pregnant... | |
| 2 or more times? | 5 |
| 1 time? | 3 |
| 7. Have you taken any birth control pills or estrogen hormones for menstrual problems or endometriosis... | |
| For more than 2 years? | 15 |
| For 6 months to 2 years? | 6 |
| 8. Have you taken prednisone, Decadron, or other cortisone-type drugs for arthritis, skin problems, asthma... | |
| For more than 6 weeks? | 30 |
| For more than 2 weeks? | 15 |
| For 2 weeks or less? | 6 |
| 9. Does exposure to perfumes, insecticides, fabric shop odors and other chemicals provoke... | |
| Moderate to severe symptoms? | 20 |
| Mild symptoms? | 5 |
| 10. Are your symptoms worse on damp, muggy days or in moldy places? | 20 |
| 11. Have you had athlete's foot, ring worm,"jock itch", vaginal yeast infections,or other chronic fungus infections of the skin or nails? Have such infections been... | |
| Severe or persistentt? | 20 |
| Mild to moderate? | 10 |
| 12. Do you crave sugar? | 10 |
| 13. Do you crave breads or wheat products? | 10 |
| 14. Do you crave alcoholic beverages? | 10 |
| 15. Does tobacco smoke really bother you? | 10 |

Total Score,Section A__________

SECTION B: MAJOR SYMPTOMS

| | MILD | FREQUENT &/OR MODERATELY SEVERE | SEVERE |
|---|---|---|---|
| 1. Fatigue or lethargy | 3 | 6 | 9 |
| 2. Feeling of being "drained" | 3 | 6 | 9 |
| 3. Depression | 3 | 6 | 9 |
| 4. Poor memory | 3 | 6 | 9 |
| 5. Feeling "spacy" or "unreal" | 3 | 6 | 9 |
| 6. Inability to make decisions | 3 | 6 | 9 |
| 7. Numbness, burning or tingling | 3 | 6 | 9 |
| 8. Headache | 3 | 6 | 9 |
| 9. Muscle aches | 3 | 6 | 9 |
| 10. Muscle weakness or paralysis | 3 | 6 | 9 |
| 11. Pain and/or swelling in joints | 3 | 6 | 9 |
| 12. Abdominal pain | 3 | 6 | 9 |

| | | | |
|---|---|---|---|
| 13. Constipation and/or diarrhea | 3 | 6 | 9 |
| 14. Bloating, belching or intestinal gas | 3 | 6 | 9 |
| 15. Vaginal burning, itching or descharge | 3 | 6 | 9 |
| 16. Prostatitis | 3 | 6 | 9 |
| 17. Impotence | 3 | 6 | 9 |
| 18. Loss of sexual desire or feeling | 3 | 6 | 9 |
| 19. Edometriosis of infertility | 3 | 6 | 9 |
| 20 Cramps and/or other menstural irregularities | 3 | 6 | 9 |
| 21. Premanstural tension | 3 | 6 | 9 |
| 22. Attacks of anxiety or crying | 3 | 6 | 9 |
| 23. Cold hands or feet and/or chilliness | 3 | 6 | 9 |
| 24. Shaking or irritable when hungry | 3 | 6 | 9 |

Total Score, Section B______________

SECTION C: OTHER SYMPTOMS

| | MILD | FREQUENT &/OR MODERATELY SEVERE | SEVERE |
|---|---|---|---|
| _1. Drowsiness | 3 | 6 | 9 |
| 2. Irritablility or jitteriness | 3 | 6 | 9 |
| 3. Incoordination | 3 | 6 | 9 |
| 4. Inability to concentrate | 3 | 6 | 9 |
| 5. Frequent mood swings | 3 | 6 | 9 |
| 6. Insomnia | 3 | 6 | 9 |
| 7. Dizziness/loss of balance | 3 | 6 | 9 |
| 8. Pressure above ears...feeling of head swelling | 3 | 6 | 9 |
| 9. Tendency to bruise easily | 3 | 6 | 9 |
| 10. Chronic rashes or itching | 3 | 6 | 9 |
| 11. Numbness, tingling | 3 | 6 | 9 |
| 12. Indigestion of heartburn | 3 | 6 | 9 |
| 13. Food sensitivity or intolerance | 3 | 6 | 9 |
| 14. Mucus in stools | 3 | 6 | 9 |
| 15. Rectal itching | 3 | 6 | 9 |
| 16. Dry mouth or throat | 3 | 6 | 9 |
| 17. Rash or blisters in mouth | 3 | 6 | 9 |
| 18. Bad breath | 3 | 6 | 9 |
| 19. Foot, hair or body odor not relieved by washing | 3 | 6 | 9 |
| 20. Nasal congestion of post nasal drip | 3 | 6 | 9 |
| 21. Nasal itching | 3 | 6 | 9 |
| 22. Sore throat | 3 | 6 | 9 |
| 23. Laryngitis, loss of voice | 3 | 6 | 9 |
| 24. Cough or recurrent bronchitis | 3 | 6 | 9 |
| 25. Pain or tightness in chest | 3 | 6 | 9 |
| 26. Wheezing or shortness of breath | 3 | 6 | 9 |
| 27. Urinary frequency or urgency | 3 | 6 | 9 |
| 28. Burning on urination | 3 | 6 | 9 |
| 29. Spots in front of eyes or erratic vision | 3 | 6 | 9 |
| 30. Burning or tearing of eyes | 3 | 6 | 9 |
| 31. Recurrent infections or fluid in ears | 3 | 6 | 9 |
| 32. Ear pain or deafness | 3 | 6 | 9 |

Total Score, Section C_______________

Total Score, Section A_______________

Total Score, Section B_______________

GRAND TOTAL SCORE_______________

# OBESITY

- Obesity occurs when the body weight is greater than 20% of standard weight for the person's height and frame.
- A triceps skinfold greater than 18.6mm for males and 28.0mm for females is also a sign of obesity.
- More than 20-25% body fat in males and 30% in females is also indicative of obesity.
- It should be noted that it is possible to be of normal weight for height and frame size, but have a higher % of body fat. Also it is possible to be obese by the height and weight charts and be of an excellent % body fat.
- It has been estimated by some researchers that over 30% of the U.S. population is obese.
- Obesity increases risk for coronary heart disease, diabetes mellitus, hypertension, gall bladder disease, intestinal disorders, respiratory disease, thrombophlebitis, back and joint pain, and cancers.

## I. Etiology

1) **Genetics**–A child has a 10% chance of becoming obese if neither parent is obese; 40% chance if 1 parent is obese; and an 80% chance if both parents are obese. Identical twins are found to have larger differences in weight when raised apart. **Greater differences were observed between fraternal as compared to identical twins.**

2) **Fat cell number** increases four fold between birth and age 2 in normal weight and obese children. From age 2 to puberty the number of fat cells gradually increase. After puberty fat cell numbers can increase but they do so more slowly. Obese children generally increase their fat cell numbers faster than normals and by adolescence they will have a greater number of fat cells.

**Fat cell size** is greatest at 6 months of age and afterward cell size gradually decreases, in normal weight children, up to the age of 6 years of age. In obese children they do not experience this gradual decline in fat cell size. In normal weight children after age 6, there is a gradual increase in fat cell size "adiposity rebound." When there is an early rebound in fat cell hyperplasia, it is a strong predictive chance of developing obesity later on, even if there is no hyperplasia at age 1. Fat cell depots around the body have the ability to expand up to 1000x! During weight loss fat cells only decrease in size not number.

> Note–because fat cells, once formed, can not decrease in number, weight loss in the adult obese patient can be very difficult. If their fat cells start to lose fat, they may feel starved, resulting in overeating. Their bodies try to maintain a certain level of fat within each cell.

STUDY–Fomon, Filler, Thomas, Zeigler, Leonard. *Food consumption and growth of normal infants fed milk-based formulas* Acta pediatr. Scand(Suppl) 223:1-36, 1971 ABSTRACT–It was found that infants fed formula diets had an **increase in average weight gain** compared to breast fed infants.

STUDY–Jelliffe & Jelliffe *Fat babies, prevalence, perils, and prevention.* Environmental child health monograph 41: 123-159,1975. ABSTRACT–It was found that infants introduced to solid foods early resulted in greater caloric consumption and an average increased weight gain.

3) **Social discrimination**–Fashion trends, insurance programs, college placements and employment opportunities all discriminate against obese people. The obese person learns self-defeating and self-denigrating responses. Low self esteem depression and overeating for consolation results in a vicious cycle.

4) **Psychological factors**–As mentioned previously, social discrimination can play a role in lowering people's self esteem leading to obesity. In one study, children were asked," If they had a choice between being obese or disabled which would they choose." Most of the children chose to be disabled over being obese.

Emotional issues can certainly play a role in obesity. Previous emotional traumas that haven't been dealt with can be obstacles that can not be overcome through diet and exercise. Many authors have written about this topic including "Bradshaw and the family, Bradshaw."

4) **Hypothyroidism**

a) Axillary basal temp 97.2 and below

b) Delayed Achilles return reflex with Signs & Symptoms–dry skin, FHK, dry hair, low blood pressure, low pulse, elevated cholesterol & triglycerides, cool body temperature, fatigue, constipation, headaches, PMS, menorrhagia etc. (see hypothyroid).

5) **Reduced BMR**–decrease in lean body mass, inactive brown fat

6) **Decreased physical activity**–Certainly this plays a big role in obesity and it has been found that next to a previous history of obesity television watching is the strongest predictor of the development of obesity. The degree of obesity is proportional to the amount of T.V. that is watched. Television watching results in a lack of physical activity, less preparation of nutritious foods, and an actual lowering of the basal metabolic rate.

STUDY–*Physical Activity of Obese and Non-obese Adolescent Girls Appraised Motion Picture Sampling* Am. J. Clin. Nutr.,14:211, 1964 ABSTRACT–Activity of obese and lean girls playing tennis showed, via time-lapse photography, a pronounced increase in inactive frames in the obese girls.

7) **Set-point theory**–Our weight may be controlled by a "thermostat" in the hypothalamus. It is postulated that our hunger and food intake are regulated by our brain which tries to keep our weight around a certain level. It is postulated that as we deplete our fat cells, we become starved, even though our weight may be above ideal. This set point is regulated in part by the activity of brown fat. Since obese children and adults have an increased number of fat cells, they will tend to get hungry if they deplete their fat cells.

8) **Hormone therapy or other medications**–especially birth control pills and cortisone derivatives.

## II. Therapeutic Considerations

1) Only 8% of people on the average weight loss program achieve short term success (i.e. meeting their ideal weight). Less than 1% maintain this weight loss after 1 year.

2) As we get older, our "set-point" goes up in part due to the decreased activity of our brown fat.

3) Obesity is a matter of consuming more than we expend energy-wise, but like our society many people tend to buy (eat) much more than they earn (energy expenditure). Obesity is a sign of our times, overweight on empty calories. Many studies indicate that obese people actually do not eat more than normal weight people and in many cases they eat less!

STUDY–Miller W., et al. *Dietary fat, sugar and fiber predict body fat content.* J Am Diet Assoc, 94:612, 1994. ABSTRACT–23 aged matched lean men, 23 obese men, 17 lean women, and 15 obese women were studied and it was found that there was no difference in energy consumption or total sugar intake. Obese subjects however eat a greater % of their calories from fat and added sugars while their fiber intake was significantly lower.

## III. Treatment

**1) Treat obese parents**–While fat cells should be stable in numbers from age 2 to puberty, it is especially important to be watchful of weight gain. Personally, I have observed that if Mom is obese or hypothyroid, there is a very high correlation of obesity in her female offspring. Since evidence indicates that both genetic and environmental factors are involved in obesity, it is important that parents are treated along with children.

**2) Hypoallergenic diet**-see diet pages 302 & 303 in the Allergies chapter. This diet may be modified over an extended period of time. Elimination of wheat, dairy and simple carbohydrates in most people will have a dramatic effect on weight loss.

**3) Emotional work**–core issues really need to be addressed. If a person is obese because they are trying to protect or insulate themselves from pain they must absolutely address these issues

**4) 70-75% CHO, 15-20% FAT, 10% PRO**–Unsaturated fatty acids tend to activate brown fat. The fat % may be up to 25% if the fats are omega 3 fatty acids. Certain blood types may require higher levels of protein (see Eat Right for Your Blood Type, D'Adamo). Make sure if high carbohydrate intake that simple carbohydrates are eliminated.

**5) Regulate thyroid**–fully evaluate thyroid function

a) Axillary basal temp

b) Be conscious and careful of heart disease, elevated BP and pulse rate, palpitations, insomnia, osteoporosis, jitteriness.

c) Start with 1/2 grain thyroid. Increase by 1/2 grain every 2 weeks. Monitor BP, pulse rate, Achilles tendon return reflex, and symptoms.

d) Tyrosine-1-3gms/day- Substrate for thyroid and epinephrine hormone synthesis. It also activates brown fat.

STUDY–Landsberg & Young, *Diet induced changes in Sympathoadrenal activity: Implications for thermogenesis & obesity* Obesity and Metabolism,1;5(1981). ABSTRACT–Tyrosine was found to stimulate epinephrine synthesis.

e) Zinc picolinate–15mg/day

f) Copper–3mg/day

g) Iodine–50-200mg/day (use with caution at this dose as may start to inhibit thyroid function)

**6) Aerobic exercise**–Make sure the patient is aerobically fit before starting an exercise program. Consider stress ECG. Maintain aerobic heart rate at 50-60% of maximum capacity for at least 20 minutes every day or every other day. The lower percentage results in greater fat catabolism and more weight control benefits. Exercise stimulates brown fat activation, increases lean body mass and encourages appetite control. It takes a minimum of 2 months to have an effect on decreasing body fat.

STUDY–Sharkey *Physiology of fitness: Rx exercise for fitness, weight control and health* Champaign, Ill.,Human kinetics publishers,1979.

**7) Thermogenesis**–Brown fat has been shown to be more metabolically active than yellow fat, the predominate fat in the body. As we grow older brown fat tends to become less active.

STUDY–Shelly, Jung, & Callingham, *Post prandial thermogenesis in obesity*, Clinical Science, 60, 519(1981). ABSTRACT–Women aged 26-67 years who could not lose weight on most diets were found to have relatively inactive fat in part related to underactive adrenal and thyroid glands.

**8) Increase fiber**–The more unrefined the carbohydrate (e.g. whole wheat berries versus whole wheat bread), the greater the time it takes to chew the food and the more time the body has to recognize the sensation of satiety. This also causes a decrease in caloric absorption of food. As part of the treatment protocol can use psyllium seed powder between meals 1 round teaspoon between meals with a large amount of water. This will tend to make the person feel more full between meals. In addition, the fiber will decrease bowel transit time and will tend to eliminate more endotoxins from the lower bowel. The fiber also will have a stabilizing effect on the blood glucose.

9) **Natural sugars**, such as fructose found in fruits, stimulate brown fat thermogenesis better than refined carbohydrate.

**10) Yohimbine**–blocks alpha receptors which seem to be especially concentrated in the areas where men and women put on the most weight. The net effect is to stimulate Beta receptors which increase the metabolic rate of the local tissues.

**11) Green tea (Camellia sinensis), Ephedra sinensis (Ma huang), and Cola nitida (cola nut)** all contain methylxanthines that can increase metabolic rate.

**12) N-acetylated glucosamines (NAGS)**–may benefit obesity by binding onto certain lectins which have insulinomimetic actions on insulin receptors. When these foods, containing lectins, are eaten the insulin-like compounds bind to the insulin receptors stimulating antilipolytic and prolipogenic effects. The net effect is to increase the obesity. These lectins are found in many healthy foods such as fish, unrefined grains, legumes and seeds By NAG binding to these lectins it makes them nonfunctional.

**13) Tryptophan**–increases serotonin levels in the brain and inhibits carbohydrate craving.

**14) Tyrosine**–precursor to norepinephrine and thyroid hormones, both of which increase metabolic activity.

**15) Protein powder**–Depending upon blood type and activity level consider protein powder supplementation. It may inhibit appetite.

**16) Omnibalance®** (with debittered Stevia)-as a sweetener can aid significantly in weight loss.

## Notes

---

| Activity | kcal/min |
|---|---|
| Handball and squash | 10.0 |
| Mountain climbing | 10.0 |
| Skipping rope | 10.0–15.0 |
| Judo and karate | 13.0 |
| Football (while active) | 13.3 |
| Wrestling | 14.4 |
| Skiing: | |
| Moderate to steep | 8.0–12.0 |
| Downhill racing | 16.5 |
| Cross-country: 3–8 mph | 9.0–17.0 |
| Swimming: | |
| Pleasure | 6.0 |
| Crawl: 25–50 yd/min | 6.0–12.5 |
| Butterfly: 50 yd/min | 14.0 |
| Backstroke: 25–50 yd/min | 6.0–12.5 |
| Breaststroke: 25–50 yd/min | 6.0–12.5 |
| Sidestroke: 40 yd/min | 11.0 |
| Dancing: | |
| Modern: moderate—vigorous | 4.2–5.7 |
| Ballroom: waltz—rhumba | 5.7–7.0 |
| Square | 7.7 |
| Walking: | |
| Road—Field (3.5 mph) | 5.6–7.0 |
| Snow: hard—soft (3.5–2.5 mph) | 10.0–20.0 |
| Uphill: 5–10–15% (3.5 mph) | 8.0–11.0–15.0 |
| Downhill: 5–10% (2.5 mph) | 3.6–3.5 |
| 15–20% (2.5 mph) | 3.7–4.3 |
| Hiking: 40-lb pack (3.0 mph) | 6.8 |
| Running: | |
| 12-min mile (5 mph) | 10.0 |
| 8-min mile (7.5 mph) | 15.0 |
| 6-min mile (10 mph) | 20.0 |
| 5-min mile (12 mph) | 25.0 |

| Activity | kcal/min |
|---|---|
| Mopping floors | 4.9 |
| Repaving roads | 5.0 |
| Gardening, weeding | 5.6 |
| Stacking lumber | 5.8 |
| Chain saw | 6.2 |
| Stone, masonry | 6.3 |
| Pick-and-shovel work | 6.7 |
| Farming, haying, plowing with horse | 6.7 |
| Shoveling (miners) | 6.8 |
| Walking downstairs | 7.1 |
| Chopping wood | 7.5 |
| Crosscut saw | 7.5–10.5 |
| Tree felling (axe) | 8.4–12.7 |
| Gardening, digging | 8.6 |
| Walking upstairs | 10.0–18.0 |
| Pool or billiards | 1.8 |
| Canoeing: 2.5 mph–4.0 mph | 3.0–7.0 |
| Volleyball: recreational—competitive | 3.5–8.0 |
| Golf: foursome—twosome | 3.7–5.0 |
| Horseshoes | 3.8 |
| Baseball (except pitcher) | 4.7 |
| Ping pong—table tennis | 4.9–7.0 |
| Calisthenics | 5.0 |
| Rowing: pleasure—vigorous | 5.0–15.0 |
| Cycling: 5–15 mph (10 speed) | 5.0–12.0 |
| Skating: recreation—vigorous | 5.0–15.0 |
| Archery | 5.2 |
| Badminton: recreational—competitive | 5.2–10.0 |
| Basketball: half—full court (more for fast break) | 6.0–9.0 |
| Bowling (while active) | 7.0 |
| Tennis: recreational—competitive | 7.0–11.0 |
| Water skiing | 8.0 |
| Soccer | 9.0 |
| Snowshoeing (2.5 mph) | 9.0 |

| Activity | kcal/min |
|---|---|
| Sleeping | 1.2 |
| Resting in bed | 1.3 |
| Sitting, normally | 1.3 |
| Sitting, reading | 1.3 |
| Lying, quietly | 1.3 |
| Sitting, eating | 1.5 |
| Sitting, playing cards | 1.5 |
| Standing, normally | 1.5 |
| Classwork, lecture (listen to) | 1.7 |
| Conversing | 1.8 |
| Personal toilet | 2.0 |
| Sitting, writing | 2.6 |
| Standing, light activity | 2.6 |
| Washing and dressing | 2.6 |
| Washing and shaving | 2.6 |
| Driving a car | 2.8 |
| Washing clothes | 3.1 |
| Walking indoors | 3.1 |
| Shining shoes | 3.2 |
| Making bed | 3.4 |
| Dressing | 3.4 |
| Showering | 3.4 |
| Driving motorcycle | 3.4 |
| Metal working | 3.5 |
| House painting | 3.5 |
| Cleaning windows | 3.7 |
| Carpentry | 3.8 |
| Farming chores | 3.8 |
| Sweeping floors | 3.9 |
| Plastering walls | 4.1 |
| Truck and automobile repair | 4.2 |
| Ironing clothes | 4.2 |
| Farming, planting, hoeing, raking | 4.7 |
| Mixing cement | 4.7 |

Listed on this page are activities and the energy required to perform each activity. Each activity will thus burn the number of Calories listed. Obviously there are different levels you can perform each activity therefore different people will expend different levels of energy performing each task. Prolonged activities can burn off a tremendous amount of energy. E.g., bicycle touring with packs can burn up to 7,000 to 10,000 Calories over the course of a day. Similar activities such as Ironman events can also burn enormous amounts of energy.

# HYPOTHYROIDISM & FATIGUE

- Hypothyroidism is a relatively common condition that may arise primarily (defect in the thyroid gland) or secondarily (defect in pituitary or hypothalamus). Primary hypothyroidism is much more common. Estimates based on blood levels of thyroid hormone are that 1-4% of the U.S. population has moderate to severe hypothyroidism and that 10% has mild hypothyroidism. Some clinicians estimate that by using multiple criteria, including history, signs and symptoms, and basal body temperatures, the incidence may rise to between 15-40% of the population!
- Blood tests are notoriously insensitive to mild or borderline cases of hypothyroidism. In many cases of hypothyroidism, blood levels may be perfectly normal but tissue levels (intracellular levels) may be low, or there may be a problem with T4 being converted into T3.
- Hypothyroidism appears to run in families. It is significantly more common in females and can sometimes be triggered by stressful events such as pregnancy, or emotional or physical trauma. When parents or grandparents have been diagnosed with hypothyroidism it appears to occur in female offspring at a very high rate, usually occurring sometime in adulthood.

## I. Etiology

Generally, the etiology of primary hypothyroidism is unknown but may be related to consumption of goitrogens (substances in foods which inhibit the normal function of the thyroid), or from lack of iodine. Most likely there is some genetic component to this condition because of its high prevalence. Some scientists, like Broda Barnes, M.D., believe that people who may not have survived certain infectious diseases in the past, due to low thyroid and a diminished immune function, are now surviving because of antibiotics and other heroic measures. Thus, he believes that we are breeding a whole host of hypothyroid individuals. Other scientists have argued that environmental conditions have lead to a diminished functioning of the thyroid gland. Alexander Schauss, Ph.D. sites a phenomenon that occurred in Nevada in the 1960's. He states in the Journal of Biosocial Publications, that certain districts in Nevada that were spending in the top ten percentile for education compared to the rest of the country, had students scoring in the lowest percentiles on national test evaluations (up until 1978-80). It was uncovered that 1963 was the last year for above ground testing for nuclear bombs. This meant that children in those areas in Nevada where above ground testing was done were consistently exposed to nuclear radiation prior to 1963. It is well known that nuclear fallout has a most pronounced effect on the thyroid gland. When the thyroid gland becomes diminished in its function, intelligence goes down. Thus when above ground testing ceased, the children were no longer exposed to nuclear fallout and their thyroids began to work normally. The end result was that their national test scores went up dramatically in a very short time.

Another researcher, a dentist in Florida, Roy Kupsinel, DDS. believes that mercury amalgams are responsible for the diminished thyroid effect and that prolonged exposure to mercury vapor from amalgams can have a dramatic effect on the thyroid gland. He believes that removal of mercury amalgams can often times allow a weakened thyroid gland to return to normal function.

In recent years another physician, Dr. Denis Wilson, has put forth the concept that in many cases it is not the thyroid gland that is malfunctioning, but rather it is the peripheral tissues which are having problems converting the less active T4 into T3. He states that this is why people often have perfectly normal blood tests when it is obvious that there is a problem with the level of thyroid hormone in the tissues. He reasons that many different types of stress can cause the peripheral tissues to shut down their conversion of T4 into T3. For example, when people go on starvation diets, their metabolism slows way down in an effort to conserve energy. Their temperature drops down and when they resume eating, weight usually comes back with a vengeance because their basal metabolism slows down in an effort to conserve.

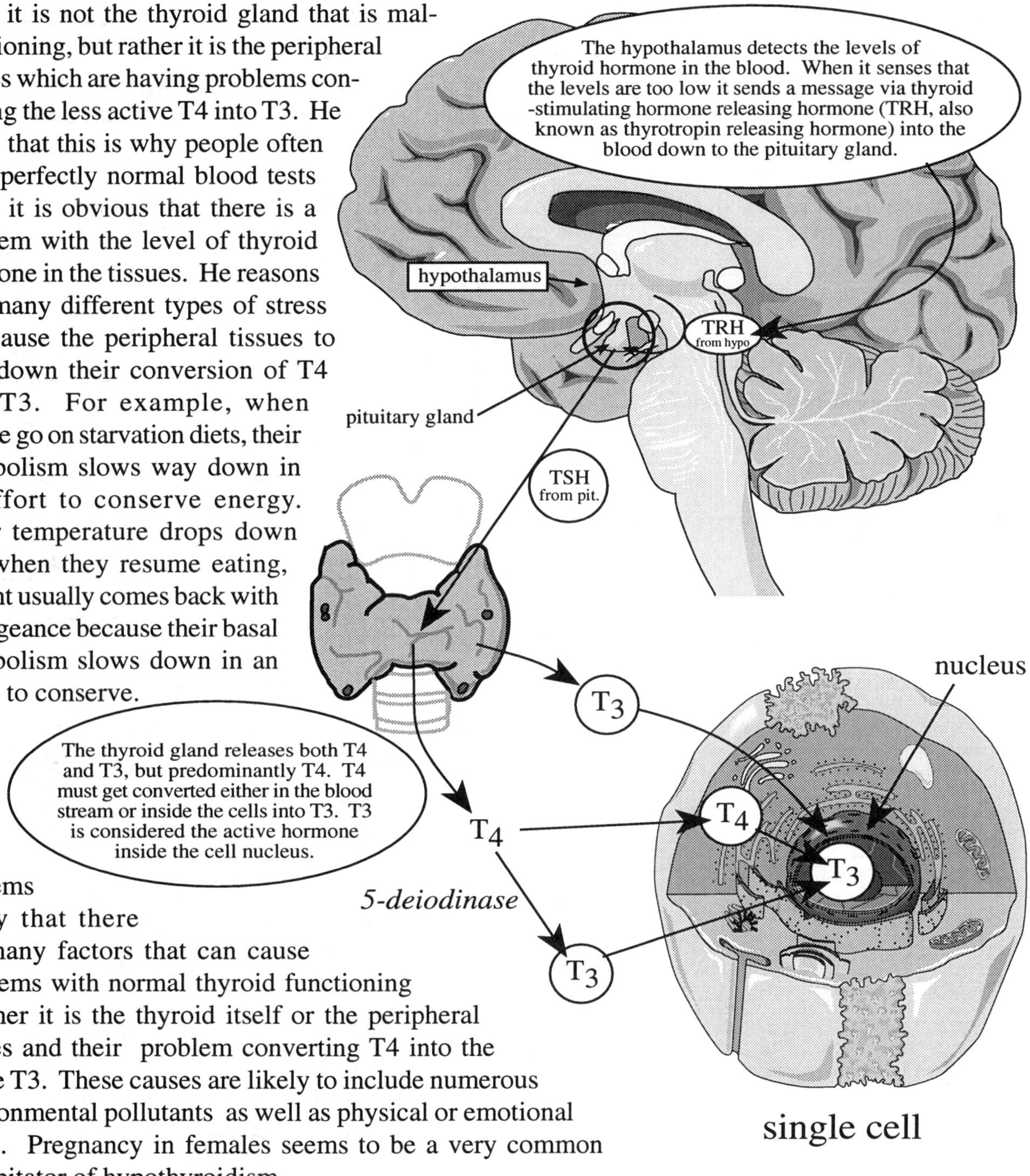

The hypothalamus detects the levels of thyroid hormone in the blood. When it senses that the levels are too low it sends a message via thyroid -stimulating hormone releasing hormone (TRH, also known as thyrotropin releasing hormone) into the blood down to the pituitary gland.
hypothalamus
TRH from hypo
pituitary gland
TSH from pit.
nucleus
$T_3$
The thyroid gland releases both T4 and T3, but predominantly T4. T4 must get converted either in the blood stream or inside the cells into T3. T3 is considered the active hormone inside the cell nucleus.
$T_4$
$T_4$
$T_3$
*5-deiodinase*
$T_3$
single cell


It seems likely that there are many factors that can cause problems with normal thyroid functioning whether it is the thyroid itself or the peripheral tissues and their problem converting T4 into the active T3. These causes are likely to include numerous environmental pollutants as well as physical or emotional stress. Pregnancy in females seems to be a very common precipitator of hypothyroidism.

Worldwide there are about one billion people who are possibly low in iodine or are eating enough goitrogens (substances in foods that either block the absorption of iodine or in some way interfere with its normal functioning) to become deficient in iodine due to antagonistic actions to that of iodine. There is also evidence that in certain parts of the world local water supplies may contain goitrogenic substances from rocks or from the organism E. coli. When this phenomenon happens during pregnancy it leads to cretinism, a syndrome characterized by mental and physical retardation. In the U.S. there is an area in the midwest that is known as the goiter belt because of the high incidence of goiters in these people. In fact in Michigan, which is part of the goiter belt, in the mid 30's over 40% of people living there developed goiters (swelling of the thyroid gland in the neck). The following are foods that contain substantial amounts of goitrogens: sweet potato, cabbage, cauliflower, turnips, rutabagas, rapeseeds, peanuts, cassava, pine nuts, mustard, millet and soybeans (see table on page 410). These goitrogenic substances are inactivated by cooking or soaking in some cases.

## II. Signs and Symptoms

Below is a list of both subjective symptoms and objective physical findings of hypothyroidism:

| | | | |
|---|---|---|---|
| Fatigue | 5 | Delayed achilles return reflex | 10 |
| Excessive sleeping (waking up still tired) | 3 | Dry skin | 3 |
| Weight gain-especially where not eating much still causes weight gain | 5 | Follicular hyperkeratosis (bumps on back of arms or front of thighs) | 2 |
| Headaches (migraines or low grade) | 2 | Coarse, very fine, thinning or loss of hair | 2 |
| Ringing in ears | 1 | Edema (swelling) in face or legs | 3 |
| Dizziness | 1 | Low body temperature | 5 |
| Joint pain, stiffness or muscle stiffness | 2 | Thick tongue | 2 |
| Depression | 2 | Cold hands and feet | 3 |
| Decreased libido (lack of sex drive) | 2 | Pallor of skin, lips or hands | 2 |
| Heart disease (murmurs, arrhythmias etc.) | 1 | High or low blood pressure | 1 |
| Cold or heat intolerance (dislike cold) | 3 | Slow heart rate (below 60 beats/min) | 3 |
| Poor memory (forgetfulness) | 2 | Brittle nails/slow growing or ridging | 2 |
| Slowness of mind; can't concentrate | 2 | **FEMALE SIGNS & SYMPTOMS** | |
| Constipation (hard stools/skipping days without bowel movements) | 3 | Long cycles (greater than 35 days apart) or shortened cycles (less than 24 days) | 2 |
| Irritability or emotional outbursts | 1 | Lack of periods or skipping periods | 3 |
| Decreased sweating/difficulty sweating | 2 | Infertiility | 2 |
| Difficulty breathing at times | 1 | Menorrhagia (heavy or long menses) | 4 |
| Hoarse voice | 1 | Chronic miscarriages or premature births | 2 |
| Loss of appetite | 1 | Pre-eclampsia (toxemia of pregnancy) | 3 |
| Changes in vision, blurriness, difficulty focusing | 2 | PMS (moody, irritable, swollen breasts, fluid retention pre-period, headaches, depression) | 4 |
| Allergies or frequent colds, flu, infect. | 3 | Painful periods (cramping) | 2 |
| | | **Score for males add both columns** | |
| | | **Score for females add both columns** | |

### How to rate the scores?

Males with a score above 40 very likely hypothyroid. Non mensturating females with a score above 50 very likely hypothyroid. Menstruating females with a score above 55 are very likely hypothyroid.

Pertaining to the above score for males, if basal temperatures average below 97.0 and total T4 levels are below 6.0ng/dl then can score 30 and have a very likely probability of hypothyroidism. Likewise for females, if they have temperatures averaging below 96.8 with T4 levels below 5.5ng/dl their score can be 10-15points lower and I would strongly consider hypothyroidism.

As with most conditions, it is necessary to use clinical judgement with signs and symptoms. Many of the conditions that are listed on the previous table can easily be ascribed to other conditions not related to the thyroid gland, but unfortunately the thyroid gland is often left out the diagnostic picture once blood tests, especially the TSH come back in the normal range. This is very unfortunate for many people including women who have hysterectomies because of menorrhagia with which no cause can be found. Hysterectomies are probably the most often performed unnecessary surgeries. Every woman who has even a slight chance of having a low thyroid and who has undiagnosed menorrhagia should have at least a trial with thyroid hormone. As pointed out in the chart, unexplained weight gain can often be traced to the thyroid gland or at least peripheral conversion problems.

## III. Diagnosis

To make an accurate diagnosis of hypothyroidism it is necessary to do a complete physical along with blood tests. There are many physicians who relay too heavily on just blood tests. Years ago gross basal metabolism tests were performed where patients came in early in the morning and they had their total oxygen consumption per minute measured. This crass technique often yielded erroneous results and often it was the physicians clinical skills which were the most important for evaluating the thyroid function. When blood tests came along, measuring protein bound iodine along with T4 and T3 later, they too gave erroneous results and physicians tended to rely more on them rather than the clinical picture. Today physicians measure TSH, T4 and free T3 and sometimes reverse T3 and T7 to give the so called "definitive diagnosis." Unfortunately again, physicians often ignore the clinical picture of the patient and tend to rely exclusively on these lab tests. This is certainly an unfortunate turn of events because there are many people who come out normal on these tests yet are still low in thyroid function, at least in terms of their symptomatology.

To make an accurate diagnosis of hypothyroidism it is vital to do a complete physical, and perform a chemistry which includes TSH, T4 and free T3, cholesterol, blood glucose, and triglyceride level. In addition, a thorough family history should also be taken as thyroid problems commonly run in families, especially among the female side. If a parent and/or sibling has been diagnosed with hypothyroidism, and the patient scores high on the table of symptoms on the previous page, they most likely have a deficiency of thyroid hormone, at least intracellularly. If I see a TSH above 4.0 (usually the normal lab values are approximately 0.5-5.5) and a T4 below 6.0 (approx. normal range is 4.5-12.5) and they have many of the symptoms of hypothyroidism along with low basal body temperatures, I will make the diagnosis of hypothyroidism. I am also looking at blood sugar, cholesterol and triglyceride levels which are often elevated in hypothyroidism.

In addition, I weight very strongly the Achilles return reflex (Physical and Clinical Diagnosis, Barbara Bates but only pictured in a few editions). Most physicians do not perform this simple test, but I believe it is crucial to the diagnosis of low thyroid function. **A delayed Achilles return reflex is considered a classic finding in hypothyroidism.** If the patient does not have a spinal lesion and they have delayed Achilles return reflexes bilaterally, then there is a very good chance that they have low thyroid function assuming they also have the symptom picture. If they have brisk Achilles return reflexes, then even if they have symptoms of low thyroid function I generally look for other causes for their symptoms. You can purchase a special device that measures the Achilles return speed (Achilliometer), but with practice you can probably get a more accurate reading doing the reflex yourself manually.

In addition to the above findings, another valuable piece of information for evaluation of low thyroid function is the basal body temperature. The basal metabolism is largely regulated by the thyroid gland and if a person's internal body temperature is very low this is strong diagnostic information regarding the function of the thyroid gland.

## How to take basal body temperatures?

Basal body temperatures (BBT) are temperatures that reflect what your basal metabolism is. They can give you valuable information concerning the function of your thyroid gland. Your basal metabolism is how much energy your body expends while it is totally at rest. There are vast differences between peoples basal metabolism. That is why two people, eating the same diet and doing the same physical activity, can have opposite changes in body weight where one gains and the other loses weight.

To accurately take your BBT, you must use a glass ( mercury filled) thermometer. Digital, tape, or ear thermometers although convenient, are too inconsistent and do not give accurate BBT measurements. Special BBT thermometers are available that show degree slash marks further apart, making small changes in temperature easier to read. However, a regular glass fever thermometer will work. To take your BBT shake your thermometer down below 96.0 degrees F the night before (fever thermometers usually only go down to 96.0). Have your thermometer handy by the side of the bed for when you awaken. Upon awakening, do not move around except to reach over and get your thermometer. Do not get up, eat anything or do anything until you take your temperature. Place the mercury bulb part of the thermometer into the deepest part of your armpit and hold it here for at least 5-10 minutes (only experience will tell you if your temperature will go up any more beyond 5 minutes). You do not have to read the thermometer immediately as the temperature will stay the same until you shake the thermometer down. Record the temperature to 1/10 of a degree. In menstruating women, the temperature will vary according to where you are in your cycle. True basal temperatures are from the first day of menses to ovulation. After ovulation both estrogen and progesterone hormones secreted in the body, cause the temperature to rise. Certain things can artificially elevate your temperature giving you inaccurate readings such as having an electric blanket or water bed heated to high level, a fever, some type of inflammation such as from a toothache, ear infection or boil on the skin, certain types of cancer, medication such as progesterone or estrogen hormones, birth control pills, steroid hormones such as cortisone, prednisone or DHEA. You should record your temperatures for at least 7-14 days and then average them out to 1/10 of a degree. It is best to chart your temperatures on a basal temperature chart (p.541). Looking at a chart of temperatures makes low or elevated temperature averages more decernable.

Basal body temperatures should be used as one piece of information concerning your thyroid function and clinical judgment is always necessary to make your final diagnosis. Just as blood work should used as a guide and not used as the final say in diagnosis.

In your differential diagnosis hypoadrenal function has a large overlap in symptoms with hypothyroidism. In hypoadrenalism usually people tend to be thin, fatigued off and on, Achilles return reflex tends to be normal and they tend to have orthostatic hypotension. In hypothyroidism cholesterol, triglycerides and glucose tend to be elevated. Exercise makes the hypothyroid person worse where in hypoadrenalism it improves the person's stress response.

What are considered low basal body temperatures?

In Hypothyroid, the Unsuspected Illness Broda Barnes, M.D. states that normal basal temperatures are between 97.8 & 98.2 degrees Fahrenheit. This range, from my clinical experience as well as others who use this technique, appears to be quite high. In fact, if we used this range for females to make the diagnosis of hypothyroidism, we would probably have 80-90% of the population diagnosed with low thyroid. I use 97.2 as my cutoff point with room for flexibility, depending upon the clinical picture. Certainly, other things can cause low basal body temperatures, such as low calorie diets, anemias, low adrenal function and low levels of lean body mass.

As previously mentioned, a Dr. Wilson, who wrote the book, *Wilson's Syndrome, 1991 (1(800)621-7006* believes that taking temperatures during the day can give information concerning how well the body is converting T4 into T3. During a personal conversation with him he has stated that the best times to take body temperatures are 12 noon, 3pm and 6pm (before eating). He believes that the average of these temperatures should be close to 98.6 degrees F. From my personal experience evaluating these temperatures in hundreds patients, I believe that this temperature average is probably too high and that if we used this as a standard, we would get a very large percent of people being low in intracellular thyroid hormone. He also recommends that you need to use a glass mercury thermometer, but, unlike the basal temperatures, it should be used under the tongue.

Other diagnostic tests can include studies for autoimmune disease such as Hashimotos thyroiditis or Graves Disease. Auto-antibodies can sometimes be found to the thyroid gland. I have seen in animals reactions to vaccinations where they develop a hypothyroid condition after a rabies vaccination. Consider the possibility of a similar reaction in people.

## IV. Treatment

1) **Armour thyroid hormone–**start with small amount 30mg (1/2 grain or less) taken first thing in morning at same time each day away from any food. It is best not to have any food with the glandular thyroid so that it can get maximally absorbed. Food could possibly bind up or interfere with thyroid hormone absorption. I find that if you start someone out with a small amount of thyroid, they will be much less likely to have any adverse reactions. Also if they slowly increase their thyroid intake, the body can adapt, and there will be less chance for the hypothalamus to think there is enough thyroid hormone in the blood. As a result, it will not decrease its production of TSHRF, and there will be an added effect to the body's own endogenous production of thyroid hormones. I always monitor patient's signs and symptoms as well as blood pressure, heart rate, Achilles return reflex and their basal body temperatures during their treatment. I gradually increase the dose of the thyroid by 1/2 grain every 2 weeks until I start to see symptom changes. If there are any signs or symptoms of too much thyroid then I stop or cut back on the dose. I like to see basal body temperatures go up, but I do not always see this happen. Broda Barnes states that the temperatures always will go up. From my experience with thousands of patients I have not found this to be true, at least not up to the desired level (many other practitioners have also had the same experience). Usually patients will get up to between 1-3 grains before they

start to experience positive benefits. I usually am cautious about going higher than this dose although I have had people up to 6 grains per day and many physicians have had patients up to 10-12 grains per day. As far as adverse effects I tell my patients to watch for symptoms that they might have if they drank too much coffee. Watch for palpitations, feeling very warm, problems sleeping, fast heart beat, feeling jittery, tense or wired and having an increase in their BP. It is also wise to check bone density before undergoing long-term treatment to establish any possible connection with osteoporosis and excessive thyroid hormone supplementation.

It is possible to have reactions with other hormones such as adrenal hormones. It is a good idea to evaluate both low adrenal and thyroid functions as they both have similar symptoms. Sometimes the thyroid dose can be lowered if the adrenals are working better.

**NOTE**–The use of the glandular form of thyroid is a controversial point. Most conventional physicians seem to share a very common belief. This belief is clearly stated in the Merck Manual under the treatment of hypothyroidism. It states, "glandular thyroid is from thyroids obtained from pig carcasses. It is very variable and unpredictable from batch to batch." I have heard this statement repeated many times. First off USP glandular thyroid is assayed to meet certain standards, so the dose can not be so varied from batch to batch. Even if that were true it does not make a difference if you are treating the patient and the patient's symptoms. Treating just blood tests until they come into the normal range does not mean that the thyroid hormones are getting into the cells. It is always best to see how the patient is responding to the treatment. Monitoring blood tests can be helpful if a patient has too much thyroid in their blood. Certainly they should be monitored carefully if they have too much and the dose lowered if they are elevated. However, many times I have seen thyroid blood tests make no sense, e.g., after increasing a dose of thyroid hormone and not seeing any changes in either TSH or T4. Certain physicians believe that when using glandular USP thyroid, i.e., Armour thyroid, blood tests do not accurately show what is really going on with thyroid hormone levels intracellularly. It has been my personal experience that many people taking synthetic thyroid hormones, such as thyroxine, often start to experience side effects before they start to derive any benefit from the hormone. I have seen many patients put on thyroxine (Synthroid®) and experience alarming side effects before they can get up to a dose that fully benefits them. Their physician usually lowers the dose back down to a level that does not fully treat their low thyroid function. The patient may even take this lower dose for an extended period of time and deteriorate because of hypothyroidism! The physician may then check blood levels of T4 and TSH, which might come back in the so called normal range, and decide everything is fine, leaving the patient at a sub-therapeutic level. Obviously if they were low to begin with and their symptoms were caused by low thyroid hormones, they should have at least experienced some sort of benefit upon taking the thyroid. Let us treat people, not blood tests!

It should be noted that there are some people who may respond well to the synthetic T4 hormone. Again clinical judgment should prevail. If someone has been taking the T4 and they have responded well you may decide to leave them on it. I would strongly consider switching if however there is little or no response. Other hormones can also be used in treatment such as Euthroid® (combination of T4 & T3) or "Cytomel©(T3). T3 is much more potent than T4 (4x more) and its half life is only 21/2 days compared to 71/2 days for T4. Uncommonly people have been known to be sensitive to the pork proteins found in the USP thyroid. In such cases the synthetic thyroid would be more indicated.

The following is a list of thyroid derivatives and their approximate equivalent doses:

| | |
|---|---|
| Armour or other USP thyroid– | 1 grain |
| L-thyroxine (T4)– | 0.1 mg or 100mcg |
| Euthroid® (T3 & T4)– | 1.0 |
| Triiodothyronine or liothyronine (T3)– (also known as Cytomel®) | 25mcg |

Many physicians who have patients on thyroid medication tell them they need to be on the thyroid hormone for life. As with any therapy this should certainly be monitored and the least dose that is effective should be used. It is possible to come off thyroid hormone, but care must be taken to come off very slowly and gradually (over a period of months). Monitor symptoms as always. The more slowly one comes off the easier the body will have a chance to adapt to the new thyroid levels and start making its own to compensate.

2) **Wilson's Syndrome treatment**–It is probably best to study Dr. Manual on Wilson Syndrome. Basically the treatment plan requires taking daytime temperatures and seeing how low they average. I use 98.2 or below as being low, again supported by signs and symptoms. Treatment best uses a timed or sustained release of T3 (this can be made up in compounding pharmacy such as (Lloyd Center Pharmacy, Port. OR., Apothecure or College Pharmacy). Dr. Wilson proposes that doses of T3 should be taken exactly 12 hours apart the same time each day. Start with 7.5mcg bid and every 2 days go up by 7.5mcg. Daytime temperatures must be taken to determine the therapeutic effect of the treatment. Temperatures should reach at least up to 98.6. If they do not then the dose should be continuously increased every two days until the temperatures have risen. Once the temperatures have risen to the desired level, the dose should be maintained for a period of 5 days and then lowered by the same increments that the dose went up except that the drop should be every 3 days on the way down. Ideally the temperature should continuously stay up. If it does not then another cycle of T3 is indicated. The goal is to keep the temperature at the ideal level 98.6. It has been my experience with 20-30 patients using this protocol that results are mixed. Temperatures often do not stay up. I believe that certainly there is something worth investigating here, but I would contact Dr. Wilson's staff to get hold of his reference manual or talk to him in person.

3) **Glandular non-USP thyroid products**–(I have used several different thyroid glandular preparations such as thyrotropin, Standard Process; Spectra 303T, NF, BMR formula, Tyler, Thyroforte, PHP). There are a number of products out there that have thyroid tissue but are not supposed to have actual thyroid hormone in them. In the past the FDA has confiscated a number of these over the counter health food preparations of glandular thyroid because they had been assayed and were found to possess actual thyroid hormones. The FDA has since tightened up what could be sold in health food stores (over the counter) but most likely many of them have minor levels of thyroid hormone still. These products would be called protomorphogens, meaning that they are the whole gland

in a more crude state and there may be a number of compounds that might stimulate the thyroid to possibly produce more thyroid hormone. I have used them in the past with considerable success.

4) **Tyrosine**–500mg 3x/day–This is the precursor amino acid for thyroid hormones.

5) **Iodine**–400-800mcg/day-If low certainly should be used to treat goiters or hypothyroidism (see p.142 for list of foods with iodine). SSKI (Scientific Bot) can be helpful 2 drops 2x per day (1 drop = 38mg iodine).

6) **Zinc**–20mg 2x/day

7) **Copper**–2 mg 2x/day

8) **Mercury (Hg) amalgam removal–**Dr. Roy Kupsinel believes that heavy metal toxicity can effect the thyroid gland, particularly Hg . He has seen many people who have had their Hg amalgams removed and their thyroid function return to normal and also their BBT go up. Removal of Hg amalgams is a complicated process and should not be done randomly without someone who is skilled in their removal (they should be set up to have good air filtration, suction and to know special techniques for amalgam removal. Grinding out the amalgams may cause much more harm than good (see chapter on Hg toxicity p. 470).

9) **Hydrotherapy, Constitutional–**(See Drs. Wade Boyle & Andre Saine; Lectures in Naturopathic Hydrotherapy) Often times doing a series of "Constitutional Hydrotherapies" can stimulate the thyroid gland to start being more active and BBT will rise (Contact the National College of Naturopathic Medicine (503)499-4343 or its teaching clinic (503)255-7355.

Note–There have been several adverse effects attributed to excessive doses of thyroid hormone. Mostly they have involved the synthetic derivatives of thyroid (T4). Bp can go up (often it goes down, especially with Armour thyroid). Osteoporosis has also been reported but the studies to support this finding are questionable. If you are not sure about your diagnosis and thyroid hormone treatment, doing bone densiometry is critical to monitoring possible deleterious long term consequences.

## Foods containing Goitrogens

cabbage family (cooking or soaking of these foods usually inactivates the goitrogenic substances)

| | | | | |
|---|---|---|---|---|
| almonds | cassava | kale | peaches | soybeans |
| broccoli | cauliflower | kohlrabi | pine nuts | sweet potato |
| brussel sprouts | collards | millet | rapeseeds | turnips |
| cabbage | horseradish | mustard greens | rutabagas | white mustard |

The following foods contain *arachidoside* that acts similarly to goitrogens

ground nuts & peanuts

Other *"goitrogen like"* substance-paraaminobensoic acid (PABA)

A diet high in fat or calcium can have a goitrogenic effect on the body also. There may be some unidentified substance found in water, indigenous to certain areas in the world, that may contain goitrogenic substances

# ECZEMA (Atopic Dermatitis)

- Eczema is a chronic inflammatory skin condition.
- Characterized by dry, hyperkeratotic skin with lesions that include excoriations, papules, scaling with small vesicles formed within the epidermis, it also may include lichenification–hyperpigmented plaques of thickened skin with accentuated furrows.
- Classically, the lesions occur in the antecubital and popliteal flexures.
- Usually there is a personal or family history of atopy (family history in 2/3rds of patients).
- Eczema is a very common condition which occurs in 2.4% of the population.

## I. Etiology

*"The cause is unknown"* - MERCK MANUAL

1) Immediate sensitivity allergy–Elevated serum IgE is found in 80% of patients and all sufferers have positive skin and RAST tests. Allergic rhinitis and/or asthma are commonly developed. Most patients improve with elimination diets.

   *"Frequently, numerous inhalants and foods produce wheal and flare reactions on scratch or intradermal tests, but these reactions are usually nonspecific. Recent studies suggest that certain foods induce erythema and itching in young individuals. Patients with atopic dermatitis usually have high serum levels of reaginic (IgE) antibodies and peripheral eosinophilia, but the etiologic significance of these findings is unknown."* Merck Manual

2) White blood cells from eczematous patients have decreased levels of cAMP due to the increased activity of cAMP phosphodiesterase. This lack of intracellular cAMP results in increased histamine release and decreased bacteriocidal activity.
3) Decreased levels of prostaglandins secondary to delta 6 desaturase.

## II. Signs and Symptoms

Atopic dermatitis may begin in the first few months of life with red, weepy crusted lesions of the face, scalp, and extremities. Itching is a constant feature. In older children or adults, it may take a more localized chronic form typically in antecubital and popliteal fossae. Other common lesional areas are the scalp, around the ears, and on the hands between the fingers. The skin often is dry, hyperkeratotic with decreased water holding capacity and a marked tendency to lichenification in response to itching or rubbing. Other aspects are Denie's lines and dermatographism, which are often a sign of hypersensitivity.

## III. Diagnosis

Diagnosis is made entirely on clinical findings and is based on the distribution of lesions, the duration, and, often, a family history of atopic allergy. It must be differentiated from seborrheic dermatitis in infancy or from primary irritant dermatitis at any age.

# IV. Therapeutic Considerations

1) Compensate underlying metabolic abnormalities:

a) Try to increase cAMP production and inhibit the action of phosphodiesterase, which reduces intracellular cAMP.

**Eczema - Figure 1**

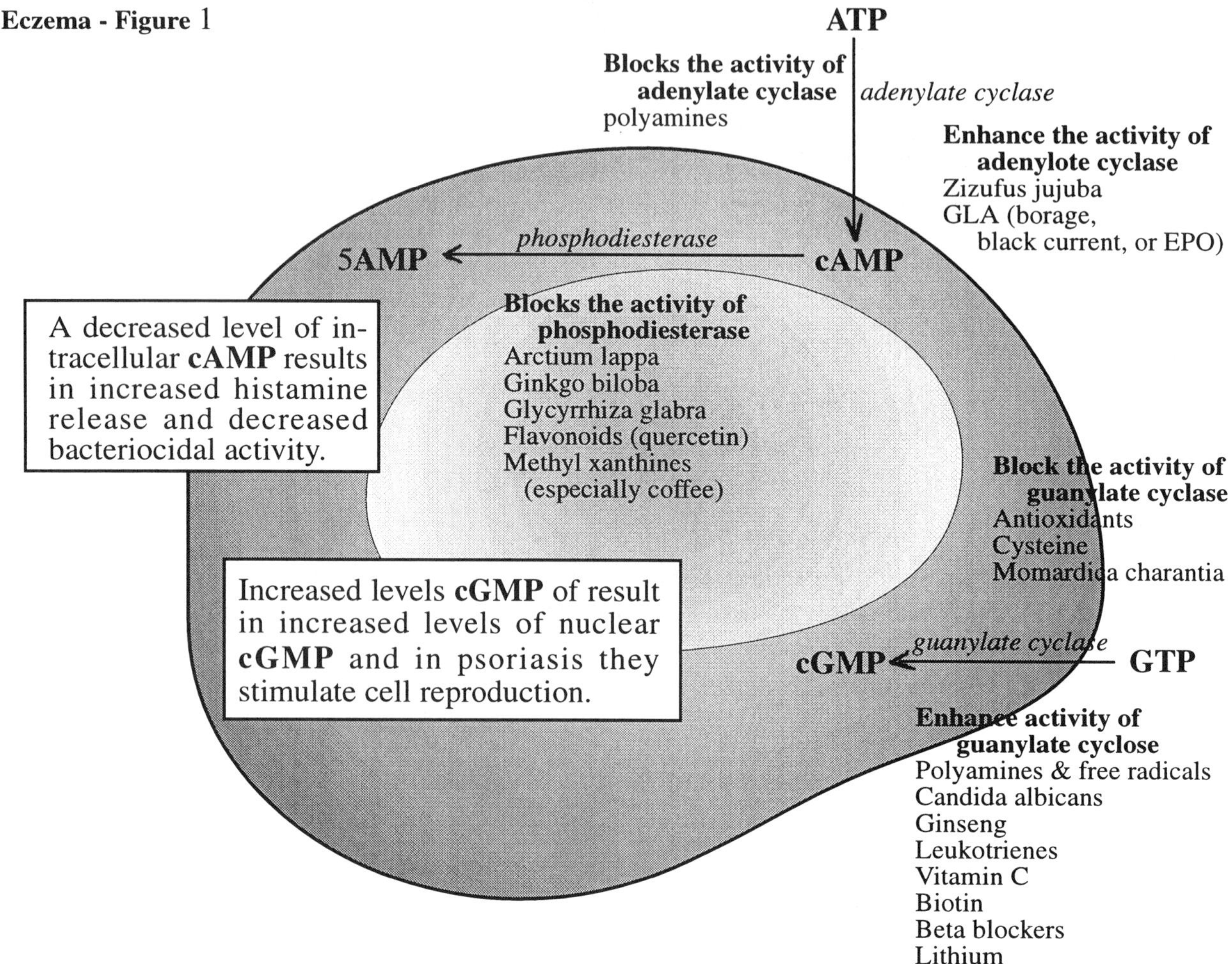


b) Stimulate production of PGE1 series and decrease the production of PGE2 series which leads to the production of inflammatory leukotrienes (LTB4). Remember, humans generally lack the enzyme to form arachidonic acid from DHGLA ($\Delta 5$ desaturase), therefore the membrane phospholipid pools of arachidonic acid are mainly from the diet.

**Note**–EPA competes for arachidonic acid binding sites which results in a net decrease in production of pro-inflammatory 4 series leukotrienes.

STUDY–Clark, William et al. *Omega 3 fatty acid dietary supplementation in SLE.* Kidney International, Vol. 36;653-60, 1989. ABSTRACT–Omega 3 fatty acid supplementation of daily doses of 6gms and 18gms. This supplementation resulted in a 16-20% reduction in platelet arachidonic acid incorporation. Neutrophil leukotriene B4 release was reduced 78-42% by the low and high doses respectively.

The production of PGE1 and PGE3 are beneficial for eczema. They are derived from omega 6 and omega 3 oils respectively. The production of PGE2 in humans is almost entirely from arachidonic acid which is derived from animal flesh. Arachidonic acid not only gives rise to PGE2 but also leukotrienes(LTB4), thromboxane A2, and PGF2α all of which promote inflammation, swelling and pain. Remember that in humans the enzyme to synthesize arachidonic acid from DHGLA (Δ5 desaturase) is largely lacking, Membrane phospholipid pools of arachidonic acid are mainly from high fat animal products(see pages 53-54 under "fats" for a more detailed diagram).

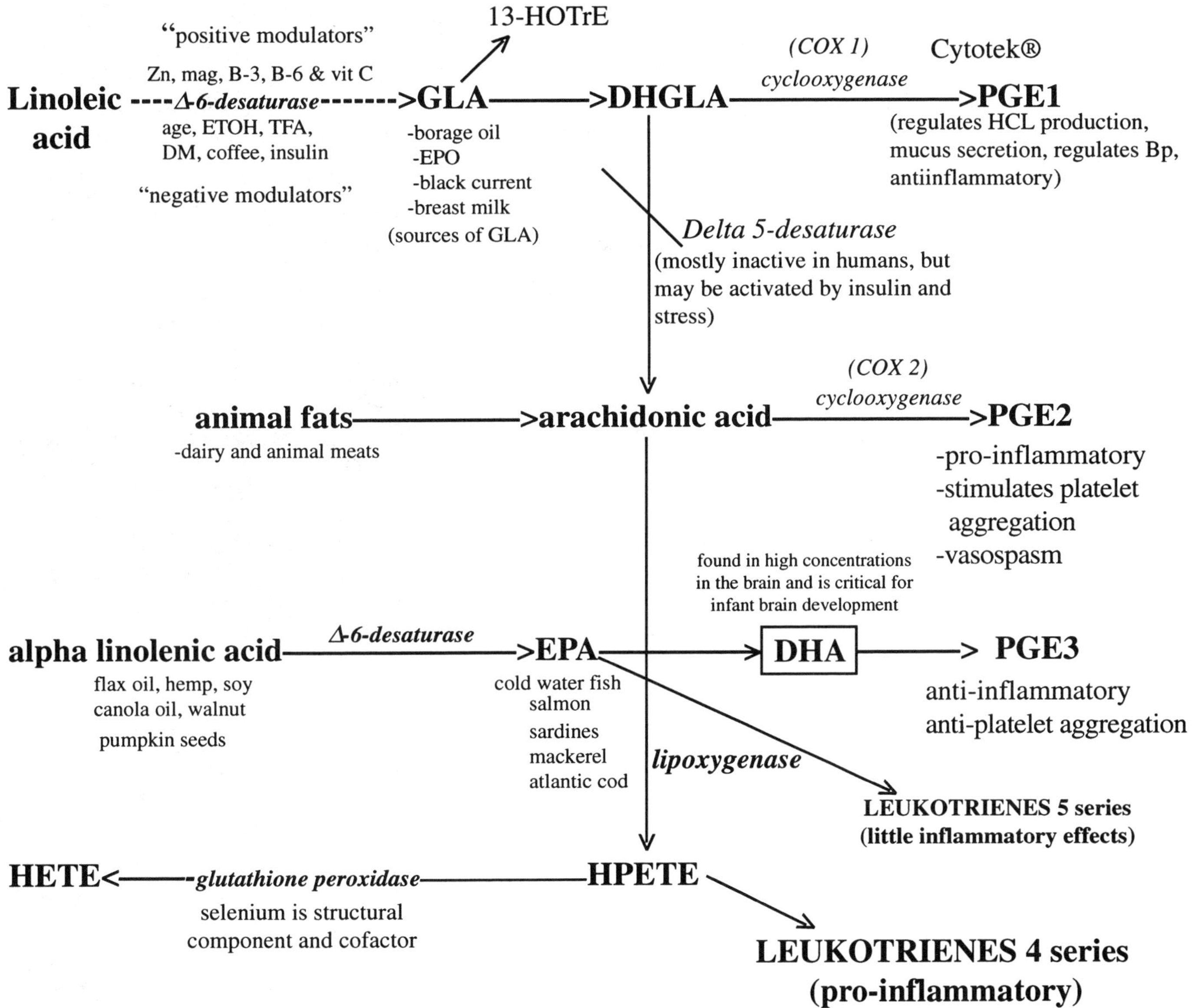


**Note-** EPA completes with arachidonic acid for lipoxygenase binding sites which results in a net decrease in production of pro-inflammatory 4 series leukotrienes. DHGLA competes with arachidonic acid for cyclooxygenase which results in a decreased production of inflammatory PGE2.

**STUDY**- Clark, William et al. *Omega 3 fatty acid dietary supplementation in SLE* Kidney International, Vol 36;653-60,1989. ABSTRACT- Omega 3 fatty acid supplementation of daily doses of 6gms and 18gms. This supplementation resulted in a 16-20% reduction in platelet arachidonic acid.

## V. Treatment

**1) Treat food sensitivities**:

STUDY–Mathew, D., Norman, A., Taylor, B. Turner, M., Soothill, J. *Prevention of eczema.* Lancet 1:321, 1977. ABSTRACT–Infants of allergic parents were divided into 2 groups. The allergen-avoidance group was breast fed for 6 months. Supplementation, when necessary, was with soy rather than cow's milk formula. All dairy products, fish, and eggs were avoided during the first 6 months. Avoidance of pets, horsehair mattresses, feather pillows and quilts was advised. Measures were taken to minimize house dust. All of these measures were discontinued at 6 months of age. Infants in the control group did not avoid the above antigens. The *allergen avoidance group had significantly less eczema at 6 months AND AT ONE YEAR than the control group.* Mean serum IgE levels were lower in the allergen-avoidance group at 6 weeks of age.

STUDY–Sampson, H., Jolie, P. *Increased plasma histamine concentration after food challenges in children with atopic dermatitis.* NEJM 311:371-6, 1984. ABSTRACT–33 afflicted children underwent a 10 day elimination of allergic foods followed by food challenges. 35 challenges elicited symptoms, 31 of which involved the skin, 17 the gastrointestinal tract, 8 the nasal passages, and 6 the respiratory tract within 10-90 minutes. All 60 placebo challenges were negative.

**2) Avoid arachidonic acid**–Found in animal foods, this substance gives rise to inflammatory leukotrienes of the four series (see diagram on previous page).

**3) Evening primrose oil (EPO)**–2-3gms/day, usually 45mg/cap of gamma linolenic acid (GLA). Use topically, especially in infants. Can use borage oil, has higher conc. of GLA.

STUDY–Wright, S. & Burton, J. *Oral evening primrose improves atopic eczema.* Lancet Nov. 20, 1982 pg 1120-22. ABSTRACT–60 adults and 39 children with moderate or severe atopic eczema received EPO or placebo (liquid paraffin), each for 12 weeks. In a randomized, double blind cross over trial adults took either 2, 4, or 6 capsules 2x per day and children received 1-2 capsules 2x per day. Each capsule contained 360mg of linoleic acid and 45mg of ÌÒA. Standard treatment was continued during the study. In the low dose groups, in adults and children, itching was the only symptom significantly improved by the EPO. At higher doses, itching, scaling and general condition was significantly better on EPO than on placebo. Overall improvement in severity was about 43% in those taking high doses of the oil. Adults responded better than children, possibly because the dosage in children was inadequate. 14 responded more favorably to the antigen-avoidance diet versus only 1 on the control diet. There was no correlation between positive prick test to egg and cows' milk antigen and response to the trial diet. No side effects were noted. In the low dose groups, there was a 30% overall improvement.

**4) Zinc picolinate**–30mg tid–Zinc oxide can also be used topically.

**5) Quercetin**–600-800mg 15 minutes prior to meals

**6) Vitamin E**–400iu/day

**7) Vitamin A**–50,000iu/day

**8) Consider thyroid**

**9) Ginkgo biloba**

**10) Zizufus jujuba**–"Sweet fruit" has a high nucleotide content which stimulates adenylate cyclase activity (from Ed Madison, ND).

**11) Arctium lappa** inhibits phosphodiesterase

**12) Glycyrrhiza glabra**

**13) HCL**

# PSORIASIS

- Psoriasis consists of sharply demarcated erythematous papules or plaques covered with overlapping silvery scales.
- A family history of psoriasis is present in 50% of the cases.
- In the U.S., prevalence is between 2-4% with only a few blacks affected. Native Americans and blacks living in tropical zones rarely have this condition.
- **The mitotic rate in psoriatic skin lesions is very high (1,000x greater than in normal skin)**, exceeding the rate in squamous cell carcinoma. Even in uninvolved skin, the number of proliferating cells is up to 2.5x greater than in non-psoriatics.

## I. Etiology

A possible genetic error in mitotic synthesis control is indicated by the increase in the incidence of psoriasis in HLA-B13, HLA-B16, and HLA-B17. **Increases in DNA turnover are associated with increases in intracellular cGMP.** This results in cell proliferation and the thickening of the skin associated with psoriasis. Increases in intracellular cAMP are associated with enhanced cell maturation and differentiation and decreased cell proliferation. Balancing the cAMP:cGMP ratio generally brings about a measurable improvement.

## II. Signs and Symptoms

Onset is usually gradual with a typical course of chronic remissions and recurrences that vary in frequency and duration. Factors that precipitate psoriatic eruptions include local trauma (lesions appearing at the trauma site–the "Koebner phenomenon"), irritation from topical medications, and, sometimes, in children after upper respiratory infections. Eruptions characteristically involve the scalp (post-auricular), the extensor surface of the extremities (particularly the elbows and knees), the back, and the buttocks.

Lesions are sharply demarcated, usually non-pruritic, erythematous plaques covered with overlapping, silvery or slightly opalescent shiny scales. Lesions heal without scarring and hair growth is not altered. Nail involvement may resemble a fungal infection, with stippling, pitting, fraying or separation of the distal margin, thickening, discoloration, and debris under the nail plate. Psoriatic arthritis often closely resembles rheumatoid arthritis, but the patient's serum contains no rheumatoid factor.

## III. Diagnosis

Signs and symptoms are usually unequivocal but may be confused with seborrheic dermatitis, squamous cell cancer in situ (when on the trunk), secondary syphilis, fungal infections, cutaneous lupus erythematosis, eczema, lichen planus, or localized scratch dermatitis. **In psoriasis, removal of the superficial scale typically shows tiny bleeding points ("Auspitz sign").**

## IV. Therapeutic Considerations

An abnormal cAMP to cGMP ratio (one-third the ratio of uninvolved skin) is noted in psoriasis. Treatment should involve the stimulation of cAMP production and the inhibition of cGMP. cGMP can be increased via free radical-induced guanylate cyclase activation (see Eczema, Figure 1). Thus, prevention of free radicals should be a part of the basic treatment.

In addition, the involved epidermis has respectively 250x and 810x greater content of free arachidonic acid and 12-HETE (a product of lipoxygenase degradation of arachidonic acid) than the uninvolved epidermal tissue. These elevations appear to be due to the presence in the plaques of an inhibitor of cyclo-oxygenase, which normally degrades arachidonic acid.

**Note**–Trauma induces the release of free arachidonic acid and may account for the common clinical observation of plaques at the site of repeated trauma.

## V. Treatment

1) **Rule out food sensitivities**–consider gluten avoidance

STUDY–Lithill, H. *A fasting and vegetarian treatment trial in chronic inflammatory disorders.* Acta Derm. Vener. Stockholm 63:397-403, 1983. ABSTRACT–Patients improved on a fasting and vegetarian regime.

STUDY–Douglass, J. *Psoriasis and Diet. Letter to the Editor.* California Med. 133(5):450, 1980. ABSTRACT–6/6 patients improved on elimination diets. One improved on a diet which avoided fruits (especially citrus), nuts, corn, milk; another improved on a diet which avoided acidic foods such as coffee, tomato, soda, and pineapple.

2) **Avoid sources of arachidonic acid**–decrease the ingestion of animal fats

3) **Limit simple carbohydrates**–Increased levels of both insulin and glucose have been noted in psoriatic patients.

4) **Weight reduction**

5) **Vitamin E**–400iu/day-an antioxidant, inhibits lipoxygenase, and promotes PGE1.

6) **Selenium**–200mcg/day–is involved with the breakdown of HPETE through glutathione peroxidase.

7) **Vitamin A**–50,000iu/day

8) **Evening Primrose Oil**–4 capsules 3x/day–In psoriasis it is especially important to avoid sources of arachidonic acid because it gets converted into inflammatory leukotrienes. GLA, because it is largely converted into the anti-inflammatory PGE1 series and little is converted into arachidonic acid, is very useful.

9) **EPA or flax seed oil**–1 tablespoon/day–This oil promotes anti-inflammatory PGE3 and not inflammatory PGE2.

10) **Zinc picolinate**–30mg/day–promotes PGE1, inhibits calmodulin receptors, which, when stimulated, increases cGMP levels.

11) **Avoid cyclo-oxygenase inhibitors** such as aspirin, NSAID's.

12) **Garlic**–2 capsules 3x/day–inhibits lipoxygenase

13) **Quercetin**–1/4 teaspoon 3x/day

14) **Folate-1-10mg per day**

15) **Avoid cGMP stimulators** such as biotin, ginseng, and vitamin C and **cAMP antagonists** such as beta-blockers (see Eczema - Figure 1).

16) **Avoid activation of the Alternate Complement Pathway** (ACP)–This pathway exacerbates psoriasis because of the promotion of PMN release and lipoxygenase products. **Herbs such as arctium lappa, Echinacea, and inula are contraindicated because they promote the ACP.**

17) **Increase fiber in diet**–Low fiber is associated with increased numbers of gram negative rods and diverticular disease, both of which contribute to endotoxemia which can activate the ACP and guanylate cyclase directly.

18) **Vitamin D**–activated forms Calcitriol®/Calcipotriol® Dovonex® topical ointment

STUDY–Kragballe, Knud. *Vitamin D analogs in the treatment of psoriasis.* Journal of Cellular Biochemistry. ABSTRACT–It has been found that 1,25-dihydroxy cholecalciferol inhibits epidermal proliferation and promotes epidermal differentiation by binding to skin receptors. Topically applied at 50 ug/g bid, it is more efficacious than betamethasone.

STUDY–Morimoto S, Yoshikawa K, Kozuka T, et al. *An open study of vitamin D3 treatment in psoriasis vulgaris.* Brit J Dermatol 15:421-9, 1986.

STUDY–Kragballe K. *Treatment of psoriasis by the topical application of the novel cholecalciferol analogue Calcipotriol (MC 903).* Arch Dermatol 125:1647-52, 1989..

STUDY–Smith EL, Pincus SH, Donovan L, Holick MF. *A novel approach for the evaluation and treatment of psoriasis.* J Am Acad Dermatol 19:516-28, 1988.

19) **Fumaric acid**–Psoriactin® from Cardiovascular Research. several studies show this oil to be helpful when used topically. They also have a capsulated product for oral consumption.

STUDY–Kolbach DN, Nieboer C. *Fumaric acid therapy in psoriasis: results and side effects of 2 years of treatment.* J Am Acad Dermatol ;27:769-71, 1992.

STUDY–Altmeyer PJ, Matthes U, Pawlak F, et al. *Antipsoriatic effect of fumaric acid derivatives.* J Am Acad Dermatol 30:977-81, 1994.

Note–Udo Erasmus (Author of Fats that Heal, Fats that Kill), during a lecture April of 1998, recommended 3-4T per day and has used as much as 30T per day. In certain unusual cases it may be beneficial to go this high on the doseage. The conversion, however, of alpha linolenic acid into EPA and DHA may be greatly diminished in some cases. In such instances consider giving fish oil instead of flax oil or maybe a combination. Consider EFA analysis available through Kennedy Krieger Research Lab at Johns Hopkins in Maryland [call BodyBio (609) 825-8338].

## Notes

# ACNE VULGARIS OR CONGLOBATA

Acne, the most common of all skin problems, usually manifests as:

- **Open comedones**–dilated follicles with central dark, horny plugs (black heads)
- **Closed comedones**–small follicular papules which are red if inflamed, or white (whiteheads) if there is no inflammation
- **Superficial pustules**–collections of pus at the follicular openings

Acne is more common in males and onset is typically at puberty, although the conglobata form may appear somewhat later.

## I. Etiology

The initial microscopic change is intrafollicular hyperkeratosis which leads to blockage of the pilosebaceous follicle with consequent formation of the comedo, composed of sebum, keratin, and microorganisms, particularly *Propioni-bacterium* (Corynebacterium) *acnes.* Most of the microbes are normal skin species. Lipases from *P.acne* break down TG's in the sebum to form free fatty acids, which irritate the follicular wall.

> "Acne is often exacerbated during the winter and improved during the summer probably because of the beneficial effect of the sun. Diet has little, if any, effect, but if a food is suspected it should be omitted for several weeks and then eaten in substantial quantities to see if eating it makes any difference."
>
> Merck Manual

## II. Related Factors

1) **Simple carbohydrates**–One researcher called acne *"skin diabetes"* because of the fact that skin glucose tolerance in acne patients was significantly impaired compared to normals. However, one study comparing GTT's of acne patients to controls showed no difference.

2) **Birth Control Pills (BCP)**

It has been shown that the local area around the plugged follicle has elevated levels of glucose. In addition, the amount of sebum that is produced is regulated by various prostaglandins, especially PGE1. These prostaglandins require certain essential fatty acids such as $\gamma$ linolenic

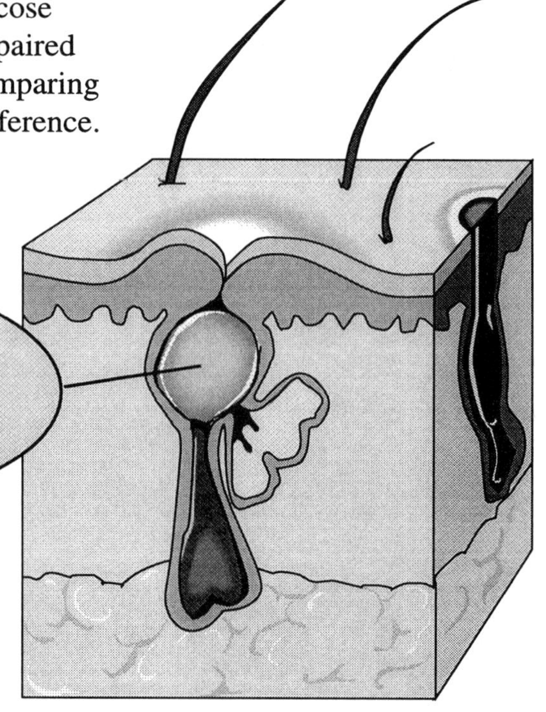

## III. Signs & Symptoms

Acne vulgaris is characterized as a pilosebaceous disease with comedones, papules, and pustules. Acne conglobata is a more severe form, with cyst formation and subsequent scarring. The lesions occur predominantly on the face and to a lesser extent on the back, chest, and shoulders.

## IV. Diagnosis

1) Signs and symptoms
2) Oral zinc sulfate test–Metagenics. Also, check fingernails for white spots.
3) Microclot generation test
4) Hair analysis
5) Stool analysis
6) Urinary indican
7) BBT–thyroid and hormonal changes
8) Peroxide serum levels
9) Glucose Insulin Tolerance Test

## V. Therapeutic Considerations

- Many dermatologists have reported that insulin is effective in the treatment of acne. This suggests impaired glucose tolerance and/or insulin insensitivity. The insulin can be given either systemically or injected directly into the lesion.
- One study showed that 50% of patients with severe acne had a "positive microclot test," indicating circulating endotoxins.
- Acne is considered to be an androgen-dependant condition. Excess androgen, either systemic or local, is associated with more severe forms of the disease. Androgens control sebaceous gland secretion and exacerbate the development of abnormal dekeratinizing follicular epithelium. The skin of acne patients shows greater activity of 5-alpha reductase, the enzyme that converts testosterone to the more active DHT. This increased activity is independent of systemic levels of androgens and may explain the poor correlation between systemic levels of androgens and the severity of the acne lesions.

## VI. Treatment

1) **Avoid simple carbohydrates**–sugar levels should be kept down as much as possible. Treatment should be similar to diabetes mellitus. Consider glycosylated Hgb for evaluation long term.

2) **Increase the amount of fiber**

STUDY–Kaufman, W. *The diet and acne. Letter to the Editor.* Arch. Dermatology 119(4): 276, 1983. Patients showed rapid clearing following supplementation with 1 oz daily of an all-bran cereal. This may be effective due to correction of constipation.

3) **HCL and digestive enzymes**–consider Heidelburg and/or stool analysis. Also, consider urine indican to detect endotoxins.

4) **Essential Fatty Acids**-EPO and alpha linolenic acid

STUDY–Wright, S. *EFA and Clinical Dermatology.* J. Nut. Med. 1, 301-313, 1990. ABSTRACT-This review hypothesized that there may be a local EFA deficiency and decreased activity of Δ 6 desaturase. Linoleic acid in the sebum falls as sebum secretion increases. This can correspond with the severity of acne.

**5) Zinc picolinate**–30mg tid for 8-12 wks then cut back

STUDY–Michaelsson, G. et al. *A double blind study of the effect of zinc and oxytetracycline in acne vulgaris.* 97:561, 1977. ABSTRACT-Effervescent zinc sulphate (135mg daily) was as effective as tetracycline (750mg daily) and showed about 70% improvement over 12 week. with fewer side effects from chronic use.

**6) Brewers yeast-**1 T 2x/day

**7) Vitamin A**–100,000-300,000iu/day for 3 months then cut back

STUDY–Kligman, A.M., et al. *Oral vitamin A in acne vulgaris.* Int. J. Dermatol. 20:78, 1981. 123 cases of acne vulgaris were treated with vitamin A. Doses below 300,000iu daily were ineffective. After 5 months there were no serious cases of toxicity. Only 1 patient. had a transient elevation of LV function tests. Two patients had transient headaches.

**8) Vitamin B-6**–especially for PMS acne–100mg tid.

**9) Vitamin E and Vitamin A**

STUDY–Mihan, R.T. *Acne vulgaris and lipid peroxidation: new concepts in pathogenesis and treatment.* Int. J. Dermatol. 17:305, 1978. ABSTRACT-Over 100 patients had conditions which were successfully controlled with average daily doses of 100,000iu of vitamin A and 800iu of vitamin E. Most responded within weeks, and results were maintained with lower doses over time.

**10) Selenium**

STUDY–Michaelsson, G., Edquist, L. *Erythrocyte glutathione peroxidase activity in acne vulgaris and the effect of selenium and vitamin E treatment.* Acta. Derm. Venereol. (Stockh.) 64,10:9-14, 1984. ABSTRACT-47 male acne patients had significant decrease in erythrocyte glutathione peroxidase levels compared to controls, while the levels of 47 female patients not on oral BCP did not differ from those of controls.

STUDY–Michaelsson ibid. ABSTRACT-29 patients with severe acne received selenium 200mcg and vitamin E 10mg 2x daily for 6-12 wks with "good" results, especially in those with pustular acne and low glutathione peroxidase activity, and improvement was usually paralleled by a slow rise in glutathione peroxidase activity.

**11) Folate**

STUDY–Callaghan, T.J. *The effect of folic acid on seborrheic dermatitis.* Cutis 3:583-88, 1967. ABSTRACT-8 patients with acne vulgaris were given oral synthetic folic acid 5-10mg daily. Six were *"much improved"* and 1 was *"improved."*

**12) Vitamin C**–1 gm/day

**13) Ultra Violet light**

**14) Bentonite masks**–topical treatment, especially for oily skin

**15) Tea Tree oil**-topical

**16) Azelaic acid** (a 9 carbon chain fatty acid)–topical from molds Cardiovascular Research

**17) Garlic**–may decrease blood glucose levels and also change gut flora

**18) Vitamin D Calcitriol** (active form 1,25 DHCC of Vitamin D)

**19) Staphage lysate**–be very careful of allergic reactions

**20) Benzoyle peroxide**

**21) Detoxification**–A general detoxification treatment is often helpful in reducing acne. Colonics may also be considered.

# HERPES SIMPLEX

- Herpes simplex is a recurrent viral infection that manifests, either singly or in multiple clusters, on the skin or mucus membranes.
- The specific type of herpes infection is determined by where the lesions appear on the body. In Type I, herpes labialis and keratitis appear around the mouth and lips. Type II manifests around the genitalia and is usually sexually transmitted.

## I. Etiology

Herpes simplex is caused by the herpes virus *hominis.* It usually lies dormant in the skin or nerve ganglia. The lesions may be precipitated by various stressors such as overexposure to sun, illness, physical or emotional stress, medications and certain foods. There seems to be a relationship to the intake of lysine to arginine. The lower the lysine intake and the greater the arginine intake the greater the growth of herpes (see arginine/lysine ratio table).

## II. Signs and Symptoms

Lesions may occur anywhere around the mouth or genital area. In women they may occur intravaginally. The first symptoms are a short period of tingling, burning or itching sensation. Vesicles are the first lesions to form and they generally begin to dry in a few days. Healing usually begins in 7-10 days and is complete by around 3 weeks. Healing may be slower within moist body areas. Recurrence is quite common. Type II may be transmitted to the fetus with development of severe viremia. It may also cause fatal encephalitis.

## III. Diagnosis

**Signs and symptoms**–Differentiate between herpes and pleurisy, trigeminal neuralgia, or Bell's palsy. The pain may also resemble appendicitis, renal colic, cholelithiasis, or colitis. Antibody titers may be measured and the fluid may be cultured to differentiate.

## IV. Clinical Considerations

Allopathic medicine has few treatments for Herpes simplex. Antibiotics may be used if secondary infections develop.

## V. Treatment

1) **Enhance immunity**–consider constitutional hydrotherapy if the patient can tolerate it.

2) **Lysine–3-6gms** per day in acute conditions. Make sure the diet is balanced with the correct ratio of lysine to arginine. Avoid foods that contain arginine. Eat foods with a high lysine to arginine ratio (see table at end of chapter).

3) **Glycyrrhiza–**Herplic–(Scientific Botanicals) can be used topically

4) **Quercetin**–500mg 3-4x per day

5) **Vitamin C**–A high dose to bowel tolerance is most effective. Vitamin C can also be given IV.

6) **AMP**–IM 2-3ml per day–**with vitamin B-12**–1000mcg

7) **Topical lithium succinate**

8) **Topical vitamin E and zinc**

9) **Selenium- 200-400 mcg**

**Best Sources of Lysine along with Arginine amounts & ratios**

| Food | amount | mg lysine | mg arginine | Ratio Arg to Lys | Food | amount | mg lysine | mg arginine | Ratio Arg to Lys |
|---|---|---|---|---|---|---|---|---|---|
| Tuna 3 oz | 1/2 can | 2400 | 1450 | .6 | Beans, red canned | 1/2 cup | 630 | 510 | .8 |
| Turkey (baked light meat) | 3 oz | 2400 | 1770 | .74 | Oatmeal flakes | 1 cup | 600 | 600 | 1.0 |
| Halibut, baked | 3oz | 2083 | 1357 | .65 | Carrot juice | 12 cup | 600 | | .8 |
| Salmon | 3 oz | 2014 | 1311 | .65 | Granola | 1 cup | 500 | 900 | 1.85 |
| Liver, beef | 3 oz | 1671 | 1363 | .82 | Wheat germ, toasted | 1/4 cup | 500 | 675 | 1.3 |
| Cheese | 3 oz | 1650 | 600 | .4 | Bacon | 3 slices | 500 | 525 | .9 |
| Cheese, ricotta | 1/2 cup | 1600 | 800 | .5 | Duck | 3 oz | 480 | 407 | .85 |
| Pork | 3 oz | 1586 | 1470 | .83 | Sausage | 3 oz | 420 | 315 | .8 |
| Cheese, cheddar | 3 Oz | 1497 | 729 | .49 | Egg | 1 med | 400 | 400 | 1.0 |
| Wild game | 3 oz | 1300 | 962 | .75 | Chicken (baked light meat) | 3 oz | 2232 | 1584 | .71 |
| Cheese, cottage | 1/2 cup | 1200 | 700 | .6 | Peanuts | 1/4 cup | 363 | 1080 | 3.0 |
| Sardines, canned in oil | 3 med | 814 | 531 | .65 | Avocado | 1 med | 200 | 100 | .5 |
| Meat, luncheon | 3 oz | 740 | 592 | .8 | Cashews | 10 nuts | 185 | 490 | 2.6 |
| Yogurt | 1 cup | 700 | 250 | .35 | Almonds | 18 nuts | 145 | 683 | 4.7 |
| Milk, whole | 1 cup | 650 | 300 | .45 | | | | | |

## Foods High in Arginine

| Food | amount | mg | | Food | amount | mg |
|---|---|---|---|---|---|---|
| Turkey (baked light meat w/o skin) | 3 oz | 1770 | | Wheat germ, toasted | 1/4 c | 675 |
| Chicken (baked light meat w/o skin) | 3 oz | 1584 | | Cashews, roasted | 1/4 c | 650 |
| Lamb, leg roasted | 3 oz | 1531 | | Oats | 1 c | 600 |
| Pork | 3 oz | 1470 | | Meat, luncheon | 3 oz | 592 |
| Tuna | 1/2 sm can | 1400 | | Soybeans, cooked | 1/2 c | 540 |
| Beef, chuck | 3 oz | 1372 | | Bacon | 3 med slices | 525 |
| Liver, beef | 3 oz | 1362 | | Kidney beans, cooked | 1/2 c | 420 |
| Salmon | 3 oz | 1311 | | Duck | 3 oz | 412 |
| Shrimp | 3 oz | 1166 | | Egg | 1 med | 400 |
| Peanuts | 1/4 c (1.3oz) | 1080 | | Sausage | 3 oz | 315 |
| Wild game | 1/4 c | 966 | | Milk, whole | 1 c | 300 |
| Almonds, whole | 1/4 c | 910 | | Chicken, white fried | 3 oz | 278 |
| Granola | 1 c | 900 | | Bread, whole wheat | 2 slices | 255 |
| Cheese, ricotta | 1/2 c | 800 | | Yogurt | 1 c | 250 |
| Walnuts | 1/4 c | 750 | | Collards, cooked | 1/2 c | 240 |
| Cheese, cottage | 1/2 c | 700 | | Rice, brown, cooked | 1 c (185g) | 183 |

Washington DC ARS USDA 1976-1986

From USDA Composition of Foods USDA handbook # 8 Washington DC ARS USDA 1976-1986

# HERPES ZOSTER (SHINGLES)

- Herpes zoster is a viral infection that invades the nerve root.
- It may occur at any age but is most common after age 50.
- *Shingles are especially prevalent in the elderly and may be chronic.*
- Lesions may disappear while the herpetic neuralgia persists.

## I. Etiology

Herpes zoster is caused by the varicella zoster virus, the same virus that causes chicken pox. It may be activated by systemic disease, immunosuppressive therapy, or by general debilitation. Inflammation of the sensory root ganglia, the posterior horn of the gray matter, the meninges and the dorsal and ventral roots may be observed. Depressed immunity may be a significant factor, especially in the elderly.

## II. Signs & Symptoms

Prodromal symptoms of fever and chills with malaise and GI disturbances can occur 3-4 days before the outbreak of the lesions. Pain may or may not occur at time of initial prodromal symptoms. Initial lesions usually appear as small vesicles with some hyperemia. The area may become hyperesthetic and the pain may become severe enough that the patient cannot stand the touch of clothing on the affected region. The thoracic area is the most common area for the lesions to occur. Sequelae can affect the trigeminal nerve and cause paralysis and corneal damage. After the lesions have disappeared the herpetic nerve pain (post herpetic neuralgia) may remain for months and even years.

## III. Diagnosis

**Signs and symptoms**–Differentiate between herpes zoster and pleurisy, trigeminal neuralgia, or Bell's palsy. The pain may also resemble appendicitis, renal colic, cholelithiasis, or colitis. Antibody titers may be measured and the fluid may be cultured to differentiate.

## III. Therapeutic Considerations

There is no allopathic treatment for Herpes zoster other than corticosteroids in more severe cases. However, this is contraindicated if there is acute ocular Herpes simplex.

## IV. Treatment

1) **Enhance immunity**–consider constitutional hydrotherapy if the patient can tolerate it.
2) **Vitamin C**–Use high doses to bowel tolerance. Vitamin C can also be given IV.
3) **Zostrix (capsaicin)**–Topical applications may be helpful in some cases. Zostrix affects the efferent nerves endings.

4) **Glycyrrhiza** topically may be helpful. It can be applied with DMSO to drive the Glycyrrhiza into the nerve root. Other botanicals may also be administered–such as aloe vera, along with vitamin E and zinc oxide.

5) **Quercetin** can inhibit the replication of various viruses and may be effective in the treatment of Herpes zoster.

6) **Selenium**–up to 800mcg per day for acute situations

7) **Consider IM or IV vitamins such as vitamin C, Echinacae, "Myers' Cocktail", Vitamin B-12 & B-1** similar to sciatica treatment. Heel homeopathics such as Herpes zoster, can be given IM around trigger points, or IV.

8) **Herpes zoster ophthalmicus**–vitamin C and A drops. Call the Tahoma clinic for recipe and Rx (206) 854-4900.

9) **Adenosine monophosphate** (AMP 25mg/ml), 2-3ml IM every day or other day as patient is responding. Can also use IV. Call the Tahoma Clinic for recipe and Rx (206) 854-4900.

10) **DHEA or low dose cortisone** may be indicated.

11) **Chinese medicine**–Consider electroacupuncture, trigger point therapy or indirect moxa to lesions.

12) **Moist Burn ointment** or Mebo burn cream: (Chinese formula from CHI's Enterprise Inc. (714) 921-1957) Phenomenal results on severe skin burns or severe Herpes Zoster lesions. Call for further information.

13) **Bee Venom Therapy** (see appendix)

14) **Homeopathics- Heel** (they have injectable homeopathic extracts of Herpes Zoster).

## Notes

---

# PREMENSTRUAL SYNDROME (PMS)

- PMS refers to recurrent signs and symptoms that develop 7-14 days prior to menses.
- PMS is not a disease in itself, but rather an imbalance in the body biochemistry resulting in decreased energy, tension, irritability, depression, mood swings, headache, altered libido, mastalgia, fluid retention, insomnia, food cravings, and increased sensitivity to foods.
- 50% of the menstruating U.S. female population have some symptoms of PMS.

## I. Etiology

It is generally believed that PMS is caused by an imbalance in various hormones at the period of time between ovulation and the onset of menses.

1) From mid to late luteal phase, plasma estrogens and prolactin are elevated and, at mid luteal phase, plasma progesterone levels are reduced
2) Allergies
3) Hypothyroid
4) **Excess lead** blocks the binding of estrogen to receptor sites, but has no effect on progesterone. It thus may be an important factor in PMS-D (see below). Decreased magnesium results in greater lead absorption and retention, while decreasing resistance to stress. Hair analysis has shown that PMS patients have higher heavy metal levels and lower magnesium.
5) Autotoxicity
6) Mental and Emotional: 40% of women who seek treatment for PMS have been sexually abused. Half of these talk about it with their therapist.

## II. Signs and Symptoms

PMS Subgroups

1) **PMS-A**–70% (high estrogen & low progesterone)–anxiety, irritability, mood swings, nervous tension (most common). In the case of PMS-A, it is thought that the elevated levels of estrogen cause an inhibition of monoamine oxidase (MAO). This results in a potentiation of the effects of catecholamines which causes mood and behavioral changes. In addition, there is also a decrease/increase in serotonin levels which leads to anxiety, nervousness, irritability, insomnia and other mood alternations (note conflicting documentation on serotonin levels). A tryptophan load test may be appropriate. **NOTE-**There is no correlation between progesterone levels and severity of symptoms.

2) **PMS-C**–35% (deficient PGE1, decreased RBC magnesium)–"increased" carbohydrate tolerance, cravings, increased appetite, headache, fatigue, dizziness, fainting, and palpitations.

3) **PMS-D**–30% (low estrogen, high progesterone and elevated androgens if there is hirsutism)–depression, crying, forgetfulness, confusion, insomnia. In this type of PMS, the decreased levels of estrogen results in decreased levels of serotonin and melatonin as opposed to PMS-A. Thus, depression is the biggest symptom.

4) **PMS-H**–70% (elevated aldosterone)–fluid retention, weight gain, breast tenderness, abdominal bloating. Estrogen excess increases production of angiotensinogen, the precursor to angiotensin II. This results in increased water retention.

## III. Diagnosis

1) See menstrual symptom questionnaire
2) Urinary estrogen quotient
3) Hair analysis for lead
4) Bowel transit time, indican, microclot, tryptophan load test

## IV. Therapeutic Considerations

General findings concerning the diets of PMS patients:

1) 63% higher in refined carbohydrates
2) 275% higher in refined sugar
3) 79% higher in dairy products
4) 78% higher in sodium
5) 53% lower in iron
6) 77% lower in magnesium
7) 52% lower in zinc

## V. Treatment

**1) Increase consumption of complex carbohydrates by 70%**

STUDY - Abraham, Guy. *Nutritional factors in the etiology of the PMS syndromes.* J. Repro. Med. 28:446-64, 1983. ABSTRACT–PMS patients were compared to normals and it was observed that PMS women ate 63% more refined carbohydrates, and 275% more refined sugar.

2) **Decrease consumption of saturated fats** - especially red meats and dairy products. PMS patients in one study were found to eat 79% more dairy products than "normals." For PMS-A, where there is an excess of estrogen, decrease any endogenous estrogens. Overweight patients must shed the extra pounds.

- **Animal fats** stimulate the growth of certain intestinal bacteria, which can hydrolyze conjugated estrogens thus rendering them active again.
- Arachidonic acid from animal fats is a precursor to PGF2, which is leuteolytic in women (decreases progesterone).

STUDY–Dennefors, B., Sjogren, A., Hamberger, L. *Progesterone and cAMP formation by isolated human corpora lutea of different ages: influence of HCG and prostaglandins.* J. Clin. Endocrin. & Metab. 55:102-107, 1982. ABSTRACT–It was found, in vitro, that PGF2 had a net effect of decreasing progesterone secretion. Thus animal fats should be avoided as much as possible.

**3) Increased fiber–Increased binding and excretion of estrogens**

STUDY–Golden, B. *Estrogen excretion patterns and plasma levels in vegetarian and omnivorous women.* N. Eng. J. Med. 307:11542-47, 1982. ABSTRACT–Fecal excretion of estrogen in 10 vegetarian and 10 omnivorous menstruating women was performed. The omnivorous women consumed an average of 12 gms fiber/day while the vegetarian women consumed an average of 29 gms/day. It was found that there was a positive correlation between fecal estrogen and fiber intake. An inverse relationship existed between blood estrogen levels and fiber intake.

4) **Decrease salt intake**–to 3gms/day or less–especially for PMS-H.

5) **Decrease sugar intake**

6) **Magnesium**–400-800mg/day (preferably aspartate)–Magnesium levels are usually normal in the serum, but intracellular erythrocyte magnesium is usually found to be lower in PMS women. Dairy and calcium interfere with magnesium absorption while sugar increases its excretion.

STUDY–Abraham, G. *Magnesium deficiency in PMS.* Magnesium Bulletin 1:68-73 ABSTRACT–It was found that women with PMS-A consume 2.5X more refined sugar than women without or with mild PMS.

STUDY–Nicholas, A. *Treatment of premenstrual syndrome with Magnesium.* First Int. Sympos. on magnesium deficiency in Human Pathology. ABSTRACT–192 patients received magnesium nitrate 4.5-6 gms daily for 1 week premenstrually and 2 days menstrually. Nervous tension was relieved in 159/179, mastalgia in 155/162, weight gain in 59/62 and headache in 16/37.

7) **Vitamin B-6**–100mg 3x/day–use two weeks before period.

STUDY–Doll, H., et al. *Pyridoxine and the PMS: A randomized crossover trial.* J. Royal College of General Practitioners 39:326, 364-68, Sept. 1989. ABSTRACT–63 women ages 18-49 were enrolled in a random double blind cross-over trial. The women received either 50mg/day B6 or placebo for 3 months. Symptoms included depression, irritability, tiredness, headache, breast tenderness, swollen abdomen/hands, etc. At this dose depression, irritability and tiredness were the only symptoms to respond and they were reduced by 50%.

STUDY–Abraham, G., Hargrove, J. *Effect of Vitamin B6 on PMS symptoms in women affected: A double blind crossover study.* Infertility, 3(2):155-65, 1980. ABSTRACT–25 patients with moderate or severe PMS symptoms were studied for 6 cycles. For 3 months half received either placebo or 500mg time release B6. They were then switched. During this time a symptom diary was kept recording 19 total symptoms. 21 of the 25 did better on the B6 than the placebo. In each of the cases the differences were statistically significant.

8) **Decrease caffeine**

STUDY–Rossignol, A. *Caffeine containing beverages and PMS in young women.* Am. J. Public Health 75(11):1335-37, 1985. ABSTRACT–295 students with moderate to severe symptoms were studied. 61% of the women who drank 4.5 to 15 caffeine containing drinks daily experienced moderate to severe symptoms, while only 16% of the women who consumed no caffeine experienced moderate to severe symptoms.

STUDY–Rossignol, A. *Tea and PMS in China.* Am J. Public Health 79:67-9, 1989. ABSTRACT-188 nursing students were questioned about tea consumption and PMS. Women consuming more than 4.5 cups per day had a relative risk of 9.7. This adds to work done by Minton regarding coffee and FBD.

9) **Treat the liver**–The liver conjugates estrogens and is involved in estradiol and estrone production.

10) **Vitamin B complex**

11) **Vitamin E**–200-600iu/day–2 studies double blind

12) **Flax oil or EPO**

13) **Tryptophan**

14) **Tyrosine**–500mg 2x/day–especially for PMS-D. Tyrosine may help catecholamine synthesis

15) **Vitamin A**

16) **Cofactors for PGE** 1–Zinc, B-3, magnesium, etc.

17) **Consider thyroid**

**18) Calcium**

STUDY–Thys-Jacobs, S. et al. *Calcium supplementation in PMS: a randomized crossover trial.* J. Gen. Intern. Med. 4:183-89, 1989. ABSTRACT–78 PMS patients were given 1 gm of Ca carbonate for 3 months in a double blind intervention trial. 33 completed the trial. Pain, bloating and "negative effect" were significantly reduced in the calcium group. Overall symptoms were cut in half, and 73% preferred the calcium to the placebo.

**19) Work on digestion**

**20) Progesterone** (orally or topically)

## Notes

---

# DYSMENORRHEA

- Dysmenorrhea may be either primary (functional) or secondary (acquired).
- In primary dysmenorrhea, the patient experiences cyclical pain associated with menses during ovulatory cycles, but without demonstrable lesions affecting the reproductive cycle.
- Secondary dysmenorrhea is pain with menses caused by a demonstrable pathology.

## I. Etiology

1) Primary dysmenorrhea is thought to be a result of uterine contractions and ischemia mediated by the effect of prostaglandins, particularly the $\mathbf{F}_2\mu$ series produced in the secretory endometrium.
2) It is almost always associated with ovulatory cycles and may be made worse by the passage of tissue through a narrow cervical os, malposition of the uterus, lack of exercise, pelvic or lumbar subluxation, congealed blood or stagnant Qi, or an imbalance of dietary fats.
3) Dysmenorrhea caused by autotoxicity must also be considered.
4) Psychological components may also be a factor in dysmenorrhea.

## II. Signs and Symptoms

Usually women experience low abdominal crampy or colicky pain or a dull constant ache which radiates to the lower back or legs. It usually starts a day before or during the onset of menses. Headache, nausea, constipation or diarrhea, and urinary frequency are often present. Other PMS symptoms may occur simultaneously, merging with the symptoms of dysmenorrhea.

## III. Diagnosis

After secondary dysmenorrhea has been ruled out, the signs and symptoms of dysmenorrhea are sufficient for a diagnosis of primary dysmenorrhea.

## IV. Treatment

1) **Alter the diet** to include a high percentage of complex carbohydrates and low fat intake, especially from arachidonic acid sources, which is the substrate for prostaglandin.

2) **Essential fatty acids**

3) **Magnesium**–500-800mg/day

STUDY–Abraham, G. *Primary dysmenorrhea* Clin. Obstet. Gynecol. 21(1):139-45, 1978. ABSTRACT–Patients received amino-acid chelated magnesium and B-6 100mg of each every 2 hrs as needed during menses and 4x daily throughout the cycle until RBC magnesium returned to normal. There was a progressive decrease in intensity and duration of menstrual cramps over 4-6 months.

4) **Vitamin B-6**

5) **Calcium**–1-1.5gms/day

**6) Vitamin E**–1200iu/day

STUDY–Butler, McKnight. *Vitamin E in the treatment of primary dysmenorrhea.* Lancet 1:844-47, 1955. ABSTRACT–100 young women 18-21 with spasmodic dysmenorrhea received either 50mg vitamin E 3x/day or placebo for 10 days premenstrually and for the next 4 days. After 2 cycles, 34/50 (68%) in the experimental group improved compared to 9/50 (18%) of the controls.

**7) Piscidia** (botanical)

## Notes

---

# MENORRHAGIA

- Excessive menstrual bleeding greater than 80ml during the regular menses cycle is considered menorrhagia. These cycles are usually, though not always, of normal duration.

## I. Etiology

1) **Local lesions**–Uterine myomas, endometrial polyps, endometrial hyperplasia, adenomyosis, and endometritis can be factors in menorrhagia. Other causes include cancer, ectopic pregnancy, IUD's, excess estrogen, failure of midcycle surge of LH, hyperprolactinemia, and polycystic ovarian disease.
2) **Abnormalities in prostaglandin metabolism**–The endometrium incorporates arachidonic acid into the phospholipid components in menorrhagia. During menses, the increased arachidonic acid release during menstruation results in increased production of PGE2 and PGI2. These prostaglandins cause vasodilation and anti-aggregating activity.

**Other contributing factors**

- Iron deficiency
- Hypothyroidism
- Vitamin A deficiency

## II. Signs and Symptoms

Excess cyclical bleeding at the time of the menses, often associated with dysmenorrhea.

## III. Diagnosis

It is very difficult to assess a greater than 80ml blood loss, since studies have shown that there is no correlation between pads used and measured blood loss. One study found that 40% of women with a menstrual blood loss exceeding 80ml considered their periods to only be moderately heavy or scanty, while 14% of those with a measured loss of less than 20 ml judged their periods to be heavy.

**Serum ferritin levels are the best indication of excess menses.**

STUDY–Lewis, G. *Do women with menorrhagia need iron?* Brit. Med. J. 284:1158, 1982. ABSTRACT–Serum ferritin of menorrhagic patients was significantly lower than that of controls despite the lack of significant differences in HgB concentration, MCV, and MCH.

- Evaluate thyroid function
- Check Prothrombin time
- Test serum vitamin A

## IV. Therapeutic Considerations

First rule out serious pathological causes.

## V. Treatment

1) **Green leafy vegetables**–The patient should consume as many green leafy vegetables as possible because of the vitamin K content.

2) **Decrease consumption of arachidonic acid**–Avoid animal fats. Remember safflower, corn, and sunflower oils may possibly get converted to arachidonic acid in times of stress. It is best to stick with omega 3 EPA.

3) **Vitamin A**–25,000iu 2x/day

STUDY–Lithgow, D. & Politzer, W. *Vitamin A in the treatment of menorrhagia.* S. Afr. Med. J. 51:191-3, 1977. ABSTRACT–Serum vitamin A was measured in 71 women with menorrhagia. Vitamin A levels were significantly lower than in controls (healthy women who attended the GYN clinic). Forty of the women with menorrhagia were given vitamin A in doses of 25,000iu 2x/day for 15 days. Of the 40 women treated, menstruation returned to normal in 57.5%, and there was a substantially diminished menstrual period or a reduction in the duration of menses or both in an additional 35%. Thus, **92% of vitamin A treated women had either complete relief or significant improvement.**

4) **Iron**–30-100mg/day

STUDIES–Taymor, M. *The etiological role of chronic iron deficiency in production of menorrhagia.* JAMA 187:323-27, 1964. ABSTRACT–In a double blind study, 75% of those on iron improved compared to 32.5% on placebo, a significant difference. ABSTRACT–74/83 patients in whom organic pathology had been excluded, responded to iron supplementation. It was also noted that when initial iron levels were high, there was a decreased response to iron therapy, and there was also a correlation of menorrhagia with depleted tissue iron stores (bone marrow or ferritin) irrespective of serum iron level.

STUDY–Samuels, AJ. *Studies in patients with functional menorrhagia: the antimenorrhagic effect of the adequate replication of iron stores.* Israel J Med Sci 1:851, 1965.

5) **Vitamin C**–1gm/day–decreases capillary fragility and increases absorption of iron.

STUDY–Cohen, J. & Rubin, H. *Functional menorrhagia: Treatment with bioflavonoids and Vitamin C:* Curr. Ther. Res. 2:539-42, 1960. ABSTRACT–Supplementation with 200mg 3x/day vitamin C and bioflavonoids reduced menorrhagia in 14 of 16 patients. Of the 2 that did not respond, one had endometriosis and the other had metrorrhagia.

6) **Vitamin K**–5-10mg/day of phytonadione

STUDY–Gubner, R. & Ungerleider, H. *Vitamin K therapy in menorrhagia.* S. Med J. 37:556-8,1944. ABSTRACT–Crude chlorophyll preparations were used in the treatment of menorrhagia with some success.

7) **Thyroid**-one of the most frequent causes of menorrhagia is hypothyroidism. There are many unnecessary hysterectomies every year that could be prevented if thyroid function was returned to normal (see hypothyroidism p.402).

STUDY–Stoffer, C. *Menstrual disorders and mild thyroid insufficiency.* Postgraduate Med. 72:75-82, 1982.ABSTRACT–It was found that patients with minimal thyroid insufficiency and menorrhagia responded dramatically to thyroxine.

8) **Vitamin E**–400iu/day–decreases capillary fragility and promotes PGE1.

STUDY–Dasgupta, P., Dutta, S., Banerjee. *Vitamin E in the management of menorrhagia associated with the use of IUD's.* Int J. Fertil 28:55-6, 1983. ABSTRACT–Patients who had IUD's were given 100iu vitamin E and at the end of 10 weeks, all patients had improved in symptoms of menorrhagia.

9) **Evening Primrose Oil**–3 caps 3x/day–promotes the production of PGE1 series.

10) **Bioflavonoids**–3 gms/day–decreases capillary fragility.

11) **Vitex**–3x per day–may decrease bleeding over extended period of time

## Notes

# FIBROCYSTIC BREAST DISEASE (FBD)

- 20-40% of premenopausal women have fibrocystic breast disease.
- The condition is often asymptomatic, although the patient may also have pain or premenstrual breast pain.
- FBD is usually cyclical and bilateral with multiple cysts of varying sizes giving the breast a nodular consistency.
- FBD, also known as cystic mastitis, is usually a component of PMS and is considered a **risk factor for breast cancer.** It is not as significant a factor as family history, early menarche, and late or no first pregnancy.

## I. Etiology

- Increased estrogen to progesterone ratio.
- Etiology is the same as PMS.

## II. Diagnosis

**Estrogen Quotient** $= \dfrac{\text{estriol}}{\text{estrone + estradiol}}$ A healthy woman should have a ratio >1.0.

The estrogen quotient is an indication of how well the liver is metabolizing estrogenic hormones. As the liver becomes compromised in its function, or if it is overburdened, the levels of estrone and estradiol go up in relationship to estriol. This appears as a decreased EQ. The incidence of breast cancer goes up significantly when the ratio drops below 0.5. The opposite is also true. As the ratio goes above 1.1, the incidence of breast cancer goes down.

- Measure bowel transit time using charcoal (as previously discussed)
- Perform an Obermeyer test (urinary indican)–see p.19
- Measure thyroid function (see chapter on hypothyroidism p.402).

## III. Treatment

1) **Increase consumption of complex carbohydrates and fiber**–it has been found that women who have fewer than 3 bowel movements per week have a 4.5x greater risk of FBD than women having at least one bowel movement/day.

**2) Avoid methylxanthines**

STUDY–Minton, J., Abou-Issa, H., Reiches, N., Roseman, J. *Clinical and biochemical studies on methylxanthine-related FBD.* Surgery 90:299-304, 1981. ABSTRACT–85 women with FBD were studied. 45 stopped all methylxanthine consumption. Of these, 37 had a resolution of their disease, 7 were improved, and 1 was unchanged. 28 women decreased consumption by more than 1/2. Of these, 7 had a resolution of their disease, 14 were improved, and 7 were unchanged. 12 women continued methylxanthine consumption as before. Two had a resolution, 1 was improved, and 9 were unchanged. **Women suffering from FBD were not found to be consuming more methylxanthines than women without the disease**. Those with the disease were more likely than controls to have a family history of breast cancer or FBD. Breast tissue from women with the disease was significantly more sensitive to adenylate cyclase than normal breast tissue. **It is thus suggested that women with FBD have a genetically determined increased sensitivity to methylxanthines.**

STUDY–Ernster. *Effects of a caffeine-free diet on FBD: a randomized trial* Surgery 91(3):263-67, 1982. ABSTRACT–158 women with FBD were randomly assigned to a diet free of methylxanthines or to a group receiving no dietary advice. Four months later there was a significant decrease in palpable breast findings in the caffeine-free group as compared to the controls. The diet was most effective in severe cases. The authors concluded that the improvement was minor and may be of little clinical significance. **However, analysis of breast fluid after 4 months on the diet showed substantial levels of caffeine in many women assigned to the caffeine-free diet.** Thus, the 25% improvement could have been better with tighter controls.

**3) Avoid exogenous estrogens** (oral contraceptives and animal products with estrogen residues).

**4) Vitamin E**–800iu/day– normalizes elevated FSH & LH levels commonly seen in FBD.

STUDY–Abrams, A. *Usef Vitamin E in chronic cystic mastitis.* New Engl. J. Med. 272:1080-81, 1965. ABSTRACT–29 women with chronic FBD which was aggravated premenstrually took vitamin E 300 or 600iu daily for 3 months. 16 had moderate to complete symptom relief, the remaining 13 had palpable breast softening, with reduction of cyst size or complete elimination of cysts.

**5) Flax oil**–2T/day

**6) Iodine SSKI** (saturated solution of Potassium Iodine)–30mg=1 drop. Give 1-10 drops/day–Wright says to start out with 6-8 drops/day, then cut back. This will have a definite effect on the estrogen quotient. **Above 300mg/day inhibits thyroid.** Dr. Myers, using Lugol's idodine intravaginally followed by 1-2 gms of magnesium sulfate IV over 5-15 minutes, had dramatic effects on FBD. Ghent in Canada, has for many years, treated FBD and recommends diatomic iodine [original formula available from Lloyd Center Pharmacy (503)281-4161].

STUDY–Ghent WR, Eskin BA, Low DA, Hill L. *Iodine replacement in fibrocystic disease of the breast.* Canadian J Surg 36:453-60, 1993.

STUDY–Eskin, B. *Mammary gland dysplasia in iodine deficiency.* JAMA 200:115-19,1967ABSTRACT–In a series of histologic studies, iodine deficiency was found to enhance responsiveness of rat breast tissue to infections of estrogen or testosterone. Breast changes in iodine deficiency rats were clearly distinguishable from those induced by sex hormones in the hypothyroid or euthyroid rat. Estrogen given to iodine deficiency rats resulted in lesions which resembled histologically human fibrocystic disease.

STUDY–Boyle CA, Berkowitz GS, LiVoisi VA, et al. *Caffeine consumption and fibrocystic breast disease: a case-control epidemiologic study.* J Natl Cancer Inst 72:1015-9, 1984.

STUDY–Vecchia C, Franceschi S, Parazzini F, et al. *Benign breast disease and consumption of beverages containing methylxanthines.* J Natl Cancer Inst 74:995-1000, 1985.

**7) Evening Primrose Oil**–1500mg 2x/day

STUDY–Pashby, N. *Clinical experience of drug treatment for mastalgia.* Lancet 2:373-77, 1984. ABSTRACT–41 patients with cyclical breast symptoms were treated with EPO. After 2 months, significant improvement was observed in patient's assessment of breast tenderness and nodularity, general well-being and irritability, and in physician's assessment of breast nodularity. There were no side-effects and responses were sustained for up to 18 months with continuing supplementation.

STUDY–Mansel RE, Pye JK, Hughes LE. *Effects of Essential fatty acids on cyclical mastalgia and noncyclical breast disorders.* in Omega-6 essential fatty acids: Pathophysiology and roles in clinical medicine, Alan R Liss, New York 557-66, 1990.

**8) Vitamin A**–150,000iu/day as trial

STUDY–Band, P. *Treatment of benign breast disease with Vitamin A.* Prev. Med. 13:549-54, 1984. ABSTRACT–10 of 12 women with moderate to severe breast pain, which had not responded to mild painkillers or caffeine withdrawal, reported reduction in breast pain following supplementation with 150,000iu/day. In 5 patients breast masses decreased at least 50%. Two patients had to stop supplementation due to severe headaches and 3 had mild reactions, while 5 had no side effects. Patients who responded showed continued benefit at follow-up 8 months later, and side effects were rapidly reversed.

9) **Lipotropic factors-**these include inositol, choline, methionine

10) **Vitamin B complex-**can use thiamin 100mg 3x per day

11) **Lactobacillus acidophilus** if bowel problems are also present.

12) **Thyroid-** if bowel problems are also present.

## Notes

---

# CERVICAL DYSPLASIA

- Cervical Dysplasia is generally regarded as a precancerous lesion with risk factors similar to those of cervical cancer.
- Approximately 16,000 cases of invasive cervical cancer (CA) and 45,000 cases of in situ CA occur yearly in the U.S. This accounts for about 7,500 deaths per year.
- Cervical Dysplasia is the second most common malignancy of women aged 15-34.
- Peak incidence of invasive lesions occurs at age 45. In situ lesions peak at age 30.

## I. Etiology

Factors associated with the onset of cervical dysplasia are:

1) Early age of intercourse
2) Multiple sexual partners
3) Herpes simplex type ll and papilloma viruses
4) Smoking
5) Oral contraceptive use
6) Nutritional factors

## II. Therapeutic Considerations

95% of cervical cancer originates in the squamocolumnar junction of the cervical os. This actively growing area is more susceptible to multiple insults and cancer-causing substances.

STUDY–Basu & Jayasri, et al. *Plasma ascorbic acid and B-carotene levels in women evaluated for HPV infection, smoking and cervical dysplasia.* Cancer Detection and Prevention 15(3): 165-69, 1991. ABSTRACT–75 women with abnormal pap smears were evaluated, and of those 45 had documented dysplasia with varying grades of severity. 53% of the dysplastic females were smokers. 66 of the subjects with dysplasia were positive for HPV. There was a mean reduction in vitamin C, retinol and B-carotene levels in the dysplastic group. There was a strong association between reduced plasma vitamin C levels and smoking history that was independent of cervical dysplasia or HPV status.

## III. Treatment

1) **Stop smoking and taking birth control pills**

2) **Cut back on fats,** especially of animal origin

3) **Cut back on consumption of toxic food sources**–fried eggs, deep fat fried foods, beef jerky, etc.

4) **Folate**–10mg/day for 3 months, then cut to 2.5mg/day. "Folarinse" from Scientific Botanicals –Cervical cytological abnormalities related to folate deficiency precede hematological abnormalities by many weeks. Folate is the most common deficiency in the world, and is quite common in women who are pregnant or taking BCPs. It is probable that many abnormal cytological smears reflect folate deficiency rather than being true dysplasia.

STUDY–Butterworth, C., et al. *Improvement in cervical dysplasia associated with folate therapy in users of BCP.* Am. J. Clin. Nut. 35:73-82, 1982. ABSTRACT–47 young women with mild or moderate dysplasia who had been on combo-type BCP for at least 6 months received either 10mg folate daily or placebo. Pretreatment RBC folate levels were lower in subjects on BCP's than in those not on BCP and lowest in subjects on BCP with cervical dysplasia. After 3 months, cervical biopsies showed significant improvement only in the women receiving folate. The dysplasia completely disappeared in 7 women receiving folate, while 4 women on placebo showed progression to carcinoma in situ.

STUDY–Whitehead, N., et al. *Megaloblastic changes in the cervical epithelium associated with BCP and reversal with folate.* JAMA 226:1421-4, 1973. ABSTRACT–115 women taking BCP had megaloblastic changes in cervical cells, compared to none of the 51 controls. 8 women with the abnormal cervical cytology took 10mg of folate daily for 3 months and all had complete remission or marked improvement!!

**NOTE**–It was found that serum levels of folate were normal in women with dysplasia and even elevated in some cases. It is believed that BCP may induce the synthesis of a protein that blocks the uptake of folate. When RBC folate levels were monitored, it was found that levels were depressed. Regression rates for patients with untreated cervical dysplasia are typically 1.3% for mild and 0% for moderate dysplasia. When treated with folate the regression rate was observed to be 20% to 100% in different studies.

5) **Beta-carotene**–200,000iu/day–as well as concentrating on beta carotene rich foods such as apricots, yams, yellow vegetables, carrots, etc.

STUDY–Wilie-Rosett, J., et al. *Influence of Vitamin A on cervical dysplasia and carcinoma in situ.* Nutrition and Cancer 6(1):49-57, 1984. ABSTRACT–Vitamin A and beta-carotene intake, as well as cellular retinol binding protein levels, were assessed for 87 women with dysplastic changes or carcinoma in situ. Women consuming less than average vitamin A and beta carotene were 3x as likely to develop severe dysplasia and 2.75x as likely to develop cancer in situ. Binding protein levels in the cervical tissue samples were inversely correlated with the severity of the dysplasia.

STUDY–Orr, J., Wilson, K., Bodifordwith, et al. *Nutritional status of patients with untreated cervical cancer. Biochemical and immunologic assessment.* Am. J. Ob. Gyn. 151:625-31, 1985. ABSTRACT–It was found that while only 6% of patients with untreated cervical CA had below normal serum vitamin A levels, 38% had stage-related abnormal levels of beta carotene.

6) **Vitamin B-6**–100mg 3x/day

7) **Vitamin C**–1gm 3x/day–Intake has been negatively correlated with the degree of dysplasia.

STUDY–Wassertheil-Smoller, S., et al. *Dietary vitamins and uterine cervical dysplasia.* Am J Epidemiol. 114(5):714-24, 1981. ABSTRACT–Dietary habits of 49 women with cervical abnormalities were compared to those of 49 matched controls. 29% of cases with dysplasia had vitamin levels to 3% of controls (less than 50% of the RDA). This resulted in a 10 fold increased risk for developing cervical dysplasia. Multiple logistic analysis indicated that low vitamin intake is an independent risk factor for the development of severe cervical dysplasia when all other factors are equal.

8) **Vitamin E**–400-800iu/day

9) **Selenium**–100-200mcg/day

STUDY–Dowson, E., et al. *Serum vitamin and selenium changes in cervical dysplasia.* Fed. Proc. 43:612, 1984. ABSTRACT-Serum selenium levels were significantly lower in patients with cervical dysplasia.

10) **Zinc picolinate**–30mg/day

**NOTE**-See *Gynecology and Naturopathic Medicine* by Dr. Tory Hudson. National College of Naturopathic Medicine bookstore (503) 255-4860. This book has a comprehensive discussion on the naturopathic treatment of cervical dysplasia.

## Notes

# BENIGN PROSTATIC HYPERTROPHY (BPH)

- Symptoms of bladder outlet obstruction, such as urinary frequency, urgency, nocturia, hesitancy, and intermittency with reduced force and caliber of urine are indicative of BPH.
- 50-60% of males between the ages of 40-59 years have BPH and by age 80 more than 80% have BPH based on autopsy studies. One study of males age 30-49 years showed the incidence of precancerous prostate gland lesions to average over 30%!
- The annual overall cost of hospital care and surgery for BPH is over 4 billion dollars per year in the U.S. alone, with over 400,000 surgeries being performed yearly.
- Pain in the prostate is not necessarily related to infection of the prostate; only 5% of all prostatitis is bacterial, usually E. coli.

## I. Etiology

- According to Merck, the etiology of BPH is "unknown but may involve alterations in hormonal balance associated with age."
- Nutrient deficiencies may play a role in BPH.
- Prostaglandin deficiency is also a suspected cause.

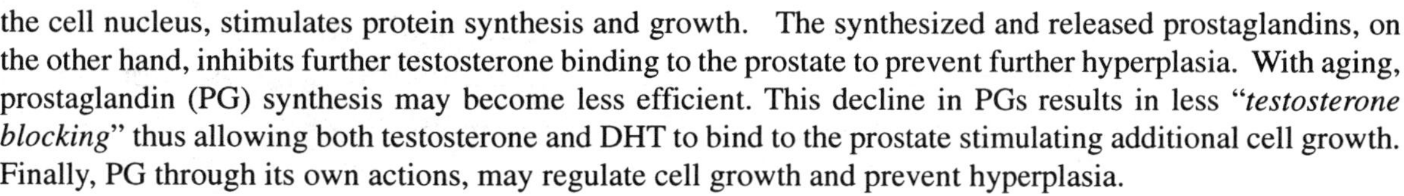


STUDY–Klein, L. & Stoff, J. *Prostaglandins and the prostate: An hypothesis on the etiology of BPH.* Prostate 4(3):247-51, 1983. ABSTRACT–It is believed that testosterone, once it enters the prostate cell, both converts to dihydrotestosterone (DHT) and stimulates prostaglandin synthesis and release. DHT, when it enters the cell nucleus, stimulates protein synthesis and growth. The synthesized and released prostaglandins, on the other hand, inhibits further testosterone binding to the prostate to prevent further hyperplasia. With aging, prostaglandin (PG) synthesis may become less efficient. This decline in PGs results in less "*testosterone blocking*" thus allowing both testosterone and DHT to bind to the prostate stimulating additional cell growth. Finally, PG through its own actions, may regulate cell growth and prevent hyperplasia.

## II. Signs and Symptoms

Classically, BPH symptoms include progressive urinary frequency, urgency, and nocturia due to incomplete emptying and rapid refilling of the bladder. Hesitancy and intermittency with decreased size and force of the urinary stream occur along with sensations of incomplete emptying, terminal dribbling, continuous overflow incontinence, or complete urinary retention.

**NOTE**–During a rectal exam the prostate may seem small, but it could still be large enough or congested enough to cause urethral obstruction or partial blockage.

## III. Diagnosis

a) Palpation of the prostate–Stony hard indicates probable cancer. Tenderness indicates prostatitis. The usual presentation for BPH is soft, amorphous, irregular, with no central sulcus.
b) Cystoscopy permits estimation of the gland size and the appropriate surgical approach. It also offers the opportunity to differentiate between vesical neck contracture, chronic prostatitis, and other obstructive phenomena.
c) Prostatic acid phosphatase should be less than 3.
d) Prostatic antigen (PSA) should normally be no higher than 3.0. If there is BPH, then a value no higher than 12.0 is acceptable. However, if no BPH is present, a value of 12 is reason for biopsy. When PSA is between 4-10, 20% of biopsies are cancerous and if a nodule is present that rate jumps to 50-60% .
e) Consider a hair analysis for cadmium toxicity. There is some evidence to show that there are higher levels of cadmium in cancerous and hyperplastic prostates. Evidence is conflicting. Cadmium inhibits zinc function and selenium, both of which are lower in men with prostate cancer.

## IV. Treatment

1) **Decrease cholesterol** (both blood levels and intake)–Cholesterol metabolites are cytotoxic and carcinogenic and have been shown to accumulate in the hyperplastic or cancerous human prostate. Epoxycholesterols initiate degeneration of epithelial cells, leading to the increased regeneration seen in BPH (LDL oxidizes the most easily).

STUDY–Hinman, F. *BPH* Springer-Verlag N.Y., 1983. ABSTRACT– Hypocholesterolemic drugs have been shown to have a favorable influence on BPH, preventing the accumulation of cholesterol in the prostatic cells and limiting subsequent formation of epoxycholesterols.

2) **Decrease animal products** that may contain DES residues.

3) **Eat foods containing zinc**–nuts, walnuts, pumpkin seeds, safflower seeds, oysters.

**Zinc picolinate**–60mg/day–Inhibits the activity of 5-alpha reductase, the enzyme that irreversibly converts testosterone to dihydrotestosterone (DHT). DHT has a 3-4X greater affinity to prostatic androgen receptors than testosterone. Zinc also has the ability to inhibit binding of androgens to prostatic receptors. Zinc, in addition, inhibits prolactin secretion. Prolactin has been shown to increase the binding of testosterone to prostatic tissue. Prolactin antagonists such as bromocriptine have been shown to reduce many of the symptoms of BPH.

**NOTE**–Do not forget copper when supplementing zinc for long periods of time, as in the treatment of BPH. It is necessary to balance zinc with copper (a minimum ratio of 30 to 1), other wise an increase in total cholesterol and a reduction in HDL can occur thus increasing the risk of cardiovascular disease.

STUDY–Fahim, M. *Zinc treatment for the reduction of hyperplasia of the prostate.* Fed. Proc. 35:361, 1976 ABSTRACT–Zinc supplementation reduced the size of the prostate and BPH symptomatology in the majority of patients in this study.

STUDY–Bush, I. *Zinc and the prostate*: presented at the annual meeting of the Am. Med. Assoc., Chicago, 1974. ABSTRACT–19 men with BPH took 150mg of zinc sulfate daily for 2 months, and then 50-100mg daily. 14 of the 19 had shrinkage of the prostate as determined by rectal palpation, X-Ray, and endoscopy. In 200 men with chronic abacterial prostatitis, 50-150mg zinc daily for 2-16 weeks relieved symptoms in 70%.

**4) Flax oil**–2 T/day–for prostaglandin synthesis

STUDY–Hart, J. & Cooper, W. *Vitamin F in the treatment of BPH.* Report #1 Lee foundation for nutritional research, Milwaukee, Wisconsin, 1941. ABSTRACT–19 men with BPH took six 5 grain tablets daily of Vitamin F complex, a concentrate containing 10mg of linoleic, linolenic and arachidonic acids. This dosage was continued for 3 days, then 4 tablets were taken daily for several weeks, then a maintenance dose of 2 tablets daily. All cases showed a diminution of residual urine. 12 of 19 had no residual urine by the end of the treatment period. Nocturia was eliminated in 13 of the 19 cases. Dribbling was eliminated in 18 of the 19. All subjects had a reduction in prostate size as determined by palpation.

**5) Amino Acid combination:**

**Glycine–200mg/day**
**Glutamic acid–200mg/day**
**Alanine–200mg/day**

"*Prostall*" (Probiologics) or *Prostex* (Levine) . Two 6 grain caps 3x/day

STUDY–Dumrau, F. *BPH: Amino Acid therapy for symptomatic relief.* Am J. Ger. 10:426-30, 1962. ABSTRACT–45 patients with BPH were supplemented with glutamic acid, alanine, and glycine. Nocturia was relieved or reduced in 95%, urgency by 81%, frequency was reduced 73%, and delayed micturition alleviated in 70%.

STUDY–Shimaya, M. & Sugiura, H. *Double blind test of PPC for prostatic hyperplasia.* Hinyokika Kiyo 16(5):231-36, 1970. ABSTRACT- Patients randomly received:

1) L-glutamic acid, L-alanine and glycine;
2) L-glutamic acid and L-alanine;
3) L-glutamic acid alone.

Outcomes showed a significant difference between the reduction in subjective symptoms in the group receiving all 3 agents versus the 2 control groups. However, in none of the patients was satisfactory improvement observed on rectal palpation or x-ray exam.

**6) Selenium**–100mcg. In studies showing cadmium induced hyperplasia in human prostates, selenium was shown to have a prophylactic effect.

STUDY–Webber, M. *Selenium prevents the growth stimulatory effects of cadmium on human prostatic epithelium.* Biochem. Biophy. Res. Commun. 127(3):871-77, 1985. ABSTRACT–When the degree of epithelial growth was examined from Cd it was found that selenium could block these effects.

**7) Vitamin E**–800-1200iu. A good rule of thumb is to give antioxidants when you supplement EFA.

**8) Prostatic tissue**–Protomorphogens

**9) Quercetin**–500mg t.i.d.

STUDY–Theoharides, T.C., et al. *Mast cell activation in sterile bladder and prostate inflammation.* International archives of allergy and applied immunology, 92:281-86, 1991. ABSTRACT–This study involves a case study of a 48 year old male who had chronic sterile hematuria dysuria and lower abdominal pain with significant number of bladder and prostate mast cells. He had significantly elevated histamine in his urine. This histamine released in the bladder wall of interstitial cystitis may be responsible for the pathophysiology of the disease. Antihistamines have had little success in interstitial cystitis, but in rat studies disodium cromoglycate has shown some benefit in chemical cystitis.

**10) Saw palmetto**–inhibits 5 alpha reductase and has been very effective in treating BPH

STUDY–Champlault G, Patel JC & Bonnard AM.. *A double-blind trial of an extract of the plant Serenoa repens in BPH.* Brit J Clin Pharmacol 18, 461-62, 1984. ABSTRACT–This double bind study showed that Pygeum extract was significantly more effective than placebo at reducing major symptoms of BPH

STUDY–Schneider HJ, Honold E, Mashur T. *Treatment of BPH. Results of a surveillance study in the practices of urological specialists using a combined plant-base preparation.* Fortschr Med 113:37-40, 1995.

STUDY–Koch E, Biber A. *Pharmacological effects of sabal and urtica extracts as a basis for a rational medication of benign prostatic hyperplasia.* Urologe 334:90-95, 1994.

STUDY– Braeckman J. The extract of Serenoa repens in the treatment of benign prostatic hyperplasia: A multicenter open study. Cur Ther Res 55(7):776-785, 1994.

### 11) Pygeum africanum–

STUDY–Dufour B & Choquenet C. *Trial controlling the effects of Pygeum africanum extract on the functional symptoms of prostatic adenoma.* Annul Urology. 18, 193-195, 1984. ABSTRACT–This double bind study showed that Pygeum extract was significantly more effective than placebo at reducing major symptoms of BPH. It was noted in this study that the placebo had a relatively high rate of improvement as well.

STUDY–Donkervoort T, et al. *A clinical and urodynamic study of Tadenan in the treatment of BPH.* Urology. 8, 218-25, 1977. ABSTRACT–This double bind study showed that Pygeum extract was significantly more effective than placebo at reducing objective symptoms such as daytime frequency, nighttime frequency, weak stream & hesitation.

## Miscellaneous Studies

## Tomato and lycopenes

Lycopenes found in tomato products particularly tomato paste, juice and sun dried tomatoes, have been shown to be quite protective against prostate cancer. In one study 10 servings per week significantly reduced the incidence of prostate cancer.

STUDY–Mills PK, Beeson WL, Phillips RL, Fraser GE. *Cohort study of diet, lifestyle, and prostate cancer in Adventist men.* Cancer 64:598-604, 1989.

STUDY–Carter HB, Coffey DS. *The prostate: an increasing medical problem.* Prostate 16:39-48, 1990.

STUDY–Hsing AW, Comstock GW, Abbey H, Polk F. *Serologic precursors of cancer. Retinol, carotenoids, and tocopherol and risk of prostate cancer.* JNCI 82:941-6, 1990.

STUDY–Levy J, Bosin E, Feldman B, Giat Y, et al. *Lycopene is a more potent inhibitory of human cancer cell proliferation than either beta-carotene or beta-carotene.* Nutr Cancer 24:257-66, 1995.

## Diet

STUDY–Mills, P., et al. *Cohort study of diet, lifestyle, and prostate cancer in Adventist men.* Cancer 64:64598-604, 1989. ABSTRACT–14,000 7th day Adventist males were studied from 1976-82. It was found that increased consumption of beans, lentils, peas, tomatoes, raisins, dates, and other dried fruit were all associated with a significant decreased prostate cancer risk. Previous prostate problems correlated with a 60% increased risk of prostate cancer, and consumption of animal products had a somewhat loose association.

STUDY–Mettlin, C., Selenskas, S., et al. *Beta-carotene and animal fats and their relationship to prostate cancer risk: A case control study.* Cancer 64:605-12, 1989. ABSTRACT–A case control study of 371 prostate cancer patients and comparable control subjects admitted to Roswell Park Memorial Institute, Buffalo, N.Y. was conducted. It was noted that there was a significant decrease in incidence of cancer in patients who had high levels of beta-carotene intake. The effect was only significant in men under the age of 68. Although overall fat content of the diet did not show increased risk, the consumption of high fat milk did. This study supports the weight of evidence which appears to favor the hypothesis that animal fat intake is related to increased risk for cancer of the prostate.

## Notes

---

# Infertility

- Infertility can be a very complex problem that has many psychological and physiological causes.
- Infertility is defined as failure to conceive after one year of unprotected intercourse.
- Infertility affects an estimated 20% of all couples

## I. Etiology

There may be a problem with either the male or female. The major factors are as follows: abnormalities in sperm (40%), abnormal tubal dysfunction (30%), ovulatory dysfunction (20%), cervical factors (5%) and unidentified factors (10%). Over the last 10 years the rate of male infertility has risen significantly. There are many theories to help explain this. Since fertility is not essential for the survival of one person, this increase in infertility may be a result of declining nutritional status, toxins in the environment or a general sign of unhealthiness in the general population. In males there can be a problem with the sperm count, motility, morphology and/or agglutination.

## II. Treatment for males

1) **Decrease cholesterol & improve cardiovascular system**
2) **Decrease animal products** that may contain DES residues.
3) **Eat foods containing zinc**–nuts, pumpkin seeds, wheat germ, oysters (see list p.121).
4) **Carnitine**–1 gm 3x per day
5) **Arginine**–2gms 2x per day
6) **Zinc picolinate**–60mg/day–inhibits the activity of 5 alpha reductase
7) **Magnesium**–check ionic magnesium or Exatest (both measure intracellular magnesium levels, see magnesium p.103)-400mg 2x/day or sustained release magnesium (Omnivite).
8) **EPO, EPA, flax oil**–increase production of PGE1 and PGE3
9) **Vitamin E**–400iu 2x per day
10) **Vitamin C**–1gm 3x per day

## II. Treatment for Females

1) **Decrease cholesterol & improve cardiovascular system** (see atherosclerosis p. 243).
2) **Decrease animal products** that may contain DES residues.
3) **Hypothyroid**–very common in women, but men can have low sperm count with low thyroid
4) **Relaxation**–meditation, yoga, prayer can all be useful tools in relaxation. In Chinese Medicine it is common for the female, because of family and societal pressures, to become tense and anxious about getting pregnant. It is a good idea not to think about having a baby if you have been trying for a while. Chinese herbs and acupuncture can be very helpful.
5) **Multi-mineral/vitamin supplement** (high in antioxidant nutrients)
6) **Adrenal insufficiency**–XS cortisol production (stress) can decrease DHEA levels. Consider adrenal supplements along with vitamins E, C, and B-5 (all concentrated in the adrenals).

# Pre-eclampsia and Nausea/Vomiting of Pregnancy

## Pre-eclampsia

**Prevention:**

1) **Diet high in protein**. Should get at least 75-100 gms of protein depending upon body weight. Follow outline p.260 "Cholesterol Lowering Diet" diet. Read Metabolic Disease of Late Pregnancy: A Disease of Malnutrition, Thomas H. Brewer, 1982
2) **Calcium**–1500 mg total (see calcium table pg 111)
3) **Magnesium**–800 mg or to bowel tolerance, consider sustained release magnesium (Omnivite) Check intracellular magnesium levels via ionic magnesium, EXAtest, (see magnesium pg 103)
4) **Vitamin B6**–50-100 mg per-day
5) **High-potency multivitamin/mineral supplement** not over 20,000 IU per day of retinol (beta carotene OK) total food and supplement level
6) **Diet high in potassium** and low in sodium (see potassium pg 129)

**Treatment**:

1) **Vitamin B6**–100 mg 3x per-day (can also use P5P form of B6)
2) **Magnesium**–consider higher oral dose or IV magnesium sulfate 2-3 gm along with vitamin B6 100-300mg (can repeat daily as needed)
3) **Dandelion tincture**–35 drops 3x per-day
4) **Consider following blood-typing diet** (Eat Right for Your Type, D'Adamo)

## Nausea and Vomiting

1) **Vitamin K with Vitamin C**–5 mg 2x per-day taken with 500 mg 2x per-day of vitamin C (see reference p.180)

STUDY–Merkel, R. *The use of menadione bisulfite and ascorbate in the treatment of Nausea and Vomiting of pregnancy.* Am. J. Ob & Gyn. Aug 416-418,1952. ABSTRACT–64 out of 70 consecutive cases were helped with complete relief of symptoms in 3 days. 3 cases had the vomiting halted but not the nausea.

2) **Ginger Root**–can use the fresh herb as a tea, add lemon and honey (I freeze fresh ginger root and then grate into hot water and let seep for 15 minutes). Also consider Reed's Ginger Brew or equivalent (available in health food stores)
3) **Vitamin B6**–100 mg 3x per-day
4) **IM Vitamin K**–5 mg along with vitamin B6–100 mg, B-complex 1 cc and B-12 1cc as needed (daily if necessary)
5) **Pill Curing**-Chinese patent formula available in Chinese herbal stores or ITM (see pharmacy list in appendix).
6) **Acupuncture**-can be particularly helpful. They make wrist bands with magnets or pressure beads to apply over pericardium 6 acupuncture point.

# SCHIZOPHRENIA

- Schizophrenia is a condition in which the person withdraws from other people into a world of unrealistic fantasies and delusions.
- Chronic schizophrenics occupy more than 1/2 of all psychiatric hospital beds in the U.S.

## I. Etiology

1) **Autoimmunity**–Anti-brain antibodies have been demonstrated in schizophrenics. It has been found that a large number of schizophrenics have antibodies to herpes, influenza and EBV. It is possible that live virus vaccinations may be increasing the number of schizophrenics by stimulating the production of anti-brain antibodies.

2) **Food sensitivities** from toxic neuropeptides - pepsin hydrolysates of wheat gluten have demonstrated opioid activity.

STUDY–Mycroft. *MIF-like sequences in milk & wheat proteins*. New Eng. J. Med. 307(14): 895, 1982. ABSTRACT–It was found that the amino acid sequence Pro-Leu-Gly is generated with the enzymatic breakdown of alpha gliadin. This amino acid sequence represents a moiety found in MIF. Casein found in milk also has the same sequence. Animal studies have shown that MIF enhances dopaminergic activity in the CNS and antagonizes both the behavioral and neurochemical effects of neuroleptic drugs. It has been found that 50mg worth of this tripeptide induces EEG changes in normal subjects and 75mg has induced mood changes in clinically depressed subjects (an average diet contains about 150mg of this tripeptide).

STUDY–Singh & Kay. *Wheat gluten as a pathogenic factor insSchizophrenia.* Science 191: 401-2, 1976. ABSTRACT–14 non-paranoid schizophrenics eliminated milk and cereal grains for 14 weeks. There was a significant improvement in 10 of these patients. When wheat gluten was introduced back into the diet improvement stopped or reversed.

3) **Nutrient deficiencies**

a) **Niacinamide**

b) **Vitamin B-6**

c) **Folate**–Folate deficiency is associated with a wide variety of psychiatric symptoms including psychosis, depression, confusion, disorientation, and dementia,as well as with neurologic symptoms of weakness, numbness, stiffness and spasticity, both with and without muscular atrophy.

STUDIES–Kallstrom. *Vit B-12 and folate concentrations in mental patients.* Acta Psychiat. Scand. 45:137-52, 1969. **and** Hunter et al. *Folate and B-12 conc. in mental patients.* Brit. J. Psychiat. 113:1292-5, 1967. ABSTRACT–**25% of all patients in state mental hospitals are deficient in folate.**

d) **L-tryptophan**

STUDY–Gilmour. *Assoc. of plasma tryptophan levels with clinical change in female schizophrenic patients.* Biol. Psychiat. 6:119, 1973. ABSTRACT–Plasma tryptophan levels was found to be low in female schizophrenics and rose during periods of improvement, while remaining low in patients who failed to improve.

e) **Zinc**–In one study of autopsies, it was discovered that various aspects of schizophrenic brains had only 50% of the Zinc content of control brains.

f) **Essential Fatty Acids–Linoleic acid, GLA, and $PGE_3$**

STUDY–Horrobin, Huang. *Schizophrenia: the role of abnormal EFA metabolism.* Med. Hypotheses 10:329-36, 1983. ABSTRACT–Schizophrenics were found to be deficient in Linoleic acid, GLA, DGLA, and $PGE_3$, but had an excess of arachidonic acid and its 2 series prostaglandins.

**g) Polysystemic candidiasis**

STUDY–Truss, *The Missing Diagnosis*, Birmingham, Ala. p. 86, 1982.

## II. Treatment

**1) Eliminate gluten and milk products**

**2) Avoid caffeine**–Caffeine has been shown to increase synthesis of epinephrine & norepinephrine in the CNS of rats.

**NOTE**–Jonathan Wright, M.D., in a personal exchange, stated that more than **50% of schizophrenics are hypoglycemic.** Thus, you may want to consider treatment with a hypoglycemic diet.

**3) Vitamin B-6**–500mg 3x/day–30% of schizophrenic patients excrete abnormal amounts of kryptopyrrole (KP). It is theorized by Dr. Pfeiffer that this compound binds pyridoxine and causes it to be excreted in the urine. This, however, only amounts to a few mgs/day. It is also possible that KP may interfere with other B6 dependant enzymes, meaning that it may take a very large amount to overcome this inhibition.

STUDY–Pfeiffer. *Treatment of pyroluric schizophrenia with large doses of B-6 and a dietary supplement of zinc.* J. Orthom. Psych. 3:4, 292-300, 1974. ABSTRACT–More than 300 pyroluric patients were treated with B-6 and zinc, with remission of psychosis in most. Upon cessation of supplements symptoms returned.

STUDY–Cruz & Vogel. *Pyroluria: A poor marker in chronic schizophrenia.* Am J Psychiat. 135(10):1239-40, 1978. ABSTRACT–9 schizophrenics taking neuroleptics and 10 healthy controls were evaluated for urinary pyrrole. Their pyrrole levels were then compared with their signs and symptoms. It was found that a poor correlation existed between these parameters. It was postulated by the authors that perhaps Pfeiffer's observations were made on *acute schizophrenics* with secondary porphyria which may be associated with psychotic symptoms and B-6 deficiency.

**4) Niacinamide**–Abram Hoffer prefers niacin. Interestingly Schizophrenics do not have the same flushing reaction to the niacin as do others. 1gm 3x/day time release from Theratech. Can use niacinhexaniacinate (Thorne Niasafe) and it appears to not have the same effect on raising liver enzymes.

**NOTE**–Watch for nausea and elevation of liver enzymes.

STUDY–Ananth. *Potentiation of therapeutic effects of nicotinic acid by pyridoxine in chronic schizophrenics.* Can. Psychiatr. Assoc. J. 18:377-83, 1973. ABSTRACT–30 chronic patients hospitalized at least 2 years received either 3gms nicotinic acid and 75mg pyridoxine for 48 weeks, nicotinic acid and placebo, and pyridoxine and placebo. There was significant improvement in each of the singly supplemented groups, but not the combined group, although, the combined group was the only group able to lower its dose of phenothiazine.

**5) Zinc**

**6) Manganese**

**7) Vitamin C**–3-6gms/day

**8) Black current oil**–3caps 3x/day (check for dry skin)

**9) Folate**–2mg/day

STUDY–Pfeiffer & Braverman. *Folate & Vit B-12 therapy for low-histamine, high-copper biotype of schizophrenia* in Botez, MI, Folic acid in Neurology, Psychiatry, and Internal Medicine. N.Y. Raven Press, 1979, 483-87. ABSTRACT–Patients who had low histamine levels and high copper levels responded favorably when supplemented with B3, Zinc, Vit. C, folate, and B-12.

**NOTE**–Folate can cause an extreme exacerbation of psychotic behavior if blood levels become elevated.

**10) Treatment for systemic candida**–see chapter on polysystemic candidiasis.

Reference-Natural Healing for Schizophrenia and other Common Mental Disorders Eva Eldelman

## Notes

---

# DEPRESSION

- Depression is the most common emotional disorder. Approximately 25% of all Americans suffer from depression at one time or another during their lifetime.
- At any given time, as many as 20 million Americans, or 13% of the population, may be suffering from serious depression. It is the leading cause of hospitalization for mental illness.

There are 3 basic types of depression:

- **Reactive**–This type arises from an external situation, such as financial difficulties, marital problems, or the death of a loved one. These people often improve with time or with the insights of a psychotherapist.
- **Endogenous**–Where no obvious event seems to trigger the illness, the depression seems to come from inside the person. These people do not respond to psychotherapy and are incapable of lifting themselves from their misery.
- **Drug induced** by birth control pills, hypertensive medications, etc.

## I. Etiology

1) **Drug induced**–Oral Contraceptives–It is thought that in a significant number of cases, depression is caused by oral contraceptives. which create a vitamin B-6 deficiency. Other nutrient deficiencies thought to be caused by oral contraceptives are folate, vitamin B-1, vitamin C, and vitamin B-2. Other drugs which can cause depression include alcohol, nicotine, cannabis, caffeine, corticosteroids, betablockers, and other anti-hypertensive medications.

2) **Hypothyroidism** is one of the most frequent causes of depression and must be ruled out.

3) **Nutrient deficiencies**

a) **Vitamin B-6**–coenzyme in the production of monoamine neurotransmitter; also cofactor for delta-6-desaturase, the rate limiting enzyme for the production of PGE1, a hormone that may be helpful in prevention of depression (Essential Fatty Acids and Immunity in Mental Health, by Charles Bates). B-6 is also a vital cofactor for the conversion of tryptophan into serotonin and melatonin.

STUDY–Russ. *Vit B-6 status of depressed and obsessive-compulsive patients.* Nutrition Reports International, 867-73, 1983. ABSTRACT–7 depressed patients were studied for plasma pyridoxal phosphate levels. It was found that 4 of 7 depressed patients were B-6 deficient, and none of the 7 controlled patients were. Using an enzyme stimulation test (EGOT), all of the depressed patients were deficient in B-6 and none of the controls were.

**EGOT TEST** (Tahoma Labs)–Erythrocyte glutamic oxaloacetic transaminase activation. Start with 100mg 3x/day. Measure the activity of this enzyme. Double the dose to 200mg 3x/day and, after 10 days, measure the enzyme activity again. If it goes up, double the dose again and see if the activity of the enzyme goes up again. Continue doubling until enzyme activity plateaus. Obviously, symptoms should be monitored as well. The dose does not need to go higher once the patient responds favorably.

b) **Folate**–often deficient in psychiatric patients

c) **Vitamin B-12**
d) **Iron**
e) **Thiamin**
f) **Vitamin C**
g) **Essential fatty acids (especially omega 6 fatty acids)–**

**4) Excessive consumption of methylxanthines such as theobromine, theophylin or caffeine from coffee, black tea, cola or chocolate**
**5) Excessive consumption of simple sugars triggering hypoglycemic reactions.**

**6) Imbalance in brain nucleotides**

**7) Higher requirement for neurotransmitters such as tyrosine and tryptophan**

The afferent nerve at the terminal button releases various chemical messengers including norepinephrine and monoamines. Anti-depressant medication such as monoamine oxidase inhibitors (MAOI) act by blocking the action of monoamine oxidase which keeps monoamines in the synapse active for a long period of time. Alternative treatments such as tyrosine and DL-phenylalanine act as precursors to norepinephrine which acts to stimulate the efferent nerve. The end result is mental stimulation and less depression.

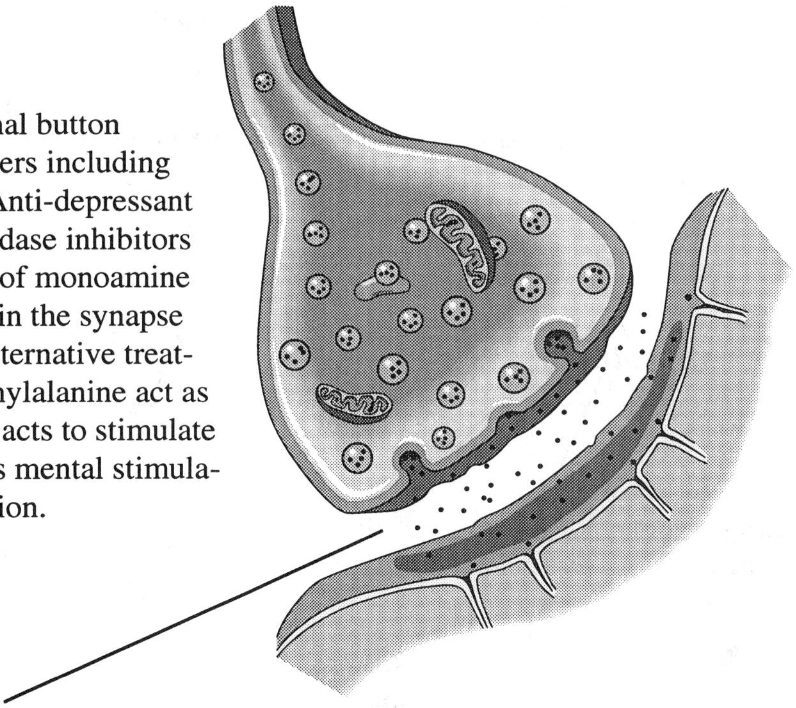

**Neurotransmitters involved in the synapse include norepinephrine, dopamine, gamma-amino-butyric acid and serotonin**

Serotonin reuptake inhibitors prevent serotonin from being taken back into the afferent nerve. This allows for more serotonin to be present in the synapse with the end result being serotonin stimulation. Various pharmaceuticals (Prozac, Paxil and Zoloft) along with St. John's Wort) are thought to work, at least in part, by this mechanism.

**TRYPTOPHAN LOAD TEST**

1) Give 2 gms of tryptophan orally
2) Collect urine for 24 hours
3) Urinary 3-hydroxykynurenine, kynurenine, and **xanthurenic acid** are measured. When high levels of xanthurenic acid are found in urine then pyridoxine is low.

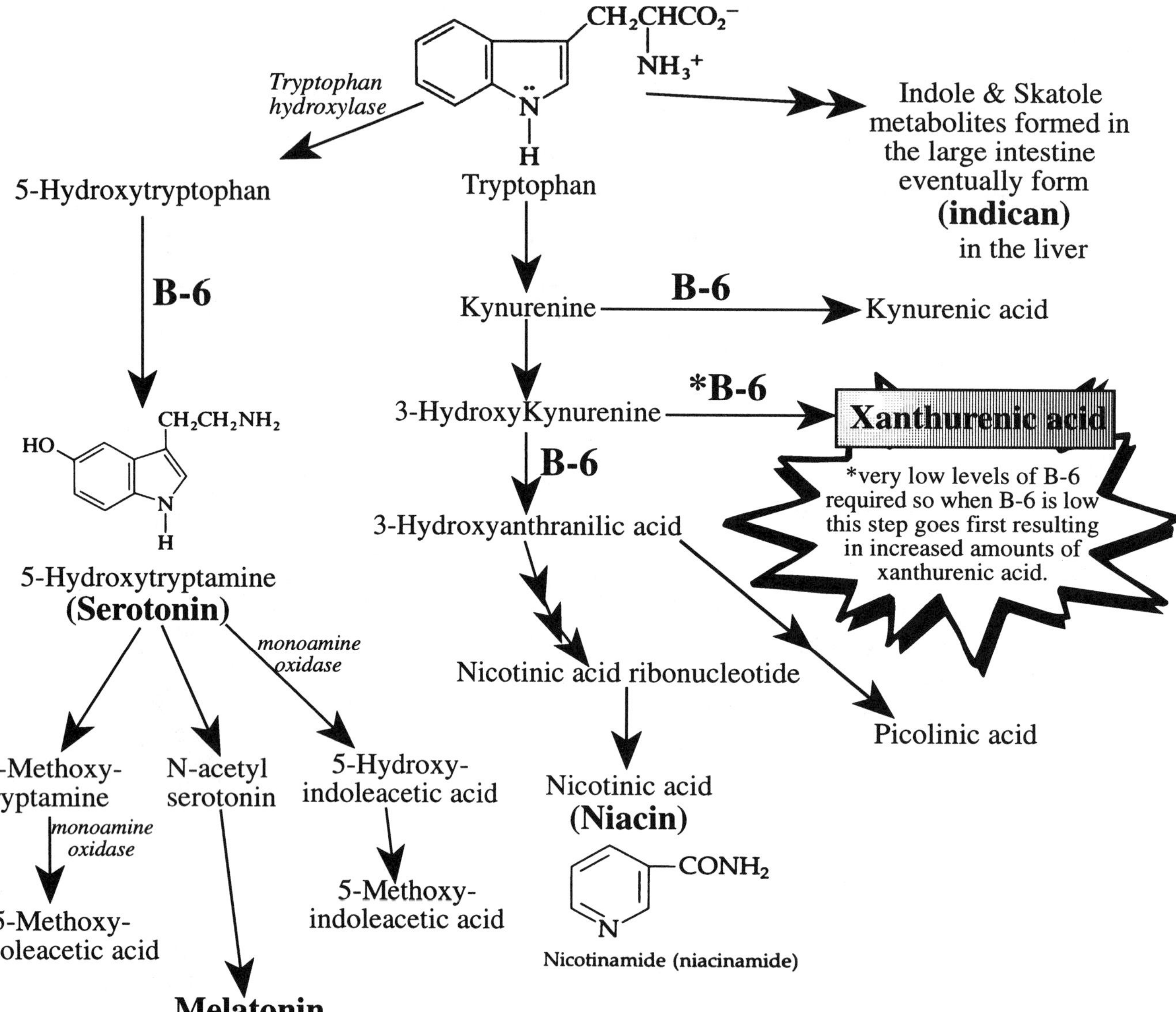


4) **Hypoglycemia**

5) **Heavy metal toxicity**–can do hair analysis to determine heavy metal toxicity.

6) **Bowel toxicity**–Constipation, abnormal bowel flora, parasites, etc. may cause depression.

7) **Toxic fumes**–Various agents can produce depression, including solvents used in paints, furniture making, and boat building etc. Cheateau, MT & Love Canal, NY are 2 places in the U.S. that toxic environmental chemical exposures have taken place.

## II. Diagnosis

This is obviously a very subjective definition, but the American Psychiatric Association in its Diagnostic and Statistical Manual of Mental Disorders gives the following 8 categories:

1) Poor appetite with weight loss, or increased appetite with weight gain.
2) Insomnia or hypersomnia.
3) Psychomotor agitation or retardation
4) Loss of interest or pleasure in usual activities, or decrease in sex drive.
5) Loss of energy and feelings of fatigue.
6) Feelings of worthlessness, self-reproach or inappropriate guilt.
7) Diminished ability to think or concentrate.
8) Recurrent thoughts of death or suicide.

It is felt that if 5 of these symptoms exist for at least 1 month then depression exists. 4 of these symptoms indicates that depression probably exists.

## III. Therapeutic Considerations

The goal should be to raise levels of brain monoamines, serotonin, melatonin, dopamine, epinephrine and norepinephrine.

1) Give precursors, substances which can be converted into active brain neurotransmitters.
2) Give cofactor or coenzyme therapy. This will allow the enzymes to work more efficient so that the patient requires less substrate (precursor).

## IV. Treatment

**1) Consider food sensitivities**

STUDY–Rippere V. *Some varieties of food intolerance in psychiatric patients: an overview.* Nutr Health,3(3):125-36, 1984. ABSTRACT–In this review it is stated that foods may cause many mental and behavioral symptoms by a variety of different mechanisms including cerebral allergy, food addictions, hypoglycemias, hyperinsulin reactions, caffeinism, hypersensitivity to chemical food additives, reactions to vasoactive amines in foods and reactions to neuropeptides formed from foods.

STUDY–King DS. *Can allergic exposure provoke psychological symptoms? a double-blind test.* Biol Psychiatry, 16(1):3-19, 1981. ABSTRACT–30 patients with depression, confusion, difficulty concentrating or other psychological symptoms noted significantly grater cognitive emotional symptoms when tested with sub-lingual antigens (foods and chemicals) compared to placebos (p=0.0001). There was also found to be the most severe reactions to the real antigens than compared to the placebo. There was also a greater variability of heart rate change was found for allergens than for placebos (p=0.008).

**2) Hypoglycemic diet–**(See under allergies)

**3) Treat hypothyroidism–**Low thyroid function is a very common cause of depression and should always be checked for (see hypothyroid, the Unsuspected Illness Broda Barnes)

**4) Chelate heavy metals–**(see heavy metal toxicity chapter).

**5) Avoid toxic fumes** including cigarette smoke. Inhaling toxic fumes results in an increased level of cortisol and may exacerbate a pre-existing hypoglycemia. Cortisol decreases the uptake of tryptophan in the brain resulting in decreased levels of serotonin.

**6) Vitamin B-6**–100mg 3x/day– is a cofactor for the conversion of tryptophan into serotonin and niacin.

STUDY–Adams. *Effect of B-6 upon depression associated with oral contraception* Lancet, Apr.28: p.897-904, 1973. ABSTRACT–22 depressed women were suspected of having B-6 deficiency depression due to BCP. 1/2 of them took a placebo for 2 months and the other 1/2 20mg B-6 2x/day. They then switched. 11 of the women were found to have decreased serum B-12 levels in the blood. Every one of these women responded favorably when on the B-6 while none of the women who were not deficient responded.

STUDY–Baumblatt, Michael, and Winston. *B-6 and the Pill.* Lancet, April 18, 1970, p.832-33. ABSTRACT–58 women who were depressed and taking the pill (BCP) were treated with 25mg B-6 2x/day at first sign of PMS depression. After 3 months of therapy, more than 75% of the women reported either complete relief or considerable improvement in their symptoms. The 44 women who seemed to respond to B-6 were then asked to discontinue treatment to see if their symptoms would return. **All the women refused to discontinue their B-6**!

**NOTE**–There are times when B-6 supplementation can make symptoms worse. One explanation is that some cases of depression are due to an imbalance of the brain amines rather than a deficiency. B-6 might accentuate an amine that is already out of balance. The other explanation is that some people may have an enzyme that is extremely sensitive to B-6 and might convert the tryptophan outside the blood brain barrier (BBB) into metabolites that can't cross the BBB.

**7) L-Tryptophan** (substrate)–3-6gms/day (give together with pyridoxine)–They may stimulate the production of serotonin and melatonin, both of which have been found to be useful for the treatment of depression. If the patient has insomnia along with depression, tryptophan seems to be even more effective. Studies generally show mixed results. There may be a specific subset of depressed people who respond very well to treatment with tryptophan.

STUDY–Chouinard. *Tryptophan in the treatment of depression and mania* Adv. Biol. Psychiat. 10:47-66,1983. ABSTRACT–8 studies on the action of tryptophan in patients who were unipolar or of uncertain polarity were reviewed. 5 of the studies showed improvement of the majority of the patients, but they all lacked controls.

STUDY–Praag HM, Lemus C. *Monoamine precursors in the treatment of psychiatric disorders.* Nutrition and the Brain, Vol. 7, New York, Raven Press, Wurtman and Wurtman, p.49-88, 1986. ABSTRACT–L-tryptophan seems to enhance the action of MAOI and Lithium in both manic and depressed patients.

**NOTE**–Be careful when giving tryptophan. If the patient is deficient in B-6, then he/she may convert tryptophan into metabolic by-products that can inhibit the transport of tryptophan into the brain. In fact it is possible to cause a net deficiency in the brain.

**8) Folate**–Check for hypersegmented neutrophils and also serum folate.

STUDY–Godfry, PSA, et al. *Enhancement of recovery from psychiatric illness by methylfolate.* Lancet, 336:392-95, 1990. ABSTRACT–24/76 pts with major depression referred as out patients or candidates for psychiatric hospitalization had borderline or definite folate deficiency according to red-cell folate levels. These 24 people who were low in folate and were proven to have normal B-12 levels, randomly received placebo or 15mg folate in addition to standard psychotropic drugs. After 3 and 6 months there were significant improvements noted in the folate supplemented group compared to the placebo group.

STUDY–Coppen A. *Folic acid enhances lithium prophylaxis.* J Affective Disorders 10:9-13, 1986. ABSTRACT–42 pts. with affective disorders on lithium therapy received either 200mcg folate or placebo. Treatment lasted for 1 year and results showed a small insignificant change in the affective morbidity index (AMI) in the folate group compared to the placebo. In the unipolar patients that received the folate a significant improvement was noted in their average Beck depression scores. Overall it was noted that there was a correlation to the degree of depression and what the level of folate was in the tissues as measured by RBC measurements.

STUDY–Carney MWP. *Psychiatric aspects of folate deficiency.* Folic Acid in Neurology, Psychiatry and Internal Medicine. Botez, Reynolds, eds., New York, Raven Press, 1979. ABSTRACT–13 of 36 patients with endogenous depression or schizophrenia were found to have low serum folate levels. They were treated with folic acid along with standard treatment. 12 of the 13 subjects treated with the folate made a full social recovery (either with or without residual symptoms vs. 16/23 controls. Of 18 patients with endogenous depression who were hospitalized 10 or more days, the 10 folate treated patients average 23.3 days while the 8 controls averaged 32.9 days, a significant difference.

9) **Avoid foods containing tyramine** if the patient is on MAO inhibitors. Cheese, chicken, liver, sardines, red wine, yeast, beer, soured cream, eggplant, and green bean pods should all be avoided.

10) **Vitamin B-12**–IM 1000mcg 1x/week

11) **Avoid Nutrasweet** which increases CNS tyrosine and phenylalanine while decreasing tryptophan availability. This results in decreased levels of serotonin in the brain.

12) **DL-phenylalanine**–Start with 500mg/day and work up to 3-4gms. This is a precursor for epinephrine and phenylethylamine (PEA). PEA has amphetamine-like stimulant properties. **Chocolate has lots of PEA** and may help explain why people respond to it.

STUDY–Beckmann. *DL-phenylalanine versus imipramine: A double-blind controlled study.* Arch. Psychiat. Nervenkr. 227:49-58,1979. ABSTRACT–20 Patients received 75-200mg of DL-phenylalanine. After 3 weeks, 8 patients had complete recovery, 4 had a good response, 4 experienced a mild-moderate response, and 4 had no response.

13) **Tyrosine-2gms 3x/day**–Precursor for epinephrine.

STUDY–Gibson & Gelenberg. *Tyrosine for the treatment of depression* Adv. Biol. Psychiat. 10: 148-59,1983. ABSTRACT–3/5 patients had at least a 50% reduction of symptoms compared to 1/4 on the placebo. The reduction in depression was positively correlated with the increases in fasting plasma tyrosine.

STUDY–Buist. *The therapeutic predictability of tryptophan and tyrosine in the treatment of depression.* Int Clin Nutr. Rev. 3:1, 1983. ABSTRACT–2 groups of depressed patients were studied. Group A, which had low urinary levels of the norepinephrine metabolite, MHPG, failed to respond to amitryptyline (Elavil), which tends to raise norepinephrine levels more than serotonin. Rather they responded to imiprimine (tofranil), which tends to raise the level of serotonin. Group B, which had high levels of MHPG, responded more to amitryptylin (Elavil) which tends to raise levels of norepinephrine. They tended to not respond to tofranil.

STUDY–Van Praag HM. *Studies in the mechanism of action of serotonin precursors in depression* Psychopharm Bull. 20(3):599-602, 1984. ABSTRACT–This review article points out that the author has apparently conducted many double-blind studies using 200mg of L-5-hydroxytryptophan, 150mg carbidopa and/or tyrosine is effective for the treatment for depression because it enhances both 5HT and catecholamine metabolism. When L-tryptophan is used by itself at 5 gms per day it only increases 5HT and tends not to work that well.

14) **S-Adenosyl-L-Methionine(SAM)**–acts as methyl group donor in numerous reactions in the brain (see chapter on methionine under amino acids). It affects the turnover rate of monoamines such as serotonin and dopamine.

15) **MYBA** (MOVE YOUR BUNS AROUND)–Exercise is essential in the treatment of depression. Daily walks or some physical activity can stimulate endorphins.

16) **Evening Primrose Oil**–See *Essential Fatty Acids and Immunity in Mental Health* by Charles Bates. It has been found that depressed people in general have lower levels of PGE1. Usually they have a decreased activity of delta 6 desaturase and their ability to make more PGE1 is compromised. This is especially true of people whose ancestry is 25% or higher of Celtic Irish, Welsh, Scottish, Scandinavian or Native Indian origin.

**17) Hypericum perforatum (botanical)**–has been shown in numerous studies to be effective in the treatment of depression. It is probably best to use the whole plant as it has been found that it is not just the hypericin that provides the benefits for depression. It appears to inhibit the enzyme monoamine oxidase and to block the reuptake of serotonin.

STUDY–Muldner VH & Zoller M. *Antidepressive wirkung eines auf den*. Lancet, 336:392-95, 1990.

STUDY–Hö J. *Constituents and mechanism of action of St. John's wort.* Zeitscrhift Phytother 14:255 64, 1993.

STUDY–Suzuki O, Katsumata Y, Oya M. *Inhibition of monoamine oxidase by hypericin.* Planta Med 50:272-4, 1984.

STUDY–Hö J, Demisch L , Gollnik B. *Investigations about antidepressive and mood changing effects of Hypericum perforatum.* Planta Med 55:643, 1989.

STUDY–Reichert RG. *St. John's Wort for depression.* Quart Rev Nat Med summer:17-18 , 1994.

**18) Negative Ions-**It has been found that negative ions, which are produced in large amounts near the ocean, around a waterfall or after a rainstorm, help make people feel better in general. Consider living in areas that can provide these or buy a machine that can generate them.

**19) Full spectrum lighting and bright lights** (Health and Light, John Ott)

## Notes

# ANXIETY/PANIC ATTACKS

- Anxiety or nervousness affects over 14 million people in the U.S. Panic attacks, which can occur independent from anxiety, are extremely common and 80 million people in the U.S. experience at least one attack in their lifetime. Over 10 million people experience frequent recurring panic attacks.
- Symptoms include nervousness, a sense of inappropriate fear, shortness of breath, heart palpitations, numbing and tingling sensations around the body, excessive sweating, dryness in the mouth and a myriad array of seemingly unrelated symptoms. Agoraphobia (generalized anxiety) is defined as an intense fear of being alone or being in public places.

## I. Etiology

Anxiety is a syndrome that has many causes. It is usually a sign that something is going on in a person's psychological makeup that needs to be addressed. People who have survived severely disturbing experiences rape victims, soldiers from war (particularly Viet Nam), abusive childhood experiences etc. all tend to be prone to anxiety attacks especially if they have not received professional psychological counseling. Patients with anxiety or panic attacks have elevated levels of lactate. Injecting patients with lactate, who have a history of panic attacks, will trigger an episode. Injecting normal people causes no such reaction.

## II. Diagnosis

Diagnosis is usually made through process of elimination.

## III. Therapeutic Considerations

Try to explore the underlying reasons for the anxiety symptoms and address the emotion issues that may be precipitating these symptoms. In addition it is important to reduce those triggers that may lead to the anxiety attacks such as stimulants, medications, stressful situations. Consider a glucose insulin-tolerance test for evaluation of blood glucose problems.

## IV. Treatment

1) **Diet**–eliminate all stimulants: coffee, chocolate, cola, black tea (see Coming off Coffee, p.518) Consider avoiding food allergies and simple carbohydrates which could cause hypoglycemic reactions. Avoid alcohol as well.
2) **Niacinamide**–500 mg - 3 gm in divided doses, watch for nausea, cut back on dose if any
3) **Calcium/Magnesium**–1000 mg/500 mg
4) **Kava Kava**–can drink as tea or take in capsules
5) **Hypericum**–standardized extract especially if anxiety mixed with depression
6) **L-tryptophan**–500 mg–3 gm/day (take away from protein foods) along with B6 100 mg 2x/day
7) **Vitamin B12**–1000 mcg 2x per-day or IM 1-3 gm or consider as an IV vitamin cocktail to include B-6, B-3 and thiamin (may also use orally 100mg each per day)
8) **Heavy metal detoxification**-First check for elevated heavy metals and chelate if high.
9) **Omega 3 fatty acids**–2-6 T per day of flax seed oil

# HEADACHES AND MIGRAINES

- Migraines are recurrent, profoundly disabling headache attacks.
- While the headache is typically pounding and unilateral, it may become generalized.
- Psychological or visual disturbances often precede the attacks which may be accompanied by nausea and gastrointestinal upset or anorexia. Drowsiness often follows.
- The highest incidence of migraines is between the ages 20-35. Family history of migraines is present in more than 50% of patients.

## I. Etiology

The cause of migraines is unknown, however, 3 theories are currently being studied:

1) **Vasomotor Instability**–It is thought that there is an inherent vasomotor instability in migraine patients. Orthostatic symptoms occur more often in migraine sufferers than in normals. It is generally believed that the vasodilatory effects of physical and chemical agents are more profoundly felt by migraine patients. It has also been found that during attacks, there is vasodilation of the superficial cerebral vessels.
2) **Platelet Disorders**–The aggregation of platelets, both spontaneously and when exposed to serotonin and/or catecholamines, occurs more readily in migraine sufferers. While the total amount of serotonin is the same in migraine platelets and normals, the amount of serotonin released from migraine platelets goes up steadily with the approach of an attack. Interestingly, it has been found that mitral valve prolapse (MVP) occurs twice as often in migraine sufferers. The MVP damages platelets and increases their aggregation.
3) **Neuronal Disorder**–In this hypothesis, the primary initiator of the vascular events in migraines is the nervous system. It is thought that the trigeminovascular neurons release substance P in response to various stress factors or to changes in the CNS. An important mediator of pain, the release of substance P into the arteries is associated with vasodilation, mast cell degranulation, and increased vascular permeability. The theory is that the endothelial cells of the arteries release vasoactive substances–such as arachidonic acid metabolites, purine compounds, or molecules containing carbonyl groups–in response to substance P. It is generally thought that the functional changes in the noradrenergic system are brought about by chronic stress .

## II. Signs and Symptoms

Headaches may be preceded by short period of depression, irritability, restlessness, or anorexia, and in some cases by scintillating scotomas, visual field defects, paresthesias, or, rarely, hemiparesis. Nausea, vomiting, and photophobia are common. Extremities are cold and cyanosed, and the patient is irritable and seeks seclusion.

## III. Diagnosis

Signs and symptoms. Diagnosis is more likely with family history and/or visual prodromal symptoms.

## IV. Treatment

### 1) Treat underlying allergies

STUDY–Grant, E. *Food Allergies and migraine.* Lancet 1:966,1979. ABSTRACT–60 patients with frequent migraines were studied. Most of them had been using oral contraceptives, tobacco or ergotamine and had failed to improve by discontinuing these substances. Mean duration of migraines was 18 years for the women and 22 years for the men. Most of the patients had other symptoms including lethargy, depression, anxiety, flushing dizziness, abdominal pain, constipation, diarrhea, or rashes. Each patient ate an exclusion diet for 5 days, consisting only of 2 low risk foods usually lamb and pears and drank only bottled spring water. **Migraines disappeared by the fifth day in most cases**. Each patient then tested 1-3 common foods per day, looking for reactions. **Mean number of foods causing symptoms was 10 per patient** (range 1-30). Foods most frequently causing symptoms and/or pulse changes were wheat (78%), orange (65%), egg (45%), tea and coffee (40%) each, chocolate and milk (37%), beef (35%), corn, cane sugar, and yeast (33% each), mushrooms (30%), and peas (28%). When offending foods were avoided, all patients improved. The number of headaches in the group fell from 402 to 6 per month, with 85% of the patients becoming headache free. Exclusion only of amine-containing foods (e.g. cheese, chocolate, citrus, and alcohol) significantly reduced the number of headaches, but only 13% became headache free. All 15 patients with hypertension at the start of the study became normotensive with diet plus avoidance of other precipitants.

STUDY–Egger, J. *Is Migraine Food Allergy?: A double blind controlled trial of oligoantigenic diet treatment* Lancet Oct 15, p.865-9, 1983. ABSTRACT–**93% of 88 children with severe frequent migraine recovered on oligoantigenic diets**; the causative foods were established by a double-blind controlled trial in 40 of the children.

**2) Avoid dietary amines**–such as chocolate, cheese, citrus and alcohol. They contain vasoactive amines, such as beta-phenylethylamine and tyramine. These amines cause vasoconstriction either directly or indirectly through the liberation of catecholamines.

**3) Avoid arachidonic acid**–This will decrease platelet aggregation, decrease histamine release, and decrease inflammation associated with migraine.

**4) Increase consumption of EFA especially omega 3 fatty acids**–This will decrease platelet aggregation and change the membrane composition to more of the unsaturated fatty acids.

**5) Increase fiber and complex carbohydrates**–This will increase the number of bowel movements and decrease bowel transit time.

**6) Quercetin**–500mg 15 minutes prior to eating

STUDY–Monro, J. *Migraine is a food-allergic disease* Lancet Sept. 29, 1984. ABSTRACT–Foods which provoked migraine in 9 patients with severe migraine refractory to medications were identified. The patients were then given either sodium cromoglycate or placebo in a double-blind manner along with provoking foods. Sodium cromoglycate exerted a protective effect on the symptoms and immune complexes were not produced in the protected patients.

**7) Magnesium**–400-800mg/day–Magnesium is helpful in mitral valve prolapse. It also prevents release of catecholamines which is an important mediator of platelet aggregation. IV magnesium is very effective in the treatment of acute migraines. 2-5 grams of magnesium sulfate can be slowly pushed causing a vasodilation response. Care should be taken with people with low blood pressure as magnesium given IV can cause a drop in Bp.

STUDY–Schoenen, J., et. al. *Blood Magnesium Levels in Migraine* Cephalalgia, 97-99,1991. ABSTRACT–88 migraine sufferers were studied with and without auras. It was found that patients without auras had a significant reduction in RBC magnesium compared to sufferers with auras. No difference was seen in serum magnesium.

**8) Niacin**–100-400mg at the first onset of symptoms and 100mg/day prophylactically.

**9) EPO** inhibits platelet aggregation.

STUDY–Arregui, A., et. al. *High Prevalence of Migraine in a High Altitude Population.* Neurology, Oct 41:1668-70,1991. ABSTRACT–205 families from a Peruvian mining town at an altitude of 14,000 feet was compared to over 1000 individuals in the same country at sea levels for the frequency of migraine. The rates of all headaches were increased 22.3% at high altitudes compared to 14.5% at the lower altitudes. For migraines it was 12.4% versus 3.6% at sea level.

**10) Garlic**–Inhibits platelet aggregation.

**11) Tanacetum parthenium** inhibits the secretion of serotonin and other platelet granule constituents, decreases smooth muscle response to endogenous substances (norepinephrine, acetylcholine, bradykinin, prostaglandins, histamine, and serotonin), and inhibits the production of inflammatory substances (leukotrienes, thromboxanes).

STUDY–Johnson, E., Kadam, Hylands, and Hylands. *Efficacy of Feverfew as prophylactic treatment of migraine.* Br Med J. 5669-73, 1985. ABSTRACT–An initial survey found that 70% of 270 migraine sufferers who had eaten feverfew daily for prolonged periods of time had both decreased frequency and severity of migraine headaches. In a double blind study, patients who believed they received help from the herb received either the herb or a placebo. Most of the patients who were on the placebo had significant increase in the frequency and severity of headaches along with nausea and vomiting during the 6 months of the study, while patients taking the feverfew showed no change in the frequency or severity of their symptoms. 2 patients in the placebo group, who had been in complete remission during self-treatment with fever few leaves, developed recurrences of incapacitating migraines and had to withdraw from the study. The resumption of the herb in these 2 patients led to renewed remission of symptoms in both patients.

STUDY–Barsby, R., et. al. *Irreversible Inhibition of Vascular Reactivity by Feverfew.* Lancet Oct. 19, 338:1015, 1991. ABSTRACT–Effects of a crude extract were found to have parthenolide and other a-methylene-lactones which inhibited the contractile response, of aortic muscle rings from rabbits, to serotonin, phenylephedrine, thromboxane A2 agent, and angiotensin ll. **These effects were not observed from dried feverfew leaves obtained commercially from a health food store.**

STUDY–Makheja AN, Bailey JM. *A platelet phospholipase inhibitor from the medicinal herb feverfew (Tanacetum* parthenium). Prostagland Leukotrienes Med 8:653-60, 1982.

**12) Consider environmental allergens.**

**13) Thyroid**–especially for chronic non-migraine type headaches.

## Notes

---

## Notes

# HUMAN IMMUNODEFICIENCY VIRUS (HIV) INFECTION ACQUIRED IMMUNODEFICIENCY SYNDROME (AIDS)

- Onset may be sudden or insidious.
- Sudden onset may present with fever, sweats, malaise, fatigue, myalgia, arthralgia, headaches, sore throat, lymphadenopathy, diarrhea, macular erythematous truncal eruption.
- Symptoms of insidious onset may be an unexplained progressive fatigue, weight loss, fever, diarrhea, and generalized lymphadenopathy.
- Pneumocystis carinii pneumonia, a nonproductive cough and dyspnea, is the first presenting symptom in 50% of patients.
- Kaposi's sarcoma, reddish brown or bluish plaques or nodules on the cutaneous or mucosal surfaces is the initial symptom in 30%. Usually the sarcomi first appear on the lower extremities.
- Opportunistic infections, such as mucosal candidiasis or progressing anal herpes lesions, are the initial presentations in 12% of patients.

## General Considerations

First described in 1981, there were 37,000 cases of AIDS in the U.S. from 1981-1987 and over 21,000 deaths in the same time period. From 1987 to 1994 more than 323,000 cases of AIDS were reported. In 1994 alone there were 441,000 people in the U.S. that tested positive for AIDS. In 1995 the CDC determined that one out of every 250 people were infected with AIDS (about one million people) and a considerably higher number of carriers. Worldwide estimates are hundreds of millions of people are carriers.

It should be noted that 50% of the AIDS cases are made up African Americans, Hispanics, Asian/Pacific Islanders, American Indians and Alaska Natives (33% blacks & 17% Hispanic). Caucasians make up 49% of all cases. As of April 1995, the CDC reported that 53% of cases of AIDS have been from male to male contact and 25% through IV drug use. Women make up an increasing proportion which is estimated, in the U.S. as of 1996, at about 20%. The number of total cases is now doubling every 2 years. The number of heterosexual-contact cases of AIDS is increasing at the rate of about 120% every year. Adolescents, young adults, women, blacks and Hispanics are at the highest risk for heterosexually transmitted AIDS.

A profound defect in cell-mediated immunity is the chief characteristic of AIDS. This results in the onset of opportunistic infections and malignant diseases. Pneumocystis carinii and Kaposi's sarcoma have been mentioned. Others include CMV, EBV, HSV, Toxoplasma gondii, Mycobacterium tuberculosis, Salmonella, and Candida albicans to name a few. There are a number of conditions related to AIDS: ARC, PGL, an acute "mono-like" syndrome, chronic fatigue syndrome, PSC and an asymptomatic state.

**The major U.S. AIDS high-risk groups are:**

Group

Homosexual/bisexual men
IV drug users
Haitians
Hemophiliacs
Transfusion or blood product recipients
Heterosexual persons who have sexual contact with AIDS, or "at risk for AIDS", people.

The time period from the initial infection of HIV and the development of AIDS is very variable and it is not known that all HIV positive people develop full blown AIDS. There are documented cases of HIV positive people still alive today who have been positive since 1982.

> **NOTE**–It should be noted that there are many conditions that may predispose individuals to developing full blown AIDS. Not included in the above statistics are life style habits and other debilitating diseases which lower one's resistance to infection. One noteworthy exception has been presented in the book by Harris Coulter, *AIDS and Syphilis the Hidden Link.* The book discusses the extremely high prevalence of syphilis in patients with AIDS.

## I. Etiology

AIDS is caused by HIV infection which invades the genetic core of the CD4+ or T-helper lymphocyte cells. The infection causes a progressive depletion of CD4+ cells which results in a compromised immune function. The compromised immunity leads to opportunistic infections and cancers. Transmission is through blood, semen and in pregnancy across the placenta. It is not transmitted in saliva or by casual contact. The virus has been discovered in breast milk. Transmission through breast milk is not known, but it is recommended that HIV positive mothers not breast feed. There are a number of predisposing factors that are involved with contracting the AIDS virus. Below is a list of some of the predisposing factors:

1) Weakened immune system
    - a) Exposure to recreational drugs (e.g. smoking, alcohol, cannabis).
    - b) Pre-existing disease (e.g. HIV, syphilis, CMV, EBV, hepatitis, Candida, STD).

    STUDIES–Various studies have shown that there is a very high percentage of syphilitic infection of HIV positive patients. It is postulated that there has been a smoldering of subclinical as well as symptomatic cases of syphilis which have been improperly treated. The result is a lowered immunity to the HIV virus.

    - c) Exposure to immunosuppressive medications, steroids, chemotherapy (study–tetracycline has adverse effects on chemotaxis, lymphocyte transformation, phagocytosis).
    - d) Malnutrition with either subclinical or clinical deficiencies of various nutrients.
2) Environmental toxin exposure
3) Malabsorption
4) Food allergies
5) Stress (both lack of and too much) exercise and sleep have a stimulating effect on interleukin and interferon production
6) HIV exposure (measured via ELISA & Western blot test).
    - a) AIDS patients 50% isolation HIV & 95-100% antibody to HIV antigens.
    - b) ARC patients 80% isolation HIV & 70-95% antibody to HIV antigens.
    - c) "At risk" with depressed T4+ cells 30% isolation HIV & 75-95% antibody to HIV antigens.
    - d) "At risk" with norm T4+ 50-70% HIV antibodies.

## II. Signs and symptoms

There are many manifestations of AIDS including classic viral like symptoms such as sore throat, fever, joint pain and rashes. Persistent lymphadenopathy is common. Seroconversion occurs within 8 weeks after infection and individuals with and without symptoms can test positive for the HIV. Other common symptoms include night sweats, chronic or intermittent fatigue and malaise, diarrhea and weight loss. Other common finding are various types of opportunistic infections, malignancies, neurological diseases, and digestive problems. Opportunistic infections include bacteria, fungi, protozoa, and or other viruses. Candida, Cryptococcus, Cryptosporidium, CMV, Herpes simplex and zoster, Mycobacterium, and Pneumocystis carinii.

Often there are intestinal symptoms that are caused by enteric pathogens known as *AIDS enteropathy.* There is often damage to the small and large intestine showing villus atrophy with chronic inflammatory cells. This causes both malabsorption and increased permeability leading to various vitamin deficiencies (especially fat soluble) and allergies to various foods.

## III. Diagnosis

1) First evaluate signs and symptoms. For the diagnosis of AIDS there are a number of criteria to be met which leads to a high degree of suspicion. If there is a documented HIV + test along with Candida infection of bronchi, trachea, lungs or esophagus, Cryptococcosis, Cryptosporidium infection with chronic intestinal symptoms, CMV disease (other than liver, spleen or nodes), chronic Herpes simplex or zoster, Kaposi's sarcoma, various lymphomas, Mycobacterium infections, Pneumocystis carinii pneumonia, wasting syndrome due to HIV, Toxoplasmosis of the brain and systemic Salmonella to name a few.
2) HIV via first ELISA and then Western blot test (Note that high risk serum negative patients have had HIV isolated from their blood). CD4+ levels below 200/mm usually have serious consequences regarding opportunistic infections, CD4+ 200-499 are fair and above 500 is considered pretty good.
3) Immune differential
4) Differentiate between **Syphilis** as well as CMV, EBV, etc.
5) Consider hair analysis for heavy metals to evaluate stress on the immune system

## IV. Treatment

**1) Strengthen the immune system**

a) Avoid recreational drugs
b) Treat underlying diseases
c) Avoid immunosuppressive medications.
d) Supplement nutrients especially immune modulating nutrients and membrane stabilizing.

**2) Avoid environmental toxins** (foods, air, water, workplace)-consider hair analysis.

**3) Correct malabsorption**–As noted above, there are often digestive problems caused by enteric pathogens. The pathogens need to treated as well as the damage to the mucosa (see ulcerative colitis and Celiac disease chapters p. 375 & 362).

**4) Treat food allergies.**

**5) Deal with stress.**-Both physical and emotional stress should be reduced.

6) **Avoid HIV exposure-**This means "safe sex",i.e., avoiding: unprotected & anal intercourse (best to use latex condom), exposure to blood constituents, and reducing sexual contacts.

7) **Diet–**(see final chapter on the "*Ideal Diet*")–consider blood typing to maximize effectiveness of diet therapy (*Eat Right For Your Blood Type*, D'Adamo). Also consider elemental diet to maintain weight (ENFOOD, Vivonex see page 290).

## V. Supplements

1) **Beta carotene**–300,000IU/day. Can do carrot juice 1 cup = 150,000IU (approximately). See section on beta carotene and foods containing p.168.

2) **Vitamin C**–Either IV or buffered 10-60gms/day (Give calcium also).

STUDY– Cathcart RF III. *Vitamin C in the treatment of AIDS).* Med Hypotheses 14:423-433, 1984.

STUDY–Harakeh S, et al. *Suppression of human immunodeficiency virus replication by ascorbate in chronically and acutely infected cells.* Proc Natl Acad Sci 87:7245-7249, 1990.

3) **Zinc picolinate**–30-50mg/day.

4) **Antioxidants**–vitamin E, selenium, glutathione etc. Vitamin E enhances AZT therapy.

STUDY–Staal FJ et al.. *Glutathione deficiency and HIV infection.* Lancet 339(8798):909-912, 1992.

5) **High potency multivitamin and mineral** with lots of trace minerals

STUDY– Ince S. *Vitamin supplements may help delay onset of AIDS.* Med Tribune, November 9, p. 18, 1993.

6) **Thymus and/or spleen extract–**B and T cell formulas (Cardiovascular Research).

7) **EFA , GLA, MCT**

8) **Botanicals: Garlic, Lomatium, Astragalus memranaceious, Echinacea, Momordica charantia (Bitter Melon), and Hypericin and Shiitake mushrooms**

STUDY–Zhang QC. *Preliminary report on the use of Momordica charantia extract by HIV patients.* J Naturopath Med 3:65-9, 1992. ABSTRACT–Bitter melon inhibits the growth of certain viruses.

9) **Germanium**–up to 1.5 mg.

10) **Quercetin-**1 gm 3x per day

11) **N-acetyl cysteine**–may enhance glutathione levels.

STUDY–Fidelus RK et al.. *Enhancement of intra cellular glutathione promotes lymphocyte & L activation by mitogen.*

STUDY–Roederer M, et al. *Cytokine-stimulated human immunodeficiency virus replication is inhibited by N-acetyl-L-cysteine.* Proc Natl Acad Sci 87:4884-4888, 1990.

STUDY–Mihm S, et al., Pessara et al.. *Inhibition of HIV-1 replication and NF-kB activity by cysteine and cysteine derivatives.* Cellular Immunol . 97:155-63, 1986. ABSTRACT–It was found that NAC increased the ratio of CD4 to CD8 and the changes were based upon dose.

12) **Silymarin–**(standardized extract 80%) 400mg 2x/day especially if intestinal symptoms.

13) **IV vitamin therapy-**use 50-100 gms vitamin C per vitamin cocktail

14) **PCM-4-**spleen & Ginseng combination

15) **Protease inhibitors**–have done wonders for maintaining and even gaining significant amounts of weight.

16) **Adrenal hormones-**Evaluate adrenal hormones cortisol and DHA (Adrenal Stress Index Diagnostechs). Supplement if appropriate.

# MULTIPLE SCLEROSIS (MS)

- Sudden transient motor and sensory disturbances–including impaired vision.
- Diffuse neurologic signs, with remissions and exacerbations.
- Zones of demyelination in nerves varying in size and location.

## I. Epidemiology

Two thirds of MS cases begin between the ages of 20-40 (rarely after 50) with 60% female and 40% male. **A higher incidence occurs at higher latitudes than tropics (5-10x higher)**. In Japan the incidence is rare in all latitudes. Development occurs early in life as people who move from low risk areas to high risk areas before the age of 15 acquire a high risk of development of MS. If they move from a high risk area to a low risk area before the age of 15 they then develop MS at a low risk rate.

## II. Diagnosis

1) Signs and symptoms:

| Type | Freq. | Symptoms |
|---|---|---|
| Motor | 42% | Feeling of heaviness, weakness, leg dragging, stiffness, tendency to drop things, clumsiness |
| Sensory | 18% | Tingling, heat, electrical sensations, numbness, a dead feeling |
| Visual | 34% | Blurring, fogginess, haziness, eye pain, blindness, double vision |
| Vestibular | 7% | Lightheadedness, vertigo, drunken sensation, nausea & vomiting |
| Genitourinary | 4% | Incontinence, loss of bladder sensation, loss of sexual function |

2) Flicker Fusion Test–as MS progresses and more neurological damage occurs vision becomes impared. The ability to discern moving multiple frames, similar to an old movie, becomes impaired. The result of the increasing neurological damage is an inabilty to destinguish the individual frames as they flashed in front of the eyes.
3) RBC electrophoresis
4) EFA analysis (Meridian Labs has a blood test that can evaluated whether or not there is a deficiency of some of the down line metabolites of the essential fatty acids.
5) MRI–can detect lesions in the cord or brain.
6) Heavy metal screen (hair analysis)

## III. Etiology

**1) Autoimmune factors**–Just before an attack, suppressor T-cell levels have been shown to decrease and then increase after the attack. This could allow a latent autoimmune condition to take hold. Autoimmune reactions can happen especially to grains, which have not been in peoples diet for very long from an evolutionary standpoint (See *Your family Tree Connection*, Reading).

**2) Diet**

a) Diets high in gluten and milk have much higher prevalence of MS

b) Diets high in animal and dairy products have a much higher incidence of MS.

STUDY–Swank, Lerstad, Strom: *MS in rural Norway: its geographic distribution and occupational incidence in relation to nutrition.* NEJM 246:7212-8,1952. ABSTRACT–It was observed that inland farming communities in Norway had a higher incidence of MS than the costal areas. It was discovered that the inland farmers had a diet that was much higher in animal and dairy products than the diets of the coastal dwellers.

c) Deficiency of polyunsaturated fatty acids

STUDIES-Bernsohn & Stephanides: *Etiology of MS.* Nature 10:523-30,1963. ABSTRACT–It was found that deficiencies of omega-3 oils produced impairment of normal myelin.

Mertin & Meade. *Relevance of fatty acids in MS.* Brit. Med. Bull 33:67-71,1977. Linoleic acid was found to be low in the blood of MS patients and to fall further during relapses.

**3) Lipid peroxidation**–Reduced glutathione peroxidase has been shown in red blood cells and white blood cells in MS patients. This decreased level is currently thought to be a genetic factor. The decreased antioxidant protection, which if shown to exist in myelin tissue, would render this tissue extremely susceptible to lipid peroxidation.

**TEST–Lipid peroxidation in body–Antibody Assay Lab & Meridian Labs**

**4) Virus**–In humans many viruses are capable of producing demyelination of nerve tissue. Post-infectious encephalomyelitis is a condition that develops 10-40 days after an acute viral infection or an immunization.

- Demyelination may be a direct result of the virus or a viral infection leading to autoimmunity.

**5) Mercury toxicity**–See Hal Huggins, DDS (800)331-2303 Box 2589, Colorado Springs CO 80901 (fax-(719)522-0563.

STUDY–Craelius. *Comparative epidemiology of MS and dental caries.* J. Epidemiol. Comm. Health 32:155-65,1972. ABSTRACT–Death rates from MS were "linearly related to the numbers of decayed, missing and filled teeth in 6 Australian and 48 American states and in 45 Asian and European countries."

STUDY–Craelius. J. Epidemiology and Community Health, 32,155-65,1978. ABSTRACT–An extremely low rate of MS was reported amount the Eskimos from 1950 to 1963. This period of time corresponds to a very low rate of caries found among Eskimos form the same area in a survey in 1960.

Another important test case not included in the correlation is that the 15 million Bantus of S. Africa are unique in the total absence among them of any reported MS. Dental surveys in 1937 and more recently in 1975 have found extremely low rates of dental caries among this population 60% of rural Bantus ages 16-17 years were entirely free from caries and 33% of urban Bantus. The average DMF for both rural and urban Bantus was 1.7 which is the lowest of almost everywhere in the world. Areas in S. Africa where there has been an increase in dental caries has showed and increase in the incidence of MS.

A study of Asians living in California and Washington showed that this group had a much lower risk of MS than Caucasians. Parallel results were found with MS.

STUDIES–Ingalls. *Epidemiology, etiology, and prevention of MS.* Am. J Forensic Med. & Path. 4:55-61,1983. ABSTRACT–Inorganic mercury in mouth from fillings can be converted to an organic neurotoxic form from the action of gingiva and oxidation.

–Ingalls, *Triggers for MS* Lancet 2:160,1986. ABSTRACT–Development of diplopia after a pulverization of an old Hg amalgam filling which was theorized to have released enough Hg vapor to be toxic to the oculomotor nerves.

# IV. Treatment

**1) Low fat diet–**10gms/day saturated fats (If 2000 calories then not more than 24 gms fat)– Total fat percentage in the diet should be less than 12% (if 2,000 cal then 4.5%).

**2) Treat food allergies**–In a study most severe patients had food sensitivities.

**3) Prevent lipid peroxidation**

**4) Supplement EFA**

a) Decreases platelet aggregation-improves microcirculation of CNS and other tissues.

STUDY–Dwarkin *Linoleic acid and MS: A re-analysis of 3 double blind trials.* ABSTRACT–Treatment with linoleic acid reduced the severity and duration of relapses at all levels of disability compared to controls.

STUDY–Simpson *Dietary supplementation with Efamol and MS.* New Zea. Med. J 98:792:1053-54,1985. ABSTRACT–16 patients had abnormal blood rheology with MS and supplementation with 4gms of EPO/day for 3 weeks improved rheology and hand grip strength

STUDY–Field and Joyce–*MS: Effect of GLA administration upon membranes and the need for extended clinical trials of USFA.* Eur. Neurol.22:78,1983. ABSTRACT–Electrophoretic mobility studies or RBC's from MS patients indicate that treatment with USFA must continue for at least 2 years before normal reactivity is restored. If treatments are to be effective in treating myelin, clinical trials need to be extended.

b) Decreasing an autoimmune response–Allergic encephalomyelitis has been shown to be greatly minimized in its severity with linoleic acid.

c) Normalizing decreased fatty acids levels in RBC's and cerebral spinal fluid.

**5) Increase fatty acids**

**a) Flax oil**–2 tsp 2x/day

**b) Maximum EPA**–3caps 2x/day

**c) Black current oil or EPO or borage oil**–2caps 2x/day EPO–has only 40mg GLA compared to borage which has up to 240mg GLA per capsule.

**6) Antioxidant nutrients Vitamin E**–800iu/day, **Selenium**–200mcg/day

**7) Lecithin**–2400mg 2x/day

**8) Vitamin B-12 IM 1-3 mg per day** Probably best to use mercury free B-12 (Apothecure).

**9) Bile salts and lipase–especially if there are problems with the patients digestion**

STUDY–Lange & Shiner. *Small bowel abnormal in MS.* Lancet 1319-22,1976. ABSTRACT–It was noted that 42% of MS patients had fat malabsorption, 42% had undigested meat fibers, and 12% had malabsorption of B-12.

6) **Adrenal supplements**–vitamin C, E and B-5 along with adrenal glandulars, Royal Jelly & DHEA. In autoimmune diseases like MS can go dramatically higher in the dosage of DHEA. For women can go as high as 50-100mg per day and up to 150mg for men.

7) **Bee Venom**–can use the live bees or collect bee venom. Work up to 30-40 BV per treatment. Can use small amount of lidocaine when administering. Contact the American Apitherapy Society (802) 436-2708. There have been some facinating and dramatic improvements in people with MS in the last 10 years.

**Resources:**

Swank Mulitple Sclerosis Clinic; school of medicine Oregon Helath Sciences University; Sam Jackson Park Rd.; Portland, OR 97201. (503) 494-8370.

## Notes

---

# HEAVY METAL TOXICITY

## MERCURY (Hg)

- The U.S. uses 400 metric tons of mercury in agriculture and the Japanese use 1600 metric tons every year.
- Mercury is used in the paper industry to prevent molds, fungus, and general "slime buildup."
- In agriculture seeds are treated with mercury to prevent any molds or fungi from growing.
- In coal burning industries and petrochemical production work 3,000 metric tons of mercury per year are released into the atmosphere worldwide.
- Dentists used 200,000 pounds of mercury in 1980, 400,000 pounds in 1990 and will use another 600,000 pounds by the year 2,000.
- 3/4 of cavities are filled with mercury amalgams.
- In 1972 the National Institute for Occupational Safety and Health set the standard for "Threshold Limit Value". This value is 5x higher in the U.S. than it is in the Russia. Studies by the World Health Organization show that a single amalgam can release 3-17mcg of mercury per day. It has been found that the level of Hg found in the brain and kidneys is directly correlated to the number of Hg fillings in the mouth.
- Most major dental schools in Tokyo, Japan no longer teach the use of amalgam fillings because their plumbing does not adequately filter the mercury waste which is subsequently dumped into the rivers, lakes, and streams. The use of Hg amalgams has been outlawed in Japan. In Sweden the country's health commission issued an advisory against the use of Hg amalgams in pregnant women. The government even pays for 50% of the cost of removal of the Hg amalgams.

**concentration of mercury in the food chain**

| Inorganic Hg——>Bacteria———>Plankton——>Small fish——> Large fish——>WO/MAN |
|---|

### Findings Concerning Mercury Toxicity

In 1953 in Japan, large amounts of mercurial containing fungicides were dumped into a bay at a costal town. This killed 43 people directly, and seriously injured another 111. The illness that people developed was named "Minamata Disease" after the bay into which the wastes were dumped. These people were poisoned by contaminated fish and shellfish from the bay.

Again in 1965 a similar epidemic occurred in riverside villages along the Agano River, Nigata, Japan. Again the poisoning was from contaminated fish from the nearby river and sea. Generally the larger the fish the higher the concentration of mercury. Water shed areas that have had a history of mining nearby usually have significantly elevated levels of mercury. The sediment toward the bottom of a water body may be particularly high in mercury levels.

# I. Etiology

1) **Contaminated fish**, especially deep sea fish who concentrate mercury (tuna & Swordfish). By law, any fish over 75lbs must be checked for Hg levels. Over 95% of the Hg in fish gets absorbed.
2) **Dental mercury amalgams**–It has been shown that when amalgams are exposed to various changes or stresses they readily "gas off". Mercury amalgams are ~50% mercury. The following are factors associated with increased gassing off of mercury:
   a) Hot and cold fluids
   b) Chewing–vaporization increases for ~20 minutes after finishing chewing
   c) Acid pH of saliva
3) **Contaminated grain seed**.
4) **Environmental waste-water**

# II. Signs and Symptoms

Symptoms associated with mercury toxicity are known as Hunter-Russell syndrome since it was first reported by Hunter, Bomford and Russell.

1) Ataxia
2) Impairment of speech
3) Constriction of visual field
4) Impairment of hearing
5) Sensory disturbance

| OBJECTIVE SYMPTOMS | SUBJECTIVE SYMPTOMS |
|---|---|
| Gingivitis with blue line at gum margin | Sore mouth |
| Atrophy of tongue | Metallic taste in mouth |
| Tremor of hands, Fasciculations | Anorexia |
| Motor weakness of limbs | Diarrhea |
| Atrophy of limb and trunk muscles | Epigastric discomfort |
| Hyper-reflexia & Hypo-reflexia | Vomiting |
| Acrodynia "Pink Disease" infants and children | Constipation |
| Fetal abnormalities and infertility | Headaches |
| Allergic reactions such as contact dermatitis | Psychic irritability |
| Elevation of white blood cells | Hyperactivity |
| ALS-like syndrome | Asthma |

STUDY–Kantarjian. Neurology ll p.639, 1961 College of Med. U. of Bagdad, Dept of Neurology. ABSTRACT–11 cases of chronic mercurialism with a neurologic picture akin to ALS were reported. All of these patients consumed bread prepared from wheat treated with a seed fungicide called Granosan M. (Dupont). The active ingredient is 7.7% ethyl mercury toluene sulfonalide. The period of consumption was about 2-3 months. One of these patients died and the presence of large amounts of mercury in the urine established the etiology in this case.

**NOTE**–It was speculated that chronic low levels of mercury can have an inhibitory effect on the hypothalamus, causing a decrease in TSH-RF and subsequent secondary hypothyroidism. Mercury blocks uptake of iodine and depresses thyroid hormone levels. Dr. Roy Kupsinel, a dentist in Florida, has found that the removal of mercury amalgams results in an increase in basal body temperatures.

## III. Diagnosis

1) **Hair analysis**-according to Dr. David Quig of Doctors Data, hair analysis is a good screening tool for the heavy metals Hg, Pb, Ar, and Cd. However, hair may not always show up high levels of mercury. For evaluating mercury, which is stored in the CNS, intravenous DMPS (250mg/5 CC) should be administered over 20 minutes followed by a 6 hour urine collection. 85% of the mercury will spill into the urine in the first couple of hours. Oral or IV Minerals should be avoided during this chelation period.

2) **Serum bio-compatibility testing–Huggins Diagnostic Center** Colorado Springs, CO (719)548-1600 has a *Serum Compatibility Test Kit* which can be used to evaluate the immunological sensitivity to the various materials that are used in dentistry. Antibodies IgM, IgA, IgG, and IgE are determined for each of the materials used in the dental structures. These tests do not take into consideration the abnormal electrical currents in the mouth. As a result this test may come out negative but yet the patient could have a reaction to the conductivity of the metal.

3) **Urine mercury-**can do a DMSA or DMPS challenge and then collect 6 hours urine (Doctors Data). As previously mentioned in #1, DMSA does not do a very good job at chelating mercury, because of its poor absorption, and DMPS should be used for Hg.

4) **Serum mercury**–There is only a temporary rise in blood mercury when mercury is released during dental work. The mercury goes into equilibrium with the tissues soon after it goes into the blood. Most of it gets stored in the CNS.

5) **Fecal mercury**–This is a relatively new test being used by Doctors Data.

**NOTE**–There is no correlation between hair, blood, and urine mercury and the degree of symptoms that a patient may experience. This is because there is such a variable sensitivity to the amount of mercury that it is impossible to predict who will or won't react. There may be a better correlation to other heavy metal levels and symptoms.

**STUDY**–Ricktersnap, Boyer, Peterson, & Svare. *The contribution of dental amalgams to mercury in blood* J Dental Research. March, 1989. ABSTRACT–10 subjects had blood mercury levels checked before and after removal of mercury dental amalgams restoration. Weekly blood samples were analyzed ultraviolet spectrophotometry to establish baseline levels. Dental amalgams were removed weekly and blood samples were taken. After removal, 9 of 10 subjects had a significant drop in blood mercury levels . This supports the concept that the presence of mercury amalgams in the mouth results in an elevated blood mercury level, but does not establish a correlation to toxic effects in the body. This is because high levels in one person may produce no symptoms and low levels in another person may result in marked toxic effects.

**NOTE**–Mercury patch tests are largely inaccurate and should not be used to evaluate mercury toxicity. This test may merely show an allergic sensitivity or direct irritation such as a burn from the mercury.

5) **The Jerome mercury vapor analyzer** measures gassing off of mercury vapor from mercury amalgams in mouth.

6) **Voles, Vega, Inter tests** can be used to evaluate the sensitivity of the body to the overall electrical or chemical imbalance that may be created in the mouth.

## IV. Treatment

1) **Avoid sources of Mercury** (see list ).

Remove mercury amalgams if necessary. It is a good idea to take some precautions upon doing dental work to remove mercury amalgams. One of the biggest problems is the large amount of vaporized mercury that can get released by a filling once it gets drilled. Dr.

Murray Vimy, of The University of Calgary in Canada (403) 266-2251, is a world expert in mercury toxicity and believes that there is a technique for removing Hg amalgams where the filling can have an etching into it and then be pulled out in large chunks. In this manner grinding is avoided and there is much less gassing off. In addition a vapor suction device, along with oxygen and a dam can be used to further reduce exposure. Contact Mike Ziff, DDS (author of *Silver Dental Fillings-The Toxic Time Bomb* Aurora Press, 1986) at (407)298-2450 for dentists who belong to the American Holistic Dental Association.

## Common Sources Containing Mercury

- Contaminated fish, especially tuna and swordfish, are high sources.
- Preparation H®
- Vegetables especially carrots and lettuce contaminated with sprays.
- Hair dyes
- Merthiolate
- Contact lens solutions
- Mercurochrome
- Laxatives
- Calomine lotion
- Toilet paper made from recycled paper
- Vaginal gels, especially contraceptives
- Mascara
- Certain perfumes
- Afrin® nasal spray
- Certain injectable B vitamins contain Phenyl Mercuric acetate (PMA) as a preservative. Injectables are available without preservatives from compounding pharmacies
- Fungicides for lawns, shrubs and trees (check occupational hazards such as working in a nursery)
- Latex paint solvents and fabric softeners
- Wood preservatives and adhesives
- Air conditioner filters
- Floor waxes
- Watch for the prefix or suffix, "Mer", listed in the ingredients

**The following is a list of precautions that can be taken 1-2 weeks prior to having mercury amalgams removed:**

1) a) **Vitamin E**–800-1200iu/day

b) **Vitamin C**–3-6gms/day

c) **Selenium**–200-300µg/day

d) **N-acetyl cysteine**–3gms/day & **glutathione (reduced)**-500-750mg per day

e) **Silybum marianum extract 80%** 3-4 days prior to chelation.

f) **2,3-dimercaptopropanosulfonic acid and 2, 4-dimercaptosuccinic acid**–This is a strong chelator compound that is much less toxic compared to British Anti-Lewisite. The day of the chelation give homeopathic Arnica montana, 30c b.i.d. The above materials can be taken for 4-7 days following the procedure. In addition, EDTA may be used during the procedure to chelate any heavy metals that may be going into the blood.

According to Mike Ziff, DDS the best materials to use are Helthco "Status," Herculite, P50. Currently there are 2nd generation composites that are superior in quality and lower in toxicity. Gold amalgams do contain some mercury, especially the ones with a lower percentage of gold. Porcelain may be bound to mercury amalgams. Porcelain contains depleted radium 300-1000ppm. One source, OBTEK, states that no depleted radium is in their porcelain and that it is just as strong, but not as abrasive. Titanium has the lowest toxicity.

2) **Increase foods containing sulfur amino acids**–eggs, beans, garlic, onions. Garlic has been especially useful for chelating heavy metals from the body.

3) **Supplement various fibers such as pectin and especially oat bran**–Bile binds onto mercury and if excreted then you can lower your body burden of mercury.

4) **Lactobacillus acidophilus**

5) **Charcoal & Bentonite clay** (I like the colloidal suspension from Springgreen) acts to bind mercury in the stool.

6) **Selenium**–200µg/day & **Vitamin E**–400-800iu/day

7) **Vitamin C to bowel tolerance.**

8) **Glutathione reduced**–50-200mcg/day–detoxifies mercury and allows it to be excreted from the body. Read Pfeifer and Braverman, *The Healing Nutrients from Within,* which is all about amino acids and their medical uses, including detoxification.

9) **Cysteine & methionine**–Cysteine increases renal mercury concentration and reduces mercury accumulation in liver, cerebrum, and red blood cells. Precursor to glutathione.

10) **Zinc**–If using zinc for an extended period of time, remember to supplement copper.

11) **Vitamin B-12**–1-3mg/day–Hydroxocobalamin form may raise tissue levels better than cyanocobalamin form. Can also use IV with other nutrients for detoxification reasons.

12) **Molybdenum**–250-500mg day

STUDY–Yanan, Toshiaki and Koizumi. *Protective effect of molybdenum on the acute toxicity of mercury* . Toxicology and Applied Pharm. 65, 214-21, 1982.

13) **2'4'-Dimercaptosuccinic acid (DMSA/Chemet®) & 2,3 Dimercaptoproprionic acid (DMPS)** –Dr. Quig recommends IV DMPS chelation 1st as DMSA is poorly absorbed. In my experience DMPS is much more effective than DMSA at decreasing urinary Hg levels. It is best to do a 6 hour urine catch following 5cc of IV DMPS ( Apothecure). 5-7 treatments reduces urinary mercury by 30%. Treatments should be spaced 2-3 weeks apart although I have done them weekly without problems. Occasionally I have gotten a flu like reaction with lymphadenopathy which lasted a couple of days. It is believed that DMPS does not cross the blood brain barrier and that after levels of urinary Hg have come down it may be necessary to do several months of DMSA chelation to pull the remaining Hg out of the CNS.

STUDY–Annual Review Pharmacology & Toxicology (Dept of Pharm. U of Az Tucson, 85721) Department of Cellular & Developmental Biology 23:193•215, 1983. First used in 1956 by the Soviet Union to treat mercury toxicity.

14) **Lipoic acid** (similar to vitamin B-1)–Improves cardiovascular function through its chelation action & also chelates heavy metals such as mercury (Cardiovascular Research).

15) **Thyroid**–It has been found that mercury inhibits thyroid function and may result in hypothyroidism which leads to a decreased metabolism and excretion of Hg.

16) **Sauna, hydrotherapy and exercise**–Mercury has been found in perspiration. Anything that promotes sweating may be beneficial in the excretion of mercury.

17) **Folate**–It has been found that mercury has an antagonistic effect on folate function.

18) **Porphyra-Zyme**–(Biotics)

19) **Chlorella**–This has been found to have significant chelating effects on mercury.

**References**-Bioprobe Newsletter–4401 Real Court, Orlando FL 32808. Mike Ziff, DDS (407)298-2450. *It's All in Your Head* by Hal and S.A Huggins; *Silver Dental Fillings-The Toxic Time Bomb* by Sam Ziff, Aurora Press, 1986.; *How Safe are Silver/Mercury Fillings* by Betsy Russell-Manning

## Lead Toxicity

- Lead toxicity is the U.S. is a major concern as exposure levels have risen dramatically over the last 300 years. In 1700 estimated worldwide production was about 100,000 tons per year. By 1930 levels had risen ten fold to 1 million tons per year and finally by 1980 that level increased to 3 million tons per year. In one study the bones of ancient Peruvians, some 1800 years ago, had lead levels 500 times less than current Americans (*Preventing & Reversing Osteoporosis* Gaby, 1994).
- The drinking water in the U.S. exceeds federal safety standards in 130 cities. In addition, it is estimated that about 32 million Americans drink water that exceeds the safety standards of 15 parts per billion!

## II. Signs and Symptoms of lead toxicity

Anemia, fatigue, muscle aches, high blood pressure, strokes, loss of appetite and body weight, poor memory, constipation, headaches, loss of cognitive function, decreased coordination, and inability to concentrate are generally associated with lead toxicity. Elevated lead levels in children have been clearly shown to decrease academic performance in school. Recent studies show a correlation between elevated lead levels and dental carries, as well as osteoporosis.

STUDY–Moss ME et al. *Association of dental caries & blood lead levels*. JAMA. Jun 23-30, 281(24):2294, 1999.

## III. Treatment for Lead Toxicity

1) **Avoid sources of Lead-**Lead is especially found in drinking water. Pipes soldered with lead easily enters into the water depending upon the pH of the water (lower pH increases lead solubility), and how long the water stays in the pipe. Always run the water, if it has been still for more than 6 hours, before drinking. Newer copper pipes don't usually use mercury solder and therefore do not present a problem. Charcoal or carbon based water filters do not necessarily take out heavy metals. Check with the manufacturer and ask for proof that their filter actually removes heavy metals including lead.

2) **DMSA (Chemet®)**-100-400mg per day for several months then recheck. FDA has approved the use of DMSA for chelation of lead. Generally well tolerated, DMSA can either be prescribed or obtained from Thorne Research as Captomer.

3) **Calcium 1-2 gms per day** preferably citrate to avoid problems with kidney stones. Lead tends to get stored in the bone and is especially found in drinking water.

4) **Porphyra-Zyme (Biotics Res.)**-4-6 caps per day. This product is a concentrated extract of Spirulina plankton. It is believed that the porphyrin ring of chlorophyll binds onto magnesium. Under acidic conditions, as in the stomach, magnesium is freed up and the central porphyrins ring is then able to bind other heavy metals such as Hg, Ar, Pb and Cd.

5) **Bentonite clay**-1-3 teaspoons per day for several months then recheck pb levels.

NOTE-Contact Doctors Data for addition information concerning heavy metals including information on cadmium and arsenic. A booklet compiled by Dr. David Quig concerning heavy metals and mineral analysis has recently been completed in 1999 (800)323-2784, extension 149.

# DOWN SYNDROME (Trisomy 21)

Down syndrome, or Trisomy 21, is a genetic defect involving an extra chromosome (95 % of cases there is an extra chromosome 21). Overall incidence is about 1 per 700 live births but the age of the mother shows an exponential increased incidence after the age of 30 years old. There is a tremendous variability depending upon the age. Women having babies in their early 20's have about 1/1600 risk and for women over the age of 40 there is a 1/40 risk (see chart at bottom). About 20% of all Down Syndrome babies come from mothers greater than 35 years of age yet they have only 8% of the babies. The percentage of women having babies over the age of 35 is greatly increasing. In about 30% of the time the extra chromosome comes from the father.

## I. ETIOLOGY

Down syndrome is attributed to an extra chromosome 21. The reason for the development of this extra chromosome is subject to debate but it appears that there is some matter of the aging process of the egg of the female or the healthiness of the sperm. There may be some association of environmental toxins triggering off this genetic defect.

## II. SIGNS AND SYMPTOMS

Infants tend to be relatively less active and cry very infrequently. They also demonstrate poor muscle tone and developmentally are physically and mentally retarded. The average IQ in the Down Syndrome child is about 50. Microcephaly, brachycephaly and a flattened occiput are classic characteristics. The bridge of the nose is usually flattened with a large tongue that is protruded from an open mouth. The tongue usually shows a furrow that lacks a central fissure. The ears are small with down folded helixes. Other classic appearances include slanted eyes with epicanthic folds (characteristic of Mongolians, hence the name "Mongolism" is also used to describe Trisomy 21) and gray /white spots around the periphery of the iris that disappear after the first year of life (Brushfield's spots). The hands are short and broad with a single palmar crease "Simian crease" and the fingers are short with an incurved 5th finger that often has only 2 phalanges. The feet have a wide gap between the 1st and 2nd toe with a plantar furrow extending backward.

Congenital heart defects such as atrioventricular canal defects and ventricular sepal defects are very common, occurring in about 35% of all Down syndrome people. Many babies born with Trisomy chromosomal abnormalities do not survive (close to 50%). However infant mortality for Down Syndrome babies has gone down drastically from 53% in 1948 to 22% in 1975. This increased survival is the result of heroic treatments of both infectious and cardiac diseases.

Life expectancy of Down syndrome people is lessened because of the high frequency of heart defects and the propensity to develop acute leukemia and severe pulmonary infections. Most Down syndrome people, that do not have major heart defects, live into adulthood, but the aging process is greatly accelerated. Life expectancy is only 30-50 years and it seems that Down syndrome people show typical findings of Alzheimer's disease (neurofibulary tangles in the brain) and symptoms as well.

Down syndrome people have areas in their body where they have increased tissue levels of SOD and glutathione peroxidase. This elevated level of antioxidant nutrients is an indication that there is a higher requirement in DS patients for antioxidant nutrients. This is supported by the increase in various accelerated aging processes that occur in DS such as cataracts, atherosclerosis, early graying and loss of hair, drying of skin, oxidative changes in the brain.

**Risk of having liveborn child with Down syndrome or other chromosomal abnormality**

| Maternal age | Risk of Down syndrome | Total risk for chromosomal damage | Maternal age | Risk of Down syndrome | Total risk for chromosomal damage |
|---|---|---|---|---|---|
| 20 | 1/1667 | 1/526 | 36 | 1/294 | 1/156 |
| 21 | 1/1667 | 1/526 | 37 | 1/227 | 1/127 |
| 22 | 1/1429 | 1/500 | 38 | 1/175 | 1/102 |
| 23 | 1/1429 | 1/500 | 39 | 1/137 | 1/83 |
| 24 | 1/1250 | 1/476 | 40 | 1/106 | 1/66 |
| 25 | 1/1250 | 1/476 | 41 | 1/82 | 1/53 |
| 26 | 1/1176 | 1/476 | 42 | 1/64 | 1/42 |
| 27 | 1/1111 | 1/455 | 43 | 1/50 | 1/33 |
| 28 | 1/1053 | 1/435 | 44 | 1/38 | 1/26 |
| 29 | 1/1000 | 1/417 | 45 | 1/30 | 1/21 |
| 30 | 1/952 | 1/384 | 46 | 1/23 | 1/16 |
| 31 | 1/909 | 1/384 | 47 | 1/18 | 1/13 |
| 32 | 1/769 | 1/323 | 48 | 1/14 | 1/10 |
| 33 | 1/625 | 1/286 | 49 | 1/11 | 1/8 |
| 34 | 1/500 | 1/238 | 50 | 1/8 | 1/6 |
| 35 | 1/385 | 1/192 | | | |

## III. DIAGNOSIS:

In evaluating the Down syndrome patient, diagnostic tests should evaluate the cardiovascular system, immune system, and brain function. These areas are most frequently affected and can cause many other problems as well. A full workup for any heart defects, such as ECG and US, along with thorough blood testing to detect any abnormalities is essential (see appendix "Evaluating cardiovascular disease"). In Down Syndrome there is always a great acceleration of the aging process that involves free radical pathology. A thorough evaluation of antioxidant status is certainly valuable. Finally brain chemistry, which is a relatively new science, could offer important clues. Studies concerning fatty and amino acids show great promise to uncovering secrets related to Down syndrome. There are some definite findings that give valuable information regarding brain function. Below are some basic tests that would be useful in assessing Down Syndrome patients:

**Down Syndrome Test Evaluations**

1) *Cardiovascular system*–Chem-screen that includes apolipoproteins, LDL, HDL cholesterols, ferritin, homocysteine, fasting blood glucose, and thyroid panel (see cardiovascular disease). It is known that hypothyroidism occurs commonly with estimated incidence of about 17% in one study. About 1/3 of Down syndrome patients also have thyroid antibodies indicating an autoimmune response. 28% have high levels of TSH. The incidence of hypothyroidism is probably higher than these conservative estimates.

STUDY–Sare, Z, et al. *Prevalence of thyroid disorder in Down syndrome* Clin Genet 14:154-158, 1973.

2) *Immune function and environmental toxins*–Hair analysis for heavy metals (these contaminants will inhibit normal immunity), CBC (to determine decreased WBC's), WBC zinc or zinc taste test can be performed in office.

3) *Brain function*–Amino acid analysis to determine imbalances in (these contaminants will inhibit normal immunity), CBC (to determine decreased WBC's),

4) *Digestive function analysis*–If there is a digestive problem, such as gas, bloating, indigestion, ulcers, diarrhea, or constipation, consider stool analysis for parasites or other pathogens.

5) *HCL analysis (Heidelberg Test)*–checks HCL production from the stomach if there is a problem with digesting proteins and nails are not growing, or hair is falling out etc.
6) *Blood Typing*–can evaluate the different blood types as well as whether someone is a secretor or non-secretor. It can show which foods may not be compatible with blood type.
7) *Salivary adrenal test to check for DHEA and also cortisol* levels throughout the day.

In addition to the above a complete nutritional physical should be performed to determine areas that might require increased amounts of certain nutrients (see appendix)

## IV. TREATMENT:

**1) Cardiovascular disease**–(see cardiovascular disease)

Antioxidant nutrients–(Oxyquench from Omnivite Nutrition Inc.)
Coenzyme Q 10–
Taurine–
Carnitine–

**2) Enhance immune function and remove environmental toxins–**Various immune enhance herbs can be used including Echinacea, Lomatia, thymus extracts, B and T Cell Formulas (Cardiovascular Research), Phytogen (Thorne), Optibiotic (Eclectic), Spleen extracts

**3) Brain function–**

a) Phosphatidyl choline–is a precursor to acetylcholine, a vital brain neurotransmitter. May be used in conjunction with other Nootropic drugs such as Piracetam.
b) Tyrosine–is a precursor to epinephrine and norepinephrine which are important neurotransmitters. In addition, it is a precursor to thyroid hormones.
c) Tryptophan–is especially useful for calming the brain to enhance concentration and also to improve sleeping.
d) Ginkgo biloba–has had a long history of improving cognitive brain function as well as memory. In addition it has marked effects on improving circulation and also acting as an antioxidant in various tissues.
f) thyroid–consider zinc, copper, tyrosine and thyroid glandulars or straight T4.

**4) Adrenal function enhancement**–The adrenal glands are considered essential for proper immune function, they are particularly involved with the prevention of aging and they have been used to treat chronic fatigue

**5) Nootropic drugs**–Piracetam–acts to increase neurotransmitters in the brain. Also acts as an antioxidant. It is quite costly however 800mg capsules are ~$1.00 per cap. Studies have used 7.2gms up to 20gms per day.

**6) Dietary–**avoid allergens and consider following blood typing recommendations

**7) Craniosacral work and BNS-**Craniosacral work is a subtle technique used to balance out the cranial bones. BNS (binasal specifics) is technique that uses balloons to expand the sinus cavities. Both techniques have been used to enhance brain function.

# Alternative Dietary Approaches to Disease

Macrobiotics-Michio Kushi

"Sickness or Disease-Sickness is nothing but the result of being out of balance with nature and the universe." It develops through the following stages:

1) *Fatigue*- This includes both physical and mental fatigue. A person who frequently changes their job, place of living, or spouse, is suffering from this stage of sickness. When healthy people work very hard, they may naturally feel exhausted, but after a good night's sleep, they will awaken the next morning feeling completely refreshed and eager for any challenge or difficulty. This is quite different from the chronic fatigue which many people presently experience. Tightness in the back of your neck and shoulders may be a sign of fatigue. The major causes are lack of physical exercise and overeating and overdrinking, in particular the consumption of meat and sugar, all of which tax the muscles and circulation.

2) *Aches and Pains*-Problems such as muscle aches, occasional headaches, menstrual cramps, stomach pains, and others occur at this 2nd stage, in which the nervous system is starting to weaken.

3) *Blood Diseases*- Sicknesses of the blood are often the result of a chronically over-acid blood condition, or of a fatty, sticky, or cholesterol filled bloodstream. The quality of everyone's blood is different. If the condition of the blood is chronically poor, illnesses such as anemia, leukemia, asthma, hemophilia, jaundice, varicose veins, mono, skin diseases, leprosy, and others can easily occur. Many of these conditions are considered incurable, however, even a sickness as serious as leukemia is relatively easy to control through proper eating, even if the person has suffered from it for several years.

4) *Emotional Disorders*- This includes irritability, impatience, upset, anger, anxiety, worry, fear, and uneasiness. A healthy person is not bothered by negative emotional states If we become angry even once a year, we are not completely healthy. Ideally, we should not become angry even once during an entire lifetime.

5) *Organ Diseases*- TB, heart disease., diabetes, emphysema, ulcers, cirrhosis of the liver, and gallstones are examples of organ sicknesses. At this stage, the organs are starting to degenerate.

6) *Nerve Diseases*- These include various types of mental illness, MS, spinal meningitis, Parkinson's disease, and different types of paralysis. Problems with the peripheral nerves are included in this category, as are disorders such as dull responses to others, forgetfulness, and social crimes.

7) *Arrogance*- This occurs when we try to separate ourselves from nature and the universe, and happens in one of 2 ways. The first is yang arrogance, and it appears in the form of

a domineering, conquering, or self insistent personality which tends to drive others away. The second type of arrogance is generally more yin. Persons who are exclusive or who confine themselves suffer from arrogance of this type. Often, when friends offer help or advice, a person with yin arrogance will refuse to listen and will withdraw. Many elderly people have this problem, as do many who consider themselves to be devout or religious. This type of person is usually not open to the opinions or suggestions of others.

Arrogance is actually the underlying cause of all human sickness and unhappiness, and is at the same time the end point of the first 6 stages. Ultimately, all people who suffer from arrogance commit suicide by dying an unnatural death, either through sickness, war, accident or other causes. The basic purpose of macrobiotic healing is to cure arrogance. Even though modern medicine can relieve a variety of symptoms, as can acupuncture and other forms of oriental medicine, it can not cure the basic disease of arrogance.

## The Seven Levels of Eating

Eating is the most important function in life and is the single most important factor in determining whether or not we are harmonious with our environment, and therefore, whether we are healthy or sick.

**99% of modern people are eating on these first 3 levels**

1) **Mechanical Eating**–Mom's womb. Auto eating-set times-set responses.

2) **Sensory Eating**–This level follows our senses and begins soon after we are born. It is based on our preference for certain tastes, odors, colors, and textures. We become trained to eat via sensory clues which can cause problems with various eating disorders if bad habits get formed.

3) **Sentimental or Emotional eating**– Going out to eat or eating with relatives or friends. Emotional eating may also lead to problems related to eating disorders under stressful conditions.

4) **Intellectual Eating**–This level of eating is based on nutritional recommendations which are advocated mostly by professional nutritionists and dieticians. At present, this represents the highest popular level of eating in America, and it is more popular among scientists and university professors. For the most part these systems and theories are unworkable. The U.S. is the richest country in the world, so some people in America may be able to practice these suggestions, yet, even among Americans, many can not afford to eat this way. As far as other countries are concerned, there are millions of people who can not afford to buy meat, milk, and other expensive food items on a regular basis.

5) **Social Eating**–At this level, one realizes that 98% of the world's people can not afford to eat according to nutritional theories, and that this type of eating is even too complicated and time-consuming for most of the people who recommend it.

6) **Ideologic Eating**–Diet customs of many religions such as the teaching of Jesus, Buddha, Mohammed, and others. Because of the decline of the specific environment from which they originally developed, they have become mostly extinct.

7) **Free Eating-**This implies eating in harmony with the universe. This implies eating the way people have been eating for thousands of years. It means eating with the ability to adapt to our surroundings, changing with the seasons.

**Standard Macrobiotic Eating**

1) 50% of the volume of every meal should be whole grain cereal grains including brown rice, whole wheat bread, buckwheat noodles, and oatmeal.

2) 5% soup, preferably seasoned with tamari or miso (one or 2 small bowls). Ingredients should include a variety of vegetables, seaweeds, beans, and grains, and the recipe should often vary. The taste should not be too salty.

3) 20-30% of each meal may include vegetables. These should be locally grown and in season, or else seasonal vegetables that can be naturally stored. 67% of these should be cooked in various ways, including sauteing, steaming, boiling, and baking, while the remaining 3rd may be eaten raw or as lightly boiled salad.

4) From 10% to 15% of daily intake should include cooked beans and seaweed. Beans for daily use are azuki beans, chick-peas, lentils, and black beans. Other beans are for occasional use only. Seaweeds such as hijiki, kombu, wakame, nori, dulse, agar-agar, and Irish moss can be prepared with a variety of cooking methods. These dishes should be flavored with a moderate amount of tamari soy sauce or sea salt.

5) Beverages should include 1) bancha twig tea, roasted; 2) Mu tea; 3) dandelion tea; 4) cereal grain tea or coffee; and 5) any traditional tea which is not artificially produced or does not have an aromatic fragrance and stimulant effect.

**These are the basic macrobiotic eating principles. The following are additional supplements:**

1) Once or 2x per week a small volume of white meat fish or shellfish may be eaten. The method of cooking should vary every week, and the volume of fish should always be less than 15% of the meal.
2) A cooked fruit dessert may also be eaten 2-3x per wk., provided the fruits grow in the local climatic zone and are in season. In a temperate zone, tropical and semitropical fruits should be avoided. Fruit juice is not advisable, although it may be used occasionally in hot weather.
3) Roasted seeds or roasted nuts, lightly seasoned with salt or tamari, may be enjoyed as a snack or supplement as well as dried fruit and roasted beans.

Lastly the following are additional suggestions:
-Cooking oil should be from vegetables origin. Corn or sesame oil is best.
-Salt should be from sea and tamari soy sauce and miso prepared traditionally.
-Condiments recommended include gomasio (12 parts roasted sesame seeds to 1 part sea salt)
-Roasted kelp (kombu) powder or roasted wakame powder.
-Umeboshi plums
-Tekka

You may eat 1,2, or 3 meals per day, or as much as you want, provided that the proportion is correct and chewing is thorough. Each mouthful should be chewed 50 times or more. Avoid eating for approximately 3 hrs before sleeping. For thirst you may drink a small amount of water, but not iced or with meals.

## **Chinese System of Food Cures** by Henry Lui

There are 2 basic differences between Chinese and Western diets. Western diet focuses almost exclusively on diet for weight loss. Chinese diet is designed not only to help you lose weight, but also to treat many other ailments, including hypertension, diabetes, common cold, gastritis, diarrhea, constipation, cough, hepatitis, psoriasis, acne, eczema, etc.

The 2nd difference between Chinese and Western diets is that in the West foods are considered for their protein, calorie, CHO, vitamin, and other nutrient content, but in Chinese diet, foods are considered for their flavors, energies, movements, and common and organic actions. (These flavors and colors may be critical for optimal health because they may contain certain flavonoid compounds that may protect our cells from oxidative damage).

### The 5 Flavors of Foods

1) **pungent**-includes green onion, garlic, grapefruit peel, green onion, red pepper, sweet basil, soybean oil, ginger, peppermint, chive, clove, parsley, and coriander-these foods can induce perspiration and promote energy circulation. Pungent flavor can act on the lungs and large intestine.

2) **sweet**-includes sugar, cherry, honey, watermelon, apple, barley, bean curd, beef, beet roots, brown sugar, cabbage, carp, carrot, celery, chicken, chicken eggs, coffee, coconut, sweet potato, wheat, wine, milk, chestnut, and banana. Sweet flavor slows down acute symptoms and neutralizes the toxic effects of other foods. Sweet flavor acts on the stomach and spleen. They cause weight gain by improving the functions of the stomach and the Spleen.

3) **sour**-includes lemon, plum, pear, sour plum, apple, apricot, crab apple, grape, grapefruit, hawthorn fruits, kumquat, litchi, loquat, mandarin orange, mango, olive, peach, pineapple plum, raspberry, small red or azuki bean, star fruit or carambola, strawberry, tangerine, , vinegar and tomato. The sour flavor can obstruct movements, and are useful in checking diarrhea and excessive perspiration.

4) **bitter**-includes apricot seed, asparagus, bitter gourd, wild cucumber, celery, cherry seed, coffee, grapefruit peel, hops, kohlrabi, lettuce, lotus plumule, radish leaf, sea grass, vinegar, wine, animal gall bladders, hops. Foods that are slightly bitter include ginseng and pumpkin The bitter flavor can reduce body heat, dry body fluids, and include diarrhea.

5) **salty**-includes kelp and seaweed and functions to soften hardenings, which explains their usefulness in treating TB of the lymph nodes and other symptoms involving the hardening of muscles or glands.

## Other classifications of Foods:

**COLD**-banana, bitter gourd, clams, crab, grapefruit, kelp, lettuce, lotus plumule, muskmelon, persimmon, salt, sea grass, seaweed, star fruit, sugar cane, water chestnut, watermelon. Slightly cold-hops, tomato.

**COOL** energy: apple, barley, bean curd, egg white, Chinese wax gourd, common button mushroom, cucumber, eggplant, Job's tears, lettuce, loquat, mandarin orange, mango, marjoram, mung bean, soy, sesame oil, spinach, strawberry, and wheat bran.

**HOT**-black pepper, cinnamon bark, cottonseed, ginger (dried), green pepper, red pepper, soybean oil, white pepper.

**WARM**-apricot seed, brown sugar, caraway, carp, cherry, chestnut, chicken, chive, clove, coconut, coffee, date, eel, fennel, garlic, fresh ginger, ginseng, guava, ham, kumquat, leaf mustard, mutton, nutmeg, peach, raspberry, rosemary, shrimp, squash, sunflower seed, sweet basil, tobacco, vinegar, walnut, wine. *Sightly warm*-asparagus, malt

**NEUTRAL**-apricot, beef, Chinese cabbage, carrot, celery, chicken egg, corn, cry mandarin orange peel, duck, fig, grape, honey, kidney bean, kohlrabi, licorice, milk, polished rice, pork, peanuts, pineapple, plum, olive, potato, pumpkin, shiitake mushroom, sour plum, string bean, sunflower seed, sweet potato, white sugar, yellow soybean.

## MOVEMENTS OF FOODS

UPWARD-These foods are good to eat in the *spring* as this is a time when living things begin to grow or move upward. They are foods that have 3 flavors: pungent, sweet, or bitter. They include apricot, beef, beet roots, black sesame seed, black soybean, Chinese cabbage, carrot, celery, cherry, chicken egg, duck, gig, grape, honey, kidney bean, licorice, milk, olive, oyster, peanuts, pineapple, plum, pork, potato, pumpkin, small red bean, azuki bean, shiitake mushroom, string bean, sunflower seed, sweet potato, white sugar, yellow soy bean.

DOWNWARD-These foods are good to eat in the "fall". Such foods have 3 energies: cold, cool, or warm and 2 flavors sweet or sour. Foods include apple, bamboo shoots, banana, barley, bean curd, chicken egg white, Chinese wax gourd, clam, common button mushroom, cucumber, eggplant, grapefruit, lettuce, mango, mung bean, peach, spinach, star fruit, strawberry, sugar cane juice, tangerine, water chestnut, watermelon, wheat, and wheat bran.

OUTSIDE-These foods are good to eat in the summer. These foods have a hot energy and are pungent or sweet. They include black pepper, cinnamon bark, cottonseed, dried ginger, green pepper, red pepper, soybean oil, and white pepper.

INSIDE-These foods are good in the winter. They have a cold energy and have 2 different flavors bitter and salty. Clams, crab, hops, kelp, lettuce, salt, and seaweed.

*Diarrhea-*

–2 cloves garlic peeled and crushed, add 2 t brown sugar boil the 2 in 1/2 glass water. Drink the hot soup 2-3x daily.

–fry fresh ginger without oil until it becomes dry and burned on the outside. Grind into powder. Take 8 gms ground ginger each time, 3x per day with warm water.

–Fry 3 bean curds in peanut oil over low heat add a little salt and 60ml rice vinegar and boil for a short while. Eat it as is.

*Coughing-*

-Peel 50g fresh ginger and cut into small slices. Boil the ginger slices with100g maltose in 2 glasses of water for 30 minutes. Drink it hot, 2x per day.

-Make a hole on the side of a pear or an apple. Pour some honey into the hole and steam the pear or the apple. Crush the apple or pear after steaming for 5-10 minutes and eat.

# Detoxification Program

Introduction–Naturopathic medicine has a long history going back to the "Nature Cure," principles espoused back in the 18th century. Even as far back as Hippocrates, the father of medicine who spoke about "leaving drugs in the chemists pot if you can cure the patient with food." He made such a statement back in 420 BC. He was acutely aware of the bodies own natural ability to heal itself if given the correct essential nutrients. Over the years since Vincent Priessnitz, who some say is the father of the Nature Cure movement, detoxification and cleansing programs have evolved and progressed through the observations and intuition of the healers of the times. Today we are in a marvelous time where the nature cure principles have melded with modern science and we are able to evaluate more thoroughly the biochemistry of the individual to determine more specifically what we are detoxifying. Modern laboratory tests have been developed to show us where we may be collecting toxins and in what organs they may be effecting. Thus we have objective criteria in which to evaluate and assess our treatment. As always the true evaluation comes from the patient, their response and how they feel.

Naturopathic medicine today has evolved to a great extent because of what we know about gastrointestinal health and how it effects other parts of the body. We understand that everything in the intestines must get absorbed, excreted or else maintain itself in equilibrium with the rest of the GI tract milieu. We have come to realize that our western culture has a very poor record of health, especially with regard to gastrointestinal health, which is only getting worse. This has mainly arisen because of the energy rich, nutrient poor, refined foods that we currently consume daily. Enormous changes have been made in a very short period of time and people have not had time to really adapt to these changes. The simple solution is to return to where our diet was hundreds, if not thousands of years ago, but incorporate some of the things that we have learned today so that we may improve upon our health to an even higher level than ever before .

The goal of the detoxification program is to eliminate foods that we have grown addicted to, This gives the body a chance to rest from its normal every day digestive and detoxification tasks, and allows it to advance to a higher level of cleansing. The cleansing involves the easing of physical and emotional addictions to foods we eat daily, as well as allowing for removal of toxins that may have been stored in the colon, or other parts of the body, for long periods of time.

## INDICATIONS FOR DETOXIFICATION

There are many reasons for detoxification. As mentioned above, our GI tracts are being exposed to a great many endotoxins which are constantly being made in the body. In addition to these toxins, our food, water and air are also a source of a great many contaminants which add to our body burden. These toxins also accumulate in many tissues throughout the body. This detoxification plan is one way to increase the excretion of these toxins and lower the body's burden of baleful xenobiotics. The following is a partial list of indications for this detoxification program:

1) Allergies
2) Arthritis
3) Fibromyalgia
4) Headaches
5) Fatigue
6) Heavy metal accumulation in tissues
7) Gastrointestinal problems
8) Cancer
9) Chronic constipation,
10) Skin afflictions
11) Chronic infections
12) Chronic fatigue syndrome
13) Chronic yeast infections
14) Obesity
15) Food addictions
16) Depression &/or anxiety
17) Autoimmune diseases including MS, scleroderma, RA, SLE, UC, Anklosing spondylitis

The list of indications for detoxification on the previous page is only a partial list. The clinician must use their own judgment concerning the particular individual and this detoxification program. Not all individuals will find this detox program suitable for them.

## ASSESSMENT

Before undergoing a detoxification program it is essential that some basic biochemical data be obtained so that you have some way to evaluate a patients overall toxin status. The following is a list of some basic tests that can be run to determine some of this basic data.

1) *Basic blood chemistry* which includes evaluation of fasting glucose, cholesterol, HDL cholesterol, LDL cholesterol, ferritin (iron status), triglycerides (fats), liver enzymes including SGOT, SGPT, alkaline phosphatase, and GGT. Depending upon risk of coronary heart disease (see cardiovascular disease assessment in appendix), which is still by far the biggest killer in the U.S., there are some critical tests that should be evaluated. Many of these tests are not evaluated for patients with high risk for coronary heart disease and that is certainly unfortunate.
2) *Hair analysis for heavy metals* indicates if there is an overexposure from food, water or other contamination such as mercury dental amalgams.
3) *Urinary indican*–is an indication of toxins in the bowel.
4) *Caffeine clearance*–evaluates whether or not the body is being exposed to an environmental toxin. The faster the caffeine is cleared from the body the greater is the body's exposure to environmental toxins. In other words enzymes have been stimulated into action because of an exposure to toxins. This is why an alcoholic can tolerate a lot of alcohol before they feel anything, their liver enzymes are on red alert for various toxins aside from just alcohol so the caffeine gets cleared quickly.
5) Consider *stress EKG* if there is a question regarding the health of the heart and cardiovascular system.
6) *Stool analysis*–If parasites or other imbalances of microflora exist in the large intestine then a complete stool analysis should be performed to see if there is an additional factor causing problems with toxins inside the intestines. Generally I like to make sure that Giardia, Cryptosporidium, Entameba histolytica and Helicobacter pylori are not present. If they are then the detoxification should include antiparasitic treatment (see page 383).
7) *Intestinal permeability*–evaluates if there is malabsorption or an excessive permeability of the GI tract.
8) *Peroxides and free radicals in the body*–These can actually be measured in the blood now. There are a number of labs including National Biotech, Great Smokies, Antibody Assay, and Diagnostechs that can evaluate these toxic substances in the body.
9) *Cytochrome 448 and 450*–C448 measures whether or not someone's body believes it is under attack from an environmental toxin while C450 shows how well the body is responding.

In addition to the above assessment, a nutritionally oriented physical is a valuable tool for evaluating mineral, vitamin and other essential and non-essential nutrient requirements (see nutritional physical p. 500-503 in appendix).

## TREATMENT PLAN

**1) Clearing diet–Juice fast, elemental or hypoallergenic diet–**can start with either a 4-7 day juice fast or elemental diet, followed by the hypoallergenic diet plan. This represents the clearing phase of the program. The program can start with a colonic or an enema. It is critical to continue to have daily bowel movements and to urinate regularly. During this period of time all medications should be discontinued (except for absolutely required medications), Required medications may be different for different people and will need to be evaluated for each person. In doing the detoxification program on people who are underweight I am usually cautious about fasting them. As an alternative to the fast an elemental diet may be used. An elemental or defined diet is a synthetic formula that has free amino acids (or hydrolyzed proteins) and other carbohydrates and fats that require little or no digestion for absorption. I recommend ENFood®, a product from Canada formulated by Dr. Gislason (see allergies p. 290). This formula tastes significantly better than many of the other elemental diets found in hospitals. The first 2-3 days of the program will be the most difficult as people may experience withdrawal symptoms from foods that they have previously consumed daily for many years. This is especially true for foods that have pharmacologic activity such as coffee, chocolate, cola and other caffeinated beverages. During the first week of detoxification the following can be added to the fast or diet:

a) psyllium powder (Fiber Flow®, Wise Women Herbal; Fiber Plus®, Yerba Prima; Medibulk®, Thorne–1 round teaspoon 2-3x per day between meals. The purpose of this is to attract water into the bowel and enhance elimination from the GI tract. This will make the stools more bulky and softer.

b) magnesium Twin Labs 400mg 1-2x per day depending upon bowel function. This will increase stimulation of the intestinal peristalsis. If stools become too loose cut back on the magnesium.

c) Bentonite Clay Springreen®–starting on the 3rd day, 1 T 2-3x per day. Bentonite clay has particularly strong adsorptive properties, which means it will bind onto various toxins throughout the small and large intestine.

**2) Reestablishing phase**–If the first week consisted of a fast, it is particularly critical to come off the fast gradually. It is best to transition a fast into a modified hypoallergenic diet. The most important part is to have an eating plan all laid out so that there is no crisis situation where the decision to eat something comes in the midst of being hungry. This will only lead to binging and possible serious repercussions.

When reintroducing foods back into the diet it is important to establish what the goal is. If it is to uncover hidden food allergies or sensitivities then high allergen foods should be introduced one at a time and in small amounts. If no reaction occurs, then the food should avoided for another 3 days and tried again in larger amounts. If still no reaction then the tested food is considered a tolerated food. If the food causes questionable or mild symptoms the food should be eliminated for another week and then rotated once every 5-7 days. At this rotation schedule the food is likely to become less reactive in the future.

If the goal is to continue to feel good as long as possible or for general detoxification purposes then low allergen foods are introduced into the diet, adding to the foods eaten on the hypoallergenic diet list. In this manner the low allergen diet is extended and people can continue to benefit from the program, experiencing little or no symptoms.

In the reestablishing phase the bentonite clay can be continued along with the psyllium powder and magnesium. Bowel function should remain active. At the end of the second week a colonic or a repeat enema to clear the large intestine of any remaining toxins may be useful. The following supplements can be added into the program:

1) **Lactobacillus acidophilus** -to restore normal bacterial flora *Superdophilus* Natren
2) **Butyrate**–This short chain fatty acid is important for optimal intestinal health, especially the colon (low levels of butyrate have been linked to colon cancer).
3) **Glutamine**–can use 3-6 gms per day. This is the preferred substrate for small intestinal enterocytes.
4) **Glycosamino glycans**–substrate material for the intestinal cells
5) **Arginine**–substrate for enterocytes, similar to glutamine
6) **GI Encap** (Thorne)–has Ulmus fulva, licorice, plantain banana,
7) **Folate** (5mg 2x per day) *Folarinse* Scientific Botanicals–especially useful for rapidly dividing cells of the intestines
8) **Essential Fatty Acids**-flax oil 1 T 2x per day
9) **Vitamin A, zinc, vitamin C, vitamin E, selenium, Beta carotene, Silymarin, quercetin**–can all be used to restore health back to the gastrointestinal tract *Oxyquench* (is a combination of the above to simplify) 2 caps 2x per day.

### Normalization of GI function

Continue to introduce foods one at a time.
Continue with the nutrients designed to build up the GI tract such as the vitamins, EFA
May try to streamline the supplements at 4-6 weeks.

### Repeat Detoxification

Can repeat detox program in 1-2 months depending upon how doing. Everyone needs to be evaluated individually. Urinary indican can be repeated to determine levels of toxins in GI tract. Other tests can also be repeated such as peroxide levels, heavy metals in the hair, intestinal permeability, liver enzymes, and cytochrome p-448 & 450. These tests can verify the improved health of the body.

# Thoughts on "The Ideal Diet"

The question, "What is the ideal diet?", has been asked for many years. In the last 20-30 years this question has been answered by many experts in the field of nutrition. Some believe that we do not get enough protein in our diets, others believe we get too much, some believe that certain food combining techniques are critical for optimal health, still others believe eating everything in moderation is the answer. The subject of food allergies and food sensitivities has been another area of intense research. Experts in the field believe health optimization can only take place if various food components form the diet are restricted. For years it has been thought that lowering fat consumption would greatly reduce the risk of cardiovascular disease, and with the studies that Nathan Pritikin and Dean Ornish have conducted, it certainly seems like they have a convincing argument. Recently there have been those who challenged this hypothesis. One popular book written by Dr. Barry Sears, *The Zone Diet, is* a remake of the old Atkins diet from the early 70s–a high fat/ high protein diet which cuts way back on carbohydrates. Sears argues that long term studies have shown that low fat diets do not decrease heart disease but rather they promote it. Macrobiotic diets have been around for a number of years and they have proven to be effective in the treatment of many common western diseases such as hypertension, diabetes, cardiovascular disease and cancer. Some experts believe, however, that macrobiotic diets are too restrictive and that people tend to become sickly when they have been on them for prolonged periods of time. Finally, there are those who believe that we should eat what was eaten many thousands of years ago because a lot of the changes that have come about in the last few thousand years are relatively recent and we have not had the chance to make the necessary evolutionary adjustments. Drs. James and Peter D'Adamo have postulated that certain blood types have evolved to the point where they are able to tolerate certain foods while other foods are either particularly detrimental or particularly beneficial.

In this last chapter I would like to discuss some of the pros and cons of these ideas and to try to present what I believe is the ideal diet based on the integration of this information. Certainly it is a difficult undertaking and there are many different points of view to consider.

**Some of my observations**

From my experience practicing medicine and through what I have studied over the last 21 years, since I began my studies in nutrition, there have been some interesting ideas put forth. I would like to briefly discuss some of them. First, I have been asked many times, "Is it possible to prescribe one diet that is ideal for everyone?" The answer that I invariably give would make a politician proud. I usually respond both "yes" and "no." I believe at this point in time that we have enough evidence to say that there are some basic tenets of an ideal diet that are common to all people. Certainly it is important to take into account a number of different factors. If we observe cultures around the world today that have little heart disease, diabetes, digestive problems, cancer and all the other degenerative diseases that kill 75% of our western population, there are some basic characteristics that stand out. Weston Price, in his classic text, "Nutrition and Physical Degeneration, " writes that as people change their eating habits into the western refined diet they develop many of the same diseases that we have here in the U.S. Even if they previously had none of these diseases, they all tend to develop the same pathologies at the same rate as we do here when they adopt our basic life-style. This is because we are all genetically alike and if we provide similar conditions then we develop what our genetic potential allows us to develop. In another famous text, "Pottinger's Cats: A Study in Nutrition", Francis Pottinger shows how it is possible to not only develop all of the western diseases, but also how to pass them down to the next generation. This is a very profound observation because we do not normally view the idea that having a poor diet can effect successive offspring. In his book, Pottinger shows how a generation of sickly cats took at least 2 or 3 generations on a good diet, to get back to being healthy again. This has some very disconcerting implications in regard to humans when we consider how we eat today.

In addition to cultures around the world today that are relatively free of the diseases of western civilization, we must look at our distant ancestors. What was the state of their health and what did they eat? There have been several books that have addressed this issue: *Paleolithic Prescription* Eaton, Shostak, and Konner; *Eat Right for Your Blood Type* Peter D'Adamo; and *Native Nutrition*, Ronald Schmid. These books present evidence that many thousands of years ago people were very healthy; meaning that they suffered from none of the degenerative killer diseases that we suffer from today. They died of acute infections, childhood mortality, and traumas. With modern medicine we have been able to overcome these killers, but now we are susceptible to all of the chronic diseases that people come down with. If we compare the types of foods that these prehistoric people ate (commonly referred to as *hunters and gatherers*) to what healthy cultures, devoid of chronic degenerative diseases, eat today there exists many common threads.

**Below is a summary of the basic tenets of an optimal diet.**

| | |
|---|---|
| **Carbohydrates** | 60-75% of total calories |
| Types of carbohydrates | complex 90% & simple 10% |
| **Proteins** | 10-30% of total calories |
| **Fats** | 20% of total calories |
| | Types of fats 80% unsaturated fats |
| | (omega 6 to omega 3---5 to 1) |
| Total calories | minimal to maintain low body weight |
| | |
| Fiber (mixed soluble & insoluble) | 50-100gms |
| Sodium | 500mg-1gm |
| Potassium | 8-10gms |
| Flavonoids and antioxidants | very high levels and a broad spectrum |
| Ellagic acid, cruciferous vegetables | daily servings when in season |
| Soy bean products | if tolerated 4-5x per week |
| Processed foods | none |
| | |
| Blood parameters "ideal" | cholesterol 125-175mg/dl; HDL over 60 |
| (see Blood Chemistry | glucose, fasting 70-90mg/dl |
| Results Explained) | uric acid below 5.0 |

The above formula is something that we know for certain. It is the basic tenet of an ideal diet that will lead to optimal health. There are some arguments as to how to best make up this breakdown. It is clear from health statistics that vegetarians in our western culture are significantly healthier than omnivores. There are probably a number of reasons for this. For one, omnivores, if eating a significant amount of meat, will not be able to consume enough fiber, nor will they be able to keep their fat intake down to the recommended levels. In addition, they will not be able to keep their fat ratio in accord with a significant amount of omega 3 fatty acids. Currently we consume a ratio of almost 20 to 1 omega 6 fatty acids to omega 3. This is very much out of balance. Thus, as an omnivore there is generally going to be a significant imbalance in one's dietary fat intake (taking into consideration what our typical meat supply is made of). If the omnivore ate a significant amount of cold water fish, they could certainly consume a better ratio of unsaturated omega 3 fatty acids. In addition, fish are generally considerably lower in fats than red meats.

There have been arguments made that we come from ancestors who ate meat as hunters and gatherers. This is true to a certain extent, however, the type of meat that was eaten then was not the stationary cow that we eat today, but rather it was wild game. The type of fat found in wild game is vastly different from the grass fed and highly processed meats that we eat today, at least in the U.S. For one, there is a considerable amount of omega 3 fatty acids in wild game and the overall level of fat is much lower. Thus, if we could eat wild game, I would say that red meat would be beneficial and I would consider it a more valuable food. ( See PBS video "The Missing Link" Don Johanson).

Another idea previously mentioned was popularized back in the early 80s by James D'Adamo and then recently expounded by his son Peter D'Adamo. The concept is based on blood types and that what you should eat is dictated by your blood type–certain foods are more suitable for certain blood types because of the way in which people have evolved. Macrobiotics espouses something both similar and different to this–eating foods in accordance with the season or with what is indigenous to the area in which you are living. In other words, macrobiotics advocates eating foods that are available in season wherever you are living. This rotating of foods with the seasons is something that clinical ecologists believe should be done with high allergen foods or foods that are known to cause reactions.

By observing the many food allergies that we see today this makes a lot of sense. The very same foods should not be eaten over and over again, day in and day out. Some of the earliest pioneers of food allergies or food intolerances have come from the "Nature Cure," practitioners back in the 1600's. More recently Dr. O.G. Carroll in the 1930's discovered that certain foods seemed to trigger off many people's pathologies. He noticed that these foods were very often strongly craved by the sickly people. He devised a method for evaluating people's food sensitivities and then had them avoid these foods. In prehistoric times the food rotation was done through the seasons, much like that of the macrobiotics. One of the concepts that the D'Adamos have presented is that some people may require considerably higher amounts of protein than other people. They claim that people with type 0 blood are most associated with the hunters and gatherers because it is the oldest blood type. This is certainly something to take note of, especially when you consider the wide requirement of amino acids in individuals (*Medical Applications of Clinical Nutrition* 1983, Jeff Bland & also p.7 introduction). Also when you consider that type O people secrete much higher levels of HCL, it just stands to reason that their digestive tract is more suited to having a higher level of protein. In addition, it seems that blood typing is something that can show incompatibilities with different foods because of the specific lectins that exist on foods that might not show up with other tests.

Looking further at the various pieces of the puzzle of the optimal diet, there have been studies done on overall caloric intake and it seems that people who consume lower levels of calories live longer. This is something that has been studied by a number of researchers. One person who has made the low calorie diet popular (well maybe not popular, but as an option) is Roy Walford author of, *Maximum Life Span*. In his book he presents information that shows that humans should live at least to 120 years. He goes on to review research that has been done on animals to show how they can live 50-100% longer if their diets were "calorie restricted." Calorie restriction leads to less oxidative reactions in the body due to less metabolism of food. In addition there are less fats that can be oxidized and as a result less free radicals. Because there are less foods going into the gastrointestinal tract, there is less chance for poor digestion to occur and thus less chance of developing allergies or putrefication by-products. Also less food going into the GI tract means less bile salts secreted, thereby producing less deleterious compounds in the colon (often they are derived from bile salts). There will also be less proteins and fats fermenting as well in the colon meaning less irritants and less chances of developing cancer.

In a book that was written a few years ago called *The Zone Diet*, Barry Sears, advocates the use of a high protein and a higher fat diet. From what I can tell, it also advocates a lower caloric intake. He states that a big problem with people's health is that they are secreting too much insulin and as a result the incidence of diabetes and other degenerative diseases has steadily risen. In his book however, he makes several false statements and false accusations concerning some of the low fat diets of Dean Ornish and Nathan Pritikin. Certainly elevated insulin levels are implicated in many degenerative diseases including obesity, diabetes, heart disease, and food cravings. However, he states that the overall consumption of carbohydrate foods has risen over the years. This is incorrect as the actual overall carbohydrate consumption has actually gone down since the early part of the century. What has gone up dramatically is the intake of simple carbohydrates. They have replaced much of the complex carbohydrates that were once eaten. In his book he claims that foods with a high glycemic index are the foods that are causing the problems with people's elevated insulin levels. He has people avoid all such high glycemic index foods. Unfortunately he does not take into account the nutritional value of the food. I believe that this is too general. His diet is also too high in fats & protein and too low in fiber.

Lets look at this issue further concerning high protein and high fat in the diet. High protein, especially animal protein, has been strongly linked to cardiovascular disease as well as to cancer. In addition high levels of protein also put a strain on the kidneys since they have to excrete all of the by-products of protein metabolism. High levels of protein in the diet have also been linked to osteoporosis, a major problem in the U.S. It seems that high levels of protein in the diet have serious drawbacks. Concerning fats, there are a number of problems to consider when eating a diet higher in fat. For one thing, fat is the one material that loves to store environmental pollutants. One example is a study done on breast milk in women in Michigan. It was found that 100% of the women had detectable levels of DDT, a pesticide that has a high affinity for fat. It has been stated that 85% of all breast cancer is environmentally caused. The reason is that breast tissue is mostly fat and therefore it tends to accumulate most of the toxins from the environment. Thus going too high on the fat, especially from animals, is very likely to lead to an increase intake of environmental pollutants, something that will certainly decrease health and longevity. Animal fats also contain arachidonic acid, a fat that has been implicated in many inflammatory processes in the body as well as cardiovascular diseases, such as stroke, heart attacks and phlebitis. An excellent book that describes in detail contaminants found in human milk, *Chemical Contaminants in Human Milk*, Alan A. Jensen & Stuart A. Slorach, 1991, points out that vegetarians, who consume significantly less fat that omnivores, have significantly less DDT, PCBs and other toxins in their milk. Some of the highest contaminants were found in marine products. One study showed that 80% of PCBs in the Japanese diet was from fish.

It seems that one big question remains, whether or not grains are healthy for you or not. Certainly refined grains are a problem, and that includes pasta made from white flour. Over 90% of pasta is made from white flour. Our ancestors did not consume wheat (if they did, it was a wild unhybridized species and in very small amounts) for over 9,000 years. Thus from an evolutionary standpoint, people have not had the chance to evolve into eating and tolerating grains. Grains have complex proteins that are difficult to digest and assimilate. In the book, "Your Family Tree Connection," J. Reading writes that because of the fact, that we have not been exposed to wheat and grains for a very long time, there are a significant number of people who have autoimmune reactions to them. Recent evidence shows that Celiac disease, a condition in which an immunological reaction is mounted to gluten, is much more common than was previously thought. Certainly, wheat is a big food allergen. Because a relatively short period of time has passed since the beginning of agriculture, it seems likely that only a relative few people have adapted to eating grains. It would seem wise to either look at your past (where your ancestry comes from), or examine your blood type to determine whether you should eat substantial amounts of grain. Certainly if they can be tolerated, they offer high nutrition if they are found in their whole natural state. Fiber is found in significant amounts along with many trace minerals and antioxidant nutrients.

For maximum health it is important to take into consideration cancer prevention. Eating a large array of fruits and vegetables is critical if one is to get a wide assortment of flavonoids and other cancer protecting foods. Ellagic acid is one compound that has been shown to be protective against cancer. It is found in cranberries, raspberries, blackberries, strawberries and loganberries contain significant amounts of ellagic acid. The cruciferous family of foods such as cabbage, broccoli, brussels sprouts and cauliflower have shown protective effects against many types of cancer that exceeds the protective effect of their known nutrients. Other fruits and vegetables that are high in carotenoid pigments are also very cancer protecting. Other compounds such as chlorogenic acid and caffeic acid which can be found in apples, other fruits, vegetables and nuts have been found to possess anticancer properties. Interestingly cooked and processed apples hardly contain any of these protective substances.

In summary, I believe the ideal diet should include a significant amount of raw fruits and vegetables along with cooked ones (depending upon digestion). Smoked, fried and barbecued foods should be avoided as much as possible. Foods that grow measurable amounts of molds that can produce toxins should be avoided (peanuts and corn grow aspergillus flavus, a mold that produces aflatoxin, one of the most carcinogenic substances known. Avoiding or keeping these foods down to a minimum would seem prudent. All food should be as organic as possible, especially if it has a significant amount of fat in it. In *The Healing Power of Foods*, Michael Murray goes into good detail on some of these ideas. Some juice is probably beneficial, especially if someone has had problems with their digestion. It is a very concentrated source of nutrients and should be diluted down to half.

All in all the key is to determine what foods are best tolerated and then to eat as many different kinds as possible to insure the wide array of cancer protecting substances, many that we know of and many of them that we have not identified yet. In particular leafy vegetables, especially ones grown wild, that offer essential nutrients in higher concentrations than most store bought items. As mentioned, fats should make up 20% of calories with a significant amount from omega 3 oils particularly flax oil which has been shown to offer protection against certain cancers.

**"Life in all its fullness is '*Mother Nature*' obeyed." –Weston Price**

# Appendix

# Health History Summary

Date______________

Name______________________________ Age_____ Birthdate_________ Blood type_____

Address______________________________ City_______________ State____ Zip_______

Phone(home)______________________ (work)______________________daytime or eve?

Occupation____________________ (full/part time?) Employer___________________

Insurance Co.____________________Policy #________________ Soc Sec #____________

Address _____________________City___________________ State_____ Zip___________

Nearest Relative____________________________________ Phone___________________
what is their relationship to you

Who else can we reach in case of emergency?____________________ Phone_____________
what is their relationship to you

How did you hear about the Tabor Hill Clinic?_____________________________________

Last physician or health practitioner seen?______________________ When?___________

When was your last blood test?_______________ What kind?_______________________

**Your Current Health Problems**

What is your **main** reason for coming in today? If you have a specific health condition please describe in detail. When was the very first time that you noticed your condition and describe carefully any factors that you suspect may have played a role in its onset and its continuation.

List in order of importance other health problems that are troubling you:

1)_________________________________________ & length of time_______________

2)_________________________________________ & length of time_______________

3)_________________________________________ & length of time_______________

4)_________________________________________ & length of time_______________

Other problems:_______________________________________________________________

How long has your **main** problem been troubling you?_________________________________

Is your current "main problem" getting *[better, worse, same]* and for how long?_____________

What kind of treatment have you received and from whom?______________________________

Have you ever seen a naturopathic physician, chiropractor, acupuncturist or other alternative health practitioner for your current problem? *(yes or no)* or for any problem? *(yes or no).*

What was the therapy and what were the results?________________________________________

_______________________________________________________________________________

**Your Health History**

The general state of your health is: **(excellent___) (good___) (avg___) (fair___) (poor___),** and on the average describe your energy level from 1-10 (10 is highest & 1 lowest) "________"

When during the day is your energy the best?_____________ worst?_____________

What is your current approximate weight?_________ height?________ Weight one year ago_____

As an adult what has been your maximum_______ and minumum weight_______ (do not include pregnancy)

Please list the 5 most significant, stressful events in your life, from the most recent to the most distant. Are any of these situations continuing to impact your life? *(yes or no) Please circle*

1) ____________________________________________________________ date__________

2) ____________________________________________________________ date__________

3) ____________________________________________________________ date__________

4)____________________________________________________________ date__________

5)____________________________________________________________ date__________

Are you currently working with a professional counselor, psychologist, social worker, pastor or other therapist?_______ Have you in the past?________ If so when?(give dates)_________

Are you currently working with a Doctor of conventional medicine?(M.D. or D.O.)*(Yes or No)*

What childhood illnesses have you had? (check off if had)

| | | | |
|---|---|---|---|
| measles ______ | mumps_________ | chickenpox_________ | whooping cough____ |
| polio ______ | diphtheria_______ | rheumatic fever_____ | scarlet fever________ |
| smallpox______ | typhoid fever_____ | tuberculosis________ | mono___ how long__ |

Previous surgeries and hospitalizations (include dates)___________________________________

_______________________________________________________________________________

Which of the following have you had and indicate "now or past";.& also how often and when.

| now or past | | year | now or past | | year | now or past | | year |
|---|---|---|---|---|---|---|---|---|
| ____ | pneumonia | ________ | ____ | diabetes | _______ | _____ | gonorrhea | _______ |
| ____ | tonsillitis | ________ | ____ | asthma | _______ | _____ | syphilis | _______ |
| ____ | ear infections | _______ | ____ | eczema | _______ | _____ | venereal disease | ____ |
| ____ | chronic infections | ______ | ____ | heart disease | ____ | _____ | epilepsy | ________ |
| ____ | canker sores | _______ | ____ | herpes | _______ | _____ | high blood pressure | ____ |
| ____ | allergies | ____________ | ____ | hepatitis | _______ | _____ | mononucleosis | ____ |
| ____ | thyroid problems | _______ | ____ | weight prob. | ____ | _____ | anemia | ________ |
| ____ | others | ____________ | | | | | | |

Do you have any allergies to any drugs, herbs, foods, animals or other? *(Y or N)* What? _______

_______________________________________________________________________________

**Which of the following do you currently use?**

amount (how often, how much & how long) amount (how often, how much & how long)

alcohol________________________________ tobacco________________________________

hormones ______________________________ coffee_________________________________

cortisone _____________________________ laxatives______________________________

sedatives _____________________________ antacids_______________________________

other medications (please give full name and doseage and how long have you been taking the medication)

______________________/ ______________________/ ______________________

______________________/ ______________________/ ______________________

______________________/ ______________________/ ______________________

vitamins\herbs_______________/ _______________/_______________/__________

__________/ _______________/ _______________/ _______________/ __________

__________/ _______________/ _______________/ _______________/ __________

**Family History**

Please list ages, health problems and if deceased, cause of death:

| | Living(age?) | Health Problems | Died (age?) | Cause |
|---|---|---|---|---|
| Your Mother | ______ | ______________________ | ____ | ______________ |
| Your Father | ______ | ______________________ | ____ | ______________ |
| Your Brothers | ______ | ______________________ | ____ | ______________ |
| | ______ | ______________________ | ____ | ______________ |
| | ______ | ______________________ | ____ | ______________ |
| Your Sisters | ______ | ______________________ | ____ | ______________ |
| | ______ | ______________________ | ____ | ______________ |
| | ______ | ______________________ | ____ | ______________ |
| Grandmom & granddad<br>Mother's Mom | ______ | ______________________ | ____ | ______________ |
| Mother's Dad | ______ | ______________________ | ____ | ______________ |
| Grandmom & granddad<br>Father's Mom | ______ | ______________________ | ____ | ______________ |
| Father's Dad | ______ | ______________________ | ____ | ______________ |

What is your nationality? *(please list all backrounds & give approximate %)*____________________

______________________________________________________________________________

You currently live with? spouse___ partner___ parents___ friends___ children___ alone____

Are you? married____ separated___ divorced___ widowed___ single___ in a supportive relationship___

What is your current level of education?____________________ Are you satisfied with this? ***(Yes or No)***

Do you have any children?______ How many? ______ Ever have Toxemia during preg. **(Y or N)**

Do they have any health problems?__________________________________________________

**Do you have any blood relative aunt uncle or grandparent who has had any of the following?**

____allergies ____arthritis ____asthma ____cancer ____diabetes

____anemia ____depression ____skin disease ____heart attack ____genetic prob

____High B.P. ____stroke ____ulcers ____cataracts ____thyroid prob

____hypoglycemia____seizures ____sickle cells ____venereal disease

What is your weakest organ system and why?__________________________________________

## Personal Habits

What do you enjoy most in your life?_______________________________________

What are your main interests or hobbies?_______________________________________

What do you worry most about in life?_______________________________________

Do you exercise? *(yes/no)* If yes what kind, how much & how often?__________________

Do you have a religious or spirtual practice? (*Yes/No* ) If yes, what?____________________

On a scale of 1-10, how would you rate the quality of your sleep (10 being great) ___________

Do you have problems (*falling or staying asleep*)? ____ How many hrs do you sleep at night?____

Do you awaken at night? ***(yes or no)*** If yes what time(s) do you usually wake up?__________

Do you ever sweat at night while sleeping? ***(yes or no)***. How frequently and how much do you sweat?____________________ Do you wake up feeling refreshed? ***(yes or no)***

Do you nap or rest horizontally throughout the day? ***(yes or no)***. For how long? ___________

What do you normally feel like temperature wise, compared to others? ***(warm or cooler or avg)***

What are the temperatures of your hands and feet generally? (***warmer or cooler or average)***

Do you enjoy your work? (***yes or no)*** Do you take vacations? (***yes or no***)

Are you currently in a happy satisfying relationship with someone? ***(Very, mostly, somewhat, not)***

How often do you get colds, flus, sore throat, yeast infections during the year?_____________

When you rise quickly from a sitting or lying position do you ever get dizzy? ***(yes or no)*** *If yes how often?**(daily; few times per week; 1x week; 2x per month; 1x per month; rarely)***

## Female reproduction

Age of first menses______ If periods have stopped at what age did they stop?_____________

Are your cycles regular ***(Y N)*** Period begins every _______ days. How long periods?______

Are your periods ***(Heavy, medium, light)*** & what color is blood?(***light red, dark red, medium, clots***)

Do you have any spotting or bleeding between periods ***(Y / N)*** Any cramps with period ***(Y / N)***

Do you have any premenstrual symptoms ?***(water retention, breast tenderness, irritability, depression, headaches, mood swings, food cravings)*** other ___________________________

Number of pregnancies_______ Number of abortions______ Number of live births?_______

Number of miscarriages_______ Any problems gettting pregnant?_______________________

Do you get yearly PAP smears?***(Y /N)*** Any abnormal PAP's? ***(Y / N)*** Breast lumps?***(Y / N)***

Are you currently sexually active?***(Y N)*** How often?________ Is this ***(more or less)*** than 1 yr ago?

Do you use birth control? ***(Y / N)*** What type of birth control do you currently use?________

Have you ever been physically or sexually abused? ***(Y/N)*** How old and how often?_________

## Male Reproduction

How often do you have to get up at night to urinate?____ Is this an increase in past few yrs?***(Y/N)***

Any problems with impotency? (getting or maintaining an erection) ***(Y/N)***. Any sores on penis? ***(Y/N)***.

Do you have any abnormal discharge from the penis? ***(Y/N)*** Any veneral diseases? (***yes or no)***

Any prostate problems? (**Y/N & *past/now)*** Ever have your prostate examined?(Y/N). When?_____

Are you currently sexually active?***(Y/N)*** How often?________ Is this ***(more or less)*** than 1 yr ago?

Do you use birth control? ***(Y or N)*** What type of birth control do you currently use?________

Have you ever been physically or sexually abused? ***(Y/N)*** How old and how often?_________

# Digestion and Elimination

**Digestion** *(circle or fill in the answer)*

Do you have any problems with gas, bloating or fullness after eating? (**Yor N**). How often do you have gas, fullness or bloating after eating? ***(often, sometimes, never)***. How severe?______
Do you have gas in ***(the upper part of the abdomen or lower part or both areas)***?

How long have you had this problem?____________

How often do you have bowel movements?__________________________

Do you ever have any (**blood, mucus, undigested food, black stools**)?

Any rectal itching? (**Y/N**) Do your stools tend to be ***(formed or loose)***? How often do you have diarrhea?_____________Do you ever have alternating constipation and diarrhea? (**Y N**)

How often do you have thin, long and narrow stools? ***(often sometimes never)***

How often do you have small & hard stools?***(often, sometimes, never)***

Do you ever have yellow or light colored stoolsS? ***(often, sometimes, never)***

How often do your stools have a strong disagreeable odor? ***(often, sometimes, never)***

Have you ever fasted? ***(yes or no; juice or water)*** For how long have you fasted?________

How did you feel while you were fasting?______________________________________

Have you traveled outside the U.S. in last 5 years? *(Y/N) Have you gone camping in last 5 yrs?* **(Y/N)**

**Kidneys and bladder**

Have you had recurrent bladder infections?***(Yes or No)*** How were they treated?___________

How many bladder infections have you had in the last 3 years?________________________

Do you have any burning sensation during or after urination? ***(Past or Present or now)***

Is your urine ***(dark yellow, bright yellow, cloudy, pale or clear)***?

Does your urine have a strong odor to it? ***(Yes or No)***

Do you have difficulty starting or stopping when urinating? ***(Yes or No)***

Do you have difficulty perspiring? ***(Y N)***.. Do you perspire when you exercise? ***(lightly, moderately, heavily)***. Do you perspire other times than when exercising? ***(Y N)*** When?

Does your perspiration have a strong smell? ***(Yes or No)***

Does your temperature tend to run ***(low or high or average)***compared to others?*(circle one)*

**Occupational/household**

How long have you lived at your present address?__________ Where have you lived previously? _____________***(Please describe location, if old or new place, i.e., new construction, damp or moldy)***

Do you have specialized air filtration at home? ***(yes or no)*** *Do you live in city?* ***(Yes or No)***

Do you work in an office building? ***(yes or no)*** Do the windows open? ***(yes or no)***

Do you have specialized air filtration at your work place? ***(yes or no)***

Do you work in the presence of toxic fumes or chemicals? ***(yes or no)***

Do any of your hobbies involve toxic materials? ***(yes or no)***

Are you exposed to second hand smoke currently? ***(yes or no)***

What do you use for your drinking water? ***(bottled, filtered, or tap water)***

**Do you have anything else you would like to comment on?** ______________________

# Nutritional Physical Exam

## 1. Blood Pressure

- Ideally below 120/80, diastolic Bp most important
- ↑Bp consider suppl. EFA, Mag, Ca & $K^+$.
- ↓Bp consider anemia, hypothyroid, hypoadrenals, dehydration, meds.
- *Orthostatic hypotension*-1st allow pt. to lie down for a few minutes w/o talking, take Bp in supine position, then have them stand with arm straight out, if Bp drops > 6pts diastolically then consider anemia, hypoadrenal, dehydration, prolonged bed rest or various meds
- *Hypoadrenals*- consider vit C, B-5, vit E, adrenal extract, DHEA, licorice or Dioscorea
- *Anemia*-consider B-12, folate, iron, B-6, Cu, B-1, biot.
- *Big pulse pressure* (> 50pts.)- consider Mg
- *Anemia*-consider B-12, folate, iron, B-6, Cu, B-1,biot.

## 2. Heart

- *MVP*- Mg & L-carnitine def., consider lax ligaments & hypermobile jts.-vit C, mang, Hawthorne, silica, boron & copper
- *Slow rate*- hypothyroid, athletic heart, ↑growth horm
- *Irregular rate*- $K^+$ def. due to diuretics, dehydration, Mg def., hypoglycemia, allergy
- *Tachycardia*- def Mag, Ca, B-3. Meds esp antidepressants, thyroid
- IHSS-murmur may be related to hypothyroidism

## 3. Chest

- *Wheezing*-allergies, B-6, quercetin, omega 3 FA's, B-12, sulfite sensitivity(Molyb), Staphage lysate
- *Barrel chested & shallow breathing*- emphysema Aspidosperma, lecithin, vit A
- *Coughing* (rales & rhonchi)-allergies, decr immunity, vit A, vit C, zinc, flavonoids
- *Pain*-costalchondral jts. costochondritis vitamin E topically along with Arnica oil & Hypericum (oil & homeopathically)

## 4. Head

- *Dry hair*, consider hypothyroidism & EFA
- *Itchy skin* consider CA, parasites, PSC, EFA def
- *Premature Greying*-PABA def, B-5
- *Hair loss*-generalized-parasites, heavy metal, vit A or other environmental toxicity, hypothyroid, chemo, BCP;consider folate & B-6, also B plex, EFA & B-5
- *Dandruff*-hypochorhydria, XS refined CHO's, def of EFA, antioxidants (esp selenium topically & orally) & B-6 & B-plex

## 5. Neck

- *Multiple pigmented skin tags* (around arms & upper back area as well) indicates glucose intolerance; consider glucose insulin tolerance test (see p.274)
- *Chronic lymphadenopathy*-allergies, depressed immunity, localized dermatitis, environmental toxins, Hodgkins and HIV.

## 6. Face

- Seborrheic dermatitis (forehead shiny & scaly, c yellow greasy look which extends into eyebrows, down nose, cheeks, chest). Tx with Bplex, PABA, B6, EFA esp GLA- can use topical B6(may make worse initially). Avoid refined CHO's consider glucose intolerance
- *Vertical creases* between eyebrows-consider duodenal ulcers esp c epigastric pain & L shoulder pain
- *Acne*- face & back - avoid sugar, incr leafy veggies, detox, √ for decr BTT (√ with charcoal & indican), suppl zinc, EFA, vit A. In adults over 22 y/o consider food allergy & ↓HCL
- *Dilated capillaries cheeks & nose*-too much alcohol, consider low HCL. Tx with GLA & herbal bitters
- *Acne Rosacea* redness of cheeks and forehead along c pimples consider allergies & simple CHO sensitivity

## 7. Nose

- *Salute Sign*-horizontal lines across bridge of nose-sinus allergies esp. dairy
- *Intra Nasal Polyps*-allergies or salicylate sensitivity
- *Anosmia*-zinc def
- *Runny nose*-allergies avoid breathing allergens, avoid pollution, tx with quercetin, Chinese herbs, Nettles, Bee pollen, B5, vit C.
- *Rash*, red over nose and under eyes-think SLE-consider EFA, antioxidants, and allergies

## 8. Ears

- *Diagonal ear lobe creases*-esp in males highly assoc with CVD (doesn't apply to Am. Indian & Asians).
- *Tophi*-gout; increase folate and ↓purines in diet
- *Ear wax*-lots of dark sticky wax or none with dry scaley hyperemic canals indicates ↓EFA
- TM-white matter may indicate yeast overgrowth-consider yeast antigen test tx with anti-yeast diet
- *Fluid behind TM*-allergies esp. to dairy
- Meniere's-allergies
- *Tinnitus*-aspirin tox, CVD, allergies

## 9. Mouth

- *Teeth*-many Hg fillings may effect thyroid or CNS. Do DMPS challenge & Hg urine collection p.472. If MS present consider replacing carefully p.472.
- *Tooth decay*-consider poor mineral absorption-such as decr boron, silica, calcium, vit B6-avoid simple CHO's and consider Pb toxicity and Stevia topically.
- *Periodontal disease*-def Ca, Co Q10, quercetin, antioxidants esp high dose vit C, folate & zinc as mouth wash and also IPSAB, Cratagus, and Sanguinaria.
- *Gums bleeding*-vit C, bioflav, poor brushing c hard bristles
- *Aphthous ulcers*-allergies, avoid gluten, simple CHO's, citrus, coffee & methylxanthines
- *Tonsils*-enlarged-allergies, depressed immunity, irritants
- *Bruxism*-xs stress, allergies, anxiety
- *Cheilosis* or angular stomatitis-B2 or B complex

### Tongue

- Glossitis-B12, folate, Zn or Fe def-.
- Geographic tongue-allergies, B vitamins
- Pale if conjunctiva are also pale think anemia ↓ Fe
- Swollen c teeth marks=weak digestion & allergies
- white patches on inner cheek-yeast, Leukoplakia-if yeast check simple fast bld glucose and CHO intake

## 10. Eyes

- *dark circles under eyes*-allergic shiners consider avoiding allergies esp dairy, suppl quercetin, vit C, Rose hips extract & cromolyn
- *Blepharitis*-think allergies and ↓EFA
- *Pale conjunctiva*-think ↓ Fe anemia
- *Denies' lines*-allergies tx with quercetin, vit C
- *Conjunctivitis*-inflammatory rx consider antioxidants & lubrication for eyes. Similisan, vit A, cromolyn drops.
- *Floaters*-def bld or def vit K, vit C, & bioflavonoids
- *Retinol Hemorrhages*-think diabetes; tx with flavonoids, vit C, antioxidants, Bilberry extract
- *Dry Eyes* (Sicca syndrome)-may indicate ↑ requirement for vit A. Give vit A and Similisan drops.
- *Xanthomas*-may indicate XS triglycerides; tx with
- *Cataracts*-opacity related to DM tx with quercetin, vit C, A, E, sel and Bilberry
- *Glaucoma*- vit C and B2
- *Pupillary Light Reflex*-if can't hold pupil fixed indicates weak adrenals. Can check ASI & orthostatic Bp.

## 11. Nails

- *flat angle & spooning*-Fe def
- *soft poor growth*-consider multiple mineral def, hypochlorhydria
- *cuticle inflammation*-Zn def
- brittle nails-hypothyroid or decr HCL or protein or mineral def
- *acrodynia* red tips c abn nail growth Hg tox
- ridging-consider ↓mineral absorption ↓HCL
- *Stunted growth with nail eaten away & thinned out*-consider yeast/fungal infection- avoid caffeine, simple CHO-apply topical antifungal/yeast agents. Can use garlic topically and orally.

## 12. Skin

- *Dry*-EFA def, hypothyroid, ↓vit A, ↓vit E, XS soap, XS chlorine, dehydration. *Psoriasis* on elbows, knees or scalp-use topical vit D, antioxidants, fumaric acid.
- *Follicular hyperkeratosis*-small red bumps on backs of arms, buttocks, and anterior thighs. Consider ↓vit A, ↓vit E, Zn, hypothyroidism, EFA, malabsorption. Consider bile salts or pancreatic enzymes to help abs.
- *Dermatographism*-↑sensitivity allergies topical & internal. Suppl. quercetin, vit E, C, Zn and selenium.
- *Generalized itching*-hypothyroid, cancer, EFA def. parasites, vit A toxicity, allergies, chlorine, ↓vit K
- *Acrodynia* red tips c abn nail growth=Hg tox
- *Ridging*-consider ↓mineral absorption ↓HCL
- *Slow Wound Healing*-R/O DM, def vit A, C, Zinc, EFA
- *Tinea*-consider bld sugar abn, R/O Candida
- *Bruising Easily*-consider ↓platelets, ↓vit K; also consider suppl. vit C , E & bioflavonoids.
- *Callous (thick) on heel*-suppl. vit E & A & EFA
- *Numbing & tingling*-R/O DM, B12 def. suppl. B6/B12
- *Skin sensitive to rolling*-panniculofibrositis esp. if they have chronic HA's, back pain, jaw pain. Tx c B6, bromelain & skin roll & acupuncture. Avoid allergies.

## 13. Hands

- *Eczema*-consider allergies, Zn, EFA, B6, GLA
- *Hang nails*-consider zinc talley taste test & give Zn
- *Skin cracking at tips*-think zinc deficiency,EFA & vit E
- *Cold*-think Raynaud's syndrome or anemia-↓stress, EFA omega 3,Ginkgo, niacin,vit E. If anemia tx.
- *Dupuytren's contracture*-fibrous thickening on ant. side of hand along 4th & 5th digits causing flexion of fingers. Consider glucose intolerance. Tx with high dose vit E orally and topically can use Arnica oil, vit E, SSKI, DMSO, bromelain, acupuncture & electrostimulation
- *Ulnar deviation with atrophy of muscles*-think RA and tx with allergy diet especially avoid grains, suppl vit E, zinc, glucosamine sulfate, bromelain.
- *Heberden's nodes*-on distal DIP joints of hands, think OA; tx c allergy diet esp try avoiding nightshade family, suppl niacinamide, vit E, Zn, glucosamine sulfate, boron, Cu salicylate, bromelain

## 14. Musculoskeletal

- *Growing pains & Osgood Schlatter ds*- Vit E & sel orally & topically along with DMSO.
- *CTS*- vit B6 & bromelain
- *Bursitis*-B12 IM & acup, topical Arnica oil
- *Sciatica*-B12 & B1 IM

## 15. Abdomen

- Ask pt. if needs to urinate, when they ate, if ticklish. Palpate least sensitive areas 1st initially going lightly. Watch face as you palpate.
- *Hiatal Hernia Syndrome*-some tenderness left of xiphoid and 4th intercostal interspace mid-axillary line
- Murphy Sign "+"-GB/LV pathology-consider food allergies, LV flush,↓fats, eval LV fx, cytochrome p-448
- *Colon* tender consider yeast overgrowth, irritations, diverticulitis, colitis, parasites, ↓HCL, sluggish bowel, CA esp if occult blood + R/O celiac ds.(endomysial)

## 16. Urogenital

- PAP abn-consider vit B6, folate &beta carotene, vit A.
- *Chronic bladder infection* in women consider yeast infection and avoid XS simple CHO's
- *Prostate* exam-make sure size of prostate is adequately determined, if big give EFA, zinc, vit A, alanine, glycine, glutamic acid, can check PSA esp if family hx and if hard c masses. Do PSA prior to exam. Hypertrophy will falsely elevate PSA.

## Nutrition Physical Exam

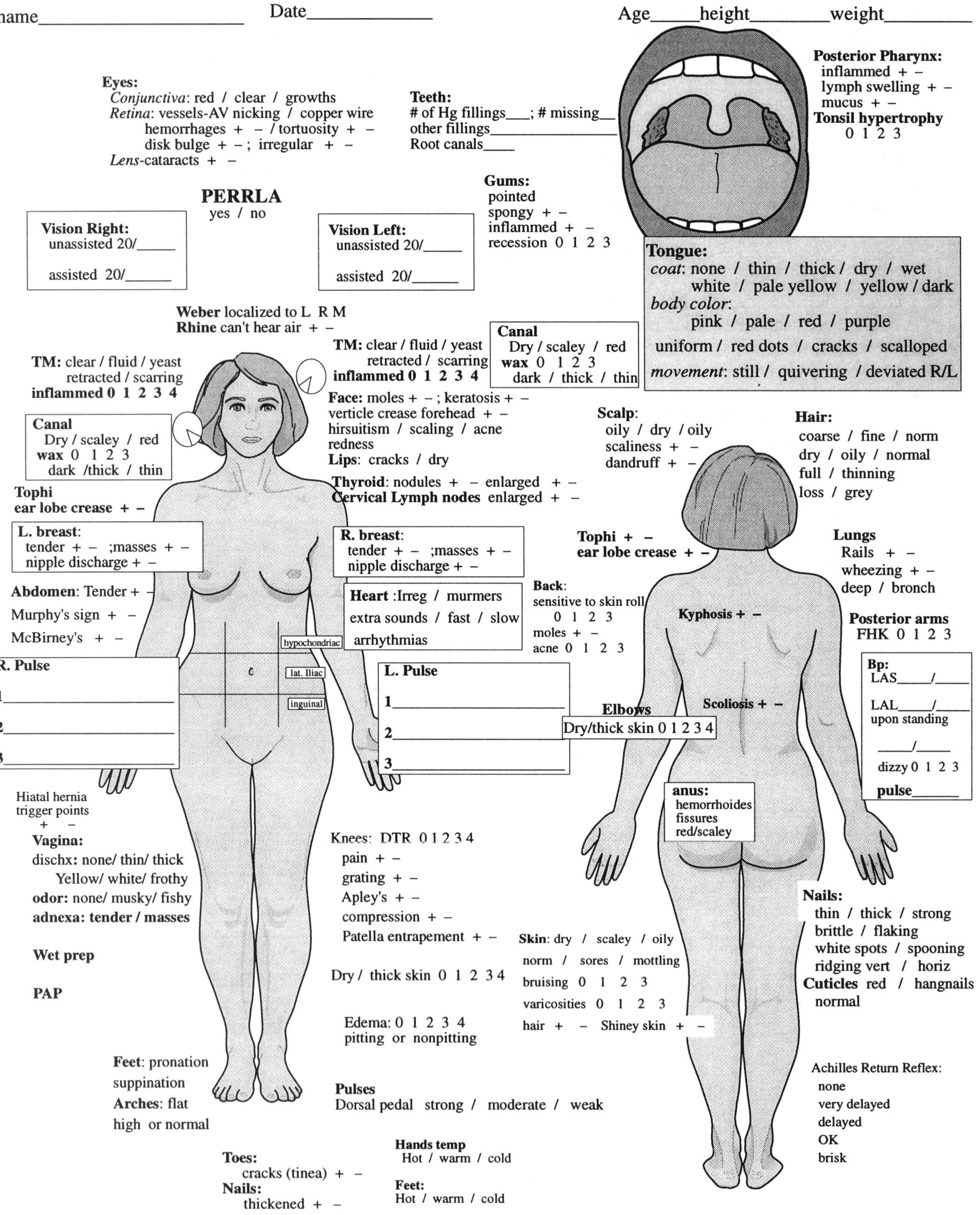

name____________________ Date____________ Age_____height________weight_________

**Eyes:**
*Conjunctiva*: red / clear / growths
*Retina*: vessels-AV nicking / copper wire
hemorrhages + – / tortuosity + –
disk bulge + – ; irregular + –
*Lens*-cataracts + –

**Teeth:**
# of Hg fillings___; # missing__
other fillings________________
Root canals____

**Posterior Pharynx:**
inflammed + –
lymph swelling + –
mucus + –
**Tonsil hypertrophy**
0 1 2 3

**PERRLA**
yes / no

**Vision Right:**
unassisted 20/_____
assisted 20/______

**Vision Left:**
unassisted 20/_____
assisted 20/______

**Gums:**
pointed
spongy + –
inflammed + –
recession 0 1 2 3

**Tongue:**
*coat*: none / thin / thick / dry / wet
white / pale yellow / yellow / dark
*body color*:
pink / pale / red / purple
uniform / red dots / cracks / scalloped
*movement*: still / quivering / deviated R/L

**Weber** localized to L R M
**Rhine** can't hear air + –

**TM:** clear / fluid / yeast
retracted / scarring
**inflammed 0 1 2 3 4**

**Canal**
Dry / scaley / red
**wax** 0 1 2 3
dark / thick / thin

**TM:** clear / fluid / yeast
retracted / scarring
**inflammed 0 1 2 3 4**

**Canal**
Dry / scaley / red
**wax** 0 1 2 3
dark /thick / thin

**Face:** moles + – ; keratosis + –
verticle crease forehead + –
hirsuitism / scaling / acne
redness
**Lips**: cracks / dry

**Scalp**:
oily / dry / oily
scaliness + –
dandruff + –

**Hair:**
coarse / fine / norm
dry / oily / normal
full / thinning
loss / grey

**Tophi**
**ear lobe crease + –**

**Thyroid**: nodules + – enlarged + –
**Cervical Lymph nodes** enlarged + –

**L. breast**:
tender + – ;masses + –
nipple discharge + –

**R. breast**:
tender + – ;masses + –
nipple discharge + –

**Tophi + –**
**ear lobe crease + –**

**Lungs**
Rails + –
wheezing + –
deep / bronch

**Abdomen**: Tender + –
Murphy's sign + –
McBirney's + –

**Heart** :Irreg / murmers
extra sounds / fast / slow
arrhythmias

**Back**:
sensitive to skin roll
0 1 2 3
moles + –
acne 0 1 2 3

**Kyphosis + –**

**Posterior arms**
FHK 0 1 2 3

hypochondriac
lat. Iliac
inguinal

**R. Pulse**
1___________________
2___________________
3___________________

**L. Pulse**
1___________________
2___________________
3___________________

**Elbows**
Dry/thick skin 0 1 2 3 4

**Scoliosis + –**

**Bp:**
LAS____/____
LAL____/____
upon standing
____/____
dizzy 0 1 2 3
**pulse**______

Hiatal hernia
trigger points
\+ –

**anus:**
hemorrhoides
fissures
red/scaley

**Vagina:**
dischx: none/ thin/ thick
Yellow/ white/ frothy
**odor:** none/ musky/ fishy
**adnexa: tender / masses**

**Wet prep**

**PAP**

Knees: DTR 0 1 2 3 4
pain + –
grating + –
Apley's + –
compression + –
Patella entrapement + –

Dry / thick skin 0 1 2 3 4

**Skin**: dry / scaley / oily
norm / sores / mottling
bruising 0 1 2 3
varicosities 0 1 2 3
hair + – Shiney skin + –

**Nails:**
thin / thick / strong
brittle / flaking
white spots / spooning
ridging vert / horiz
**Cuticles** red / hangnails
normal

Edema: 0 1 2 3 4
pitting or nonpitting

**Feet**: pronation
suppination
**Arches**: flat
high or normal

**Pulses**
Dorsal pedal strong / moderate / weak

Achilles Return Reflex:
none
very delayed
delayed
OK
brisk

**Hands temp**
Hot / warm / cold

**Toes:**
cracks (tinea) + –
**Nails:**
thickened + –

**Feet:**
Hot / warm / cold

Notes:

# Nutrition Physical Exam

name____________________ Date______________ Age_____height________weight_________

**Posterior Pharynx:**
inflammed + –
lymph swelling + –
mucus + –
**Tonsil hypertrophy**
0 1 2 3

**Eyes:**
*Conjunctiva*: red / clear / growths
*Retina*: vessels-AV nicking / copper wire
hemorrhages + – / tortuosity + –
disk bulge + – ; irregular + –
*Lens*-cataracts + –

**Teeth:**
# of Hg fillings___; # missing__
other fillings________________
Root canals____

**PERRLA**
yes / no

**Gums:**
pointed
spongy + –
inflammed + –
recession 0 1 2 3

**Vision Right:**
unassisted 20/______
assisted 20/______

**Vision Left:**
unassisted 20/______
assisted 20/______

**Tongue:**
*coat*: none / thin / thick / dry / wet
white / pale yellow / yellow / dark
*body color*:
pink / pale / red / purple
uniform / red dots / cracks / scalloped
*movement*: still / quivering / deviated R/L

**Weber** localized to L R M
**Rhine** can't hear air + –

**Canal**
Dry / scaley / red
**wax** 0 1 2 3
dark / thick / thin

**TM:** clear / fluid / yeast
retracted / scarring
**inflammed 0 1 2 3 4**

**TM:** clear / fluid / yeast
retracted / scarring
**inflammed 0 1 2 3 4**

**Canal**
Dry / scaley / red
**wax** 0 1 2 3
dark /thick / thin

**Face:** moles + – ; keratosis + –
verticle crease forehead + –
hirsuitism / scaling / acne
redness
**Lips**: cracks / dry

**Scalp**:
oily / dry / oily
scaliness + –
dandruff + –

**Hair:**
coarse / fine / norm
dry / oily / normal
full / thinning
loss / grey

**Tophi**
**ear lobe crease + –**

**Thyroid**: nodules + – enlarged + –
**Cervical Lymph nodes** enlarged + –

**Tophi + –**
**ear lobe crease + –**

**Lungs**
Rails + –
wheezing + –
deep / bronch

**Heart** :Irreg / murmers
extra sounds / fast / slow
arrhythmias

**Back**:
sensitive to skin roll
0 1 2 3
moles + –
acne 0 1 2 3

**Kyphosis + –**

**Abdomen**: Tender + –
Murphy's sign + –
McBirney's + –

**Posterior arms**
FHK 0 1 2 3

**Elbows**
Dry/thick skin 0 1 2 3 4

**R. Pulse**
1______________
2______________
3______________

hypochondriac
lat. Iliac
inguinal

**L. Pulse**
1______________
2______________
3______________

**Scoliosis + –**

**Bp:**
LAS_____/_____
LAL_____/_____
upon standing
_____/_____
dizzy 0 1 2 3
**pulse**______

**anus:**
hemorrhoides
fissures
red/scaley

Hiatal hernia
trigger points
+ –

**Penis:**
dischx: none / thin / thick
yellow / white / frothy

**Knees:** DTR 0 1 2 3 4
pain + –
grating + –
Apley's + –
compression + –
Patella entrapement + –

**Skin**: dry / scaley / oily
norm / sores / mottling
bruising 0 1 2 3
varicosities 0 1 2 3
hair + – Shiney skin + –

**Nails:**
thin / thick / strong
brittle / flaking
white spots / spooning
ridging vert / horiz
**Cuticles** red / hangnails
normal

**Prostate:** tender / masses + –
central sulcus + – irregular + –
hard / firm / spongy / soft

Size_________cm

Dry / thick skin 0 1 2 3 4

Edema: 0 1 2 3 4
pitting or nonpitting

Achilles Return Reflex:
none
very delayed
delayed
OK
brisk

**Feet**: pronation
suppination
**Arches**: flat
high or normal

**Pulses**
Dorsal pedal strong / moderate / weak

**Toes:**
cracks (tinea) + –
**Nails:**
thickened + –

**Hands temp**
Hot / warm / cold

**Feet:**
Hot / warm / cold

Notes:

**Alan Mandell Center for Bio-Ecologic Diseases**
Theron G. Randolph Ecologic Unit
New England Foundation for Allergic and Environmental Diseases
3 Brush Street – Norwalk, Connecticut 06850
Phone 203 – 838-4706

Marshall Mandell, M.D., DABP, DABAI, FACA, FSCE, FIAM, FIAPM
Medical Director

FOR RELIEF OF ALLERGIC SYMPTOMS (FROM TESTING, TREATMENT OR AT HOME)

1. DR. MANDELL'S ALKALINE SALTS (available at Center)
   a. 1/3 potassium bicarbonate
   b. 2/3 sodium bicarbonate
   Take 1 level tsp. of this mixture in a tall glass of spring water; may be followed with additional glass of water. May repeat 2-3 times in one day - NOT TO BE USED CONTINUOUSLY FOR MORE THAN 2-3 DAYS. IF SXS. PERSIST, PLEASE CONTACT THE OFFICE.

2. ASCORBIC ACID OR SODIUM ASCORBATE
   ¼ tsp. in spring water = 1 Gram (1000 Milligrams). REPEAT EVERY HOUR IF NECESSARY. If cramping or diarrhea develops, increase interval between each dose.

3. PLAIN SODIUM BICARBONATE (Arm and Hammer is O.K.)
   Take 1 level tsp. in glass of water. Dosage as above.

4. ALKA-SELTZER GOLD*
   One tablet in water as above. (*same as salts - use Gold as it does not contain aspirin: however, it does contain citric acid).

5. MILK OF MAGNESIA - As an ANTIACID
   1-2 Tbsps. NO WATER.
   Take 2-4 Tbsps. as a LAXATIVE in spring water

6. SPRING WATER ENEMA
   Use 1 qt., may repeat if necessary. May add 1 tsp. Vit. C if desired or 1 tsp. SALTS to replace Minerals lost due to enema.

7. EPSOM SALTS - As a LAXATIVE
   Take 1 tsp. in tall glass of water.

8. OXYGEN
   6 liters for 5 minutes, may repeat during day as necessary. DO NOT USE CONTINUOUSLY.

9. MAGNESIUM CITRATE - As a LAXATIVE
   Directions are on bottle.

10. FLEETS PHOSPHO SODA
    Take 2-4 tsps. on arising, 30 mins. before a meal or at bedtime. Dilute with water, then follow with another glass of water.

11. ANTIHISTAMINE (if tolerated) as a last choice.
    (Benadryl, Bromophen, Chlortrimeton, Actified, Allernade, etc.)

# Foods containing Milk or Dairy

**Foods Containing Milk**

- cheese
- cottage cheese
- yogurt
- ice cream
- butter
- most margarines
- creamed soups and sauces
- chocolate
- pudding
- custard
- baked goods
- mashed potatoes
- some "non-dairy" products
- baked goods
- pancakes & waffles
- doughnuts
- meatloaf
- gravies
- many breads have whey
- calcium supplements may have casein
- protein powders
- check vitamins

**May be listed on label as the following ingredients:**

- casein
- caseinate
- whey
- lactalbumin
- sodium caseinate
- lactose
- cream
- non-fat milk solids
- calcium caseinate

**Milk Free**

- Eden soy
- Soy Moo
- Ah soy
- Rice Dream (brown nut milks)
- coconut milk
- Rice Dream (ice cream substitute)
- try cereals with dilute fruit juice instead of milk e.g. apple
- Soy margarine (health food store)
  - Spectrum Margarine
  - Fleischmans
- Silken
- Oat Milk
- Great Harvest Bread

# FOODS CONTAINING WHEAT & WHEAT SUBSTITUTES

### FOODS CONTAINING WHEAT

crackers
corn pasta
spaghetti
noodles
soy sauce
breads(rye,sourdough etc.)
hot dogs with wheat filler
batter fried foods
some sausage
baking mixes
gravies & cream sauces
beer
gin
barley malt
liverwurst
Ovaltine
postum
whiskies
may be found in the following:
soups
yeasts
vitamin E
pepper (synthetic)
ice-cream (thickening agents)
matzos
hamburger
candy

### MAY BE LISTED ON FOOD LABELS AS:

flour
graham
wheat germ
wheat bran
wheat starch
gluten
food starch
vegetable starch
vegetable gum

### RECOMMENDED WHEAT SUBSTITUTES:

sorba buckwheat noodles macaroni

rice bread "ENER-G" (2Js)
rice cakes (round)
rice cakes (square)
*Norwegian Crisp Bread (Kavli)
FLOURS
- brown rice
- oat
- quinoa
- amaranth
- potato

buckwheat
- *rye
- *barley

CEREALS
- cream of brown rice cereal
- brown rice crunchies (Lundberg)
- Nutty rice (Perky's)
- Oatios (New Morning)
- *Oat Bran Flakes (Health Valley)
- *Amaranth Flakes (Health Valley)
- Fruite-O's (New Morning)
- Corn Nutrigain (Kellogg)
- Almond Raisin Nutrigrain (Kellogg)
- Puffed Rice (Malto Meal)
- Puffed Corn (Pure & Simple)
- *Rye Flakes
- some granola's (check label)

# Gluten & Non-Gluten Containing Foods

**Foods Containing Gluten**

| | |
|---|---|
| Wheat | Rye |
| Barley | Oats |
| Spelt | Kamut |
| Triticale | Crackers |
| Spaghetti | Noodles |

Soy Sauce
Breads:rye,sourdough etc.
Hot Dogs with wheat filler
Batter Fried Foods
Some Sausage
Baking mixes
Gravies & Cream sauces

| | |
|---|---|
| Beer | Gin |
| Barley Malt | Liverwurst |
| Ovaltine | Postum |
| Inka | Caffix |
| Pero | Roastaroma |

Whiskies

**MAY BE FOUND IN THE FOLLOWING:**

| | |
|---|---|
| Soups | Yeasts |
| Vitamin E | Pepper (synthetic) |
| Matzos | Hamburger |
| Candy | Granola's |

Rye Flakes
Fruite-O's (New Morning)
Ice-cream (thickening agents)

**MAY BE LISTED ON FOOD LABELS AS:**

Flour
Graham
Wheat Germ
Wheat Bran
Wheat Starch
Gluten
Modified Food Starch
Vegetable Starch
Vegetable Gum

**Foods Free of Gluten**

| | |
|---|---|
| *Rice | Buckwheat |
| Amaranth | Quinoa |
| Teff | *Corn |
| *Millet | *Wild Rice |

*Polenta
Arrowhead Corn Grits
Wheat Free Tamari
Health Valley Rice Bran Crackers
Subahdar Poppadums
Grey Owl Wild Rice
Corn TortillaTaco Shells
Mochi (a type of rice bread)
Dragon Toast & Toast Pizza
Arrowhead Quick Brown Rice
Soba Buckwheat Noodle
(100% buckwheat- make sure not mixed)
Patariso Rice Pasta
Corn Pasta bulk
Ancient Harvest Pasta (quinoa)
Deboles Pasta (various types)
Rice Cakes (Westbrae, Lundberg, Hain, Quaker) make sure not mixed
U.S. Mills Poppets
Nature's Path Mesa Sunrise
(corn, amaranth, flax)
Health Valley Amaranth Flakes
Erehwhon Aztec Cereal (corn &
Arrowhead Apple or Maple Corns
Arrowhead or Maltomeal Puffed Rice
Arrowhead Puffed Millet
Maltomeal Puffed Corn Cereal
Perky Nutty Rice or Nutty Corn
Corn Nutrigain (Kellogg)
Almond Raisin Nutrigrain (Kellogg)
Cream of Rice (Lundberg)
Col. Sanchez Tofu-Green
Chili Cheese Tamales
Tumaro's Blue Corn Tamales
Tumaro's Black Bean Enchilada
Tumaro's tofu Enchilada Verde
Tumaro's Cheese Enchilada
Rice Bread "ENER-G"
Tapioca bread "ENER-G"
Whole Rice Works Sandwiches
Brown Rice Snaps Edward & Sons
Garlic & Onion,Tamari Seaweed & Plain

**Flours Free of Gluten**

*Brown rice
Teff
Quinoa
Amaranth
Potato
Soy
Pinto Bean
Tapioca
buckwheat
garbonzo bean

*Indicates grains in the grass family.

Please note that flours are often contaminated with traces of gluten due to the milling of grains previously with the same miller. Unless the mill is thoroughly cleaned of the previous grinding it is impossible to tell if a food has been contaminated.

*NOTE-Always double check your label to make sure the food your are eating is indeed gluten free. The information on this page is meant as a guide and we can not assume responsibility for any inaccuracies.*

Gluten Intolerance Group
of North America
P.O. Box 23053
Seattle WA 98102

Jeanne Huffstuter
9525 S.W. 12th Drive
Portland, OR 97219

Joanne Galloway
3707 Nicolson Rd.
Vancouver, WA 98661

# ANIMAL & AIR ALLERGY TREATMENT PROTOCOL

**Take the following:**

1) Vitamin C 2 gms 4-6x/day (cut back if you get diarrhea). Best to use buffered vitamin C.
2) Quercetin 2 capsules before eating. (6 per day). Citrus bioflavonoids 2 tabs 3x/day. (this should be taken before any significant size meal). May try other flavonoids such as pycnogenol, hesperidin or citrus bioflavonoids.
3) Pantothenic acid- 500mg 2x per day
4) Vitamin B-6- 100mg 3x per day
5) OxyQuench- 2 caps 2x per day
6) Homeopathic for allergies can use antigens or general homeopathic.
7) Nettles 3 capsules 2x per day
8) Nasalcrom®- 1 spray in each nostril 2x per day. (this is a compound that is similar to quercetin but in a nebulizer form) The purpose of this Nasalcrom® is to stabilize your mast cells so that don't release histamine and other substances that cause allergic symptoms).
9) Bee pollen *Aller Bee-Gone*
10) Bi Yan Pian (patent)-5 tablets 4x per day. Can also make up other Chinese herb formulas
11) Air purification or filtration. I recommend Alpine Air purifiers.

In addition if due to animals can bath the cat or dog in a product called Allerpet®, available at veterinarian offices or other pet/animal supply stores.

# ANIMAL ALLERGY PROPHYLACTIC PROTOCOL

Below is a protocol for preventing or minimizing allergic reactions that someone may experience either traveling to an area that might cause problems for someone. It could be to someones house that has a pet or other thing that might trigger off a reaction.

**Take the following starting 5-7 days before traveling to the high risk area:**

1) Vitamin C 2 gms 4x/day (cut back if you get diarrhea).
2) Quercetin 2 capsules before eating. (6 per day).
   (this should be taken before any significant size meal).
3) Pantothcnic acid- 500mg 2x per day
4) Vitamin B-6- 100mg 3x per day
5) OxyQuench- 2 caps 2x per day
6) Homeopathic for allergies can use antigens or general homeopathic.

**Starting 3-5 days before exposure:**

3) Nettles 3 capsules 2x per day
4) Nasalchrome- 2 spray in each nostril 3x per day. (this is a compound that is similar to quercetin but in a nebulizer form). Make sure you take a nice size inhale. The purpose of this Nasalchrome is to stabilize your mast cells so that don't release histamine and other substances that cause allergic symptoms).

In addition if due to animals can bath the cat or dog in a product called Allerpet®, available at veterinarian offices or other pet/animal supply stores.

## TRAVELING ESSENTIALS TO FOREIGN PLACES: VIRAL/BACT GI PROTECTION

**For protection against parasites**

Garlic-3-8 cloves per day eaten raw chopped up
*Charcoal 3-4 capsules 3-4x per day
Artemesia Annua 3-6 capsules per day
Lactobaccilus acidophilus powder or capsules 3-6 per day

**Viral infection**

*Echinacae tincture 25 drops 4-5x per day in water
*Golden Seal tincture 20 drops 4-5x per day
*Optibiotic
EHB- Echinacae and Hydrastis 7 Berberis
Yin Chiao San for early flu with fever & chills 8 tabs 4-5x/day

**Gastrointestinal problems**

Nux vomica homeopathic 30c
Colocynths homeopathic 12x or 30c take every 2 hours or 3x/day
*Charcoal- for cramping, gas, or other GI symptoms
*Oil of peppermint (Scientific Botanicals) 2-3 caps every 2-3 hours
Bao He Wan 5 tabs 3-4x per day

**Trauma-**

*Arnica montana 1M
30c-take 3-4x per day
Rhus tox 30c- take 3 pellets 3x per day for sprains
Traumeel Ointment apply topically to bruises, sprains & strains
*Herbal Ed Salve- apply topically to cuts, abrasions, open sores
*Viavi or Succus Cineraria maritima- eye drops
*Jin Bu Huan-for pain & can't sleep 1-2 tabs 1-3x per day max
also for headaches
Skin afflictions-
charcoal
white oak bark- use topically (hot poultice) and internally
Herbal Ed Salve-
neosporin c lidocaine
stop sting- for stings, bites, and other
(*) denotes basic essential first aid for travel kit.

# EYE ALLERGIES PROTOCOL

**Take the following:**

1) Vitamin C 2 gms 4x/day (cut back if you get diarrhea).
2) Quercetin 2 capsules before eating. (6 per day). This should be taken before any significant meal.
3) Pantothenic acid- 500mg 2x per day
4) Vitamin B-6- 100mg 3x per day
5) Nettles 3 capsules 2x per day
6) OxyQuench- 2 caps 2x per day
7) Similasan eye drops #2- This you can also take alternately with the cromolyn. Everyone responds a bit differently so you will have to see what works best for you.
8) Sodium Cromolyn (Opticrome)- 2 drops in each eye every 4-5 hours. (this is a compound that is similar to quercetin but in drops form). This may sting your eyes like your other medication but should really help with the swelling and itching is to stabilize your mast cells so that don't release histamine and other substances that cause allergic symptoms)

## RECOMMENDED READING CONCERNING ALLERGIES

| | |
|---|---|
| Allergies and Your Family | Doris J. Rapp, M.D. |
| Allergies and the Hyperactive Child | Doris J Rapp, M.D. |
| Allergy self Help Book | Sharon Faelten & ed. of Prevention |
| An Alternative Approach to Allergies | Theron Randolph, M.D. |
| Antioxidant Adaptation: Role in Free Rad. Pathol. | S.Levine, Ph.D. & Paris Kidd Ph.D. |
| Are You Allergic | William Crook, M.D. |
| Brain Allergies the psychonutrient connection | W.Philpott, MD.& D. Kalita, Ph.D |
| Coping with Your Allergies | N. Golos, F.G. Golbitz, & Leighton |
| Detecting Your Hidden Allergies | William Crook, M.D. |
| Diet, Crime, and Delinquency | Alex Schauss, Ph.D. |
| Dr. Berger's Immune Power Diet | Stuart Berger, M.D. |
| Dr. Wright's Book of Nutritional Therapy | Jon Wright, M.D. |
| Dr. Wright's Healing with Nutrition | Jon Wright, M.D. |
| Dr. Mandell's 5 Day Allergy Relief System | Marshall Mandell, M.D.Dr. Mandell's |
| Lifetime Arthritis Relief System | Marshall Mandell, M.D. |
| Dr. Mandell's It's Not Your Fault Your Fat | Marshall Mandell, M.D. |
| Feed Your Kids Right | Lendon Smith, M.D. |
| Food Allergies | Thom, Dickson, N.D., DDS |
| Food Intolerance/Food & Chemical Sensitivity | Robert Buist, Ph.D. |
| Seven Weeks to a Settled Stomach | Ron Hoffman, M.D. |
| Why You Child Is Hyperactive | Ben Feingold, M.D. |
| The Yeast Connection | William Crook, M.D. |
| The Yeast Syndrome | J.Trowbridge, M.D. & M.Walker,DPN |
| If This Is Tuesday, Then It Must Be Chicken | Golos, Natalie |

## ALLERGY COOKBOOKS

| | |
|---|---|
| Coping with Candida Cookbook | Sally Rockwell, B.S. |
| Beyond the Staff of Life | Kief Adler |
| Dr. Mandell's Allergy Free Cookbook | Marshall Mandell, M.D. |
| Wheat-Free, Milk-Free, Egg Free Cooking | Rita Greer |
| The Allergy Self Help Cookbook | Marjorie Hurt Jones, R.N. |
| Super Foods: Allergy Recipes | Jones, Marjorie Hurt Jones |
| Quinoa the Supergrain | Wood, Rebecca |

## OTHER BOOKS

| | |
|---|---|
| Clinical Ecology | Laurance Dickey, M.D. |
| Basics of Food Allergy | John. Breneman, M.D. |
| Clinical Allergy | Harris Hosen, M.D. |
| Textbook of Natural Medicine | J.Pizzorno, N.D. & M.Murray, N.D. |
| One Man's Food...is someone else's poison | James D'Adamo, N.D. |
| Eat Right for Your Blood Type | Peter D'Adamo, N.D. |
| Food Allergy Its Manifestations & Control and the Elimination Diets-A Compendium | Rowe & Thomas |
| Allergy Cookbook | Shattuck, Ruth R. |
| Good Food, Gluten Free | Hills, Hilda Cerry |

## HYPOALLERGENIC DIET OMNIVOROUS

NAME: ____________________

| MONDAY | TUESDAY | WEDNESDAY | THURSDAY | FRIDAY | SATURDAY | SUNDAY |
|---|---|---|---|---|---|---|
| Watermelon | Pears | Pineapple or Papaya | Peaches or Plums | Kiwi Fruit | Strawberries or Raspberries | Blueberries or Figs |
| | | drink plenty of water | drink plenty of water | drink plenty of water | | |
| Sweet Potato (baked) and Pecans | Cream of Brown Rice and Brown Rice Syrup | Steamed Squash and Lentils | Rice Cakes and Almond Butter | Buckwheat, Peas, Cashews, and Toasted Sesame Oil (sauté buckwheat groats and cashews in sesame oil for 5-10 min. add peas then steam with 2x as much water for 10 min. - do not stir while steaming - turn over & serve) | Oatmeal and Banana | Tuna and Carrots |
| | | drink plenty of water | drink plenty of water | drink plenty of water | | |
| Salmon and Steamed Broccoli | Cod and Asparagus (if wild game such as elk, deer or buffalo is available can substitute for fish) | Lamb and Zuchini | Baked Halibut and Spinach | Flounder and Steamed Spinach | Chicken and Wild Rice | Shrimp, Brown Rice, Steamed Peas & Toasted Sesame Oil |

SPECIAL INSTRUCTIONS;

1: Use only SEA SALT as a spice.
2: Drink only spring, filtered or distilled water.
3: Use only fresh vegetables and fruits, ideally organic. Frozen is next best.
4: If you must switch meals around it is best to switch the entire day.

Notes:

**HYPOALLERGENIC DIET VEGETARIAN** **NAME:**________________

| MONDAY | TUESDAY | WEDNESDAY | THURSDAY | FRIDAY | SATURDAY | SUNDAY |
|---|---|---|---|---|---|---|
| Watermelon | Pears | Pineapple or Papaya | Peaches or Plums | Kiwi Fruit | Strawberries or Raspberries | Blueberries or Figs |
| | | drink plenty of water | | | | |
| Sweet Potato (baked) and Pecans | Cream of Brown Rice and Brown Rice Syrup | Steamed Squash and Lentils | Rice Cakes and Cashew Butter | Buckwheat, Peas, Onions and Toasted Sesame Oil | Oatmeal and Banana | Spli Pea Soup and Vegetables: steamed zucchini, acorn squash, green beans, etc. |
| | | **drink plenty of water** | | | | |
| Quinao and Steamed Broccoli | Mixed Salad Greens with Kidney Beans and Lemon | Amaranth and Zucchini | Beets and Spinach | Millet and Steamed Spinach | Beans of choice: black beans, pintos, red, etc. & Wild Rice | Brown Rice, Steamed Peas & Toasted Sesame Oil |

SPECIAL INSTRUCTIONS;
1: Use only SEA SALT as a spice.
2: Drink only spring, filtered or distilled water.
3: Use only fresh vegetables and fruits, ideally organic. Frozen is next best.
4: If you must switch meals around it is best to switch the entire day.

Notes:

**HYPOALLERGENIC DIET OMNIVOROUS** ***"GLUTEN & GRAIN FREE"*** **NAME:**________________

| MONDAY | TUESDAY | WEDNESDAY | THURSDAY | FRIDAY | SATURDAY | SUNDAY |
|---|---|---|---|---|---|---|
| Watermelon | Pears | Pineapple or Papaya | Peaches or Plums | Kiwi Fruit | Strawberries or Raspberries | Blueberries or Figs |
| | | drink plenty of water<br>may have bentonite clay or psyllium seed powder | | | | |
| Sweet Potato (baked) and Pecans | Quinoa and Steamed Chard | Steamed Squash and Lentils | Salad Greens with Kidney and Garbanzo Beans | Buckwheat, Peas, Cashews, and Toasted Sesame Oil (sauté buckwheat groats and cashews in sesame oil for 5-10 min. add peas then steam with 2x as much water for 10 min. - do not stir while steaming - turn over & serve) | Broccoli, Carrot and Yellow Squash Soup (cut veggies into small peices and cook 40 minutes | Tuna and Carrots |
| | | drink plenty of water | | | | |
| Salmon and Steamed Broccoli | Cod and Asparagus (if wild game such as elk, deer or buffalo is available can substitute for fish) | Lamb and Zuchini | Baked Halibut and Kale | Flounder and Steamed Spinach | Chicken, Zuchini and Green Peppers | Shrimp, Quinoa, Steamed Peas & Toasted Sesame Oil |

SPECIAL INSTRUCTIONS;

1: Use only SEA SALT as a spice.

2: Drink only spring, filtered or distilled water.

3: Use only fresh vegetables and fruits, ideally organic. Frozen is next best.

4: If you must switch meals around it is best to switch the entire day.

Notes:

**HYPOALLERGENIC DIET VEGETARIAN** ***"GLUTEN & GRAIN FREE"*** **NAME:**________________

| MONDAY | TUESDAY | WEDNESDAY | THURSDAY | FRIDAY | SATURDAY | SUNDAY |
|---|---|---|---|---|---|---|
| Watermelon | Pears | Pineapple or Papaya | Peaches or Plums | Kiwi Fruit | Strawberries or Raspberries | Blueberries or Figs |
| | | drink plenty of water<br>may have bentonite clay or psyllium seed powder | | | | |
| Sweet Potato (baked) and Pecans | Apple Slices with Almond Butter | Steamed Squash and Lentils | Mixed Salad Greens with Kidney Beans and Lemon | Buckwheat, Peas, Onions and Toasted Sesame Oil | Banana and Black Beans | Spli Pea Soup and Vegetables: steamed zucchini, acorn squash, green beans, etc. |
| Pinto Beans, Quinoa and Celery | Broccoli, Carrot and Yellow Squash Soup (cut veggies into small peices and cook 40 minutes | Amaranth and Zucchini | Beets and Spinach | Acorn Squash and Steamed Chard | Baked Potato and String Beans | Quinoa Zuchini and Green Peppers with Toasted Sesame Oil |

SPECIAL INSTRUCTIONS;
1: Use only SEA SALT as a spice.
2: Drink only spring, filtered or distilled water.
3: Use only fresh vegetables and fruits, ideally organic. Frozen is next best.
4: If you must switch meals around it is best to switch the entire day.

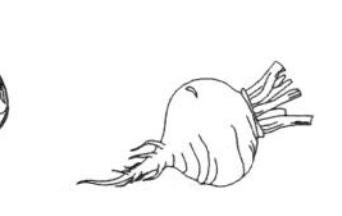
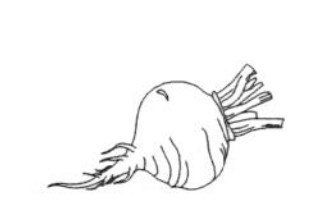

Notes:

**NUTRITION (general reading)**

Diet and Nutrition, Rudolph Ballentine, M.D.
Nutrition Against Disease Roger Williams, Ph.D.
The Healing Power of Foods Michael Murray, N.D.

Aerobic Nutrition, David Mannerberg, M.D.
Diet for a New America Robbins
Dr. Wright's Book of Nutritional Therapy Wright, M.D.
Dr. Wright's Healing with Nutrition Jon Wright, M.D
Eating Alive Matson, N.D.
Eating for a Healthy Heart Yudkin Jr. 1997
Fats that Heal Fats that Kill Erasmus
Formula for Life The Definitive Book on Correct Nutrition, Antioxidants, and Vitamins, Disease Prevention, and Longevity by Kronhausen, Ed. D. & Demopolis, M.D.
Infant Nutrition; Mark Percival, D.C. N.D.
Mental Health & Illness: Nutrition Connection Holford & Pfeiffer
Native Nutrition; Eating According to Ancestral Wisdom,Schmid
Natural Healing thru Macrobiotics, Michio Kushi
Nutrition and Evolution Crawford & Marsh 95
Omega 3 Oils A Practical Guide Rudin 1996
The Omega Plan Simopoulos, Artemis 1998
Paleolithic Prescription Eaton SB, Shostak M, & Konner
Prescription for Nutritional Healing Bach and Bach, M.D.
Staying Healthy with Nutrition Elson Haas, M.D.
Sweet and Dangerous Yudkin, M.D

Nutra-aerobics Jeff Bland, PhD
Your Health Under Siege:Using Nutrition Bland, PhD

The Complete Food Handbook Doyle and Redding
Treating and Reversing Heart Disease Dean Ornish, M.D.

**NUTRITION (more technical reading)**

Advanced Nutrition & Human Metabolism Hunt, Groeff
Antioxidant Adaptation: It's role in Free Radical Pathology by Kidd & Levine, Ph.D
Fasting Signs and Symptoms Salloum, N.D.
Handbook of Diabetes Medical Nutrition Therapy M. Powers
Handbook of Preventive & Therapeutic Nutrition J GerberD.C.
Krause's Food Nutrition & Diet Therapy Mahan & Arlin
Medical Nutrition from Marz 2nd edition '97 Marz, N.D., L.Ac.
Nutrition & Physical Degeneration Weston Price DDS
Nutrition in Health and Disease Goodhart & Young
Nutrition in Infancy & Childhood by Pipes & Trahms
Nutrition in Pregnancy & Lactation Worthington, PhD
Nutritional Biochemistry and Metabolism with Clinical Applications Maria Linder, Ph.D.
Nutritional Influences on Illness Werback, M.D.
Nutritional Influences on Mental Illness, Werback
The Healing Nutrients Within, Braverman & Pfifer

**MEDICINAL HERB BOOKS**

Advanced Herbology Willard
Botanical Compendium of dosages & Products,Peg Wolf, N.D
Botanical Influences on Illness Murray & Werbach
Complete Botanical Prescribe /Botanical Medicine Sherman, N.D.
Formulas for Healthful Living, Brinker, N.D.
From the Shepard's Purse Max Barlow
Healing Power of Herbs Murray, N.D
Herbal Medicine Weiss
Indian Herbology Guide to Medicinal Plants Keats
Naturopathic Handbook of Herbal Formulas Scalzo
Nutritional Therapy/ Fislason, M.D.
Scientific Validation of Herbal Medicine Mourey
The Healing Herbs Castleman
The Herb Doctors, Boyle
The McDougal Plan MacDougal
Toxicology of Common Botanicals, Brinker, N.D.

**FOOD ALLERGIES & SENSITIVITIES**

Surviving the 90's Coping with Food Allergies; Thom, Dickson
The None Toxic Home and Office Debra Jo Dadd
Your Family Tree Connection;Reading, M.D. & Meillor

*Basics of Food Allergy Breneman, M.D.
An Alternative Approach to Allergies, Randolph & Moss
Beyond the Staff of Life (wheat free)
Brain Allergies The Psychonutrient Connect Philpott, M.D.
Candida Albicans Chaitow
Clinical Ecology Dickey, M.D.
Diet, Crime and Delinquency Schauss, Ph.D.
Food Allergies made Simple Thrash
Food and Chemical Sensitivity Robert Buist, Ph.D.
Food intolerance William Buist, PhD
Food for Thought Saul Miller
*Good Food, Gluten Free, Hilda Cherry Hills*
Impossible Child, The Dorris Rapp, M.D.
Quinoa the Supergrain, Rebecca Wood
*Sally Rockwell's Allergy Recipes Rockwell*
Super Foods Quinoa, amaranth, Teff, Kamut
Yeast Connection William Crook, M.D
Your Home, Your Health, & Well Being Rousseau/ Rea
Dr. Mandell's 5 day Allergy Relief System, Mandell,
Dr. Mandell's Lifetime Arthritis Relief System "
The Pritikin Program for Diet & Exercise, Pritikin

Yeast Syndrome Trowbridge & Walker
The Homocysteine Revolution McCully 1997

Fit or Fat Target Diet Covert Bailey
Functional Dietetics Mark Percival, D.C., N.D..

**GENERAL HEALTH AND HEALING**

3rd Line Medicine, Werbach
7 Weeks to a Settled Stomach, Ron Hoffman, M.D.
Alternative Medicine; Burton Goldberg Group
Anatomy of an Illness perceived by Patient, Cousins
Eat Right 4 Your Blood Type, Peter D'Adamo
Feed Your Kids Right Lendon Smith, M.D.
High Blood Pressure Solution with the K factor Moore
Home Remedies, Hydrotherapy, Massage, Charcoal, and Other Simple Treatments Thrash & Thrash, M.D.
How to Get Well / There is a Cure for Arthr. Paavo Airola, N.D.
HypoAdrenoCorticism, Tintera, M.D.
Hypothyroidism the Unsuspected Illness, Barnes,M.D.
Longevity Fullfilling our Bio Potential Pelletier, Ph.D
Magical Mind Magical Body Deepak Chopra, M.D.
Maximum Immunity , Weiner, Ph.D.
Maximum Lifespan Walford, Ph.D.
Mega Nutrition, Richard Kunin
Mind as Healer, Mind as Slayer, A Holistic Approach to Preventing Stress Disorders, Pelletier, Ph.D.
Natural Healing through Macrobiotics, Michio Kushi
Natural Health, Natural Medicine Andrew Weil, MD
Natural Rememdies / More Natural Remedies Thrash
Naturopathic Hydrotherapy Boyle & Saine, N.D.'s
Naturopathic Treatment Notebook, compiled by John Bastyr Students
One Man's Food is someone else's Poison, D'Adamo, ND 1980
Optimal Health, Deepak Chopra, M.D
Philosophy of Natural Therapeutics , Lindlahr, M.D.
Pottingers Cats by Francis Pottinger
Preventing and Reversing Osteoporosis, Gaby, M.D.
Quantum Healing Depak Chopra
Rudolph Steiner & Holistic Medicine Francis King
Staying Helathy with the Seasons Hass
The D'Adamo Diet, J. D'Adamo, N.D.
Wilson Syndrome, Wilson, M.D.

**COOKBOOKS**
Laural's Kitchen, Robertson
The Vegetarian Epicure 1 & 2 Wendy Esco
The Enchanted Broccoli Forest, Molly Katzen
The New Vegetarian Cookbook Gary Null
The Golden Temple Vegetarian Cookbook, Y.Bhajan
Nutrition for Vegetarians Thrash & Thrash, M.D.'s
The Gradual Vegetarian Lisa Tracy
Transition to Vegetarianism Rudoph Ballentine, M.D.
All Natural Allergy Cookbook Martin

**VITAMINS**
The Healing Factor, Vit C against Disease Irwin Stone
The Drs Guide to Vitamin B-6 Alan Gaby, M.D.
Vitamin E and the Ailing Heart, Wilfred Shute, M.D.
Essential Fatty Acids & Immunity in Mental Health, Bates, Ph.D
Vitamin B-6: The Doctors Report Ellis, MD & Presley
Your Personal Vitamin Profile Michael Colgan
Mental and Elemental Nutrients Pfeiffer, M.D., Ph.D
Encyclopedia of Nutritional Supplements Mike Murray, N.D.
Healing Nutrients Patrick Quillin, Ph.D.

**EXERCISE**
Fit or Fat Covert Bailey
Aerobics Ken Cooper, M.D.
The Sports Medicine Book William Southmayd, M.D.
Sports & Exercise Injuries Steven Subotnick
Sports Medicine Prevention, Evalulation, management, and rehabilitation Roy/Irvin
Optimal Sports Nutrition Michael Colgan
Stretching Anderson
Mind Body Sport John Douillard
The Zone Diet Barry Sears, Ph.D.

**HOMEOPATHY**
HomeopathicMedicine at Home Panos, M.D.
Homeopathic Treatment of Children Herscu, ND
Science of Homeopathy George Vithoulkas
A New Model in Health & Disease Vithoulkas
Homeopathy and Your Child/& ..for Child & InfantsDana Ulman
Everybody's Guide to Homeopathy Dana Ullman
Divided Legacy Coulter
Homeopathy and the Family Rose
Bach Flower Therapy Scheffer
Homeopathic Emergency Guide Tom Kruzel, N.D.
Homeopathic Medicine for Sports Injuries Morgan
Homeopathic Women for Pregnancy and Childbirth Moskowitz
Healing the Body Naturally with Cell Salts Weintraub, N.D.

**CHINESE MEDICINE**
The Web that has no Weaver, Ted Kupchek
Healing with Whole Foods Oriental Traditions & Modern Nutrition; by Paul Pitchford
Chinese Herbalists Handbook Dagmar Eling
Chinese System of Food Cures Henry C. Lu
Fundamentals of Chinese Medicine, Wiseman, Ellis Zmiewski
Chinese Herbal Medicine-Formulations and Strategies, Bensky & Bartlet
The Organ Systems of Trad. Chinese Medicine, J Ross

**CANCER**
Breast Cancer: What your Dr. May Not Tell You about Prevention, Diagnosis, and Treatment lHitchcock & Austin, N.D.
Cancer & Nutrition Patrick Quillen
Cancer 50 Case Studies Max Gerson, M.D.
Cancer and Vitamin C Cameron and Pauling, Ph.D's
Cancer a New Breakthrough Livingston
The Conquest of Cancer Livingston & Wheeler
The Complete Book of Cancer Prevention Rodale
The Macrobiotic Approach to Cancer Michio Kushi

**CHINESE MEDICINE (more technical reading)**
The Practice of Chinese Medicine Giovanni Maciocia
Chinese Acupunc. and Moxibustion, Qui Mao-liang
Treatment of Disease with Acupuncture
Essentials of Chinese Medicine unknown
A Comprehensive Textbook of Chinese Acupuncture Bensky, D.O
Bag of Pearls S. Dharmananda
Foundations of Chinese Medicine Giovanni Maciocia
Extraordinary Vessels Matsumoto
Yellow Emporer's Classic of Medicine Maoshing Ni

**WOMAN'S HEALTH**
Women's Health Paavo Airola
Women & the Crisis in Sex Hormones Seaman, M.D's
Alternative Health Care for Women Westcott /Black, N.D.
The Yeast Connection and the Woman Crook, M.D.
Gynecology and Naturopathic Medicine, Hudson, N.D.
Zinc and Eating Disorders Schauss A and Costin,
Nutrition in Pregnancy & Lactation WorthingtonR/Williams
PMS Self Help Book Lark
Menopausal Matters Hall

**ARTHRITIS**
Dr.Mandell's Lifetime Arthritis Relief System, Mandell
Overcoming Arthritis & Other Rheumatic Diseases by Max Warmbrand, N.D.
Free of Pain: A proven & Inexpensive Treatment for Specific Types of Rheumatism John Ellis, M.D
Bees Don't get Arthritis, Fred Malone
Seven Health Secrets from the Hive, Charles Robson

**ADDICTION**
From Morphine to Chocolate Andrew Weil, M.D.
Many Roads One Journey Kasl
Anatomy of Food Addiction; Anne Kathrine, M.D

**AIDS**
Surviving with AIDS Calloway, M.D.
Healing AIDS Naturally Bagley

Tissue Cleansing Through Bowel Mangement B. Jensen
Charcoal Startling new facts about the World's Most Powerful Absorbent Agatha & Calvin Thrash, MD's

**MISCELLANEOUS**
Guess what came to Dinner parasites & your health Gittleman
The Ion Effect Fred Soyka Alan Edmondz
Health and Light John Ott, Ph.D.
Safe Uses of Cortisone Jeffries
Victory Over Diabetes William Philpott, M.D.
Nutrition and Mental Illness Pfeiffer, Ph.D.. , M.D
Enzyme Nutrition Howell

Love, Medicine & Miracles Bernie Siegel, MD
Nature Doctors Friedh. Kirchfield & Wade Boyle,ND
It's All in Your Head (Diseases caused by Silver-Mercury Fillings) Huggins, DDS
The Body Ecology Diet Donna Gates
E.I. Syndrome An Rx for Environmental Illness Rogers'
Tired or Toxic Rogers
Scientific Basis of EDTA Chelation Therapy B. Halstead, M.D
Survival of Civilization John Hamaker
The Book of Floating Hutchison
Body Mind Purification Program Leon Chaitow, N.D.

## COMING OFF COFFEE AND OTHER CAFFEINE CONTAINING BEVERAGES

One of the most ingrained habits that eventually becomes a physical and biochemical addiction is the daily consumption of coffee. Seeing people lined up early in the morning at coffee shops such as "Starbucks", is a vivid reminder of some peoples dependency for caffeine. Since people benefit so greatly from taking a stimulant, this would be an indication that their adrenal function is probably not functioning optimally. People drink coffee for many reasons including some that are emotionally based. These emotional issues certainly need to be addressed while attempting to come off coffee.

The following are beverages that may ease the burden of side effects of coming off of coffee. They are meant as general helpful adjuncts to coming off of coffee and are not meant as a full scale program for coming off of coffee and caffeine. Some people find it easier to come off coffee by substituting another form of caffeine which is at least healthier, (such green tea).

**<u>Coffee-like drinks void of caffeine</u>**

Caffix
Inka
Roma
Pero
Roastaroma
Chia
Postum

**Drinks that have caffeine or caffeine-like properties, but also have additional health benefits:**

Green tea (Camelia sinensis), Chai tea (Tazo), Black tea, Coca cola (only kidding!), and Gota cola. Some people may need additional help to overcome their fatigue. Acupuncture and IM/IV vitamin Therapies can be very helpful.

**Protocol for coming off coffee:**

1) Hypoallergenic diet–2 weeks–include bentonite clay Springreen®, 1 T 3x per day.
2) Calcium/magnesium citrate–1200mg/800mg can do 400mg additionally of magnesium.
3) DHEA–5-15mg 2x per day for women and 10-25mg 2x per day for men depending upon the length of time that they have been drinking coffee (can do blood or saliva test to check for both DHEA and DHEA sulfate.
4) Oxyquench–2 caps 2x per day
5) B complex # 5 (Thorne Research)–1 capsule 2x per day
6) Vitamin E 400iu 2x per day
7) Acupuncture especially in the ears daily or every 2-3 days.
8) Vitamin B-12 (hydroxycobalamin1500mcg, B complex 1/2-1cc and pantothenic acid (100mg) IM every 2-3 days for 3-4 weeks.

The above treatment protocol can be very helpful a easing the withdrawal symptoms that may be experienced when coming off coffee. If migraine HAs or severe muscle spasms or aches develop IV magnesium can be used. Some people may need additional help to overcome their fatigue. Acupuncture and IM/IV vitamin therapies can be very helpful.

# ATHLETIC INJURIES: TREATMENTS TO SPEED HEALING

The following is a treatment protocol to repair damaged muscle tissue:

1) **Acupuncture**–In acute situations, treatment should be given every day, or, minimally, every second day. Acupuncture works very well, especially in conjunction with deep muscle therapy, to reduce swelling and inflammation and to decrease muscle spasms.

2) **Arnica 1M homeopathic**–Take once on empty stomach for acute situations. For longer term injuries, use Arnica 30C. Place 3-5 pellets under the tongue and let dissolve 3x/day

3) **Magnesium aspartate**–400mg 2x per day. This may cause stools to be loose. Reduce the dosage if diarrhea develops.

4) **Bromelain/Curcumin**–2100mcu (milk clotting units is the potency of the bromelain. The higher the mcu the stronger the anti-inflammatory effect). 1200mg 3-4x per day. Take the bromelain away from food to maximize its anti-inflammatory effects. Bromelain, an enzyme which is absorbed into the bloodstream, acts by breaking down the inflammatory proteins that prevent muscle from healing as quickly.

5) **Epsom salt soak**–At least 4 lbs epsom salts per 20 gallons of water. Epsom salts are composed of magnesium and get absorbed through the skin directly into the muscles.. This helps the muscle relax . Epsom salt baths are especially useful for strained or tight muscles.

6) **Arnica oil compound mixed with small amount of DMSO**–Apply topically to injury 3-5x per day

7) **"Traumeel"**–(from Heel)–Apply topically to injured area. This is especially effective in overnight treatments.

8) **Splinting or taping or wrapping in neoprene**–This should be done upon awakening when swelling is least severe.

## WHAT TO DO BEFORE & AFTER SURGERY TO HEAL FASTER AND SPEED RECOVERY

**1-2 weeks prior to surgery**

1) Vitamin C - 2 grams 3x per day
2) Zinc picolinate - 30mg 2x per day after eating (watch for nausea)
3) Vitamin A - 20,00iu 2x per day
4) Beta Carotene - 30,000iu 2x per day
5) High Potency B Complex - 1-2x per day
6) Vitamin E - 400iu 1x per day

**NOTE**–If will be taking antibiotics (especially broad spectrum antibiotics such as penicillin, tetracycline, erythromycin, etc.) it would be beneficial to start taking Lactobacillus acidophilus, Bifidobacterium bifidum, Lactobacillus casei, Streptococcus faecium, or any other normal intestinal flora to help prevent gastrointestinal problems associated with the killing off of the natural flora by the antibiotic. Children under age 7 should take Bifidobacterium infantis which is more specific for their normal flora. This should be given away from solid foods. I usually recommend Natren® cultures because they are refrigerated. They generally come in powder form that can be mixed with different liquids.

**Immediately following surgery**

1) Continue supplements initially recommended adding Vitamin E - 400iu 2x per day. Can also apply the Vitamin E directly to the surgical incision along with the juice of the Aloe vera plant.
2) Bromelain - 4 capsules of 250mg (2100mcu potency) 4x per day on empty stomach (at least 20 minutes before eating or 1 hour after eating). Continue for at least 5-7 days depending upon swelling and bruising.
3) Citrus bioflavonoids - 2 grams 3x per day with food.
4) Arnica Montana - 1M potency taken ASAP after surgery. Following this initial dose a 30c potency can be taken - 3 pellets 3x per day for the next 7 days. Other homeopathics may also be used to speed healing. With different homeopathics being indicated for different conditions. See *Homeopathic Medicine at Home*, Panos.

## BONE FRACTURE PROTOCOL

Depending upon what type of fracture is present and to what extent there is other tissue damage aside from the fracture of the bone itself the following are nutritional supplements that will help the bone heal, usually considerably faster than the normal rate. The following supplements should be taken:

**INITIALLY TAKE THE FOLLOWING:**

1) Arnica 1M as soon as the injury occurs
2) Hypericum 30c 3 pellets 3x per day
3) Bromelain and curcumin (Scientific Botanicals)
4) Omnivite– 2 tabs 3x per day
5) Vitamin K-5mg 2x per day (Scientific Botanicals)
6) Calcium/ magnesium citrate malate–300mg 3x per day

Effervescent Cal Mag plus boron 2 teaspoons 2x per day from Priority plus.

Discontinue #1 and 3 after the initial trauma (maybe for 4-7 days).

If there is additional cartiledge damage add the following:

1) Glucosamine sulfate 500mg 3x per day
2) Ligaplex 3 tabs 3x per day ( Standard Process)

## NUTRITIONAL TREATMENT FOR ABNORMAL HAIR LOSS IN FEMALES

1) **HCL** 10-60grains with each meal if found to be deficient by Heidelberg or clinical symptoms
2) **Protein formulation**- free amino acids especially high in arginine
3) **Folate**- 1-10mg/day especially if on birth control pills or hormones
4) **Vitamin B-6**- 50-300mg per day especially if on birth control pills or hormones
5) **Essential fatty acids** - flax oil 2 teaspoons 2x per day
6) **Amino acids**- arginine 1-6gms per day and cysteine 1-6 gms per day
7) **B vitamin complex**-50-100mg/day
8) **Consider IV or IM vitamin therapy**
9) **Topical rubifacients**-capsicum and/or bee venom

## Blood Test Results Explained

The following substances are found in the serum or liquid part of the blood.

**Glucose**–Fasting blood glucose levels, where the patient has not eaten for at least 6 hours, ideally should be between 70-90mg/dl. 90-100mg/dl is a borderline value that may need further evaluation depending upon family history. Levels over 100mg/dl should be further evaluated via the Glucose Insulin Tolerance Test, especially if there is any family history of diabetes.

**BUN**–Blood Urea Nitrogen levels indicate how much nitrogen is in the blood. Nitrogen comes from dietary protein. If you eat lots of protein, you will have more nitrogen in the blood. High nitrogen levels may also indicate that the kidneys are not properly filtering the blood. It is best to have nitrogen levels below 15.0.

**Creatinine**–A waste material from muscular function, creatinine constantly comes into the blood. The kidneys filter creatinine from the blood . Thus, if creatinine levels are elevated, it means that the kidneys are not filtering properly.

**BUN/Creatinine ratio**–should be within the reference range.

**Sodium & Chloride**–These electrolytes are important for maintaining fluid balance inside and outside your cells. If the sodium level is too high, blood pressure may rise because of the increase in fluid volume.

**Potassium**–This mineral is often deficient since most people don't consume nearly enough to balance out their sodium intake. If blood levels of this mineral are too high or too low, the heart could start to beat irregularly.

**Total protein**

**Albumin**–One of two proteins measured in a standard blood screen, albumin functions to hold fluids in the blood vessels. It also buffers the pH levels.

**Globulin**–The other protein measured in blood, globulin is responsible for synthesizing all the antibodies for the immune system.

**Albumin/Globulin ratio**–This ratio may become abnormal if there is a malabsorption problem in the gastrointestinal tract or if there is insufficient intake.

**Calcium**–If blood levels of this mineral are too high, it can cause ossification of soft tissues. If calcium levels are too low, it may indicate osteoporosis or osteomalacia.

**Phosphorus** is involved in bone metabolism. Blood levels should be in the middle range.

**SGOT (AST), SGPT (ALT), LDH, Alkaline phosphatase, GGT**–These liver enzymes are found, usually in small quantities, in the cells of the liver. If the liver becomes damaged due to a virus such as hepatitis or to a toxin such as a drug or other poisonous substance, cells from the liver will become damaged and they will spill these enzymes into the serum where they can then be measured. Thus, high liver enzymes indicate liver damage. Ideally you want your liver enzymes to be in the mid to low normal range.

**Total Bilirubin**–Bilirubin is a breakdown product of your red blood cells. After their life cycle, 120 days, RBC's are recycled by the reticuloendothelial system in the body. One of the recycled materials is bilirubin which is sent to the liver to be metabolized. If bilirubin levels are on the high side of the range, or over the upper limit, it means that you are breaking your red blood cells down too quickly.

**Uric acid**–This is a breakdown product of the purines that are consumed in the diet. Certain foods have high levels of purine. If these foods are consumed, uric acid levels will be high in the blood. When uric acid reaches high enough levels in your blood, it precipitates into crystals which causing joint and kidney damage.

**Cholesterol**–Cholesterol levels, ideally, should be below 170mg/dl. As cholesterol starts to rise above 150mg/dl, the rate of heart disease slowly rises. As levels exceed 200mg/dl the rate of CVD goes up more rapidly. Very low cholesterol levels have been linked to increases in cancer. This association has been made primarily with people who consume unhealthy diets. If a person's diet is healthy, lower cholesterol levels do not increase the risk of cancer.

**HDL cholesterol**–High density cholesterol is the good cholesterol. HDL levels are best above 60mg/dl. The higher the HDL cholesterol level, the lower the rate of heart disease. HDL cholesterol transports cholesterol out of the blood vessels and back to the liver where it is removed from the body.

**Cholesterol/HDL risk ratio**–The lower the total cholesterol to HDL ratio, the lower the incidence of heart disease. Ideally, the ratio should be 3 to 1.

**LDL cholesterol**–Low density lipoprotein is atherogenic. It transports cholesterol from the liver to the blood vessels where it causes fatty plaques to build up inside blood vessels by . LDL cholesterol levels are best below 90mg/dl.

**Triglycerides(TG's) or fats**–Triglycerides tend to make platelets stick together. Ideally, triglyceride levels should be below 100mg/dl on a fasting (at least 4 hours) blood sample. When levels exceed 200mg/dl the serum starts to get a milky color which becomes progressively whiter as the levels rise. High TG's decrease oxygen and prevent other nutrients from getting to the tissues. In addition, as TG's stay high, they can cause muscles fatigue, trigger migraine headaches, and increase requirements for insulin.

**Total iron level** does not really indicate anything in regard to how much iron is in your tissues.

**% transferrin saturation**–Transferrin is a protein that carries iron around your blood. When % transferrin saturation is below the lower limit, then iron stores are low. When it exceeds the upper limit of the range, it means that iron in the tissues is too high.

**Ferritin**–Ferritin levels reflect how much iron is stored in your tissues or inside your cells. A low serum ferritin (below 30 in females & below 20 min. males) is an indication of iron deficiency. If Hct, HgB, MCV and RBC count are also low, then iron deficiency anemia is present. If ferritin levels rise to high levels, especially in males, the risk of heart disease, cancer, diabetes, arthritis and chronic infections may go up. Athletes who over-train may have low ferritin levels and should increase levels above 30. Ferritin may be high in certain pathological states such as chronic infections and inflammation. Ideally, ferritin levels in non-pregnant females should be 30-60mg/dl and 20-50mg/dl in males. Levels in the high normal range are not considered ideal and efforts to avoid excessive iron intake should be taken.

**Thyroid T-4**–Levels are best in the middle reference range. If symptoms of low thyroid are present and levels are below 6.5mcg/dl, then further evaluation is indicated. Levels in the mid-range are <u>not</u> always normal.

**TSH**–Thyroid stimulating hormone is secreted from the pituitary gland. If it is above the reference range, it indicates that the body wants more thyroid hormone. If low, it indicates that thyroid hormone levels <u>may</u> be too high.

**CBC (Complete Blood Count)**–This is the cellular component of the blood. This moiety of blood contains the red and white blood cells. The RBC's are responsible for carrying oxygen while the WBC's are responsible for the defense system of the body. It is composed of several different types of cells. The counting the different types of WBC's is called the differential.

**RBC**–Ideally, the red blood cell count should be within the normal range. If levels are low, it indicates anemia. If they are too high, blood may be too thick. This indicates dehydration or other problems.

**HgB**–This measurement should be in the mid range. It represents the color of the RBC"s and is an indication of how well they can carry oxygen. Too high a value means too thick blood.

**Hct**–This is the percentage of the blood that is made up of RBC's. Females are ideally above 37% and males above 39%. As this level gets too low, it means that the blood can not be supplied with enough oxygen to the tissues. Too high means that the blood is too thick.

**MCV**–Mean cell volume indicates the size of your RBC's. Ideally the MCV should be mid-range. Above 95 indicates larger RBC's, indicating folate or B-12 deficiency. An MCV of below 84 indicates smaller RBC's due to copper, thiamin, B-6 and or iron deficiency.

**WBC's**–These are your body's defensive cells. If levels are too low, it indicates a diminished immunity. If too high, above 8 or 9, it indicates active infection. WBC's are made up of neutrophils and monocytes which fight bacterial infections, lymphocytes which fight viruses, eosinophils and basophils which are involved with allergies or parasites.

# Book Companies & Environmental Allergy Companies & Products

| Book Companies | | |
|---|---|---|
| **Biosocial publications** | (206) 272-0530 | PO Box 1174<br>Tacoma, WA 98401 |
| **Blue Poppy Press** | 1(800) 487-9296q | Linden Ave<br>Boulder, CO 80304 |
| **Bookpeople** | 1-800-999-4650 | 7900 Edgewater Drive<br>Oakland.CA. 94621 |
| **J.A. Majors Company**<br>Distributes Medical/Scientific Books | | 1220 W. Walnut St.<br>Compton, CA 90220 |
| **Moving Books** | 1-800-762-1750<br>(206) 777 6683 | 948 South Doris St<br>Seattle, WA, 98108 |
| **Nutri-books** | 1-800-279-2048 | Box 5793, Denver, CO, 80217 |
| **Price- Pottinger Nutrition Foundations**<br>offers slides, books and videos | 1-619-582-4168 | P.O. Box 2614<br>La Mesa, CA. 92041 |

| Allergy Supplies | | |
|---|---|---|
| **AFM**<br>a custom formulating and manufacturing company that offers products for the chemically sensitive | (714) 781-6860 | 1140 Stacy Court<br>Riverside, CA. 92507 |
| **Allergy Relief Shop**<br>Air & water fitlers, cotton bedding, air exhangers, vacuums, paint sealers | (615) 52-2795 | 2932 Middlebrook Rk.<br>Knoxville, TN 37921 |
| **Allergy Resource**<br>Foods products all types of flours such as from different beans, quinoa, teff, millet, potato, milk subs, baking mixes, non wheat pasta (quinoa, buckwheat, seeds, oils, cerals, air filters, mattress covers, magnets,suppl, books, flea products, radon test kits etc | (719) 488-3630 | 745 Powderhorn, Monument, Colorado 80132 |
| **Allergy Resources**<br>Staples for the chemically sensitive | 1-800-USE-FLAX | PO Box 888<br>Palmer Lake, CO, 80133 |
| **AllerMed Corporation**<br>Sells air purifiers | (214) 442-4898 | 31 Steel Rd.<br>Wylie, TX 75099 |
| **American Environmental Health Foundation, Inc.**<br>Sell ecological masks, cleaning solutions, airl Filters and Purifiersbooks & suppl | (214)361-9515 | 8345 Walnut Hill Lane, # 200<br>Dallas, TX 75231 |

# Book Companies & Environmental Allergy Companies & Products

| | | |
|---|---|---|
| **Auro Products** imported by Sinan Company offers all natural lacquers, paints, cleaners from West Germany | (707) 427-2325 | P.O. Box 181<br>Suisun City, CA 94585 |
| **Baubiologie Hardware** specializes in alternative building, redecorating and gardening products | (408) 372-8626 | 207B 16th St.<br>Pacific Grove CA. 93950 |
| **Berner Air Products, Inc.** Sell Air heat exchangers with filters | (412) 658-3551 | P.O. Box 5410<br>New Castle, PA 16137 |
| **BioGreen** enviromentally friendly products for home and office | 1-800-39-EARTH | 10956 E. Calle Vaqueros,<br>Tuscon ,Arizona, 85749 |
| **Dust Free Inc** Offers air test equipment, air purifiers, filters | (214) 635-9565 | P.O Box 519<br>Royse City, TX 75089 |
| **E.L. Foust Co Inc** Offers air filters | (708) 834-5104 | P.O. Box 105<br>Elmhurst, IL 60126 |
| **Eco Source** Air filters, water filters, home productsClothes Light bulbs, cleaning products | (800)688-8345 | 9051 Mill Station Rd. Building E<br>Sebastopol, CA 95472 |
| **Environmental Helath Center** Directors William J.Rea, M.D. State of the art clinical ecology clinic | (204) 368-4132 | 8345 Walnut Hill Lane # 205<br>Dallas, TX 75231 |
| **Environmental Purification Systems** Water filtes and air filtration systems masks | (415) 284-2129<br>(800) 829-2129 | P.O. Box 191<br>Concord, CA 94522 |
| **EPS Environmental Purification Systems** | | |
| **Free Free Ecopaper** | (503) 295-6705 or<br>Fax 464-2299 | 121 S.W. Salmon, Suite 1100<br>Portland, OR 97204 |
| **Greening of Medicine** Theron Randolph, M.D. Info resource | (708) 844-9898 | 161 S. Lincolnway<br>North Aurora, IL 60542 |
| **Healthmed** | (16) 924-8060 | 1 Scripps Dr. # 201<br>Sacramento, CA 95825 |
| **Healthy House** by John Bower, Lyle Stuart. | Provides detailed descriptions of conventional and nontoxic alternative building products. | 1989 |
| **Healthy Household** by Lynn Marie Bower | a guide ot less toxic cleaning and household products | The Healthy House Instituite<br>(812) 332-5073 |
| **Light Energy Co** | 1(800)LIGHT CO<br>or 1(800) 544-4826 | 1056 N.W. 179th Pl.<br>Seattle, WA 98177 |

## Book Companies & Environmental Allergy Companies & Products

| | | |
|---|---|---|
| **Livos Plant Chemistry**<br>Offers finishes. waxes, art products | (505) 988-2288 | 2641 Cerrillos Rd.<br>Santa Fe NM, 87501 |
| **N.E.E.D.S., Inc.** | (800)634-1380 | 527 Charles Ave. #12-A<br>Syracuse, NY 13209 |
| **Natural Choice**<br>natural paints and finishes and hypoallergenic body products | (505) 438-3448 | Eco Design Co.<br>1365 Rufina Circle,<br>Santa Fe, NM, 87501 |
| **Practical Allergy Research Foundation** Info, audio tapes, video tapes for Dr. parents and educators and some books on allergies and ecologic ds | (716) 875 5578 | P.O Box 60<br>Buffalo, NY 14223 |
| **Priorities**<br>**Allergy relief and a healthy home**<br>offers a variety of products for the home | 1-800-553-5398 | 70 Walnut Street<br>Wellesley, MA, 02181 |
| **Real Good Store**<br>(many solar & environmental products) | (800)919-2400<br>(707) 468-9486<br>(541) 334-6960 in Eugene, OR | 555 Leslie St.<br>Ukiah, CA 95482<br>1679 W. 7th Ave. |
| **Safe Shoppers Bible** by David Steinman and Samuel Epstein M.D. | The authors rate the toxicity of many brand-name products, foods and beverages | Macmillan, 1995 |
| **Self Care Catalog**<br>offers anti-allergy bedding protection | 1-800-520-9924 | P.O.Box 182290<br>Chattanooga, TN, 37422 |
| **Sierra Group for Environmental Products Inc.** Air filters & other prods | (219) 256-6909 | 433 Rivers Edge Ct<br>Mishawaka, IN 46544 |
| **To Your Health Catalog, The Glass Bubble**<br>source of nontoxic household products including cookware, vacuum cleaners | 1-800-233-2606 or<br>(214)-939-9080 | 2815 Elm St.<br>Dallas TX, 75226 |
| **Vita.lite**<br>Duro-lite Lamps Inc | | Duro-Test corp<br>2321 Kennedy Blvd.<br>N. Bergen, NJ 07047 |
| **Tools for Exploration (many new age products)** | (888) 748-6657 | 47 Paul Dr.<br>San Rafeal, CA 94903 |

### Radiation VDTs screens

| | |
|---|---|
| **Biflyx/ Design West,** | 2532 Dupont Dr. Irvine, CA 92715 |
| **I-Protect** | 301 N. Prarie Ave # 510 |

## Alternative Laboratories Specializing in Nutritional Medicine

| | | |
|---|---|---|
| **Acu-Chem Labs**<br>**Environmental toxins** | (800451-0116 & (800)747-2878<br>(214)234-5412 | 990 N. Bowser, #800<br>Richardson, TX 75081 |
| **Antibody Assay Labs**<br>(environmental medicine) | (800) 522-2611<br>(714)-972-9979 | 1715 East Wilshire, #715<br>Santa Ana, CA 92705 |
| **BALCO**<br>(essential & toxic mineral anal) | (800) 777-1722<br>(415) 697-6708 | 1520 Gilbreh Rd.<br>Burlingame, CA 94010 |
| **Diagnostechs**<br>(stool, hormone, & altern) | 1(800)878-3787 | 620 South 192nd Pl. #J-104, Kent WA98032 |
| **Doctors Data**<br>(hair analysis & environ toxins) | (800) 323-2784<br>(630)-231-9190 fax | P.O. Box 111<br>Chicago, IL 60186 |
| **Great Smokies Diagnostic Labs**<br>(Stool analysis & detox) | (800) 542-3526<br>(828) 253-0621 | 63 Zillicoa St.<br>Asheville, NC 28801 |
| **Intracellular Diagnostics** Exatest (for minerals esp **mg**) | (800)874-4804 | CA<br>Dr. Burton Silver |
| **Labcorp**<br>(general lab & some alternative) | (800) 676-8033<br>(206) 395-4235 | 21093 68th Ave. S.<br>Kent WA 98032 |
| **Meridian Valley Clinical Lab** | (206) 631-8691 | 21093 132nd Ave. SE<br>Kent, WA 98042 |
| **Metametrix Medical Lab**<br>(amino acidanalysis & more) | (800) 221-4640<br>(404)-441-2237 fax | 5000 Peachtree Ind. Bld.<br>Norcross, GA 30071 |
| **Monroe Medical**<br>(alternative & conventional) | see Townsend Newsletter | |
| **National BioTech Lab**<br>(stool & alternative lab) | (800) 846-6285<br>(206)-363-2025 fax | 3212 NE 125th St.<br>Seattle, WA 98125 |
| **National Health Lab** | (800) 676-8033<br>(206) 395-4000 (503) 254-2339 | 21903 68th Ave S.<br>Kent, WA 98032 |
| **Practical Allergy Research**<br>Foundation Dorris Rapp, M.D. | (716)875-5578 | P.O. Box 60<br>Buffalo, N.Y. 14223-0060 |
| **Spectra Cell Labs Inc.** | (800) 227-5227<br>(713)-621-3101 | 515 Post Oak Bld. # 830<br>Houston TX 77027 |
| **Trace Minerals International,**<br>Inc.(clinical & environ chem) | (800) 530-5228<br>Fax (303) 530-5296 | 6545 Gunpark Dr. Suite 240<br>Boulder, CO 80301 |
| **Unilab Corp** | (800)422-4244 (billing)<br>(800)824-0985 (lab) | P.O. Box 600<br>San Francisco,CA 94160 |
| | | |
| **ORGANIZATIONS FOR ALTERNATIVE AND COMPLIMENTARY MEDICINE** | | |
| **International Society for Orthomolecular Medicine (ISOM)** | (433) 733-2117<br>(416) 733-2352 | 16 Florance Ave,<br>Toronto, Ontario Canada, M2N 1E9 |
| **American Association of Naturopathic Physicians (AANP)** | (206) 298-0126<br>(206) 298-0129 | P.O. Box 20386<br>Seattle, WA 98102 |
| **American Academy of Environmental Medicine (AAEM)** | (316) 684-5500 | |
| **American College for the Advancement of Medicine (ACAM)** | (949) 583-7666 | |
| **American Holistic Medical Association (AHMA)** | (202) 986-0850<br>(919) 787-5181 | |
| **International & American Assoc. of Clinical Nutritionists (IAACN)** | (972) 407-9089 | |
| **American Association of Acupuncture & Oriental Medicine** | (919) 787-5181 | |
| **American Botanical Council** | (512) 331-1924 | Austin, TX 78720 |
| **American Herb Association** | (916) 265-9552 | Nevada City, CA 95959 |
| **Herb Research Foundation** | (303) 449-2265 | 1007 Pearl St. #200 |

## Dr. Marz' Pharmacy Company List

| | | |
|---|---|---|
| **A.C. Grace Company**<br>unesterified vitamin E | (903) 636-4368 & fax (903) 636-4051 | 1100 Quitman Rd, PO Box 570; Big Sandy TX 75755 |
| **Acme Vial & Glass Co, Inc.** | (805)239-2666 | 1601 Commerce Way<br>Paso Robles, CA 93446 |
| **Allergy Research Group**<br>**Emerson Ecologics, Inc** | (800) 782-4274 (orders)<br>(510) 639-4572(800) 545-9960(info) | 400 Preda Street<br>San Leandro, CA 94577 |
| **Allergy Resources** | (800) USE-FLAX<br>(719) 488-3630 | Box 888, 264 Brookridge<br>Palmer Lake, CO 80133 |
| **Alpine Air Industries**<br>**George Binum in OR** | (800) 486-4994 (612) 785-9140<br>(fax)(503) 256-5092 | 9199 Central Ave. NE<br>Blaine, MN 55434 |
| **American Biologics**<br>**(Robert W. Bradford)** | (800) 227-4473 & (800)969-6601<br>(619) 429-8200 | 1180 Walnut Avenue<br>Chula Vista, CA 91911 |
| **AMNI-Advanced Medical Nutrition, Inc.** | (800) 437-8888<br>(415) 783-6969 | 2247 National Avenue<br>Hayward, CA 94540 |
| **Apothe' Cure Inc.** | (800) 969-6601 (214) 960-6601<br>(800) 687-5252 (fax) (214) 960-6921 | 13720 Midway Rd.Ste.109<br>Dallas,TX 75244 |
| **Arizona Natural Products (ANP)** | (800) 255-2823<br>(602) 991-4419 | 8281 E. Evans Road #104,<br>Scottsdale, AZ 85260 |
| **Bach Flower Remedies**<br>**Essence Services:Ellon USA, Inc.:** | (800) 548-0075 (516) 593-9668 (fax)<br>(800) 4BE-CALM (516) 593-2206 | Nevada City, CA 95959<br>644 Merrick Rd,Lynbrook, NY 11563 |
| **Bee Products see High Desert** | | |
| **Bezwecken** | (503) 644-7800 | 15495 SW Millikan Way 97006 |
| **BHI-Heel** | (800) 621-7644 (505) 293-3843<br>(505) 275-1672 (fax) | 11600 Cochiti S.E.<br>Albuquerque, NM 87123 |
| **Bio Force** | (800) 645-9135 | P.O Box 507<br>Kinderhook, NY 12106 |
| **Bio Pulse** | (800) 453-2483 | 2855 Midland Dr.<br>Ogden, UT 84401 |
| **BioGreen** | (800) 39-EARTH | 10956 E. Calle Vaqueros<br>Tucson, AZ 85749 |
| **Biotics Research W.W. Inc.** | (800)636-6913 & (800)863-9613 fax | Box 7027, Olympia, WA 98507 |
| **Blaine Pharmaceuticals Inc.**<br>(magnesium specialists) | (800) 633-9353 & (606)283-9437 | 1515 Productions Dr.; Burlington, KY 41005 |
| **Boericke & Tafel** | (800) 876-9505<br>(215) 922-2967 (707) 571-8202 | 1011 Arch Street<br>Philadelphia, PA 19107 |
| **Boiron/Borneman & Sons** | (800) BLU-TUBE<br>(805) 582-9094 | 98C West Cochran St.<br>Simi Valley, CA 93065 |
| **Brion Herbs Corp**<br>**Sun Ten Herbs** | (800) 333-HERB (order)<br>(800) 777-2309 (consult)<br>(714) 587-1238 (714) 587-1260 (fax) | 9250 Jeronimo Rd.<br>Irvine, CA 92718 |
| **Bronson Pharmaceuticals** | (800) 776-8308 | 600 E. Quality Dr.<br>American Fork, UT 84003 |
| **Cardiovascular Research, Ltd.(Ecological Formulas)** | (800) 888-4585<br>(510) 827-2636 | 1061-B Shary Circle<br>Concord, CA 94518 |
| **Carlson, JR Labs Inc.** | (800)323-4141 (847)255-1605 fax | 15 College, Arlington Hts, Il 60004 |
| **College Pharmacy** | (800) 888-9358 | 833 N. Tejon<br>Colorado Springs, CO 80903 |
| **Darrow Labs (Natural Law)** | (503) 625-6502 | P.O. Box 338<br>Sherwood, OR 97140 |
| **Dixie Health, Inc.** | (800) 288-9232<br>(770) 951-9232 (Cust. Serv.) | 2161 Newmarket Pky, #222<br>Marietta, GA 30067 |
| **Dixon-Shane** | (215) 673-7770 | Philadelphia PA |
| **Doctor's Data (Hair Analysis)** | (800) 323-2784 | 170 W. Roosevelt Rd<br>West Chicago, IL 60185 |
| **Douglas Laboratories** | (800) 245-4440 | 600 Boyce Road<br>Pittsburgh, PA 15205-9010 |

## Dr. Marz' Pharmacy Company List

| | | |
|---|---|---|
| **Eastern Currents** (see Helio Medical) | | |
| **Eclectic Institute** | (800) 332-HERB(4372)<br>(503) 668-4120 | 14385 S.E. Lusted Rd.<br>Sandy, OR 97055 |
| **Edom Laboritories** | (800) 723-3366<br>(516) 586-2266 | 860 Grand Blvd.<br>Box 780 Deer Park, NY 11729 |
| **Emerson Ecologics, Inc.**<br>(they distribute many companies -Allergy Research Group and Gaia Herbs) | (800) 654-4432 (info) | 436 Great Rd.<br>Acton, MA 01720 |
| **Enfood (Liv-N-Well Dist.)** | (604) 270-8474 | #1-7900 River Rd.<br>Richmond, BD V6X 1X7 |
| **Environmental Building Supplies** | (503) 222-3881<br>(503) 222-3756 (fax) | 1314 NW Northrup St.<br>Portland, OR 97209 |
| **Flora, Inc** | (800) 498-3610 | Box 950, E. Badger Rd.<br>Lynden, WA 98264 |
| **For Your Health, Inc.** | (800) 456-4325<br>(206) 365-8488 | 3212 NE 125th St<br>Seattle, WA 98125 |
| **Frieda** | (800) 545-9960<br>(212) 662-3329 | 36 East 41st Street<br>New York, NY 10017 |
| **Gaia Herbs**<br>**/Emerson Ecologics, Inc** | (800) 831-7780<br>(800) 717-1722 (fax) | 108 Island Ford Rd.<br>Brevard, NC 28712 |
| **Health Concerns** | (206) 343-7446 | 8001 Caswell Dr<br>Oakland, CA 94621 |
| **Heel See BHI** | (800) 621-7644 | |
| **Helio Medical Supplies acupunct** | (800) YIN-YANG<br>(408) 479-8625 (408) 476-6688 (fax) | 3040 Childer Lane<br>Santa Cruz, CA 95062 |
| **Henry Shein** (big medical supplier)<br>**(formerly Veratex)** | (800) 356-5788<br>(800) 772-4346 | 135 Duryea Rd.; Melville, N.Y 11747 |
| **Herb Pharm** (excellent products and great resource of organic herbs; Ed Smith extremely knowledgable) | (541)846--6262 (800)545-7392 fax<br>E-mail HerbPharm @aol.com<br>(800)348-4372 & (800)599-2392 | P.O. Box 116<br>Willliams, OR 97544 |
| **Herbal Products & Development (organic oils hemp, herbs salves)** | (408) 688-8706 | PO BOX 1084;<br>Aptos, CA 95001 |
| **Heritage Store** | (800) 862-2923 | Box 444-W<br>Virginia Beach, VA 23458 |
| **High Desert Bee Products** | (800)875-0096 | 3627 E. Indian School Rd<br>Phoenix, AZ 85018 |
| **Hollister-Stier** | (800) 992-1120<br>(509) 489-5656 | P.O. Box 3145<br>Spokane, WA 99220 |
| **Institiute for Traditional Medicine (ITM)** | (800) 544-7504<br>(503) 233-4907 (503) 233-1017 (fax) | 2017 S.E. Hawthorne,<br>Portland, OR 97214 |
| **Interplexus, Inc.** | (800) 875-0511<br>(206) 251-0511 (425)868-5393fax | 6620 S. 192nd Pl. J-105,<br>Kent, WA 98032 |
| **Karuna Co.** | (800)826)-7225 | Novato, CA |
| **Klaire Labs, Inc.** | (206) 836-3309<br>(800)533-7255 | 21101 NE 108th St<br>Redmond, WA 98053 |
| **Kripps Pharmacy**<br>**(Dr. Thorp)** | (604) 325-0025 | 994 Granville Street<br>Vancouver, BC V6Z 1L2<br>CANADA |
| **Levine Health Products** | (800) 426-6763<br>(206) 836-3309 | 21101 NE 108th St<br>Redmond,WA 98053 |
| **Lintec "Travacid"** | (800) 323-3842 | |
| **McGuff Company Med Sup** | (800) 854-7220<br>(714) 540-5614 fax | 3524 W Lake Center Dr<br>Santa Ana, CA 92704 |
| **Merit Pharmaceuticals**<br>**(Rich Anter - NW contact)** | (800) 538-0150<br>(206) 938-4429 | PO Box 16625<br>Seattle, WA 98116 |

**Dr. Marz' Pharmacy Company List**

| | | |
|---|---|---|
| **Merit Pharmaceuticals** | (213) 227-4831 | 2611 San Fernando Rd; LA, CA |
| **Metabolic Maintenance** | (503) 549-7800 | 68994 N Pine St<br>Box 3600 Sisters, OR 97759 |
| **Metagenics** | (800) 338-3948<br>(503) 345-0511 | 1030 Tyinn St Unit 9<br>Eugene, OR 97402 |
| **Montana Naturals** | (800) 872-7218 | 19994 Hwy 93<br>Arlee, MT 59821 |
| **Mountain Peoples Warehouse (used to be Nutra Source)** | (206) 467-7190 | PO Box 81106<br>Seattle, WA 98108 |
| **Natren** | (800) 992-3323<br>(805) 371-4737 | 3105 Willow Ln<br>Westlake Village, CA 91361 |
| **NF Formulas, Inc.** | (800) 325-9326 OR (503) 682-9755<br>(800) 547 4891 outside OR | 9775 SW Commerce Circle<br>Wilsonville, OR 97070 |
| **Omega Nutriton** | (800) 745-8580 | 720 E. Washington<br>Sequim, WA 98382 |
| **Omniopathy Products** | (714) 538-1540<br>(800) 745-1540 | 414 N. State College Blvd.<br>Anaheim, CA 92806 |
| **OMNIVITE Nutrition Inc.**(time release magnesium & debittered Stevia) | (800) 424-OMNI<br>(503) 239-9192 (fax)<br>(503) 233-9553 | Tabor Hill Clinic<br>2002 S.E. 50th Avenue<br>Portland, OR 97215 |
| **Oregon Health Sciences University: Bookstore & Library** | (503) 494-7708<br>(503) 494-3462 | |
| **Phyto-Pharmica (Enzymatic Therapies)** | (800) 553-2370<br>(414) 469-9099 (414) 469-4418 (fax) | P.O. Box 1745<br>Green Bay, WI 54305 |
| **Pioneer Nutritional Formulas, Inc** | (800) 458-8483<br>(413) 625-8212 | P.O. Box 259,<br>Shelburne Falls, MA 01370 |
| **Priorities (Allergy Relief Products)** | (800) 553-5398 | 70 Walnut St.<br>Wellesley, MA 02181 |
| **Priority One** | (800) 443-2039<br>(360) 671-8503 (fax) | 715 W. Orchard St, Ste 4<br>Bellingham, WA 98225 |
| **Probiologic** | (800) 678-8218<br>(206) 881-8218 | 8707 148th Ave NE<br>Redmond, WA 98052 |
| **Professional Botanicals** | (800) 824-8181<br>(801) 479-1903 (fax) | 2554 E. Woodland Dr.<br>Box 9822; Ogden, Utah 84409 |
| **Professional Health NW (Seroyal)** | (800) 952-2219<br>(503) 641-5510 | P.O. Box 1396<br>Beaverton, OR 97075 |
| **Professional Health Products** | (800) 952-2219<br>(503) 245-2720 Portland | 5112 SW Garden Home Rd<br>Box 80085 Portland, OR 97280 |
| **Progena** | (800) 545-8900<br>(505) 292-0700 | P.O. Box 14493<br>Albuquerque, NM 87191 |
| **Pure Encapsulations** | (800) 753-2277<br>(508) 443-1999 | 490 Boston Post Rd.<br>Sudbury, MA 01776 |
| **Real Goods (environmental products)** | (800) 762-7325<br>(707) 468-9486 (fax) | 555 Leslie St.<br>Ukiah, CA 95482 |
| **Rexall** | (888) 22 REXALL<br>(561) 994-2090 | 853 Broken Sound PkyNW<br>Boca Raton, FL 33487 |
| **Sandoz Nutrition Corp.** | (800) 777-8103<br>(612) 925-2100 | 5320 West 23rd St.<br>P.O. Box 370<br>Minneapolis, MN 55440 |
| **Scandinavian Pharmaceuticals, Inc.** | (215) 453-2510 | 13 N. Seventh St.<br>Perkasie, PA 18944 |
| **Scientific Botanicals Co., Inc.** | (206) 527-5521 | P.O. Box 31131<br>Seattle, WA 98103 |
| **Scientific Consulting Service** | (800) 333-7414<br>(510) 632-2370(510) 632-2370 (fax ) | 466 Whitney St.<br>San Leandro, CA 94577 |

## Dr. Marz' Pharmacy Company List

| | | |
|---|---|---|
| **Seacure** | (800) 247-5656 (orders)<br>(800) 555-8868 (610) 372-3655 | PO Box 13905<br>Reading, PA 19612 |
| **Similasan Corp.** | (800) 426-1644 -(206) 859-9072<br>(206) 859-9102 (fax) | 1321 S. Central Ave., Ste. D<br>Kent, WA 98032 |
| **Source Naturals, Inc.**<br>**(Threshold carries this co.)** | (800) 777-5677<br>(408) 438-1144 (408) 438-7410 (fax) | P.O. Box 2118<br>Santa Cruz, CA 95063 |
| **Spectrum Naturals** | (800) 955-6445 (orders)<br>(702) 227-0102 | 133 Copeland St.<br>Petaluma, CA 94952 |
| **Spectrum/Microgon** | (800) 634-3300<br>(800) 445-7330 (fax) | 23022 La Cadena Dr.<br>Laguna Hills, CA 92653 |
| **Springreen Products** (bentonite clay) | (800) 544-8147 | Kansas City, MO |
| **Standard Homeopathics** | (800)6249659<br>(213) 321-4284 | P.O. Box 61067<br>Los Angeles, CA 90061 |
| **Standard Process Labs N.W.** | (425)882-0700 | 12521 - 131 St Ct NE<br>Kirkland, WA 98034-3113 |
| **Standard Process West** | (800) 321-9807<br>(303) 223-6262 | P.O. Box 8857<br>Ft. Collins, CO 80525 |
| **TE Neesby** | (209)261-3080 | 340 W Fallbrook, Suite 106<br>Fresno, CA 93711 |
| **Thera Tech** | (800) 448-4372<br>(714) 898-6554 | 11642 Knott St #18<br>Garden Grove, CA 92641 |
| **Thorne Research, Inc.** | (800) 228-1966<br>(208) 263-1337 | 901 Triangle Drive<br>Box 3200Sandpoint, ID 83864 |
| **Threshold** | (800) 777-5677 | 23 Janis Way<br>Scotts Valley, CA 95066 |
| **Transition for Health Inc** | (800) 648-8211 | Portland OR |
| **Twinn Labs** | (800) 645-5626 | 2120 Smithtown Ave.;<br>Ronkonkoma, N.Y.. 11779 |
| **Tyler Encapsuolations** | (800)634-1051 (503)661-5401 OR<br>(800)869-9705 outside OR | 2204-8 NW Birdsdale<br>Gresham, OR 97030 |
| **Tyson** | (800) 367-7744<br>(213) 452-7844 | 12832 Chadron<br>Hawthorne, CA 90250 |
| **Ultra Life, Inc.**<br>*(Travacid X )* time release HCL | (800)323-3842 | P.O. Box 489<br>Palatine, IL 60078 |
| **Vital Nutrients (vitamin Coop)** | (888) 328-9992 (860) 638-3675<br>888)328-9993 | 50 Silver St.;<br>Middletown,CT 06457 |
| **Vitamin Research Products Inc.**<br>(Ward Dean, M.D. director) | (800) 877-2447 fax (702) 887-7517 | 3579 Hwy 50 E.<br>Carson City, NV 89701 |
| **Vitanica** | (800) 572-4712 625-7192 | Sherwood OR |
| **Western Herbs** | (206) 793-1033 | 21627 Bridal Veil Creek Road;<br>Index, WA 98256 |
| **Willner Chemists, Inc.** | (212) 685-0448 | 330 Lexington Avenue<br>New York, NY 10157 |
| **Wise Woman Herbals, Inc.** | (800) 532-5219<br>(541) 895-5152 541) 895-5174 (fax) | P.O. Box 279<br>Creswell, OR 97426 |
| **Womens International Pharmacy** | (800)279-5708 | Madison, WI |

## Boys: Birth to 36 months; Physical Growth NCHS Percentiles

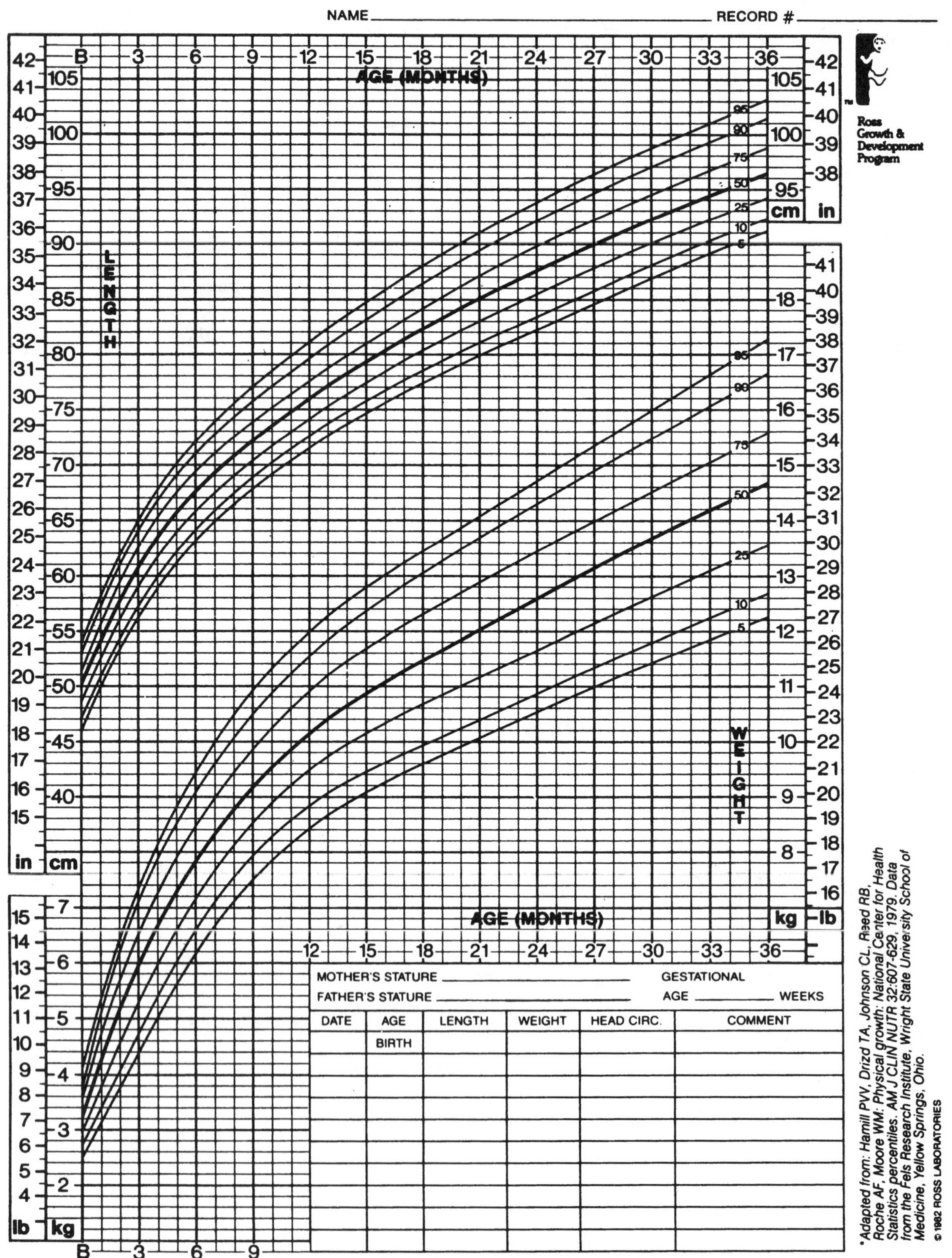

## Boys:2 to 18 Years; Physical Growth NCHS Percentiles

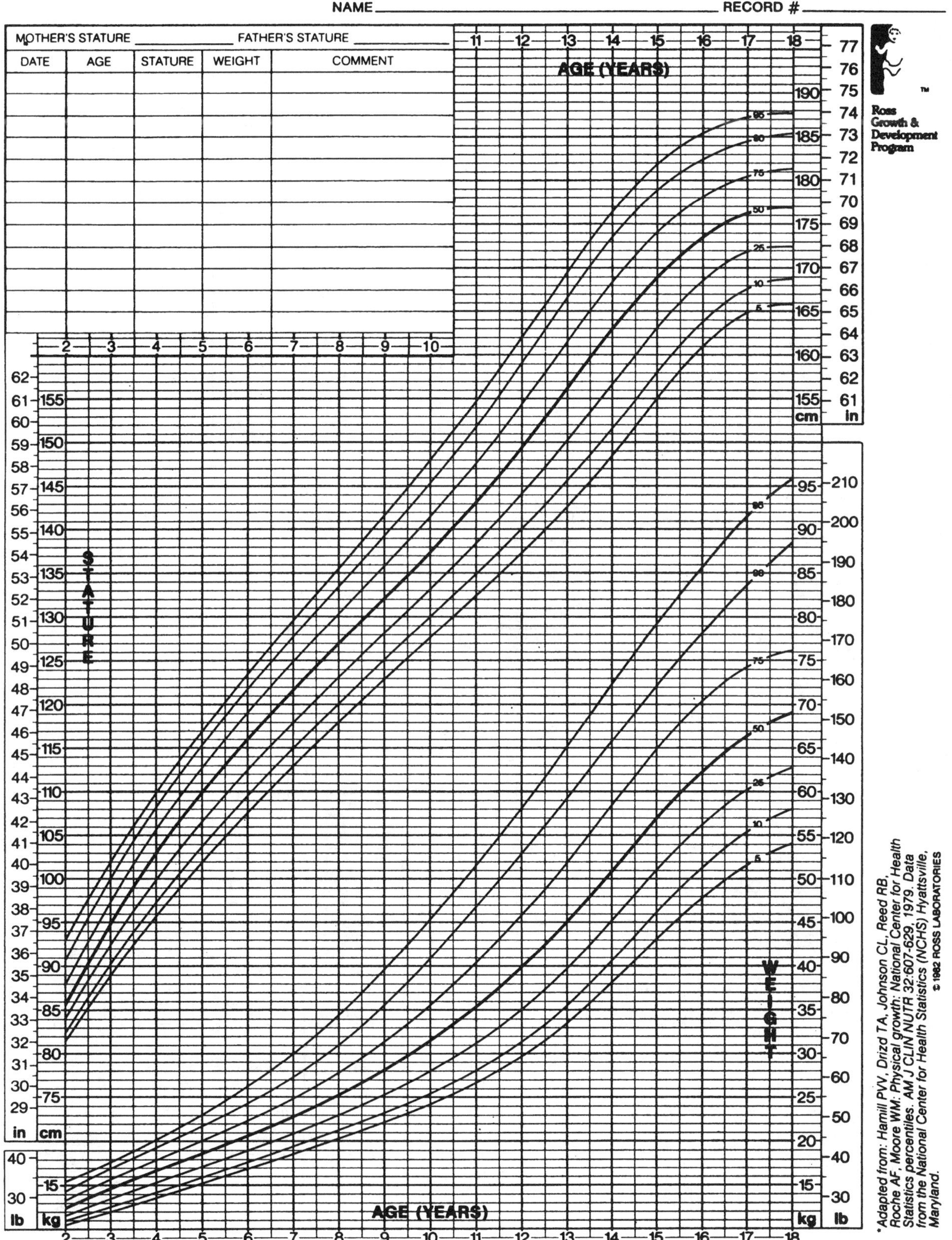

**GIRLS: BIRTH TO 36 MONTHS; PHYSICAL GROWTH NCHS PERCENTILES***

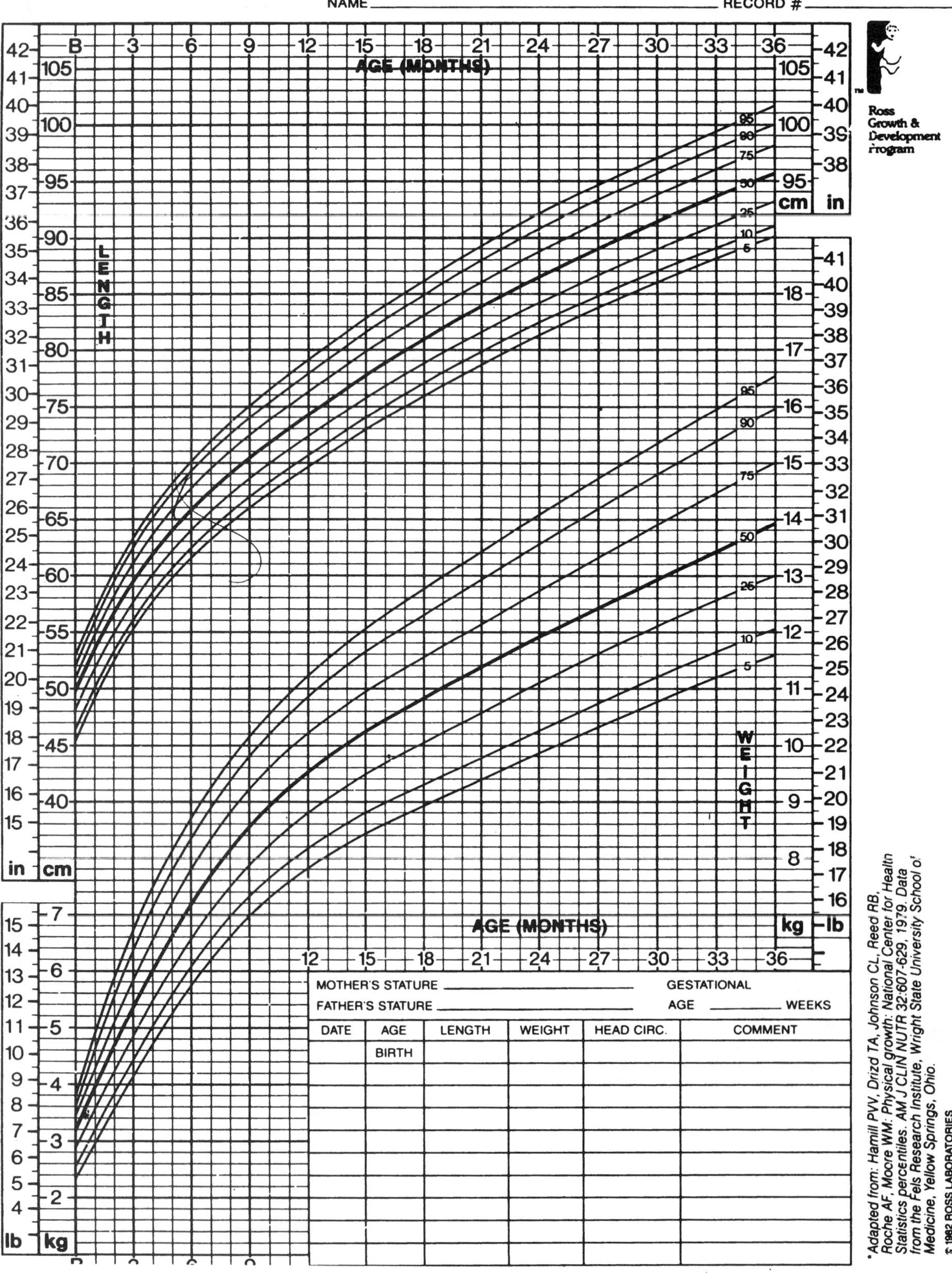

## APPENDIX 12.
## Girls: 2 to 18 Years; Physical Growth NCHS Percentiles*

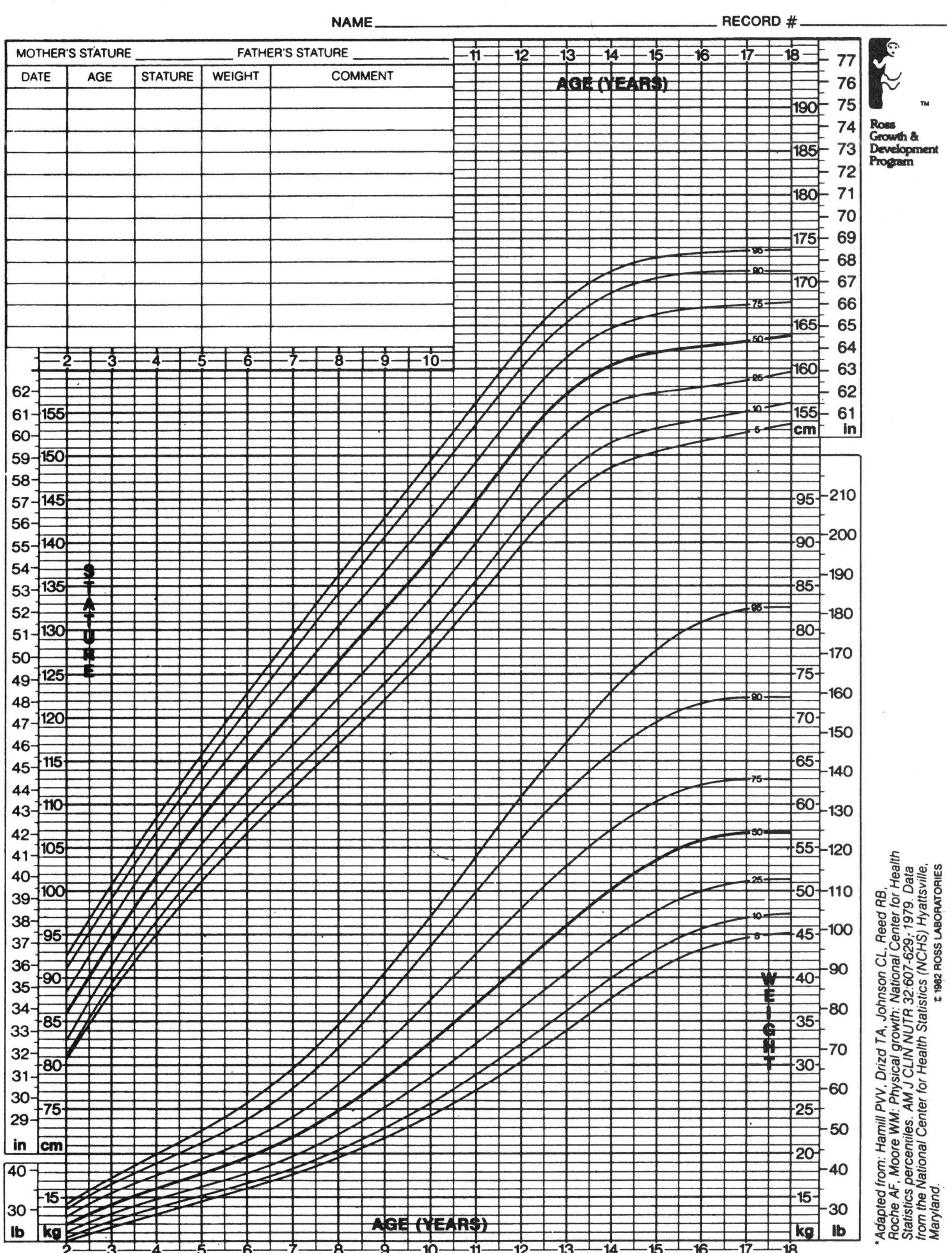


*Adapted from: Hamill PVV, Drizd TA, Johnson CL, Reed RB, Roche AF, Moore WM: Physical growth: National Center for Health Statistics percentiles. AM J CLIN NUTR 32:607-629, 1979. Data from the National Center for Health Statistics (NCHS) Hyattsville, Maryland.

© 1982 ROSS LABORATORIES

## Compostion of Human Colostrum and Mature Breast Milk

| Constituent (per 100 ml) | Colostrum, 1-5 Days | Mature Milk, >30 Days |
|---|---|---|
| Energy (kcal) | 58 | 70 |
| Total solids (g) | 12.8 | 12.0 |
| Lactose (g) | 5.3 | 7.3 |
| Total nitrogen (mg) | 360 | 171 |
| Protein nitrogen (mg) | 313 | 129 |
| Nonprotein nitrogen (mg) | 47 | 42 |
| Total protein (g) | 2.3 | 0.9 |
| Casein (mg) | 140 | 187 |
| α-Lactalbumin (mg) | 218 | 161 |
| Lactoferrin (mg) | 330 | 167 |
| IgA (mg) | 364 | 142 |
| Amino acids (total) | | |
| Alanine (mg) | — | 52 |
| Arginine (mg) | 126 | 49 |
| Aspartate (mg) | — | 110 |
| Cystine (mg) | — | 25 |
| Glutamate (mg) | — | 196 |
| Glycine (mg) | — | 27 |
| Histidine (mg) | 57 | 31 |
| Isoleucine (mg) | 121 | 67 |
| Leucine (mg) | 221 | 110 |
| Lysine (mg) | 163 | 79 |
| Methionine (mg) | 33 | 19 |
| Phenylalanine (mg) | 105 | 44 |
| Proline (mg) | — | 89 |
| Serine (mg) | — | 54 |
| Threonine (mg) | 148 | 58 |
| Tryptophan (mg) | 52 | 25 |
| Tyrosine (mg) | — | 38 |
| Valine (mg) | 169 | 90 |
| Taurine (free) (mg) | — | 8 |
| Urea (mg) | 10 | 30 |
| Creatine (mg) | — | 3.3 |
| Total fat (g) | 2.9 | 4.2 |
| Fatty acids (% total fat) | | |
| 12:0 lauric | 1.8 | 5.8 |
| 14:0 myristic | 3.8 | 8.6 |
| 16:0 palmitic | 26.2 | 21.0 |
| 18:0 stearic | 8.8 | 8.0 |
| 18:1 oleic | 36.6 | 35.5 |
| 18:2, n-6 linoleic | 6.8 | 7.2 |
| 18:3, n-3 linolenic | — | 1.0 |
| $C_{20}$ and $C_{22}$ polyunsaturated | 10.2 | 2.9 |

Casey CE, Hamidge KM: Nutritional aspects of human lactation. In Veveille MC, Neifert MR, editors: Lactation: physiology, nutrition and breast feeding, New York, 1983, Plenum Press.

**Compostion of Human Colostrum and Mature Breast Milk-continued......**

| | | |
|---|---|---|
| Cholesterol (mg) | 27 | 16 |
| Vitamins | | |
| Fat soluble | | |
| Vitamin A (retinol equivalents) (μg) | 89 | 47 |
| β-Carotene (μg) | 112 | 23 |
| Vitamin D (μg) | — | 0.04 |
| Vitamin E (total tocopherols) (μg) | 1280 | 315 |
| Vitamin $K_1$ (μg) | 0.23 | 0.21 |
| Water soluble | | |
| Thiamine (μg) | 15 | 16 |
| Riboflavin (μg) | 25 | 35 |
| Niacin (μg) | 75 | 200 |
| Folic acid (μg) | — | 5.2 |
| Vitamin $B_6$ (μg) | 12 | 28 |
| Biotin (μg) | 0.1 | 0.6 |
| Pantothenic acid (μg) | 183 | 225 |
| Vitamin $B_{12}$ (ng) | 200 | 26 |
| Ascorbic acid (mg) | 4.4 | 4.0 |
| Minerals | | |
| Calcium (mg) | 23 | 28 |
| Magnesium (mg) | 3.4 | 3.0 |
| Sodium (mg) | 48 | 15 |
| Potassium (mg) | 74 | 58 |
| Chlorine (mg) | 91 | 40 |
| Phosphorus (mg) | 14 | 15 |
| Sulphur (mg) | 22 | 14 |
| Trace elements | | |
| Chromium (ng) | — | 39 |
| Cobalt (μg) | — | 1 |
| Copper (μg) | 46 | 35 |
| Fluorine (μg) | — | 7 |
| Iodine (μg) | 12 | 7 |
| Iron (μg) | 45 | 40 |
| Manganese (μg) | — | 0.4,1.5 |
| Nickel (μg) | — | 2 |
| Selenium (μg) | — | 2.0 |
| Zinc (μg) | 540 | 166 |

The above table represents the average composition of breast milk. Certain nutrients in human milk remain relatively stable and are not as affected by the nutritional status of the mom. Other items tend to be quite variable. This variation has left to speculation just what is the optimal composition of breast milk. Studies have revealed that certain fats, namely docosahexenoic acid (DHA), can have profound effects on mental development and visual acuity. In many countries around the world DHA has been added to infant formulas because of this finding. Here in the U.S. the FDA has been slow to endorse such a mandate and manufacturers are certainly not in any hurry to have to change around their formulas. On the next page are some interesting studies revealing the effects of certain dietary changes and how it effects the breast milk in humans.

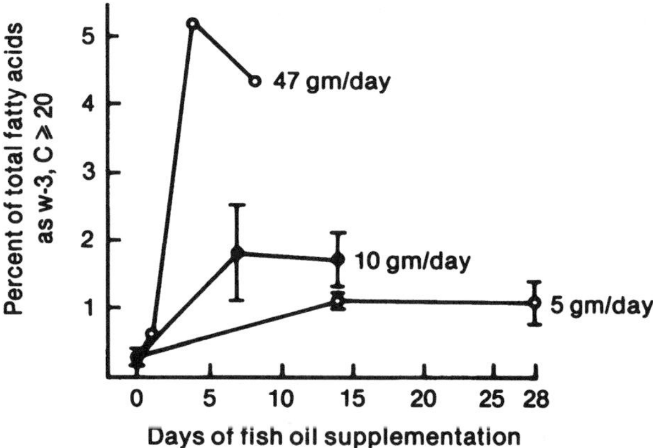


*FIG. 10-7* Effects of various levels of fish oil on levels of ω-3 fatty acids of chain length $C_{20}$ and above in human milk. Respective intake levels are indicated adjacent to the curves.

Modified from Harris WS, Connor WE, Lindsey S: Will dietary ω-3 fatty acid change the composition of human milk? *Am J Clin Nutr* 40:780, 1984.

Mean Breast Milk Fatty Acid Concentration in Vegetarians (Vegans) and Omnivores (Controls)

| Methyl Esters | Vegans* | Controls* |
|---|---|---|
| Lauric ($C_{12:0}$) | 39 | 33 |
| Myristic ($C_{14:0}$) | 68 | 80 |
| Palmitic ($C_{16:0}$) | 166 | 276 |
| Stearic ($C_{18:0}$) | 52 | 108 |
| Palmitoleic ($C_{16:1}$) | 12 | 36 |
| Oleic ($C_{18:1}$) | 313 | 353 |
| Linoleic ($C_{18:2}$) | 317 | 69 |
| Linolenic ($C_{18:3}$) | 15 | 8 |

Modified from Sanders TAB et al: Studies of vegans: the fatty acid composition of plasma cholinephosphoglycerides, erythrocytes, adipose tissue and breast milk and some indicators of susceptibility to ischemic heart disease in vegans and omnivore controls, *Am J Clin Nutr* 31:805, 1978.
*Mean values expressed as milligrams per gram total methyl esters detected for four vegans and four controls (nonvegetarians).

Above are a couple of studies demonstrating how simple dietary changes effect the composition of the breast milk. Since we know that the average diet in the U.S. is probably not optimal, the question remains, how can we improve the quality of the breast milk by supplementation and improving the diet.

Fatty acid Composition of Human milk in 1953 compared to 1977.

| Fatty Acid | 1953* | 1977† |
|---|---|---|
| Lauric ($C_{12:0}$) | 5.5 | 3.8 |
| Myristic ($C_{14:0}$) | 8.5 | 5.2 |
| Palmitic ($C_{16:0}$) | 23.2 | 22.5 |
| Palmitoleic ($C_{16:1}$) | 3.0 | 4.1 |
| Stearic ($C_{18:0}$) | 6.9 | 8.7 |
| Oleic ($C_{18:1}$) | 36.5 | 39.5 |
| Linoleic ($C_{18:2}$) | 7.8 | 14.4 |
| Linolenic ($C_{18:3}$) | — | 2.0 |

*From Macy IG et al: *The composition of milks*, pub no 254, Washington, DC, 1958, National Research Council.
†From Guthrie HA, Picciano MF, and Sheehe D: Fatty acid patterns of human milk, *J Pediatr* 90:39, 1977.

The two studies here show how significantly breast milk has changed, particularly the fatty acids which have many diverse functions in the body producing various hormones and other important compounds.

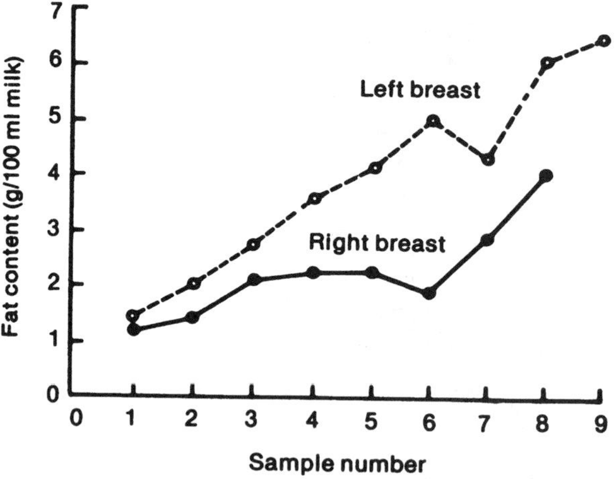


*FIG. 10-5* Variation in fat content of human milk during a single feeding. Data are from successive samples from one woman obtained by breast pump.

From Neville MC, Allen JC, Watters C: *The mechanisms of milk secretion*. In Neville MC and Neifert MR, editors: *Lactation: physiology, nutrition, and breast-feeding*, New York, 1983, Plenum Press.

The above study was something that was not expected. It seems that the milk composition from breast to breast changes very significantly and that milk production in each breast is independant of the other.

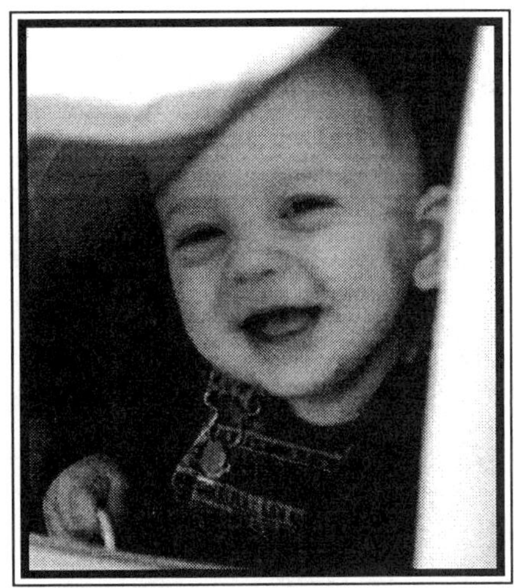

***A Happy Breast Fed Kid!***
***Emil Tristan Marz***

# TABOR HILL CLINIC

*Dr. Russell B. Marz, Naturopathic Physician*

## T3 Tracking Report

***DIRECTIONS:*** *Take one capsule in the AM and one in the PM for TWO DAYS beginning with 7.5 mcg and* ***ascending*** *to 52.5 mcg. Beginning with 60.0 mcg and* ***descending*** *to 7.5 mcg, take one capsule in the AM and one in the PM for THREE DAYS.* ***To aid in keeping on schedule, write in dates and days of week before you start the regime. Cross out AM's and PM's as you progress.***

| Date | Day | Dose | Time | Temp |
|---|---|---|---|---|
| | | 7.5 mcg | AM PM | |
| | | | AM PM | |
| | | 15.0 mcg | AM PM | |
| | | | AM PM | |
| | | 22.5 mcg | AM PM | |
| | | | AM PM | |
| | | 30.0 mcg | AM PM | |
| | | | AM PM | |
| | | 37.5 mcg | AM PM | |
| | | | AM PM | |
| | | 45.0 mcg | AM PM | |
| | | | AM PM | |
| | | 52.5 mcg | AM PM | |
| | | | AM PM | |
| | | 60.0 mcg | AM PM | |
| | | | AM PM | |
| | | | AM PM | |
| | | 52.5 mcg | AM PM | |
| | | | AM PM | |
| | | | AM PM | |

| Date | Day | Dose | Time | Temp |
|---|---|---|---|---|
| | | 45.0 mcg | AM PM | |
| | | | AM PM | |
| | | | AM PM | |
| | | 37.5 mcg | AM PM | |
| | | | AM PM | |
| | | | AM PM | |
| | | 30.0 mcg | AM PM | |
| | | | AM PM | |
| | | | AM PM | |
| | | 22.5 mcg | AM PM | |
| | | | AM PM | |
| | | | AM PM | |
| | | 15.0 mcg | AM PM | |
| | | | AM PM | |
| | | | AM PM | |
| | | 7.5 mcg | AM PM | |
| | | | AM PM | |
| | | | AM PM | |

*NOTES:* Temperature: Axillary ☐

Basal ☐

Take temperature at: ________a.m. ________ p.m.

*This medication must be taken EXACTLY as prescribed. If you have any questions please call us at (503) 233-0585 before beginning the regime.*

© TABOR HILL CLINIC

## Basal Body Temperatures

Days of Cycle →

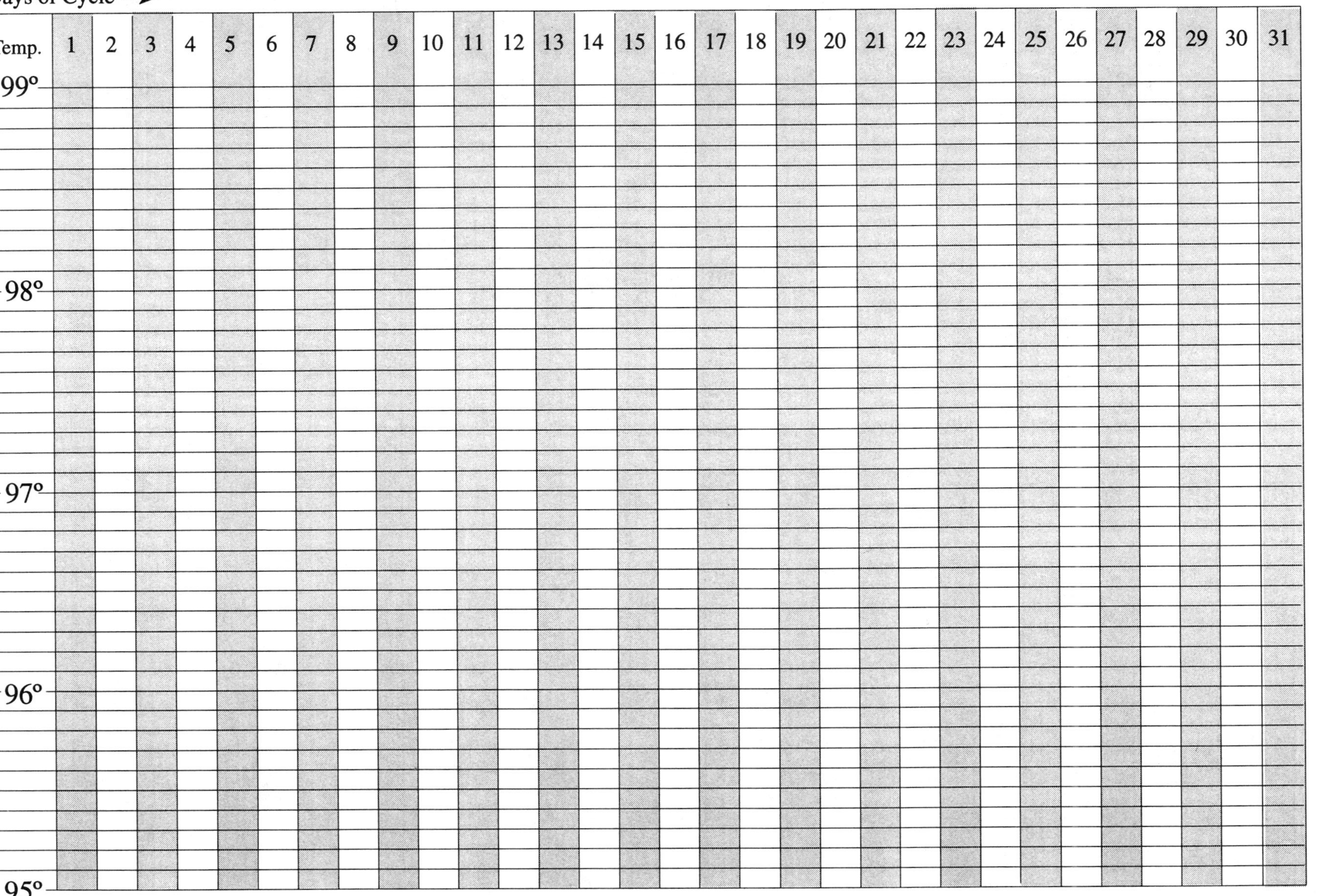

# RECOMMENDED DIETARY ALLOWANCES 1989

| Category | Age (years) or Condition | Weight[b] (kg) | Weight[b] (lb) | Height[b] (cm) | Height[b] (in) | Protein (g) | Fat Soluble Vitamins: Vitamin A (μg RE)[c] | Vitamin D (μg)[d] | Vitamin E (mg α-TE)[e] | Vitamin K (μg) |
|---|---|---|---|---|---|---|---|---|---|---|
| Infants | 0.0–0.5 | 6 | 13 | 60 | 24 | 13 | 375 | 7.5 | 3 | 5 |
| | 0.5–1.0 | 9 | 20 | 71 | 28 | 14 | 375 | 10 | 4 | 10 |
| Children | 1–3 | 13 | 29 | 90 | 35 | 16 | 400 | 10 | 6 | 15 |
| | 4–6 | 20 | 44 | 112 | 44 | 24 | 500 | 10 | 7 | 20 |
| | 7–10 | 28 | 62 | 132 | 52 | 28 | 700 | 10 | 7 | 30 |
| Males | 11–14 | 45 | 99 | 157 | 62 | 45 | 1,000 | 10 | 10 | 45 |
| | 15–18 | 66 | 145 | 176 | 69 | 59 | 1,000 | 10 | 10 | 65 |
| | 19–24 | 72 | 160 | 177 | 70 | 58 | 1,000 | 10 | 10 | 70 |
| | 25–50 | 79 | 174 | 176 | 70 | 63 | 1,000 | 5 | 10 | 80 |
| | 51+ | 77 | 170 | 173 | 68 | 63 | 1,000 | 5 | 10 | 80 |
| Females | 11–14 | 46 | 101 | 157 | 62 | 46 | 800 | 10 | 8 | 45 |
| | 15–18 | 55 | 120 | 163 | 64 | 44 | 800 | 10 | 8 | 55 |
| | 19–24 | 58 | 128 | 164 | 65 | 46 | 800 | 10 | 8 | 60 |
| | 25–50 | 63 | 138 | 163 | 64 | 50 | 800 | 5 | 8 | 65 |
| | 51+ | 65 | 143 | 160 | 63 | 50 | 800 | 5 | 8 | 65 |
| Pregnant | | | | | | 60 | 800 | 10 | 10 | 65 |
| Lactating | 1st 6 months | | | | | 65 | 1,300 | 10 | 12 | 65 |
| | 2nd 6 months | | | | | 62 | 1,200 | 10 | 11 | 65 |

| Age (years) or Condition | Vitamin C (mg) | Thiamin (mg) | Ribo-flavin (mg) | Niacin (mg NE)[f] | Vitamin $B_6$ (mg) | Folate (μg) | Vitamin $B_{12}$ (μg) | Calcium (mg) | Phos-phorus (mg) | Mag-nesium (mg) | Iron (mg) | Zinc (mg) | Iodine (μg) | Sele-nium (μg) |
|---|---|---|---|---|---|---|---|---|---|---|---|---|---|---|
| 0.0–0.5 | 30 | 0.3 | 0.4 | 5 | 0.3 | 25 | 0.3 | 400 | 300 | 40 | 6 | 5 | 40 | 10 |
| 0.5–1.0 | 35 | 0.4 | 0.5 | 6 | 0.6 | 35 | 0.5 | 600 | 500 | 60 | 10 | 5 | 50 | 15 |
| 1–3 | 40 | 0.7 | 0.8 | 9 | 1.0 | 50 | 0.7 | 800 | 800 | 80 | 10 | 10 | 70 | 20 |
| 4–6 | 45 | 0.9 | 1.1 | 12 | 1.1 | 75 | 1.0 | 800 | 800 | 120 | 10 | 10 | 90 | 20 |
| 7–10 | 45 | 1.0 | 1.2 | 13 | 1.4 | 100 | 1.4 | 800 | 800 | 170 | 10 | 10 | 120 | 30 |
| 11–14[g] | 50 | 1.3 | 1.5 | 17 | 1.7 | 150 | 2.0 | 1,200 | 1,200 | 270 | 12 | 15 | 150 | 40 |
| 15–18[g] | 60 | 1.5 | 1.8 | 20 | 2.0 | 200 | 2.0 | 1,200 | 1,200 | 400 | 12 | 15 | 150 | 50 |
| 19–24[g] | 60 | 1.5 | 1.7 | 19 | 2.0 | 200 | 2.0 | 1,200 | 1,200 | 350 | 10 | 15 | 150 | 70 |
| 25–50[g] | 60 | 1.5 | 1.7 | 19 | 2.0 | 200 | 2.0 | 800 | 800 | 350 | 10 | 15 | 150 | 70 |
| 51+ | 60 | 1.2 | 1.4 | 15 | 2.0 | 200 | 2.0 | 800 | 800 | 350 | 10 | 15 | 150 | 70 |
| 11–14[h] | 50 | 1.1 | 1.3 | 15 | 1.4 | 150 | 2.0 | 1,200 | 1,200 | 280 | 15 | 12 | 150 | 45 |
| 15–18[h] | ·60 | 1.1 | 1.3 | 15 | 1.5 | 180 | 2.0 | 1,200 | 1,200 | 300 | 15 | 12 | 150 | 50 |
| 19–24[h] | 60 | 1.1 | 1.3 | 15 | 1.6 | 180 | 2.0 | 1,200 | 1,200 | 280 | 15 | 12 | 150 | 55 |
| 25–50[h] | 60 | 1.1 | 1.3 | 15 | 1.6 | 180 | 2.0 | 800 | 800 | 280 | 15 | 12 | 150 | 55 |
| 51+[†] | 60 | 1.0 | 1.2 | 13 | 1.6 | 180 | 2.0 | 800 | 800 | 280 | 10 | 12 | 150 | 55 |
| Pregnant | 70 | 1.5 | 1.6 | 17 | 2.2 | 400 | 2.2 | 1,200 | 1,200 | 320 | 30 | 15 | 175 | 65 |
| Lactating[i] | 95 | 1.6 | 1.8 | 20 | 2.1 | 280 | 2.6 | 1,200 | 1,200 | 355 | 15 | 19 | 200 | 75 |
| Lactating[j] | 90 | 1.6 | 1.7 | 20 | 2.1 | 260 | 2.6 | 1,200 | 1,200 | 340 | 15 | 16 | 200 | 75 |

b Weights and heights of Reference Adults are actual medians for the U.S. population of the designated age, as reported by NHANES II. The median weights and heights of those under 19 years of age were taken from Hamill et al. (1979) The use of these figures does not imply that the height to weights ratios are ideal.

c Retinol equivalents. 1 retinol equivalent = 1 μg retinol or 6 μg β-carotene (See chapter on vitamin A for further calculations).

d As cholecalciferol. 10 μg cholecalciferol = 400iu of vitamin D.

e alpha tocopherol equivalents. 1 mg d-alpha tocopherol = 1 alpha-TE. (See under vitamin E for further discussion and clarification).

**Source: Recommended Dietary Allowances 10th ed, 1989 by the National Academy of Sciences , National Academy Press, Washington, DC.**

# Cholesterol metabolism

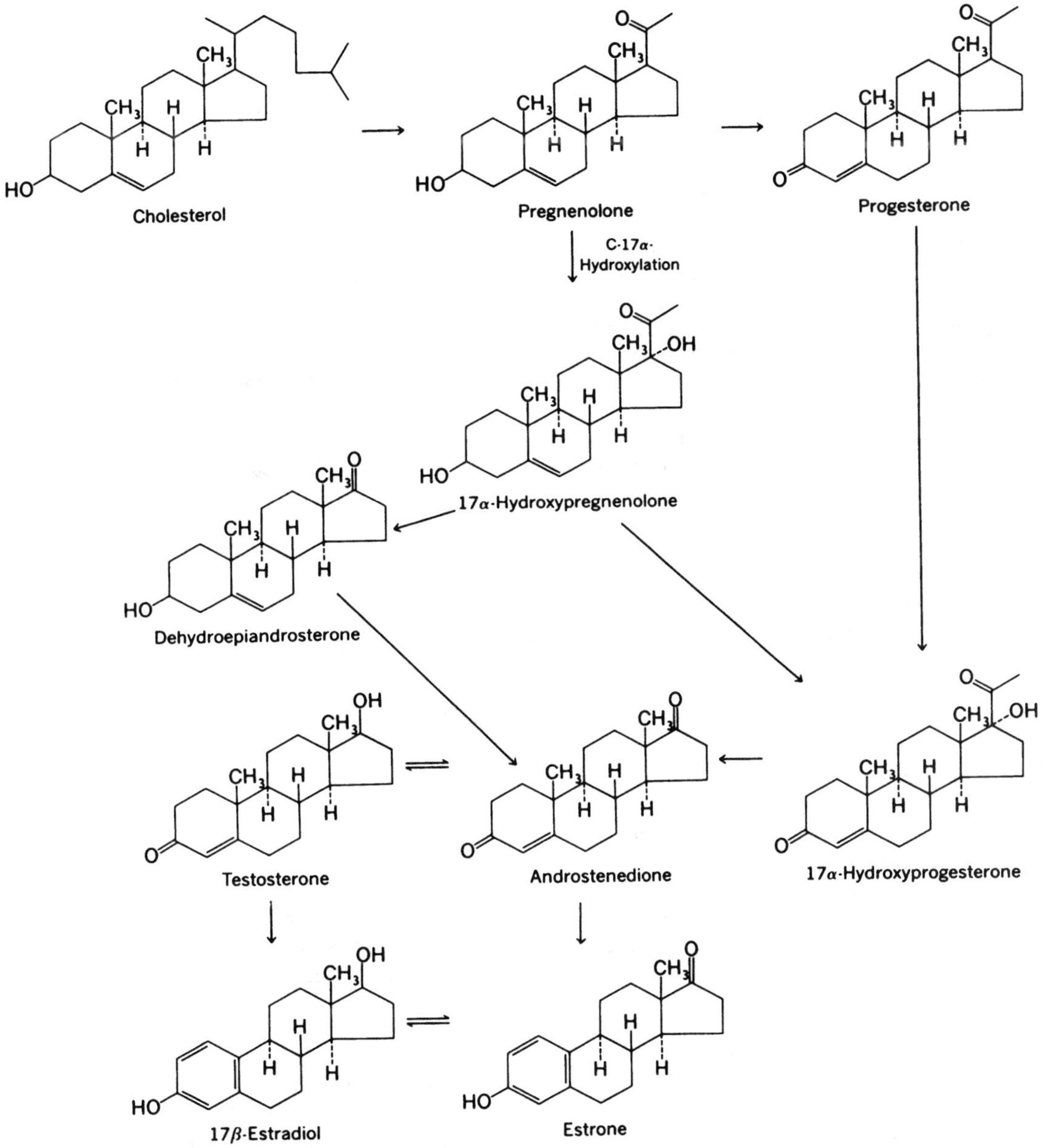

Cholesterol → Pregnenolone → Progesterone

Pregnenolone → (C-17α-Hydroxylation) → 17α-Hydroxypregnenolone

17α-Hydroxypregnenolone → Dehydroepiandrosterone

17α-Hydroxypregnenolone → 17α-Hydroxyprogesterone

Progesterone → 17α-Hydroxyprogesterone

Dehydroepiandrosterone → Androstenedione

17α-Hydroxyprogesterone → Androstenedione

Testosterone ⇌ Androstenedione

Testosterone → 17β-Estradiol

Androstenedione → Estrone

17β-Estradiol ⇌ Estrone

Note–It is important to note that there are different pathways for the cholesterol metabolites such as dehydroepiandrosterone (DHEA) and pregnenolone. Where pregnenolone gets converted into progesterone and 17 alpha hydroxyprogesterone, DHEA being further down the metabolic pathway, gets converted into androstenedione. This in turn gets converted into testosterone and estrone.

# BIBLIOGRAPHY

*Adler, Kief, Beyond the Staff of Life* (The wheat less dairyless cookbook), 1984.
Airola, Paavo., *How To Get Well*, Health Publishers, Pheonix, AR. 1974.
Anagnostides, Hodgson & Kirsner, *Inflammatory Bowel Disease* Chapman & Hall Medical, Van Nostrand Reinhold, N.Y., N.Y. 10003, 1991.
Bach and Bach *Prescription for Nutritional Healing* Avery Pub., N.Y., 1990.
Bailey, Covert., *The Fit-Or-Fat Target Diet*, Houghton Miffin, Boston, MA. 1984.
Ballentine, Rudolph., *Diet and Nutrition*, Himalayan International, Honesdale, PA. 1978.
Barnes, Broda and Galton, Lawrence., *Hypothroidism, The Unsuspected Illness*, Harper and Row, New York, N.Y. 1976.York, N.Y. 1986
Bastyr, John., *Notes of Natural Therapeutics*, 1977.
Bates, Charles, *Essential Fatty Acids, Immunity and Mental Health*, 1986.
Beasley, Joseph, The Kellogg Report
Berdanier, *Advanced Nutrition: Macronutrients*, CRC Press , 1995
Berkow, Robert and Fletcher, Andrew., *The Merck Manuel*, Merck Sharp and Dome, Rahway, N.J. 1987
Bland, Jeffrey., *Medical Applications of Clinical Nutrition*, Keats, New
Bland, Jeffrey., *Nutraerobics*, Harper and Row, San Francisco, CA. 1983.
Bland, Jeffrey., *Your Health Under Siege*, Stephen Greene Press; Brattleboro, VT. 1981.
Blaylock, Russell L. *Excitotoxins: The Taste That Kills*, Health Press, Santa Fe, NM 1992
Bove M. *An Encyclopedia of Natural Healing for Children & Infants*, 1996.
Boyle, Wade The Herb Doctors, Buckeye Press, 1988
Braverman, Eric & Pfeiffer, Carl., The Healing Nutrients Within, Keats Pub, New Canaan, CT.1987
Breneman, James C., *Basics Of Food Allergy*, Thomas, Springfield,IL. 1984.
Brewer T, Metabolic Toxemia of Late Pregnancy 1982.
Brinker *Toxicology of Common Botanicals*, .
Buist Robert *Food and Chemical Sensitivity* ,1988.
Buist, William *Food intolerance* 1984
Burton Golderg Group, Strohecker, James*Alternative Medicine* Future Medicine Publish Inc., Puyallup, WA 1994
Cameron, Ewan and Pauling, Linus., *Cancer And Vitamin C*, Norton & Co
Castleman *The Healing Herbs*
Cataldo, DeBruyne & Whitney *Nutrition and Diet Therapy* West Pub., St. Paul MN 1995.
Chaitow *Candida Albicans*
Charles, J , *Neurobiology of Down Syndrome*
Coca, Arthur., *The Pulse Test*, Arc Books, New York, NY. 1977.
Cohn R and Roth K, *Biochemistry and Disease Bridging Basic Science and Clinical Practice'* Williams and Wilkins A Waverly Comp, 1996.
Consumer and Food Economics Institute, Washington, D.C. 1978.
Crook, William G., *The Yeast Connection*, Professional Books, Jackson, TN. 1984.
Crook, Wlliam, *Chronic Fatigue Syndrome and the Yeast Conncetion* Professional Books, 1992
D'Adamo James *One Man's Food is someone else's Poison*, Richard Marek Pub., 1980
D'Adamo, James *The D'Adamo Diet* 1992.
D'Adamo, Peter *Eat Right 4 Your Type*, Putnam, N.Y. 1996
Dadd, Debra Lynn *The None Toxic Home and Office* Putnam, N.Y. 1992 & *Nontoxic, Natural & Earthwise* 1990
Dickey, Laurence, editor.*Clinical Ecology* Charles C. Thomas Pub., Springfield Ill., 1976.
DiPalma, Joseph., *Basic Pharmacology In Medicine*, McGraw-Hill, New York, N. Y. 1976
Doyle, P.Rodger and Redding, James.,*The Complete Food Handbook*, Grove Press, New York, N.Y,1976.
Eaton SB, Shostak M, and Konner M *Paleolithic Prescription* Harper & Row Pub., N.Y. 1988.
Ellis, John and Presley, James., *Vitamin B-6 The Doctor's Report*, Harper and Row; San francisco, CA, 1973
Erasmus Fats that Heal Fats that Kill
Feingold, Ben F., *Why Your Child Is Hyperactive*, Random House, New York, N.Y. 1975.
Foye, *Principles of Medicinal Chemistry* 3rd ed., Lea & Febiger Philadephia, 1989
Gaby A & Wright J, *Nutritional Therapy in Medical Practice* Wright Gaby Seminars 1996, (206)854-4900 ext 166
Gaby Alan *Preventing and Reversing Osteoporosis*, Prima, 1994..
Gerber, Jim. *Handbook of Preventive & Therapeutic Nutrition* Aspen Pub. Mayland, 1993.
Germano C & Cabot *The Osteoporosis Solution* Kensington Books, 1999.
Gislason *Nutritional Therapy* , 1992.
Gittnick Current *Gastroenterology Vol 12* Mosby Year Book, St. Louis, MO 1992
Golos, Natalie., *Coping With Your Allergies*, Simon and Schuster, New
Goodhart & Young Nutrition in Health and Disease , 1993.
Goodhart, Robert and Shils, Maurice., *Modern Nutrition In Health and Disease*, Lea and Febiger, Phil, PA. 1980.
Gottlieb, Lowe, Bricklin, Zarrow, *The Complete Book of Vitmains*, Rodale, 1984.
Guthrie, Helen A., *Introductory Nutrition*, Times Mirror/Mosby, Saint Louis, MI. 1986.

Goodhart, Robert and Shils, Maurice., *Modern Nutrition In Health and Disease*, Lea and Febiger, Phil, PA. 1980.
Gottlieb, Lowe, Bricklin, Zarrow, *The Complete Book of Vitmains,* Rodale, 1984.
Guthrie, Helen A., *Introductory Nutrition*, Times Mirror/Mosby, Saint Louis, MI. 1986.
Haas, Elson *Staying Healthy with Nutrition*
Hamaker, Donald., *The Survival Of Civilization*, Hanmaker-Weaver, Michigan, 1982.
Hamilton, Kirk., *Clinical Pearls*, Joan Howell, Sacramento, C.A. 1991.
Hilda Cherry Hills *Good Food, Gluten Free* Keats, New Canaan, CT. 1983
Hilda Cherry Hills *Good Food, Milk Free, Grain Free, Gluten Free* Keats, New Canaan, CT. 1980
Hills, Christopher *The Secrets of Spirulina*, University of the Trees Press, Donally & Sons,1980.
Hobbs, Chris Medicinal Mushrooms An Exploration o Tradition, Healing & Culture, 1995.
Hoffman, Ronald, *Seven Weeks To A Settled Stomach*, Simon and Schuster, New York, NY 1990.
Holford P *Nutrition and Mental Illness*, UK 1997.
Howard, Rosanne and Herbold, Nancie Harvey., *Nutrition in Clinical Care*, McGraw-Hill, New York, N.Y. 1978.
Huggins, Hal and S.A.., *It's All In Your Head,* Colorado Springs, CO. 1985.
Hunt & Groeff *Advanced Nutrition & Human Metabolism* 1995
Hunt, Groeff Advanced Nutrition & Human Metabolism 2nd ed.
Jacobson, Michael F., *Eater's Digest- The Consumer's Factbook of Food*
Jeffries W *Safe Uses of Cortisone* 1981
Johnson, L 4th ed.,Mosby Year Book, 1985
Kronhausen & Demopolis *Formula for Life The Definitive Book on Correct Nutrition,, Antioxidants, and Vitamins, Disease Prevention, and Longevity* William Morrow & Comp., N.Y. 1989.
Kunin, A. Richard., *Mega-Nutrition,* McGraw Hill, New York, N.Y. 1981.
Kushi, Michio *Natural Healing thru Macrobiotics*,
Kushi, Michio., *Natural Healing through Macrobiotics*, Japan Publications, Tokyo, Japan. 1978.
Levine, Stephen and Kidd, Parris., *Antioxidant Adaptation; Its role in free Radical Pathology*, Biocurrents Division, San Leandro, CA. 1985
Linder Maria Nutritional Biochemistry and Metabolism with Clinical Applications .3rd Lin Press,
MacDougal The McDougal Plan
Mahan, Kathleen, Estcott-Stump, *Krause's Food, Nutrition, & Diet Therapy*, W.B. Saunders, Montreal, CA.1996.
Mandell, *Dr. Mandell's Lifetime Arthritis Relief System*
Mandell, Marshall & Scanlon, et al., *Marshall' Mandell's 5-Day Allergy Relief System*, Nutri-Books, Denver, CO 1979.
Mannerberg *Aerobic Nutrition 1983.*
Markell, Edward; Voge, Marietta; John, David.,*Medical Parasitology,* W.B. Saunders, Philadelphia, PA. 1992
Marz, Russell *Medical Nutrition from Marz* 2nd ed. 3rd printing Omni-Press, Portland, OR 1997-99.
Marz, Russell Medical Nutrition from Marz 2nd edition 'Omni-Press, Portland, OR 1997
Mathews & Van Holde *Biochemistry*
Matsen, John., *Eating Alive*, Crompton Books, Vancouver, B.C., CA. 1987.
Miller, Saul *Food for Thought*
Miller, Saul., *Food For Thought,* Prentice-Hall, Englewood Cliffs, N.J. 1979.
Moore R. *The High Blood Pressure Solution: Natural Prevention and Cure with the K factor.* Healing Arts P1993
Murray & Werbach *Botanical Influences on Illness* Third Line Press, 1994.
Murray *Healing Power of Foods* Prima, Rocklin, CA. 1993
Murray *Healing Power of Herbs* Prima, Rocklin, CA. 1991
Murray, Granner, Mayes, Rodwell, *Harper's Biochemistry* Appleton & Lange , 1993.
Murray, Michael and Pizzorno, Joseph., *Encyclopedia of Natural Medicine*, Prima, Rocklin, CA. 1991
Murray, Michael and Pizzorno, Joseph., *Textbook of Natural Medicine*, Portland. 1984
Murray, Michael *Encyclopedia of Nutritional Supplements* Prima, Rocklin, CA. 1996
National Research Council., *Diet And Health*, National Academy Press; Washington, D.C. 1989.
Newbold, H.L., *Mega-Nutrients For Your Health*, Berkeley Publishing Co., New York, N.Y. 1978
Ornish, Dean *Dr.Dean Orninsh's Program for Reversing Heart Disease* Ballentine, N.Y., 1990.
Percival Mark *Infant Nutrition*; Dynamic Essentials, Canada, 1991.
Pfeiffer, Carl., *Mental And Elemental Nutrients*, Keats, New Canaan, CT. 1975.
Pfeiffer, Carl., *Zinc and other Micro-Nutrients,* Keats, New Canaan, CT,1978.
Philpott Brain *Allergies The Psychonutrient Connection* , M.D.
Philpott, William and Kalita, Dwight., *Brain Allergies*, Keats, New Canaan, CT. 1980
Philpott, William H., *Victory Over Diabetes*, Keats, New Canaan, CT. 1983.
Pipes, peggy & Trahms, Cristine, *Nutrition in Infancy & Childhood* 5th ed.Mosby, 1993.

## Bibliography continued

Pizzorno, Joseph E. and Murray, Michael T., *A Textbook Of Natural Medicine*, Volume 2, John Bastyr Publications, Seattle, WA. 1987
Pottenger, Francis M., *Pottenger's Cats, A Study in Nutrition*, Price-Pottenger Nutrition La Mesa, CA. 1983.
Powers M *Handbook of Diabetes Medical Nutrition Therapy* M.Aspen, 1996
Prevention Magazine editors, *The Complete Book of Vitamins*, Rodale,Emmaus, PA. 1984.
Prevention Magazine editors., *Understanding Vitamins and Minerals*, Rodale Press, Emmaus, PA. 1984.
Price, Weston., *Nutrition And Physical Degeneration*, Price-Pottenger Nutrition Foundation, La Mesa, CA. 1979
Pritikin Nathan, The Pritikin Program for Diet & Exercise, 1977.
Quillin, Patrick, Healing Nutrients Vintage Books, New York 1987
Quillin, Patrick, Nutrition and Cancer
Randolph & Moss *An Alternative Approach to Allergies*, 1979.
Rapp *Impossible Child, The*
Rapp, Doris J Allergies and the HyperActive Child; Fireside Simon & Schuster, Inc. N.Y.,1979
Reading & Meillor *Your Family Tree Connection;* Keats, New Canaan, CT 1984 Reprinted in U.S. 1988
Rinkel, Randolph & Zeller, *Food Allergy*, Charles C Thomas Pub Springfield Ill USA, 1951.
Robbins *Diet for a New America*
Robertson, Laurel; Flinders, Carol; Godfrey, Bronwen., *Laurel's Kitchen,* Nilgiri Press, Petaluma, CA. 1976.
Rockwell *Sally Rockwell's Allergy Recipes*
Rogers, Sherry, *Chemical Sensitivity & E.I. Syndrome Revised.*Prestige Pub., 1992
Rogers, Sherry, *Scientific Basis for SelectedEnvironmental Medicine Techniques* Prestige Pub., 1990.
Rogers, Sherry, *Tired or Toxic: A Blue print For Health Prestige Pub.*, 1990.
Rogers, Sherry, *Wellness Against All Odds* Prestige Pub., 1994.
Rosenberg, Harold and Feldzamen, A.Z., *The Doctor's Book of Vitamin*
Rousseau/ Rea *Your Home, Your Health, & Well Being* Hartly & Marks Pub.; Vancouver Canada, 1989.
Rudin D *Omega 3 Fatty Acids*, 1996
Salloum Fasting Signs and Symptoms , N.D.
Schauss A & Costin C *Zinc and Eating Disorders,* Self Care Health Library Keats Pub, New Canaan, CT.1989.
Schauss, Alexander., *Diet, Crime and Delinquency*, Parker House, Berkeley,CA. 1981.
Schmid, Ron *Native Nutrition; Eating According to Ancestral Wisdom*, 1987.
Seaman, Barbara and Gideon., *Women and the Crisis in Sex Hormones*, Bantam, New York, N.Y. 1977
Sherman Complete Botanical Prescribe /Botanical Medicine ,
Simopoulos, A. Omega Plan, The Harper & Collins, 1998
Smith, Lendon., *Feed Your Kids Right,* Dell, New York, N.Y. 1970.
Soyka, Fred., *The Ion Effect,* Bantam, New York, N.Y. 1977.
Stone,Irwin., *The Healing Factor; Vitamin C Against Disease* Grosset and Dunlap, New York, NY. 1972.
*Super Foods Quinoa, amaranth, Teff, Kamut*
Thom *Surviving the 90's Coping with Food Allergies*; 1993
Thomas, Clayton L., editor., *Taber's Cyclopedic Medical Dictionary*, F.A. Davis Co., Philadelphis, PA. 1970.
Thrash *Food Allergies made Simple*
Trowbridge, John and Walker, Morton., *The Yeast Syndrome*, Bantam, NewQuQ York, NY. 1986.
United States Department of Agriculture Handbook No. 8-4., Fats and Oils
Warmbrand, Max., *Overcoming Arthritis & Other Rheumatic Diseases,*
Weiner, Micheal *Maximum Immunity* Houghton, Mifflin Comp.
Werbach, Melvyn R., *Nutritional Influences on Illness,* Third Line Press, Tarzana,CA. 1988.
Werback B*otanical Influences on Illness*, Werbach & Murray
Werback *Nutritional Influences on Mental Illness*, Third Line Press, 1991.
Whitaker, Julian, *Reversing Heart Disease* Warner Books, N.Y., 1985.
Willard *Advanced Herbology*
Williams, David Health Secrets You Were Never Supposed to Have-Special Report
Williams, R & Kalita, Dwight. ed. *A Physician's Handbook on Orthomolecular Medicine*, Keats, New Canaan, CT 1977.
Williams, Roger J., *Nutrition Against Disease,* Bantam, New York, NY. 1971.
Williams, Sue Rodwell., *Nutrition and Diet Therapy,* Saint Louis, MI. 1977.
Willis, AL CRC Handbook of Eicosanoids: Prostaglandins and Related Lipids, 1989
Wilson, Denis, *Wilson Syndrome,* Cornerson Pub.; Orlando, Florida, 1991.
Wood R *Quinoa the Super Grain* 1988.
Worthington-Roberts, B and Williams, Sue R, *Nutrition in Pregnancy & Lactation* 5th ed.Mosby, 1993.
Yudkin, J. *The French Paradox*, 1997.

# Index

## A

## D

## E

## G

## H

# I

## J

# M

## N

## O

## P

# T

## U



## V

## W



X



## Y

## Z

# LABCORP

## STATE OF THE ART EVALUATION FOR CARDIOVASCULAR HEALTH

It is clear to ideally evaluate cardiovascular health one must know not just total cholesterol levels but rather the amounts and ratios of the different forms of cholesterol. This would include the different forms of cholesterol such as HDL cholesterol (high density lipoprotein) and LDL cholesterol (low density lipoprotein). In people over 50 the single most powerful predictor of coronary heart disease is HDL cholesterol.

William P. Castelli, M.D.
Director Framingham Heart Study
Lecturer Depart of Preventive Medicine
Harvard Medical School in Current Rx
June 1977

## CHOLESTEROL AND LIPOPROTEINS

In patients with premature coronary artery disease, serum levels of low-density lipoprotein cholesterol (LDL) are generally higher than normal, whereas serum levels of high-density lipoprotein cholesterol(HDL) are generally lower than normal. LDL is considered to be atherogenic (causing fatty plaques to develop inside arteries), by carrying cholesterol from the liver out into the walls of your arteries. **HDL cholesterol is thought to protect against atherosclerosis by removing cholesterol from the artery walls and transporting this cholesterol to the liver to be removed from the body.**

Epidemiologic data shows that there is a strong relationship between lower levels of HDL cholesterol and an increased risk of heart disease. Data has also shown that higher levels of HDL cholesterol have been found to be protective against atheroslerosis and have been strongly associated with longevity.

## INTERPRETATION OF HDL RESULTS

| serum HDL cholesterol (mg/ dl) | RISK OF CORONARY HEART DISEASE |
|---|---|
| 25 OR LESS | Risk at dangerous level, needs prompt attention with diet, supplements and exercise |
| 26-35 | High risk; diet & appropriate supplements and exercise needed |
| 36-44 | moderate risk diet intervention and moderate supplementation |
| 45-59 | Average risk (in the U.S. this is not a good risk) diet changes and moderate exercise indicated. |
| 60-74 | Below average risk; mild dietary changes along with mild exercise indicated depending upon family history. |
| above 75 | Protection probable associated with longevity |

**NOTE**- Ideally on your blood chemistry you should have a ratio of cholesterol to HDL of 3 to 1 or lower. This means for example if your cholesterol is 180 your HDL should be 60 or higher.

### Cardiovascular Disease Risk factors and what you can do about them.

If you have a history of heart disease, stroke, diabetes, or other cardiovascular disease related condition in your family you may want to consider a more thorough and complete evaluation by your health care provider. On the back of this handout is a guide-line to the ultimate diagnostic evaluation of your cardiovascular system. Your family history of cardiovascular disease, your age, your diet and level of exercise will determine how extensive your testing should be.

## Evaluating your cardiovascular risk factors; How to thoroughly assess your risks:

–If you have had one or more relatives ( sister, brother, parent, grandparent, uncle, aunt or other blood relative) that died of a heart attack, had a heart attack, had coronary bypass surgery or was diagnosed with diabetes before the age of 70 you should be aware of the following tests to evaluate your condition more thoroughly.

**1) Basic blood chemistry including cholesterol, HDL, LDL, TG's, ferritin and fasting glucose. If fasting blood glucose on 2 or more occasions is above 100 mg/dl then a glucose insulin tolerance test is strongly advised especially if there is any history of diabetes in family**.

–If you have 2 or more relatives (sister, brother, parent, grandparent, uncle or other blood relative) that died of a heart attack, had a heart attack, had coronary bypass surgery or was diagnosed with diabetes before the age of 70 you should have:

**2) Apolipoproteins A & B along with Lipoprotein A added to #1.**

–If one family member (sister, brother, parent, grandparent, uncle, aunt or other blood relative) died of a heart attack, had a heart attack or had coronary bypass surgery before the age of 60 you should consider the following tests to evaluate this condition more thoroughly: Also have a stress EKG done.

**3) Apolipoproteins A & B and Homocysteine added to #1 (When premature coronary heart disease is found in a family there is a good chance that they have elevated levels of homocysteine in the blood. This is a simple test that if abnormal can easily be corrected through nutrition & vitamin intervention).**

–If two or more family members (sister, brother, parent, grandparent, uncle, aunt or other blood relative) died of a heart attack, had coronary bypass surgery or was diagnosed with diabetes before the age of 60 you should consider the following tests to evaluate your condition more thoroughly: Also have a stress EKG done.

**4) Apolipoproteins A & B, lipoprotein A and Homocysteine added to #1.**

–If one family member (sister, brother, parent, grandparent, uncle, aunt or other blood relative) died of a heart attack, had a heart attack, had coronary bypass surgery or was diagnosed with diabetes before the age of 50 your should consider the following tests to evaluate your condition more thoroughly: Also have a stress EKG done.

**5)** Apolipoproteins A & B and Homocysteine and Ionic magnesium levels added to #1. ***(Most people who have early age angina or heart attacks have low tissue levels of magnesium).***

–If two or more family members (sister, brother, parent, grandparent, uncle or other blood relative) died of a heart attack, had a heart attack, had coronary bypass surgery or was diagnosed with diabetes before the age of 50 you should consider the following tests to evaluate your condition more thoroughly: Also have a stress EKG done.

**6)** ***Apolipoproteins A & B, Homocysteine and Ionic magnesium levels added to #1.***

–If one or more family members (sister, brother, parent, grandparent, uncle, aunt or other blood relative) died of a heart attack, had a heart attack, had coronary bypass surgery or was diagnosed with diabetes before the age of 40 you should consider the following tests to evaluate your condition most thoroughly: Also have a stress EKG done.

**7) Apolipoproteins A & B, Homocysteine and Ionic magnesium levels added to #1 along with a hair analysis for heavy metals especially cadmium and lead which could damage blood vessels. In addition platelet aggregation tests could also be done.**

Apoliprotein A is the more valuable component of HDL so it is possible to have a good level of HDL cholesterol and the apolipoprotein A is low showing a high risk of coronary heart disease. The same is true with apolipoprotein B and LDL cholesterol. You could have a lower level of LDL, but if the apolipoprotein B level is high then this could be an ominous sign.

**For more copies of this book contact:**
**Omni-Press**

**2002 S.E. 50th Ave.**
**Portland, OR 97215**
**(503) 233-9553 or (800) 424-OMNI**

**Dr. Marz is also available for lecturing and can be contacted through the above address and phone number.**

## About the Author

Russell B. Marz, N.D., M.Ac.O.M. is a naturopathic physician and a licensed acupuncturist. He received his B.S. degree in nutrition from Buffalo University College in New York in 1979 and his doctorate degree from the National College of Naturopathic Medicine in 1983 in Portland Oregon. Upon graduating from medical school he bicycled 10,000 miles around the North American continent with a small group of newly graduated naturopathic physicians and their spouses presenting over 120 lectures on nutrition and naturopathic medicine. During his bicycle trip he appeared on radio and television numerous times throughout 16 states in the U.S. He is a competitive athlete who participates in many sports including biathlons and triathlons. He has won numerous biathlons in his age group and is also a two time winner of the "Mountain Man" triathlon competition in Montana in 1986 and 1987. In 1994 he also received a masters in acupuncture and Chinese medicine.

Dr. Marz is currently an assistant professor of nutrition at the National College of Naturopathic Medicine in Portland, OR. He also teaches at the Oregon College of Oriental Medicine in Portland and has taught at the Western States Chiropractic College in Portland and the South West College of Naturopathic Medicine in Scottsdale, AZ. He has been in private practice since 1984 and is currently the medical director at the Tabor Hill Clinic in Portland, OR. Lastly he in the president and founder of Omnivite Nutrition Incorporated, a company specializing in high quality custom nutritional supplements.